Janet Wilkie

Obstetric Anaesthesia
and Analgesia

To Neil and Ian

Obstetric Anaesthesia and Analgesia

Donald D. Moir

MD, FFARCS, DA, DObstRCOG
Consultant Anaesthetist to the Queen Mother's Hospital
and the Western Infirmary, Glasgow
and Honorary Clinical Lecturer at
the University of Glasgow

and

John Thorburn

MB, ChB, FFARCS, DObstRCOG
Consultant Anaesthetist to the Queen Mother's Hospital
and the Western Infirmary, Glasgow
and Honorary Clinical Lecturer at
the University of Glasgow

With a contribution by *Martin J. Whittle*

MD, MRCOG
Consultant Obstetrician and Gynaecologist to
the Queen Mother's Hospital and the Western Infirmary, Glasgow
and Honorary Clinical Lecturer at
the University of Glasgow

Baillière Tindall

LONDON PHILADELPHIA TORONTO

MEXICO CITY RIO DE JANEIRO SYDNEY TOKYO HONG KONG

Baillière Tindall   1 St Anne's Road
W.B. Saunders   Eastbourne, East Sussex BN21 3UN, England

West Washington Square
Philadelphia, PA 19105, USA

1 Goldthorne Avenue
Toronto, Ontario M8Z 5T9, Canada

Apartado 26370—Cedro 512
Mexico 4, DF Mexico

Rua Evaristo da Veiga 55,20° andar
Rio de Janeiro—RJ, Brazil

ABP Australia Ltd, 44–50 Waterloo Road
North Ryde, NSW 2113, Australia

Ichibancho Central Building, 22–1 Ichibancho
Chiyoda-ku, Tokyo 102, Japan

10/fl, Inter-Continental Plaza, 94 Granville Road
Tsim Sha Tsui East, Kowloon, Hong Kong

First published 1976
Second edition 1980
Third edition 1986

Portuguese edition (Editora Guanabara Koogan, Rio de Janeiro) 1979

Typeset by Scribe Design, Gillingham, Kent
Printed and bound in Great Britain by Mackays of Chatham

British Library Cataloguing in Publication Data

Moir, Donald D.
    Obstetric anaesthesia and analgesia.—3rd ed.
    1. Labor (Obstetrics)   2. Analgesia
    3. Anesthesia in obstetrics
    I. Title   II. Thorburn, John   III. Whittle,
    Martin J.
    617′.9682   RG732
    ISBN 0–7020–1154–1

Contents

Preface

Earlier editions of this book appeared in 1976 and 1980 with a single author and, like the present edition, were written primarily for anaesthetists in training and for their senior colleagues who administer obstetric anaesthesia and analgesia and who are responsible for the provision of a service for the obstetric unit or hospital. Obstetricians, paediatricians and senior midwives should also find something of interest within these pages. The needs of the examination candidate have not been forgotten. The restructured FFARCS examinations emphasize safety in clinical anaesthesia from the earliest stages of training. The Faculty of Anaesthetists of the Royal College of Surgeons of England now requires that the period of general professional training for anaesthetists must include at least two months full-time experience in obstetric anaesthesia and analgesia under appropriate supervision and must embrace the use of epidural analgesia in obstetrics. This is an important and enlightened step forward. Although written primarily for a British readership, practices in North America and the various Commonwealth countries do not differ greatly from those in the United Kingdom, and most of the content of this book is applicable throughout the English-speaking medical world.

This edition has again been thoroughly updated and the entire text has been reviewed. Much new material has been added and important sections, such as those on the control of gastric acidity, failed or difficult intubation, epidural anaesthesia for caesarean section and the use of spinal anaesthesia in obstetrics, have been entirely rewritten. Obsolete material has been deleted and this process has been assisted by the National Council for Nursing, Midwifery and Health Visiting in withdrawing approval for the use of trichloroethylene and methoxyflurane by midwives.

The substantial task of preparing this edition has been shared by Dr John Thorburn. It is hoped that the advantages of single authorship in terms of uniformity of style and avoidance of overlap have not been lost and that the involvement of a fresh mind has stimulated a new look at older ideas. Dr Thorburn has been a consultant anaesthetist at the Queen Mother's Hospital, Glasgow, since 1974 and has contributed substantially to practice teaching and research in obstetric anaesthesia. He has been particularly interested in the management of pre-eclampsia and in regional analgesia. Dr Martin Whittle has entirely rewritten the chapter on the modern management of pregnancy and labour and has produced an exposition of great clarity for the anaesthetist who requires a basic working knowledge of modern obstetrics and the management of labour.

Women are often quite well-informed about labour and delivery and will often express, sometimes forcefully, opinions on the management of their own labours including a preference for a method of analgesia. Some will wish to eschew all pain relief. These wishes should be listened to with care and consideration. There will be situations in which a woman's wishes may be inappropriate or even dangerous for herself or her child. It is then the clear duty of all in attendance to point out these risks. Information on new regimens, alternative positions for labour and delivery, birthing chairs and rooms is included in this edition.

Effective and reliable techniques of general anaesthesia and regional analgesia have been developed and refined to a high degree of safety when properly used by anaesthetists with appropriate knowledge and skills. In the pursuit of even greater safety there has been a shift away from general anaesthesia towards epidural and spinal anaesthesia for caesarean section. At the time of writing it is believed that there have been no deaths in the United Kingdom for many years as a direct consequence of the use of regional anaesthesia for caesarean section. Is it admissable to conclude that regional anaesthesia is safer than general anaesthesia? Perhaps it is, but the conclusive answer awaits accurate national statistics on the types of anaesthesia used for caesarean section. These figures may be available in the future. Perhaps general anaesthesia may become less hazardous as rational failed intubation drills are taught and implemented and new methods of raising gastric pH are instituted on a wide scale.

Epidural analgesia has been less safe when used during labour. A few much publicized tragedies have followed top-up injections which had been given by non-anaesthetists. A consequence of these disasters has been an interest in the use of epidural infusions in place of top-up injections and in the use of fractionated top-up injections in the hope of avoiding a very extensive neural blockade. Spinal anaesthesia now enjoys greater popularity, thanks in part to the ready availability of isobaric and hyperbaric solutions of bupivacaine. Disturbing accounts of unusually rapid and extensive spread of spinal anaesthesia call for caution.

Gaps remain in the provision of satisfactory obstetric anaesthesia services throughout the United Kingdom and elsewhere. The recommendation of the Obstetric Anaesthetists Association (OAA) that a resident anaesthetist of at least one year's experience be provided for every obstetric unit where more than 2000 or 2500 babies are delivered annually has been widely agreed, but not yet universally implemented. A resident anaesthetist can offer more than emergency anaesthesia and an epidural service for labour. He, or she, can assist in the care of the critically ill mother and can often anticipate and prepare for emergencies by instituting epidural analgesia, and by taking measures to raise gastric pH and restore fluid balance. In this way, that most dangerous of anaesthetics, the emergency general anaesthetic for urgent caesarean section, will be less frequently required. A continuing problem is the provision of adequate consultant cover for obstetric units. The OAA recommends one consultant session for every 400 annual deliveries. The consultant anaesthetist should be present in the obstetric unit and should take overall responsibility for training, for the provision of satisfactory equipment and for the institution of regimens for diet and gastric pH control in labour. Small and isolated obstetric units may be impossible to staff satisfactorily, not only with anaesthetists, but with obstetricians and paediatricians, and closure may represent the safest course of action.

Donald D. Moir
John Thorburn

1

History of Obstetric Anaesthesia

Childbirth before anaesthesia

Labour has always been painful for many women. The Old Testament contains many allusions to the pain of childbirth. In *Jeremiah* 30, 6 it is written: 'wherefore do I see every man with his hands on his loins, as a woman in travail, and all faces are turned into paleness?' King David, a man with much experience of women, wrote: 'Fear took hold upon them there, and pain, as of a woman in travail' (*Psalms* 48, 6). Women sought relief from the sources available to them. Until the eighteenth century doctors seldom practised midwifery and relief had to be provided by the woman herself or her ignorant attendants.

Medicinal herbs were used. Ancient Chinese literature mentions the use of opiates in labour and opium, henbane, hemp and mandragora (mandrake) were used in many societies, perhaps with some benefit. Acupuncture has been practised as a system of medicine in China and other countries of South-East Asia for some 5000 years, although it was probably not used extensively in childbirth. Alcohol was regularly imbibed by women in labour in mediaeval times. Other prescriptions can have exerted only a placebo effect. Zerubhabel Endecott, a seventeenth century physician of Salem, Massachusetts, recommended for 'sharp and difficult travel in women with child' a mixture of powdered virgin's hair and dried ant's eggs in the milk of a red cow.

Pain was sometimes attributed to evil spirits or witches and incantations and charms were used for its relief. In 1591 Euphame MacCalzean was burned at the stake in Edinburgh, without the mercy of previous strangling. She had sought the aid of a witch to ease her labour pains onto a dog which ran away and was never seen again. Christianity and other religions have sometimes in the past seen pain as a divine punishment, through which grace might be achieved, and analgesia was consequently denied to women in pain.

Primitive peoples have at times used brutal physical violence to expedite delivery. Jumping upon the maternal abdomen was a practice in several communities. Apache squaws were sometimes suspended from a tree by a rope under the armpits. Braves then grasped the woman above the uterine fundus and swung against it. Women in the Serang islands were also delivered standing and bound to a tree by the arms held above the head. Less barbaric and more physiological was the method used in the Pago Pago islands of Samoa. The woman knelt while a strong man sat behind her and pushed his heels against her lower ribs during each painful contraction. In this way

1

pressure anaesthesia was applied to the area of skin supplied by the nerves concerned in the transmission of uterine pain.

Chloroform and Simpson

The first obstetric anaesthetic was administered by Dr (later Sir) James Young Simpson of Edinburgh on 19th January 1847. The agent used was ether, which had been demonstrated on 16th October 1846 at the Massachusetts General Hospital, Boston, by William T. G. Morton, but was not used in America for obstetric anaesthesia until administered by Keep of Boston on 7th April 1847.

The operation for which Simpson gave the first obstetric anaesthetic was typical of the age, being the delivery of a dead fetus after internal podalic version in a woman with a severely contracted pelvis. Simpson was much affected by the misery and death so often associated with childbirth in the mid-nineteenth century. In 1848 he wrote: 'the distress and pain which women often endure while they are struggling through a difficult labour are beyond description and seem to be more than human nature would be able to bear under any other circumstance'.

Simpson, son of a baker in Bathgate, near Edinburgh, became Professor of Midwifery at Edinburgh at 29 years of age and had held the chair for seven years in 1847. Simpson soon realized that open ether was far from ideal for the induction and maintenance of anaesthesia and he spent much of the year 1847 evaluating a large number of chemicals in the hope of discovering a better anaesthetic. In this he was aided by his assistants, Matthews Duncan and George Keith, and by his family. On 4th November 1847, acting on a suggestion of David Waldie, a Scottish chemist working in Liverpool, a test was made with chloroform. The experiment was, as usual, performed at the dinner table and the results were dramatic. 'Immediately an unwarranted hilarity seized the party—they became bright-eyed, very happy and very loquacious—expatiating on the delicious aroma of the new fluid. The conversation was of unusual intelligence and quite charmed the listeners, some ladies of the family and a naval officer brother-in-law of Dr Simpson. But suddenly there was a talk of sounds being heard like those of a cotton-mill louder and louder; a moment more and then all was quiet—and then crash! On awakening Dr Simpson's first perception was mental; "This is far stronger and better than ether", said he to himself. His second was to note that he was prostrate on the floor and that among the friends about him there was confusion and alarm. Hearing a noise he turned round and saw Dr Duncan beneath a chair—his jaw dropped, his eyes staring, his head bent half under him, quite unconscious and snoring in a most determined and alarming manner. More noise and still much motion. And then his eyes overtook Dr Keith's feet and legs making valorous attempts to overturn the supper table, or more probably to annihilate everything that was on it. By and by, Dr Simpson having regained his seat, Dr Duncan having finished his uncomfortable and unrefreshing slumber, and Dr Keith having come to an arrangement with the table and its contents, the sederunt was resumed. Each expressed himself delighted with this new agent and its inhalation was repeated many times that night—one of the ladies gallantly taking her place and turn at the table—until the supply of chloroform was fairly exhausted.' The lady was Simpson's niece who fell asleep crying 'I'm an angel! Oh, I'm an angel!' As the result of these happy experiments, Simpson administered chloroform to an obstetric patient on 8th November.

It is well known that anaesthesia was not immediately accepted in obstetrics, although few objected to its use for other purposes. Many clergymen and some physicians too held that pain in labour was the will of God and even in some way beneficial to the sufferer. This belief was based mainly on the text from *Genesis* 3, 16: 'In sorrow thou shalt bring forth children.' In the New English Bible this takes the form: 'I will increase your labour and your groaning and in labour you shall bear children.' A clerical opponent of anaesthesia wrote: 'Chloroform is a decoy of Satan, apparently offering itself to bless women, but in the end it will poison society and rob God of the deep earnest cries which arise in time of trouble for help!' A contemporary doctor believed that 'pain is the mother's safety, its absence her destruction'. Pain was also seen as a valuable guide to progress in labour and as a promoter of healing.

It was Simpson's contention that a Hebrew word which had, after passage through the Greek, been translated as sorrow in the curse on woman should in reality have the meaning of effort rather than suffering. Simpson's views are in general accord with those of the compilers of the New English Bible more than 100 years later and his views on anaesthesia became more generally accepted in 1853 when Queen Victoria was given chloroform at the birth of her eighth child, Prince Leopold. The anaesthetist was John Snow and chloroform was administered intermittently with the uterine contractions. This was Simpson's technique of inhalational analgesia which thereafter became known as chloroform *à la reine*.

Simpson's powerful advocacy of chloroform over ether did much to ensure its place in obstetric anaesthesia over the next 100 years. A product of an age of great medical men, Simpson was a man of dominant personality, possessed of great humanity.

It is interesting to record that in the USA in 1848 Charles Delucina Meigs, Professor of Obstetrics in Philadelphia and a man of comparable stature to Simpson, was fiercely opposed to anaesthesia and regarded pain in labour as a 'salutory and conservative manifestation of the life force'.

Nitrous oxide

Nitrous oxide was first used in obstetric analgesia by Klikovich of St Petersburg in 1880. Klikovich combined nitrous oxide with oxygen and appreciated the safety of the mixture when inhaled intermittently with contractions. He even demonstrated that uterine contractions were uninhibited by using a manometer attached to a tube passed through the cervix (Richards et al, 1976). In America an apparatus for the self-administration of nitrous oxide in labour was designed by Guedel in 1910, the year in which McKesson evolved his intermittent flow apparatus. These early techniques required a fairly complex apparatus for the administration of nitrous oxide and oxygen and were not available to most women. The great need was for a simple technique, suitable for use by unsupervised midwives. In 1933 Minnitt, a Liverpool anaesthetist, developed his apparatus for the administration of approximately equal parts of nitrous oxide and air. The Minnitt apparatus was approved by the Central Midwives Board in January 1936. The apparatus was frequently inaccurate, being capable in some cases of delivering as little as 3 or 4% of oxygen (Cole and Nainby-Luxmore, 1962; Nainby-Luxmore, 1964; Moir and Bissett, 1965), although, perhaps partly because of its inherently hypoxic characteristics, a fair degree of analgesia was often obtained. The Talley, Amwell, Jecta and Walton–Minnitt machines were all later used by midwives. An even more hypoxic technique was available to doctors who could use the 'C.M.' attachment to the Minnitt apparatus. This device, often erroneously attributed to Chassar Moir of Oxford, supplied 2.5 litres of pure nitrous oxide from a bag before continuing to supply nitrous oxide and air augmented by further 1 litre/min flow of nitrous oxide.

It is easy now to condemn totally those hypoxic techniques, yet they were the only form of analgesia available to millions of British women. The end of an era of hypoxic analgesia was signalled in 1962 when Tunstall of Aberdeen reported the use in obstetrics of premixed nitrous oxide and oxygen from a single cylinder. In 1965 the Central Midwives Board authorized the use of the Entonox apparatus for the administration of 50 : 50 nitrous oxide and oxygen and in 1970 the authorization for the use of nitrous oxide and air was finally withdrawn.

Trichloroethylene and methoxyflurane

Trichloroethylene was first used in anaesthesia by Dennis Jackson and by Striker in Cincinnati in 1934 and 1935. The agent was popularized in the UK by Langton Hewer in 1941. The Freedman inhaler developed in 1943 facilitated the administration of analgesic concentrations to women in labour. Accurate drawover inhalers, automatically temperature-compensated and relatively unaffected by variations in respiratory minute volume, were approved for midwives' use in 1955. These were the Emotril and Tecota Mark 6 machines and they made non-hypoxic inhalational analgesia available for use by midwives.

Methoxyflurane was introduced in 1959 and was quite widely used for obstetric analgesia in the USA. In 1970, after extensive trials in south Wales, midwives were permitted to use 0.35% methoxyflurane from the Cardiff inhaler.

Inhalational analgesia is now less often used and the period of inhalation is usually quite brief. This reflects current trends towards shorter labours, the greater use of regional analgesia and a more effective use of systemic analgesics and sedatives. Methoxyflurane in particular seems to have suffered from the present anxiety about a possible adverse effect on renal function, although this has not been demonstrated after intermittent inhalational analgesia in labour. In 1984 the National Board for Nursing, Midwifery and Health Visiting withdrew its approval for the use of trichloroethylene (Trilene) by British midwives and the manufacture of methoxyflurane (Penthrane) ceased. Entonox then became the only inhalational agent available to midwives.

Systemic analgesics

Morphine had been isolated from crude opium by Serturner in 1806 but drugs were rarely injected before the invention of the hypodermic syringe and hollow needle by Alexander Wood of Edinburgh in 1853. At that time it was the custom to attempt to inject morphine alongside painful nerves and its general analgesic properties were not fully appreciated. Morphine was not extensively used in labour until von Steinbuchel of Graz introduced the combination of morphine and scopolamine in 1902. This was developed by Gauss of Freiburg in 1906 into the regimen known as twilight sleep (*Dämmerschlaf*) in which a single injection of morphine and scopolamine was followed by repeated injections of scopolamine alone. Twilight sleep was extensively used in the 30 years after its introduction although it had major drawbacks. Labour was protracted, the neonate often suffered from respiratory depression and the mother was often very restless and difficult to control owing to the action of scopolamine in the absence of adequate analgesia. The patients were often satisfied by the inability to recall the events of a prolonged and painful labour.

Pethidine was synthesized in Germany in 1939 and was first used in labour in 1940. Since 1950 midwives have been authorized to prescribe and administer pethidine in domiciliary practice. Pentazocine is favoured in some centres as an alternative to pethidine and midwives have recently also been authorized to prescribe pentazocine. The introduction of levallorphan (1950) and nalorphine (1952) reduced some of the hazards of narcotic analgesics for mother and especially for her infant, although unfortunately the narcotic and narcotic antagonist combination of Pethilorfan has failed to live up to its early promise of analgesia without respiratory depression.

Regional analgesia

It was Sigmund Freud's suggestion which led Koller to use cocaine for topical anaesthesia of the cornea in 1884 and, had Freud not been absent when

Koller first used cocaine, the psychiatrist might well have had the further distinction of administering the first local anaesthetic. In the following year Halsted, the Baltimore surgeon, performed nerve blocks upon himself. This practice was to turn Halsted into a cocaine addict. In 1910 Stiasny applied cocaine topically to the vagina and vulva in an attempt to relieve pain in labour. In 1927 Gellhorn described the infiltration of the perineum with local anaesthetic solutions; this procedure has been authorized for the use of midwives.

Spinal subarachnoid analgesia was accidentally produced by Corning in 1885 while attempting to inject cocaine near the spinal cord of a dog. He later performed the technique in man as a 'therapeutic' procedure in a patient with 'spinal irritation' and in a man suffering from decompression sickness associated with working on the Hudson river tunnel! Corning's technique of lumbar puncture was unreliable and it was Quincke in 1891 who made lumbar puncture a practicable procedure. It remained for August Bier of Kiel in 1899 to use spinal analgesia for surgery. Although successful, the patients suffered severely from headaches and vomiting, attributable no doubt to the use of unsterile tap water to dissolve the cocaine crystals and to the free leakage of cerebrospinal fluid. Macintosh (1957) described how Bier and his assistant performed spinal anaesthesia on each other and then went on to eat dinner with wine and cigars.

By 1901 Tuffier had extended the scope of spinal anaesthesia to intra-abdominal surgery. From these European beginnings the use of spinal anaesthesia spread to the USA. Barker, the London surgeon, seems to have been the first to use spinal anaesthesia in the UK in 1907; it was his description of the influence of the curves of the spine and the effect of gravity on the spread of solutions that made spinal anaesthesia a more precise technique. The first to use spinal anaesthesia for operative vaginal delivery was Kreis in Germany in 1901. Spinal anaesthesia was popularized for obstetric use by Pitkin in the USA when he introduced a hyperbaric technique in 1928. The saddle block technique of very low spinal anaesthesia for forceps delivery was developed by Adriani and Parmley in 1946. Spinal anaesthesia remains popular for obstetrics in the USA although it has been partly replaced by caudal and lumbar epidural analgesia; spinal analgesia is now quite extensively used in Great Britain.

Working independently in Paris in 1901 Sicard and Cathelin introduced caudal analgesia, and Cathelin, although a urologist, envisaged the use of caudal analgesia in painful labours. In 1909 von Stoeckel of Marburg reported on 134 caudal blocks in obstetrics, but with rather unsatisfactory and shortlived analgesia attributable to the limitations of the local anaesthetics then available and the lack of a continuous technique. Schlimpert of Freiburg improved the technique in 1913. Lumbar epidural block was first performed by Fidel Pages of Spain in 1921 and the technique was developed by Dogliotti of Turin in the 1930s. Eugen Bogdan Aburel of Rumania used a silk catheter in 1931 to produce a continuous block of the lumbo-aortic nerve plexus. He did not use continuous epidural analgesia.

The now classic description of the sensory innervation of the birth canal and the report of lumbar paravertebral and caudal blocks in obstetric analgesia by John G. P. Cleland of Oregon in 1933 put obstetric conduction analgesia on a rational basis. The introduction of a continuous technique of caudal analgesia into obstetric practice in America by Hingson and Edwards in 1942 made the relief of pain throughout the whole of labour and delivery practicable. Continuous lumbar epidural analgesia was used by Curbello of Cuba and by Hingson and his associates in 1946. Although Galley reported a small series of obstetric caudal blocks in 1949 and lumbar epidural analgesia was used by Dawkins and by Steel, the development of epidural analgesia in obstetrics in Great Britain on any scale was delayed until quite recently. A series of continuous lumbar epidural blocks was reported by Moir in 1968 as the result of a 24-hour obstetric epidural service introduced in 1964, and since then, Crawford and others have recorded series of several thousand blocks. There has been a welcome increase in the number of centres in which epidural analgesia is practised in obstetrics. This has been associated with an increase in the number of consultant anaesthetists working in and specially committed to obstetric anaesthesia and the provision of 24-hour resident anaesthesia services for many major maternity units. In the last four to five years epidural analgesia has been increasingly used for caesarean section as well as for the relief of pain in labour and vaginal delivery.

Paracervical block had been used in France and Germany and was revived by Freeman in the USA in 1956. Widely used in the USA and in Scandinavia in the 1960s, the technique was only moderately popular in Great Britain. Serious misgivings about the safety of the fetus have resulted in the abandonment of paracervical block in many centres.

The importance of the correct mental attitude to pregnancy and labour was advanced by Grantly Dick-Read in his book *Natural Childbirth* in 1933, and later in *Childbirth Without Fear* in 1944. Read believed passionately that the triad of fear, tension and pain were interlinked and that a simple and fearless approach to labour could render it painless. Read overstated his case and present psychological preparation for labour is usually based on the technique of psychoprophylaxis advocated by Lamaze and Vellay over the last 20 years. Instruction in the elementary physiology of pregnancy and labour reduces the element of fear which stems so often from ignorance, and a series of breathing exercises is taught for use during labour along with techniques of relaxation. The knowledge gained is always valuable and the ability to relax is useful. Painless labour is rarely achieved and should not be expected by the patient or her attendants. Leboyer introduced his method of 'birth without violence' in 1977, and the early 1980s have seen the use of acupuncture, transcutaneous electrical nerve stimulation and the adoption of alternative positions for labour and delivery. These techniques and the work of Michel Odent and others have created a less rigid attitude towards the management of labour and delivery.

Professional organizations

In the UK the Obstetric Anaesthetists Association (OAA) was constituted in Glasgow in the Spring of 1969. Dr J. S. Crawford was elected president and the host was Dr D.D. Moir. The OAA arose from an informal gathering of interested anaesthetists in Liverpool in the Autumn of 1968 convened by Drs T.H.L. Bryson (Liverpool) and M. Lewis (Belfast). The OAA now has almost 700 members and meets twice yearly. A European meeting is held every three years.

In the USA the Society for Obstetric Anesthesia and Perinatology (SOAP) was constituted in Nashville, Tennessee in September 1970 as the outcome of a preliminary meeting in Kansas city in 1969. The OAA and SOAP are flourishing and exert considerable influence over the clinical and organizational aspects of obstetric anaesthesia and have been instrumental in raising the standards of obstetric anaesthesia services.

REFERENCES

Cole, P.V. and Nainby-Luxmore, R.C. (1962) The hazards of gas and air in obstetrics. *Anaesthesia*, **17**, 505.
Dick-Read, G. (1933) *Natural Childbirth*. London: Heinemann.
Dick-Read, G. (1944) *Childbirth Without Fear*. London: Heinemann.
Macintosh, R.R. (1957) *Lumbar Puncture and Spinal Analgesia*, 2nd ed., p. 5. Edinburgh: Livingstone.
Minnitt, R.J. (1934) Self administered analgesia for the midwifery of general practice. *Proc. R. Soc. Med.*, **27**, 1313.
Moir, D.D. and Bissett, W.I.K. (1965) An assessment of nitrous oxide apparatus used for obstetric analgesia. *J. Obstet. Gynaec. Br. Commonw.*, **72**, 264.
Nainby-Luxmore, R.C. (1964) Further hazards of gas and air in obstetrics. *Anaesthesia*, **19**, 421.
Richards, W., Parbrook, G.D. and Wilson, J. (1976) Stanislav Klikovich (1853–1910). Pioneer of nitrous oxide analgesia. *Anaesthesia*, **31**, 933.

2

Physiology of Pregnancy and Labour

There are many changes associated with pregnancy and childbirth which are of fundamental importance to the anaesthetist. Ignorance of these changes has in the past resulted in potentially serious errors in the conduct of general and regional analgesia and in the misinterpretation of observations made on the pregnant woman. In illustration of this point one may consider the erroneous impression formerly gained of apparent alterations in cardiac output and blood volume in late pregnancy which were largely spurious because they resulted mainly from occlusion of the inferior vena cava in the supine position. Ignorance of the normal respiratory changes of pregnancy will lead to misinterpretation of blood gas values and there are many changes which influence the action of anaesthetic drugs.

THE BLOOD AND ITS CONSTITUENTS

There are major alterations in the blood, the heart and the circulation in pregnancy. They are compensatory changes, designed to cope with the growing fetus, uterus and placenta and probably also with the anticipated loss of blood at delivery. It is desirable that studies of changes in physiological values should be longitudinal; that is to say that they should involve serial measurements throughout pregnancy within a group of mothers. The making of measurements in different women at various stages of pregnancy accounts for many discrepancies between certain studies.

Blood volume in pregnancy. Both the plasma volume and the red cell mass increase in pregnancy. The increased blood volume is accommodated in the dilated vessels of the uterus, placenta, kidneys, skeletal muscle and skin and there is no evidence that the circulation is overloaded in the pregnant woman without heart disease. The rise in plasma volume exceeds the rise in red cell mass, resulting in a lower concentration of red cells. The size of the red cells is increased by only a small extent and their haemoglobin content is unaltered so that the haemoglobin concentration and haematocrit of the blood usually fall in line with the red cell count.

The plasma volume. The plasma volume begins to increase between week 6 and week 12 of pregnancy and eventually rises to about 50% above the non-pregnant value. In primigravidae the rise averages 1.25 litres so that the

9

mean plasma volume in the last weeks of pregnancy is about 3.85 litres (Hytten and Leitch, 1971). The increase is slightly greater in multigravidae and in multiple pregnancy. In twin pregnancy the plasma volume averaged 1.96 litres at term and in two women with triplets the mean value was 2.4 litres. In the past it was frequently noted that the maximum rise in plasma volume occurred at 34 weeks gestation and that thereafter the plasma volume declined. This apparent fall in the last weeks of pregnancy is almost certainly an artefact resulting from occlusion of the inferior vena cava in the supine position (Chesley and Duffus, 1971). Lund and Donovan (1967) did not observe this preterm fall in plasma volume in their large series of measurements. A well conducted study by Pirani et al (1973) confirmed that plasma volume rises progressively until 32 weeks and thereafter remains unchanged. Measurements were made serially throughout pregnancy in the left lateral position. Plasma volume returns to pre-pregnancy levels six weeks after delivery. There is a further sharp increase of up to 1 litre in plasma volume 24 hours after delivery (Taylor et al, 1981). Oxytocin enhances this increase because of its antidiuretic action. Measurements have usually been made by the Evans blue dye dilution technique.

In severe hypertensive diseases of pregnancy the normal increase in plasma volume may not occur and there is a relationship between hypovolaemia, chronic placental insufficiency and neonatal birth weight (Soffronoff et al, 1977).

The red cell mass. It is thought that the red cell mass increases in an approximately linear fashion throughout pregnancy. Average values measured by various workers vary widely. This variation may be due to differences in technique (for example the making of direct estimations using tagged red cells or by indirect calculation from plasma volume and haematocrit values), the non-longitudinal design of some studies and failure to allow for the influence of iron therapy during pregnancy in some series. The use of ^{51}Cr-labelled red cells taken from the subject is the preferred technique of measurement. Isotopes of iron have a long half-life and cross the placenta.

In the absence of a supplementary intake of iron and folic acid the red cell mass increases by 200–250 ml towards term. The ingestion of iron and folic acid during the pregnancy increases this figure to 350–400 ml (Paintin, 1962; Lund and Donovan, 1967; Taylor and Lind, 1979). The red cell mass is abnormally low in severe pre-eclampsia (Soffronoff et al, 1977) and is higher in multiple pregnancy.

The changes in plasma volume and total blood volume during pregnancy are illustrated in Figure 1. The total blood volume increases by about 40% in normal pregnancy. Estimations have usually been made by measuring either the plasma volume or the red cell mass and calculating the other component from the haematocrit. Ideally both components should be measured simultaneously.

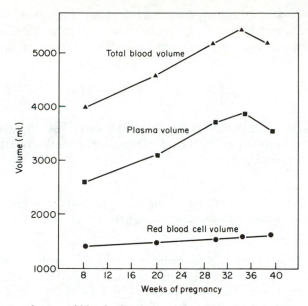

Figure 1. Plasma volume, red blood cell volume and total blood volume changes in pregnancy. The terminal falls are probably spurious and are attributable to caval occlusion in the supine position; they do not occur in the left lateral position.

Normal haematological values. It is now believed that a healthy pregnant woman who takes a proper diet and receives iron and perhaps also folic acid supplements should have haematological values which differ little or not at all from those of a healthy woman who is not pregnant. With this in mind it may appear that the following widely quoted values for haemoglobin concentration and red cell count are rather low by today's standards.

Haemoglobin concentration. There are wide racial and dietary variations and well recognized inaccuracies in many clinically used methods of measuring haemoglobin concentration. In normal pregnancy the haemoglobin concentration should not fall below 12 g/dl. There is a small increase in the number of cells containing fetal haemoglobin (HbF) which is of maternal origin.

The fall in haemoglobin concentration which is common (but by no means inevitable) in pregnancy is due in part to the relatively large increase in plasma volume in comparison with the red cell volume and is the so-called 'physiological anaemia' of pregnancy. The term is unfortunate because the anaemia can be largely prevented by prophylactic iron therapy during pregnancy. In the presence of anaemia, iron therapy promotes haemopoiesis. In the absence of anaemia the iron is absorbed, serum ferritin concentration rises, but haemopoiesis is not stimulated (Taylor et al, 1983).

Haematocrit (packed cell volume). The haematocrit usually falls to about 34% in pregnancy from a non-pregnant value of 40–42% in women who do not receive iron supplements.

Red cell count. This is usually reduced to about 3.8 million/mm^3 (3.8 × 10^{12}/litre) if iron is not given. The production of erythrocytes occurs more rapidly during pregnancy and the stimulus is thought to be erythropoietin.

Mean cell haemoglobin concentration. This is unchanged in pregnancy.

Mean cell volume and cell shape. Volume increases slightly and the erythrocytes become more spherical. Diameter decreases but thickness increases (Bolton and Street, 1983).

Platelets. There is no significant change in the platelet count in normal pregnancy and platelet adhesiveness is unaltered.

White cells. The total white cell count increases to a peak of about 9.0 × 10^9/litre at 30 weeks and there is a further sudden leucocytosis to around 40 × 10^9/litre during labour. The increase is due to a neutrophilia; the white cell count becomes normal by day 6 after delivery.

Plasma proteins. The total concentration of proteins in the plasma is reduced in pregnancy. This is accounted for mainly by a reduction of about 10 g/litre in the plasma albumin concentration to a value of about 35 g/litre. The total concentration of plasma globulins and of fibrinogen is increased by about 2 g/litre at term. In particular the α-1-, α-2- and β-globulins rise progressively during pregnancy while the concentration of γ-globulin falls slightly. The fibrinogen concentration rises substantially from about 3.5 g/litre to about 5.5 g/litre at term. New proteins are found in pregnancy. α-Fetoprotein of fetal origin and lactogen of placental origin appear in maternal serum.

The total colloid osmotic pressure of the plasma is reduced in pregnancy, although this is probably unrelated to the frequency with which oedema develops in pregnancy.

The alterations in the plasma proteins influence the binding capacity of the plasma in pregnancy. The binding to plasma proteins of many anaesthetic agents (general and local) and of many other drugs is affected. Drugs may be bound to albumin and to one of the globulin fractions. The fraction of drug which is bound to plasma protein is temporarily inactive and unavailable for placental transfer. A reduction in plasma α-acid glycoprotein concentration reduces the capacity to bind lignocaine in pregnancy (Wood and Wood, 1981). It should be recalled that the concentration of albumin in the plasma is reduced but the total mass of albumin in the expanded plasma volume is little changed. In general there is diminished binding of drugs to serum proteins during pregnancy because receptor sites are occupied by pregnancy hormones.

Plasma lipids. The total concentration of lipids in the plasma is substantially increased in pregnancy. Neutral fat, cholesterol, phospholipid and non-esterified fatty acids are all present in increased concentration and are present in the blood as lipoproteins. Darmady and Postle (1982) noted a reduction in serum cholesterol and triglyceride levels in the first trimester and an increase in the third trimester. Lactation accelerated the puerperal return to normal. The peripheral utilization of non-esterified fatty acids is increased in pregnancy and this results in a higher concentration of ketone bodies in the blood.

Plasma cholinesterase. Towards term the concentration of pseudocholinesterase in the plasma is reduced by about 28% (Shnider, 1965; Robertson, 1966). This reduction would not normally be sufficient to prolong the action of suxamethonium (Blitt et al, 1977). Later work by Evans and Wroe (1980) has shown that cholinesterase activity falls during the first trimester and reaches its lowest level in the puerperium when some prolongation of suxamthonium apnoea is most likely. Hazel and Monier (1971) have shown that the enzyme is not qualitatively altered. The incidence of muscle pain after suxamethonium infusion is reduced to about 20% in pregnancy (Datta et al, 1977). Afterpains are also relatively uncommon after a single dose of suxamethonium (Thind and Bryson, 1983).

The erythrocyte sedimentation rate (ESR). The ESR is much increased in pregnancy. Values of 55–80 mm in the first hour are normal. This phenomenon may be related to the clumping of red cells which is induced by the increase in the fibrinogen and globulin fractions in the plasma. The ESR is of little diagnostic value in pregnancy.

Blood viscosity. In normal pregnancy the blood viscosity increases at low shear rates as term approaches but is unaltered at high shear rates (Thorburn et al, 1982). Viscosity may be greatly increased in severe pre-eclampsia, which may be viewed as a hyperviscosity state. Plasma volume expanders reduce viscosity.

Extravascular fluid water and electrolytes. The extravascular and the intravascular water content increases in pregnancy. The increase is most noticeable after week 30 of gestation and by term the extravascular water volume has risen by about 1.7 litres in women without oedema or with local ankle oedema. Water retention decreases abruptly, shortly before the onset of labour. Plasma water also increases and blood viscosity decreases. The increase in extracellular water in women with generalized oedema averages almost 5 litres. Water and sodium are retained together. Although hypoproteinaemia and increased venous pressure in the legs may predispose to oedema it is believed that the chief cause of oedema in pregnancy is an increased affinity for water by the connective tissue ground substance.

Plasma electrolyte concentrations are slightly reduced throughout pregnancy, but these changes have no clinical importance. The lower concentration of electrolytes is associated with a reduction in plasma osmolality by about 10 mosmol/kg (Robertson, 1968). The level of ionized and unionized calcium rises slightly towards term.

Blood coagulation in obstetrics

There is normally a dynamic balance between the haemostatic mechanisms and the fibrinolytic systems in the blood so that haemostasis is confined to the site of bleeding by the fibrinolytic systems. During pregnancy the blood is hypercoagulable and fibrinolytic activity is reduced. Although these changes may be viewed as a precaution against excessive bleeding from the placental site after delivery they probably make the pregnant woman more liable to thrombosis, both local and generalized (Scott, 1968, 1969). After separation, the placental site is rapidly covered by a fibrin mesh and approximately 10% of the circulating fibrinogen is consumed. Coagulation is more than usually likely to occur in response to minor damage to a blood vessel and when intravascular coagulation has occurred then clot lysis may be less efficient. It is likely that the hypercoagulability of the blood in pregnancy is related to the occurrence of deep venous thrombosis in the calf and perhaps also to severe pre-eclampsia and to disseminated intravascular coagulation. There is evidence of a further increase in fibrinogen and a further decrease in fibrinolysis and sometimes also of intravascular coagulation in the form of thrombocytopenia and fibrin degradation products in the serum in severe pre-eclampsia (Bonnar et al, 1971).

In pregnancy the plasma fibrinogen concentration rises from non-pregnant values of about 3.0 g/litre to about 5.5 g/litre at term and the total circulating fibrinogen is increased from about 10 to 20 g. Clotting factors VII, VIII (antihaemophilic factor), IX (Christmas factor) and X are all increased in pregnancy. Reported alterations in the platelet count are contradictory but it is probable that the platelet count is unaltered and that platelet adhesiveness is normal. The concentration of plasminogen activator is reduced in pregnancy, although the plasminogen concentration is increased. Fibrinolytic activity returns to normal within an hour after delivery of the placenta. Diminished fibrinolytic activity in pregnancy may influence the concentration of fibrinogen degradation products (FDP). The concentration of FDP may less accurately reflect the extent of intravascular coagulation in pregnant women.

The concentration of antithrombin III is reduced and the concentration of other antithrombins is unchanged with a resulting increase in these enzymes in the already expanded plasma volume (Teisner et al, 1982). Coagulation is not inhibited and may be promoted by this additional mechanism.

Bonnar and his colleagues (1970) observed that the clotting mechanisms in the blood draining from the placental site were strongly activated after placental separation at caesarean section. The coagulability of a peripheral venous blood sample taken at the same time was unaltered. This is a clear indication that the failure to detect a coagulation defect in the peripheral blood does not exclude the possibility of localized changes in an organ.

The ability to neutralize heparin is increased and the dose requirements for heparin are slightly greater during pregnancy.

Blood loss at delivery

There is now available a good deal of fairly accurate information on the quantity of blood shed at various types of delivery and on the influence of factors such as the length of labour, the oxytocic drug used and the anaesthetic technique upon blood loss. Haemoglobin dilution techniques have been used for these estimations. Most of the values quoted in the following discussion were obtained from women in the supine or dorsal position and there is a clinical impression that compression of the inferior vena cava in these positions may have raised the pressure in the uterine veins and increased the loss of blood.

At spontaneous vertex deliveries with pethidine and nitrous oxide analgesia and ergometrine at delivery the average blood loss is about 200 ml. A further 150 ml of blood are lost if an episiotomy is performed (Wallace, 1967). With the now routine use of oxytocic drugs, excessive bleeding is perhaps more often due to episiotomy or to trauma to the cervix, vagina or perineum.

The range of blood loss is wide and, in Wallace's substantial series, 20% of patients who had a spontaneous delivery with episiotomy lost more than 500 ml of blood. It is of course customary to regard a blood loss in excess of 500 ml as a postpartum haemorrhage. Intravenous ergometrine 0.5 mg and oxytocin 5 units are equally effective at spontaneous delivery with episiotomy (Moir and Amoa, 1979). This dose of ergometrine is now considered to have been unnecessarily large.

At mid-cavity forceps deliveries the loss of blood is strikingly influenced by the method of anaesthesia (Moir and Wallace, 1967):

General anaesthesia	average blood loss 520 ml
Pudendal nerve block	average blood loss 410 ml
Epidural analgesia	average blood loss 270 ml

The general anaesthetic used consisted of thiopentone, D-tubocurarine and unsupplemented nitrous oxide.

At lower uterine segment caesarean section under modern light general anaesthesia in which only nitrous oxide is used to maintain anaesthesia, the external blood loss averages between 750 ml and 1 litre (Brant, 1966; Wallace, 1967; Toldy and Scott, 1969; Moir, 1970). Blood loss at caesarean section is almost halved when the operation is performed under lumbar epidural analgesia (Moir, 1970).

When ^{51}Cr-labelled red cells are used to measure red cell mass changes, the mean loss is 1.29 litres for first caesarean sections and 1.012 litres for repeat sections, and these higher values are said to be due to the ability of this technique to estimate blood lost into the peritoneal and uterine cavities and the vagina (Read and Anderton, 1977).

Blood loss is increased at delivery after prolonged labour (Moir and Wallace, 1967). Blood loss at forceps delivery is uninfluenced by the use of intravenous ergometrine or intramuscular Syntometrine (ergometrine 0.5 mg with Syntocinon 10 units) according to Moir and Wallace (1967), and Moodie and Moir (1976) found intravenous ergometrine and intravenous Syntocinon equally effective.

The evidence concerning the alterations in blood volume occurring at delivery is conflicting. Pritchard et al (1960) and Quinlivan and Brock (1970) found that the reduction in circulating blood volume equalled the measured external blood loss at vaginal delivery. Other workers have observed that the reduction in circulating blood volume exceeded the external blood loss, indicating sequestration of blood in the tissues (Bhatt, 1965; Pritchard et al, 1962). One may question the accuracy of some of these estimations, and the types of delivery and the oxytocic used are not always clearly stated. The haemodynamic changes at delivery are complex and of major extent. The blood volume at term is increased, the blood expelled from the uterus into the general circulation at delivery is of uncertain quantity but may be of the order of 500 ml (Hendricks, 1958) and the vasoconstrictor action of ergometrine may be expected to diminish the volume of the vascular compartment. Ueland (1976) recorded a mean reduction in blood volume of 610 ml in 1 hour after forceps delivery and there were further reductions over the subsequent three days. The mean decrease in blood volume after caesarean section was 1.03 litres, but there was no further decrease in these patients.

It is clear that blood loss at all types of delivery is much greater than is traditionally taught. Simple measurements of the quantity of blood in the placenta bowl are likely to indicate a blood loss which is approximately 50% of the true loss (Moir and Wallace, 1967). The current tendency to use epidural or spinal analgesia for forceps delivery and caesarian section can be expected to reduce the average volume of blood loss.

The pregnant woman can tolerate considerable blood loss. Because her blood volume is increased by 40% on average, she can lose up to 30% blood volume without change in haematocrit in the puerperium (Pritchard, 1965) and often without major alterations in blood pressure and heart rate. Blood transfusion is rarely required at elective caesarean section, although cross-matched blood should be available. Transfusion is not advocated unless changes in vital signs indicate hypovolaemia and this does not usually occur until the loss exceeds 1.2–1.5 litres. Blood is given together with plasma volume expanders.

The most recent available information (Department of Health and Social Security, 1982) revealed a disturbing increase in the number of maternal deaths from postpartum haemorrhage. Blood loss was sometimes underestimated by junior staff and a coagulation disorder was often present. Obstetric units should have an agreed plan for the management of major haemorrhage. Experienced obstetricians, anaesthetists and a haematologist should be involved at an early stage. Simple measures such as bimanual compression of the uterus and direct compression of the aorta may save lives.

HAEMODYNAMIC CHANGES OF PREGNANCY

Of all the many aspects of obstetric physiology it is the haemodynamic changes of pregnancy which are perhaps of greatest concern to the anaesthetist.

Heart rate. By the third month of pregnancy the heart rate has already increased to 78 beats/min on average and in late pregnancy the average rate is 85 beats/min. The increased cardiac output of pregnancy is due to an increase in heart rate and in stroke volume.

Blood pressure. The systolic blood pressure usually falls slightly in mid-pregnancy and rises again to non-pregnant levels towards term. The diastolic blood pressure is usually considerably lowered in mid-pregnancy and returns to non-pregnant levels in the last two or three months. Studies in pregnancy have almost always relied on sphygmomanometer estimations of brachial artery pressure but such measurements may overestimate systolic and diastolic pressures by about 7 mmHg (1.0 kPa) and 12 mmHg (1.7 kPa) respectively (Ginsburg and Duncan, 1969). Observer error and individual technique may vary widely.

Blood pressure in the pregnant woman is greatly influenced by posture and by occlusion of the inferior vena cava and the abdominal aorta by the gravid uterus. Supine hypotension from caval occlusion may be observed in about 10% of women when the supine position has been maintained for four or five minutes. The abdominal aorta may also be occluded by the gravid uterus in the supine position in the last months of pregnancy and this may produce a temporary rise in blood pressure above the site of occlusion and a reduction in blood flow to the uterus and the lower limbs with a fall in femoral arterial pressure (Eckstein and Marx, 1974). Blood pressure is usually highest in the sitting position. In the supine position the femoral arterial pressure may fall during contractions. This is the Poseiro effect and is due to more extensive aortic compression between the contracting uterus and the vertebral bodies (Poseiro, 1967). In normal labour the systolic blood pressure rises by 5–10 mmHg (0.7–1.3 kPa) during the first stage contractions and by 30 mmHg (4.0 kPa) during contractions in the second stage (Wiederman et al, 1965). In pre-eclampsia there is often a progressive rise in blood pressure during painful labour.

Peripheral resistance. Because the blood pressure is usually normal or slightly below normal in pregnancy and cardiac output increases substantially, the peripheral resistance is considerably reduced in pregnancy. Pyörälä (1966) has calculated that average peripheral resistance in pregnancy is 979 dyn/cm^{-5} (0.979 N). This may be compared with a non-pregnant value of 1700 dyn/cm^{-5} (1.700 N). Vasodilation and the formation of new vessels account for the widely accepted reduction in peripheral resistance in pregnancy. If the contradictory data of Atkins et al (1981) on cardiac output are used to calculate peripheral resistance then there is an apparent increase in late pregnancy.

The hypotensive response to autonomic blockade is exaggerated in pregnancy. Assali and his colleagues (1952) recorded a fourfold increase in the hypotensive effect of tetraethylammonium chloride in pregnancy.

Venous pressures. In the absence of compression of the inferior vena cava by the gravid uterus, in the supine position, right atrial pressures and pressures in the arm veins are normal in pregnancy. Central venous pressure in the supine position averages 3.8 cmH$_2$O (0.4 kPa) but this figure is influenced by occlusion of the inferior vena cava and consequent reduction in venous return (Colditz and Josey, 1970). In the lateral position the pressure in the inferior vena cava ranges from 10.6 to 15 mmHg (1.4 to 2.0 kPa) and in the supine position the pressure increases to between 20 and 30 mmHg (2.7 and 4.0 kPa) (Scott, 1963). Pressures in the femoral veins are greatly increased in pregnancy if caval occlusion exists and this may contribute, along with the increased coagulability of the blood, to the predisposition to thrombosis in the veins of the leg. In the supine position the femoral venous pressure is 20–25 cmH$_2$O (2.0–2.5 kPa) (McLennan, 1943). These substantial rises in venous pressure in the lower limbs are associated with normal pressures in the veins of the upper limbs and right atrium. Occlusion of the inferior vena cava is the principal cause of high pressure in the leg veins, although a minor contributory factor may be the emergence of blood from the uterus at relatively high pressure.

In labour the expulsion of up to 500 ml of blood from the uterus into the general circulation with each uterine contraction (Hendricks, 1958) produces a rise of 4–6 cmH$_2$O (0.4–0.6 kPa) in the central venous pressure (Wiederman et al, 1965). The central venous pressure rises occur even when contractions are painless and are therefore due to the temporary increases in blood volume and not to muscular movement or rigidity associated with pain. Expulsive efforts in the second stage of labour create enormous rises in the central venous pressure of up to 50 cmH$_2$O (4.9 kPa) (Moir, unpublished data, 1970). Central venous pressure usually falls to normal values immediately after delivery of the child. The intravenous injection of ergometrine 0.25 mg after delivery produces a rise of 8 cmH$_2$O (0.8 kPa) in the central venous pressure and this rise persists for up to 60 minutes (Williams et al, 1974).

Circulation times. Circulation times in the upper parts of the body are probably unchanged in pregnancy. The flow of blood in the lower limbs is greatly slowed in the supine position in late pregnancy. The leg blood flow accelerates on turning from the supine position to the lateral position and the improvement is greater in the left than in the right lateral position (Drummond et al, 1974). It is concluded that caval occlusion is more effectively relieved in the left lateral position.

Heart size and position. The heart enlarges by about 12% in pregnancy and the enlargement is due to an increase in the thickness of the heart muscle and to an increase in the volume of the chambers of the heart. The elevation of the diaphragm which occurs in late pregnancy pushes the heart upwards and rotates it forwards. The apex beat is felt in the fourth intercostal space and may be displaced to the left. X-ray examination may show straightening of the upper left border of the heart. This is normal and is not indicative of mitral stenosis.

Electrocardiographic changes. The ECG changes observed in normal pregnant women are mainly the result of the rotation of the heart's electrical axis to the left (left axis deviation). The T wave is often flattened or even inverted in lead III. Innocent depression of the S-T segment has been reported in pregnancy. Ectopic beats are more frequent and supraventricular paroxysmal tachycardia may occur.

Heart sounds. Phonocardiography has demonstrated that most pregnant women develop a loud and sometimes split first heart sound. A third sound is common. In the majority a systolic murmur is audible and a few develop a diastolic murmur along the left sternal border. In pregnancy these changes are normal.

Cardiac output. The changes in cardiac output which occur in pregnancy and the major influence of posture upon cardiac output are of the greatest significance in general and regional anaesthesia. There can now be no doubt that failure to prevent the drastic reduction in cardiac output which may suddenly occur in the supine position has contributed to maternal and fetal morbidity and mortality in the past and even in the present. The facts are now well documented, but regrettably there is reason to believe that they are too often not applied by anaesthetists and obstetricians for the benefit of their patients.

Many workers have measured cardiac output in pregnancy and not all of their findings are in agreement. This is because various techniques of measurement have been used, studies were not always longitudinal and because earlier workers did not understand the major influence of posture on cardiac output. Early studies involved invasive, dye-dilution techniques.

Various non-invasive techniques of questionable accuracy have been used in some recent studies.

It was formerly held that cardiac output rose steadily until about week 32 of pregnancy and thereafter declined to non-pregnant levels. It is now clear that this statement is only applicable when measurements are made in the supine position and that the apparent reduction in cardiac output in the last eight weeks of pregnancy is due to the reduction in venous return which results from occlusion of the inferior vena cava by the gravid uterus in the supine position. Occlusion of the vena cava occurs in most pregnant women in the supine position (Kerr et al, 1964) and venous return must then be maintained by the paravertebral and azygous veins. This alternative vertebral venous route is relatively long, tortuous and narrow and venous return is impeded. A sudden fall in venous return and cardiac output occurs in at least 8% of normal pregnant women after a few minutes spent in the supine position and, probably in association with reflex vasovagal bradycardia, produces a severe fall in arterial pressure—the supine hypotensive syndrome (Lees et al, 1967a,b). When serial measurements are made in the lateral position the cardiac output rises from a non-pregnant value of about 4.5 litres/min to about 6.0 litres/min by week 10 of pregnancy and remains at this level until term (Figure 2). There is an increase in stroke volume and in heart rate (Lees et al, 1967b). The increase of about 33% in cardiac output is due mainly to the demands of the uterus and its contents (Clapp, 1978).

Position greatly influences cardiac output by alleviating or augmenting caval occlusion. Turning from the lateral to the supine position causes a sharp fall in cardiac output and the converse is true. The cardiac output may be reduced by as much as 50% in the supine position (Lees et al, 1967b; Ueland

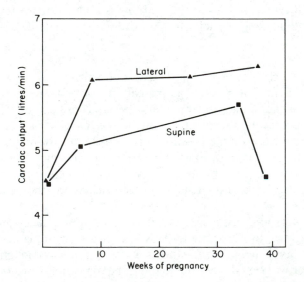

Figure 2. Cardiac output in pregnancy in the supine and lateral positions.

et al, 1968). It is this reduction in cardiac output, especially if it is accompanied by bradycardia of vagal origin, which causes the supine hypotensive syndrome. Crawford et al (1972) introduced the useful term 'revealed caval occlusion' for this syndrome and the associated term 'concealed caval occlusion' recognizes that blockage of the inferior vena cava occurs in most pregnant subjects near term but that hypotension need not always occur. The maintenance of arterial pressure and cardiac output above the critical level at which caval occlusion becomes 'revealed' probably involves an increase in the peripheral resistance in an effort to compensate for the reduced venous return and cardiac output. A reduction in the peripheral resistance caused by general anaesthesia or a subarachnoid or epidural block may result in a disastrous fall in cardiac output. No patient who has received, or is about to receive, a general anaesthetic or an epidural or subarachnoid block should remain in the unmodified supine position. A lateral or laterally tilted position should be assumed and the left lateral position is preferable to the right lateral position (Drummond et al, 1974; Buley et al, 1977). Changes in cardiac output were measured by Newman et al (1983) using transcutaneous aortvelography and showed that a left lateral tilt was associated with the highest cardiac output. There is evidence that the dorsal position is harmful to the fetus in the unanaesthetized woman (Humphrey et al, 1974) and there are good grounds for advocating a lateral or semilateral position for all patients in labour. A reduction in intervillous blood flow has been demonstrated using the ^{133}Xe clearance technique when the mother turns from the lateral to the supine position (Kauppila et al, 1980).

Vorys et al (1961) measured cardiac output in various positions. In comparison with the supine position, cardiac output rose by 13.5% in the left lateral position, but fell by 17% in the lithotomy position. In a steep (claimed 45°) Trendelenberg position the cardiac output fell by 18%. It is thought that these observations are all explicable by variations in the magnitude of the pressure of the uterus on the vena cava in the various positions.

The isovolumetric contraction time or pre-injection period is shortened in pregnancy and the left ventricular ejection time is slightly prolonged. These alterations are due to a greater stroke volume and are therefore less apparent in the supine position (Rubler et al, 1973; Burg et al, 1974).

In striking contrast to the now generally accepted view that cardiac output continues to increase until term when the woman is in the lateral position, Atkins and others (1981) in a longitudinal study using impedance cardiography observed a rise in cardiac output by week 12 and a steady decline from week 20 until term. The accuracy of impedance cardiography is open to question.

During uterine contractions there is a transient rise in cardiac output and central venous pressure and this is almost certainly due mainly to the expulsion of blood from the uterus into the general circulation which accompanies each contraction (Hendricks, 1958). Even when epidural analgesia is used, there is an increase in cardiac output of between 20 and

30% with contractions and a rise in central venous pressure of between 3 and 5 mmHg (0.4 and 0.7 kPa) (Lees et al, 1970) and these observations would imply that pain and muscular movement are not the cause of the variations in cardiac output.

The expulsive efforts of the second stage are in effect a series of Valsalva manoeuvres and are associated with high intra-abdominal and intrathoracic pressures. Cardiac output falls and arterial pressure decreases. Weaver et al (1977) have shown that the pattern of the arterial pressure changes is the same in the lateral and supine positions but that epidural analgesia and the supine position tend to cause greater reductions in arterial pressure, and recovery is then slower. Intrauterine pressures rise by about 20 mmHg (2.8 kPa) during pushing.

During caesarean section under general anaesthesia with lateral tilt, the cardiac output rose in response to surgical stimulation and increased greatly after delivery of the infant as a result of the transfer of blood from the uteroplacental to the systemic circulation and probably also to the relief of partial caval occlusion (Newman, 1982). When spinal anaesthesia was used for caesarean section and adequate hydration was maintained, the cardiac output was unchanged (Abouleish et al, 1982).

Regional blood flow

The blood flow to most organs increases during pregnancy and this is accompanied by an increase in cardiac output and a reduction of peripheral resistance. Vasodilatation is the outstanding feature and the mechanism may involve a diminished response to angiotensin II. In pre-eclampsia the response to angiotensin II is unimpaired (Gant et al, 1973). Vasoconstriction is a feature of pre-eclampsia. The greatest percentage increase occurs in the flow of blood to the uterus.

Uterine and placental blood flow. Measurement of uteroplacental blood flow is extremely difficult in the human subject for both anatomical and ethical reasons. The blood supply of the uterus is unsuitable for measurements based on the Fick principle and the application of electromagnetic flowmeters to the uterine arteries is confined to animal experiments. Using nitrous oxide, measurements have been made in human subjects with the Fick principle. The collection of venous blood from the uterus is very difficult, although a sample of blood from any artery gives acceptable values for the nitrous oxide content of the blood entering the uterus. It appears that the blood flow through the uterus at term is of the order of 500 ml/min or one-twelfth of the cardiac output (Metcalfe et al, 1955; Romney et al, 1955) and that there has been a tenfold increase in uterine blood flow from the 50 ml/min recorded at 10 weeks gestation (Assali et al, 1960). Recently uteroplacental blood flow has been measured in women by the intravenous injection of a radio-isotope such as ^{133}Xe and measuring radioactivity at the placental site with a gamma camera (Lippert et al, 1973; Rekonen et al, 1976). A biphasic curve is obtained, representing myometrial and intervillous blood flow. Approximately 80% of the uteroplacental flow goes to the placenta. The ^{133}Xe clearance technique gives a rather wide scatter of results, but it is at present the only feasible method for use in human mothers. The accuracy of the absolute values obtained may be debated, but major percentage changes in intervillous blood flow are demonstrable.

Blood reaches the maternal portions of the placenta principally by the uterine arteries. Maternal blood enters the relatively stagnant intervillous spaces by the uterine arterioles in which the pressure is 80 or 90 mmHg (10.6 or 12.0 kPa). This pressure is sufficient to drive the incoming stream of fresh maternal blood through the intervillous spaces towards the chorionic plate (the fetal surface) where placental transfer takes place. The flow of maternal blood into the intervillous spaces is uneven and takes the form of intermittent and irregular spurts from the spiral arteries. The distribution of blood to the various cotyledons is therefore erratic and seems to follow no set pattern. Gradual mixing of blood occurs in the intervillous space where the pressure is only 15 mmHg (2.0 kPa) and blood eventually leaves the intervillous space to enter the uterine veins. During contractions in labour the pressure in the intervillous space rises to perhaps 38 mmHg (5.1 kPa) and blood is temporarily squeezed out of the placenta and uterus. The powerful uterine contractions may partly occlude the uterine arteries and reduce the flow of blood into the uterus and placenta during contractions. It is thus likely that placental transfer is reduced temporarily with each contraction. This may be expected to impair the transfer of oxygen and carbon dioxide to the detriment of the fetus if contractions are powerful and labour is prolonged. The transfer of harmful substances, such as depressant drugs, may be diminished during contractions. Less powerful contractions and the pre-labour Braxton Hicks' contractions may actually promote placental transfer by occluding venous outflow from the intervillous space while not reducing arterial inflow. The time available for transfer would then be prolonged.

An important feature of the placental vasculature is the apparent absence of any intrinsic autoregulating mechanism. Spiral arteriolar flow depends almost entirely on pressure and these vessels have no nerve endings. The myometrial vessels do not possess adrenergic receptors (Greiss, 1966, 1972). Using the ^{133}Xe clearance method a group of Finnish workers demonstrated that intervillous blood flow falls during labour and that epidural analgesia increases intervillous blood flow during labour and caesarean section (Jouppila et al, 1978a,b). There is a simple, direct relationship between maternal arterial blood pressure and intervillous blood flow.

Fetal blood enters the placenta by the two umbilical arteries at a systolic pressure of 60–70 mmHg (7.9–9.3 kPa) and is distributed to the hundred or so cotyledons or placental units, each of which contains many fetal villi. Within the villi blood flows through a capillary loop, returning to the fetus by the single umbilical vein. The fetal blood in villous capillaries is separated from the maternal blood in the intervillous spaces by the 'placental barrier' of the capillary wall and the syncitial trophoblast. Fetal blood flow into the placenta is approximately 100 ml/kg fetal wt./min and flow is probably erratically distributed to the many cotyledons after the erratic pattern of flow of maternal blood.

Renal blood flow. The flow of blood through the kidneys increases early in pregnancy and probably remains at this level for most of the pregnancy, falling slightly in the final weeks, even in the lateral position (Dunlop, 1981). The increase averages 400 ml/min (Chesley and Sloan, 1964). Glomerular filtration rate and effective renal plasma flow increase during pregnancy.

Hepatic blood flow. Liver blood flow is not altered to any important extent in pregnancy.

Cerebral blood flow. It is thought that cerebral blood flow is unchanged in pregnancy.

Skin blood flow. The skin blood flow is much increased in pregnancy. This increase is especially pronounced in the hand where cutaneous blood flow is six times greater than that of the non-pregnant woman (Ginsburg and Duncan, 1967). Venepuncture is, in consequence, usually easy in the obstetric patient and Raynaud's phenomenon usually improves during pregnancy. Blood flow in the muscles of the leg and forearm is probably unaltered (Ginsburg and Duncan, 1967) but this study can be criticized for inappropriate selection of subjects and because it was not longitudinal throughout pregnancy.

Mucous membranes. The mucous membranes of the upper respiratory tract are often congested and swollen in pregnancy and some oedema of the false cords is often present. These changes may be more apparent in patients with pre-eclampsia, and tracheal intubation may occasionally be made difficult by oedema of the larynx.

RESPIRATION

Respiratory function undergoes several important modifications in pregnancy. These modifications are the result of hormonal influences (principally the high concentration of progesterone in the blood) and anatomical changes which result from the presence of the greatly enlarged uterus. The increased metabolic needs of the growing fetus, uterus and placenta increase the requirement for oxygen and the production of carbon dioxide.

Anatomical changes

The enlarging uterus displaces the diaphragm upwards in the later weeks of pregnancy but the internal volume of the thoracic cavity is unchanged. There is a compensatory increase in both the transverse and the anteroposterior diameters of the thorax so that the external circumference of the chest increases by 12.5–17.5 cm. These changes are accompanied by flaring of the ribs and an increase in the substernal angle. Flaring of the ribs begins early in pregnancy and is therefore not entirely due to pressure from the enlarging uterus.

The popular concept of an elevated and splinted diaphragm is erroneous, at least in the upright position. Radiological studies have demonstrated that the respiratory excursion of the elevated diaphragm is actually increased (von Möbius, 1961). It is, of course, possible that splinting of the diaphragm may occur in the anaesthetized pregnant woman in the horizontal or Trendelenberg position.

Lung volumes and capacities

Tidal volume. The tidal volume increases from week 10 or week 12 of pregnancy onwards. The respiratory rate is unchanged. According to Cugell et al (1953) the mean tidal volume at term is 678 ml, representing an average increase of about 40% over non-pregnant values. The minute volume in late pregnancy is about 10.5 litres. Shortly after delivery the tidal volume falls to a mean of 487 ml. The anatomical dead space is almost certainly unchanged in pregnancy; the physiological dead space is increased by only about 60 ml (Pernoll et al, 1975b). Consequently there is alveolar hyperventilation with a reduction in arterial blood partial pressure of carbon dioxide ($P_a\text{co}_2$) during the second and third trimesters. The cause of this hyperventilation of pregnancy is believed to be progesterone which probably exerts its respiratory stimulant action on the carotid body receptors (Zwillich et al, 1978). The dead space/tidal volume ratio is unchanged (Templeton and Kelman, 1976).

Functional residual capacity and residual volume. The functional residual capacity (FRC) is reduced by up to 500 ml at term. The reduction is progressive from about week 20 and is due to the upward growth of the uterus. Residual volume falls by about 300 ml according to Baldwin et al (1977), although Russell and Chambers (1981) detected no change in residual volume.

The quite substantial reduction in FRC, together with the increase in tidal volume, result in relatively large volumes of inspired air mixing with a smaller volume of air in the lungs. In consequence the composition of the alveolar gas mixture can be altered with unusual rapidity. It is thus possible to induce inhalational anaesthesia more rapidly in the pregnant woman at term. Alveolar and therefore arterial hypoxia will develop more swiftly during apnoea, respiratory obstruction or the inhalation of a hypoxic gas mixture. Archer and Marx (1974) have convincingly demonstrated that the anaesthetized mother becomes hypoxic with greater rapidity than the non-pregnant woman.

Inspiratory capacity. The inspiratory capacity (inspiratory reserve volume plus tidal volume) is increased by 5–10% in the last trimester. The increase is attributable to the increase in tidal volume. The inspiratory reserve volume is usually unchanged (see Table 1 and Figure 3).

Table 1. Representative values (ml) for lung volumes and capacities in pregnant and non-pregnant women

	Non-pregnant	Term pregnancy
Tidal volume	450	650
Respiratory rate	16/min	16/min
Vital capacity	3200	3200
Inspiratory reserve volume	2050	2050
Expiratory reserve volume	700	550
Functional residual capacity	1600	1300
Residual volume	1000	800

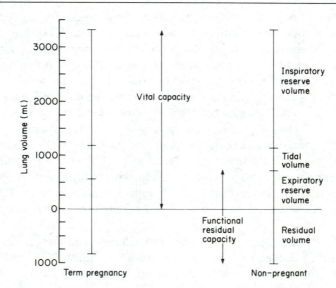

Figure 3. Representative changes in lung volumes and capacities in pregnancy.

Vital capacity and total lung capacity. The increases in the inspiratory reserve volume and the tidal volume are almost exactly cancelled out by the reductions in the expiratory reserve volume and the residual volume. Consequently the vital capacity and the total lung capacity are essentially unchanged in pregnancy, although there are modifications in their component parts (Prowse and Gaensler, 1965; Novy and Edwards, 1967; Russell and Chambers, 1981).

The foregoing changes in lung volumes and capacities are mainly due to elevation of the diaphragm and widening of the thorax and develop in the second half of pregnancy. The increase in tidal volume is probably a progesterone effect and is present from week 10 or week 12 of pregnancy. The various alterations are illustrated in Figure 3.

Forced expiratory volume. The forced expiratory volume (1 second) is unchanged in pregnancy (Cugell et al, 1953; Cameron et al, 1970). Peak expiratory flow rate is also unaltered.

Airway resistance. There is a reduction in the airway resistance and this is probably due to progesterone-induced relaxation of the bronchial muscles (Gee et al, 1967). The airway specific conductance is unaltered (Milne et al, 1977a) and this may represent a balance between the bronchodilator action of progesterone and the bronchoconstrictor effect of the hypocapnia of pregnancy.

The work of breathing. Despite the increase in minute volume, the work of breathing is unchanged in pregnancy. The explanation may be the reduction in airway resistance (Novy and Edwards, 1967).

Compliance. Lung compliance is unaltered in pregnancy. Immediately after delivery a 25% increase in chest wall compliance was observed by Marx et al (1970) and this was attributed to descent of the diaphragm. The reduced pressure of the abdominal contents on the diaphragm and perhaps also a reduction in pulmonary blood volume produce a 20% increase in total respiratory compliance after delivery by caesarean section (Farman and Thorpe, 1969). When performing intermittent positive pressure ventilation the inflation pressure can often be reduced after the delivery of the infant.

Closing volumes. In late pregnancy closing volume often exceeds the functional residual capacity and airway closure occurs within the tidal volume range in about 50% of pregnant women (Bevan et al, 1974; Craig and Toole, 1975; Holdcroft et al, 1977). This would account for the observation that arterial Po_2 falls slightly as pregnancy advances (Stenger et al, 1964; Templeton and Kelman, 1976). It is probable that the reduced FRC of late pregnancy produces the apparent increase in closing volume which, in turn, produces impaired distribution of pulmonary ventilation and a fall in arterial blood partial pressure of oxygen (P_aO_2). Russell and Chambers (1981) found no change in closing volume and closing capacity in pregnancy, but observed airway closure during tidal breathing in over half of their subjects at term. This was attributed to the reduction in FRC and was observed in the supine but not when seated. Russell and Chambers suggested that alterations in cardiac output may be more important than apparent changes in closing volume in the causation of arterial hypoxaemia in pregnancy.

Gas transfer (pulmonary diffusing capacity). Gas transfer is reduced by about 15% from mid-pregnancy (Milne et al, 1977b). This reduction may be due to the lowered haemoglobin concentration of many mothers or to an alteration in the mucopolysaccharide of the alveolar capillaries. Efficient alveolar gas distribution and a high alveolar partial pressure of oxygen (P_AO_2) may minimize the effect of reduced gas transfer.

Oxygen consumption. Studies of basal metabolism are particularly difficult in pregnancy, but according to Pernoll and others (1975a), the basal oxygen consumption is probably increased by about 15% at term in order to cope with the demands of the uterus, placenta, fetus and an increased cardiac output and respiratory minute volume. The increased oxygen requirements of pregnancy have been thought to result in an unusually rapid decline in P_aO_2 in the apnoeic, anaesthetized patient at term (Archer and Marx, 1974). This is almost certainly not the only explanation for this observation. As Sykes (1975) pointed out it is likely that the reduced FRC of late pregnancy predisposes to a rapid reduction in P_aO_2 during apnoea, and the FRC may be further reduced by anaesthesia (Hewlett et al, 1974). The reduced FRC also promotes more rapid uptake of inhalational anaesthetic agents (Palahniuk et al, 1974). Airway closure within the tidal volume range is common at term (Bevan et al, 1974). In practice a hypoxic or apnoeic episode during anaesthesia is more likely to have disastrous consequences if the patient is pregnant. Hypoxia which may leave the mother without permanent harm may prove fatal to the fetus. This hazard is greater for the fetus whose safety is already compromised.

Pulmonary circulation. The pulmonary blood flow is greatly increased in pregnancy and there is a greater volume of blood contained within the pulmonary vessels at any time. The normal woman is able to cope with these changes and the pressures in the right ventricle, pulmonary artery and pulmonary capillaries are not raised (Bader et al, 1955). If pulmonary vascular resistance is high and fixed, as it is in Eisenmenger's syndrome, then the increased pulmonary blood flow of pregnancy further increases pulmonary vascular resistance until it may exceed the now reduced systemic resistance. Lung perfusion will then be inadequate and hypoxaemia ensues.

Dyspnoea in pregnancy. About 60% of normal pregnant women experience dyspnoea, in that they become conscious of the need to breathe. Dyspnoea is therefore not usually an indication of organic disease in a pregnant woman. It is thought that the sensation of dyspnoea is the result of a lowering of the P_aCO_2 which normally occurs in pregnancy. The level of ventilation has become 'inappropriate to the needs of the patient' who therefore becomes aware of her own breathing (Campbell and Howell, 1963).

Blood gases and acid–base balance in pregnancy

The fundamental alteration in respiratory blood gas tensions in the pregnant woman is a reduction in the $P_a\text{co}_2$. By the twelfth week of pregnancy the $P_a\text{co}_2$ has fallen to a mean of about 31 mmHg (4.1 kPa) and this carbon dioxide tension persists until the onset of labour. The reduction in $P_a\text{co}_2$ is the result of the alveolar hyperventilation which is the consequence of the increased production of progesterone which occurs in pregnancy. It is of interest that progesterone can stimulate pulmonary ventilation in normal and in hypercapnic males (Goodland et al, 1953; Tyler, 1960). Hyperventilation probably starts even before implantation of the fertilized ovum and a reduction in the alveolar partial pressure of carbon dioxide ($P_A\text{co}_2$) has been recorded in the premenstrual phase of the normal menstrual cycle (Goodland and Pommerenke, 1952; Bouterline-Young and Bouterline-Young, 1956). It is presumed that progesterone enhances the response of the respiratory centres to carbon dioxide. The pregnant woman increases her ventilation by about 6 litres/min for every 1 mmHg (0.13 kPa) rise in $P_a\text{co}_2$ (Prowse and Gainsler, 1965; Pernoll et al, 1975b). The equivalent value for non-pregnant women is only 1.5 litres/min.

The reduction in the $P_a\text{co}_2$ which exists throughout pregnancy results in various compensatory adjustments in an effort to maintain a normal pH. The base excess in pregnancy usually lies between 0 and -3.5 mEq/litre (3.5 mmol/litre) (Sjøstedt, 1962; Macrae and Palavradji, 1967).This relative metabolic acidosis is affected by a reduction in the total quantity of buffer bases in the blood—serum sodium concentration and osmolality are reduced. Compensation for the respiratory alkalosis of pregnancy is not always quite complete and the arterial blood pH is usually about 7.44 (36.4 nmol/litre). The relative deficiency of blood buffer bases must reduce the ability of the pregnant patient to compensate for the metabolic acidosis which tends to develop in prolonged labour and other states in which tissue perfusion may be inadequate.

The purpose of the respiratory alkalosis of pregnancy is uncertain, but is believed to be the facilitation of the placental transfer of carbon dioxide from fetal to maternal blood.

Although Blechner and others (1968) found essentially normal values for $P_a\text{o}_2$ in pregnancy other workers have found a rather wide scatter of values around a mean of 80 mmHg (10.6 kPa), an observation which could be accounted for by the increase in closing volume known to occur in about 50% of women at term (Bevan et al, 1974). Lucius and others (1970), in contrast, found a small rise in $P_a\text{o}_2$ from about 85 mmHg (11.3 kPa) at 10 weeks to 92 mmHg (12.3 kPa) at term. An important study has been made by Templeton and Kelman (1976) in which many variables were standardized. Serial measurements were made throughout pregnancy in normal mothers in a semi-recumbent position with lateral pelvic tilt. $P_a\text{o}_2$ rose slightly in the first trimester to 106 mmHg (14.1 kPa) and then declined to 102 mmHg (13.6 kPa).

Posture also influences $P_a o_2$ at term. Caval occlusion reduces $P_a o_2$ (Jassir et al, 1973). An average increase of 13 mmHg (1.7 kPa) occurred on changing from the supine to the sitting position (Ang et al, 1969). The arteriovenous (A-V) oxygen difference is reduced throughout most of pregnancy to an average of 34 ml/litre because oxygen consumption does not greatly increase, whereas cardiac output increases substantially from week 10 onwards. Only in the final month of pregnancy does the A-V oxygen difference reach a non-pregnant value of about 44 ml/litre (Bader et al, 1955). The effect on oxygen saturation of the $P o_2$ changes discussed will be small. The oxyhaemoglobin dissociation curve is shifted progressively to the right and the P_{50} increases from 26.7 to 30.2 in normal pregnancy (Kambam et al, 1983). The value for the fetus of maternal oxygen therapy has long been debated. Recently direct measurements on monkey fetuses in utero have shown that increasing the maternal fractional inspiratory oxygen ($F_I o_2$) consistently increases the fetal $P o_2$ after an interval of about 50 seconds and that reducing the placental blood flow reduces the fetal $P o_2$ (Myers et al, 1977). Increasing the $F_I o_2$ at caesarean section increases the $P o_2$ of the umbilical venous and arterial blood (Ramanathan et al, 1982).

Effect of smoking during pregnancy on the fetus

It is now clear that smoking during pregnancy is associated with the birth of smaller and lighter babies, a higher perinatal mortality and an increased risk of spontaneous abortion and premature labour (Butler et al, 1972; Cole et al, 1972; Hardy and Mellitus, 1972; Harlap and Shiono, 1980). The harmful effects of smoking are in proportion to the number of cigarettes smoked. The precise mechanism by which smoking causes these effects is uncertain. Fetal oxygenation may be impaired by the existence of carboxyhaemoglobin levels of 4.1% on average in smoking mothers and 1.2% in non-smokers. Levels in the infants at birth were almost twice those recorded in their mothers owing to the high affinity of fetal haemoglobin for carbon monoxide (Cole et al, 1972). The exposure of fetal blood to carbon monoxide not only reduces its oxygen-carrying capacity directly but shifts the oxygen dissociation curve to the left. It is probable that nicotine can act as a vasoconstrictor upon the placental circulation. Using the ^{133}Xe clearance technique, Lehtorvita and Forss (1978) demonstrated that smoking a cigarette produces an immediate decrease in intervillous blood flow. Manning et al (1978) have demonstrated that nicotine causes fetal hypoxaemia for up to 30 minutes and a reduction in fetal breathing movement by a sympathomimetic vasoconstriction of the placental circulation. Rush (1974) suggested that the appetite suppression which accompanies smoking could explain the reduction in fetal size and weight on a nutritional basis. This theory is refuted by Meyer (1978), who believes that hypoxaemia resulting from the increase in fetal and maternal carboxyhaemoglobin is the cause of the retarded growth.

Alcohol abuse during pregnancy. A fetal alcohol syndrome is recognized in the infants of alcoholic mothers and includes microcephaly, micrognathia, microphthalmia, heart lesions and growth retardation. Thirty-two per cent of the children of heavy drinkers (at least 45 ml of absolute alcohol every day) had congenital anomalies (Ouellette et al, 1977). No safe quantity of alcohol consumption is recognized and total abstinence is usually advised. There has been an interesting suggestion that the fetal alcohol syndrome may be due to high levels of acetaldehyde in mothers whose ability to metabolize this substance is impaired by alcohol. If this is so then disulphiram (Antabuse) would expose the fetus to an increased risk.

RESPIRATION AND METABOLISM IN LABOUR

The onset of labour superimposes further biochemical changes upon those just described as occurring in normal pregnancy. In the account which follows it should be remembered that the changes described have usually been recorded in painful labour and that the effective relief of pain minimizes many of the undesirable changes in painful labour.

Ventilation in labour. Hyperventilation is obvious, even to the casual observer, when uterine contractions are painful and this hyperventilation occurs mainly in response to pain. When pain is relieved by lumbar epidural analgesia in established labour, the hyperventilation formerly associated with uterine contractions is much reduced (Fisher and Prys-Roberts, 1968).

Crawford and Tunstall (1968) measured tidal volumes and respiratory rates in patients who breathed from an Entonox apparatus during painful labour. During painful contractions in the first stage the mean tidal volume was 750 ml but the range of values was from 227 ml to 2.258 litres. The mean rate of breathing during contractions was 34 breaths/min (range 3–47). The mean ventilation during contractions was 42 litres/min while inhalation analgesia was not being given. Mean peak inspiratory flow rates ranged from 22 to 340 litres/min. Davies et al (1974) recorded a mean ventilation of 18.8 litres/min during painful contractions in patients who were receiving inhalational analgesia. It is clear that ventilation varies widely in labour but that hyperventilation of a considerable extent is the rule in painful labour. It appears that pain is the major cause of this hyperventilation but anxiety, drugs, the application of a face mask and the over-enthusiastic performance of breathing exercises may all contribute. Oxygen consumption V_{O_2} was 2.2 ± 0.3 ml/kg/min between contractions and rose to 4.4 ± 0.6 ml/kg/min during painful contractions. Epidural analgesia reduced V_{O_2} to 3.1 ± 0.4 ml/kg/min. Pain and the resulting hyperventilation, and not the uterine contractions, are the main cause of the increased oxygen requirements of painful labour (Hagerdal et al, 1983) and the importance of effective analgesia in patients with cardiac and respiratory disease is obvious. Spontaneous overbreathing occasionally results in tetany in the labouring patient.

In the second stage of labour tidal volumes may be even higher than those recorded in the first stage and there will be episodes of breath-holding during expulsive efforts.

Blood–gas tensions in labour. The direct result of the hyperventilation which accompanies painful uterine contractions is a substantial and often progressive reduction in $P_a co_2$ (Fisher and Prys-Roberts, 1968; Fadl and Utting, 1969, 1970; Pearson and Davies, 1973a). A representative value for the $P_a co_2$ in the first stage of labour would be 25 mmHg (3.3 kPa) but there are wide variations. Fadl and Utting noted that there was a further, transient fall in $P_a co_2$ during each painful uterine contraction for which intermittent inhalational analgesia was administered. A $P_a co_2$ of less than 17 mmHg (2.3 kPa) was recorded in 6 out of 20 women during painful contractions (Miller et al, 1974). When labour is managed throughout under continuous lumbar epidural analgesia there is little or no reduction in $P_a co_2$ (Pearson and Davies, 1973a), and when epidural analgesia is instituted in the course of a painful labour there will usually be an increase in the $P_a co_2$ towards normal (Fisher and Prys-Roberts, 1968). The $P_a co_2$ may be viewed as an indicator of the effectiveness of analgesia in labour. In contrast to the findings of other workers in this field, the lowest values for $P_a co_2$ in Fadl and Utting's series were recorded in patients who received epidural analgesia. The explanation for this surprising finding is not readily apparent. Crawford (1972) speculates that there may have been differences in intravenous fluid regimens (if any) and failure to prevent caval occlusion in some studies.

The oxygen tension of the arterial blood is generally believed to be normal during the first stage of labour. In many patients the $P_a o_2$ rises during painful contractions, due to the associated hyperventilation (Andersen and Walker, 1970). Huch and others (1974) measured subcutaneous $P o_2$ during labour and they also observed increases in $P o_2$ during painful contractions. In some patients who had received intramuscular pethidine there were substantial reductions in subcutaneous $P o_2$ in the intervals between contractions. The effect of maternal oxygen therapy on fetal subcutaneous $P o_2$ has been examined by Willcourt et al (1983). When oxygen was breathed from a close-fitting simple mask at a flow rate of 10 litres/min the fetal subcutaneous $P o_2$ increased by 5 mmHg (0.5 kPa). A flow rate of 6 litres/min produced an increase of only 2 mmHg (0.3 kPa).

The respiratory alkalosis which usually develops during the first stage of labour is normally accompanied by a reduction in base excess and sometimes by a fall in arterial blood pH (Andersen and Walker, 1970; Fadl and Utting, 1969, 1970; Pearson and Davies, 1973a). A progressive rise in blood lactate, pyruvate and excess lactate was observed during the first stage of labour by Marx and Greene (1964). The metabolic acidosis of the first stage of labour has usually been attributed solely to anaerobic metabolism in the uterus and other tissues. Metabolic acidosis is minimized or absent when pain in the first stage is completely relieved by epidural analgesia (Pearson and Davies, 1973a; Maltau et al, 1975) and there is the intriguing possibility that pain can promote metabolic acidosis. Certainly the uterine contractions can be eliminated as a major cause of acidosis in the first stage. Aerobic metabolism may also be increased in labour and an oxygen debt may be incurred at delivery (Marx and Orkin, 1969). An increase in the fetal scalp blood lactate concentration correlates well with pH change, Apgar score and abnormalities of the fetal heart-rate (Smith et al, 1983).

In the second stage of labour there is a sharp and substantial fall in pH and base excess and a further rise in blood lactate concentrations (Marx and Greene, 1964; Pearson and Davies, 1973b). This sudden exacerbation of the maternal metabolic acidosis in the second stage of labour is due mainly to the activity of the voluntary muscles during expulsive efforts because the changes are much less severe if expulsive efforts are not performed in patients who have received epidural analgesia and are of intermediate severity when pushing takes place with epidural analgesia (Pearson and Davies, 1973b). Uterine contractions are not the principal cause of maternal metabolic acidosis in labour. The P_aCO_2 is variable in the second stage of labour. Andersen and Walker (1970) found that the P_aCO_2 fell to a mean of 22 mmHg (2.9 kPa) between contractions and 15 mmHg (2.0 kPa) during contractions. The P_aCO_2 is likely to rise during bearing-down efforts (Fadl and Utting, 1969). In the series of Pearson and Davies (1973b) the P_aCO_2 was unchanged in the second stage.

GASTROINTESTINAL FUNCTION IN PREGNANCY AND LABOUR

The changes in gastric emptying time and in the competence of the gastro-oesophageal sphincter are of supreme relevance to the safety of the mother who receives a general anaesthetic during pregnancy or labour. The smooth muscle of the gastrointestinal tract is relaxed in pregnancy. Transit times in the small intestine are prolonged and absorption is delayed (Parry et al, 1970).

Gastric emptying. Studies of gastric emptying times in pregnancy and in labour often appear to have reached widely differing conclusions. This may be explained by the technique of measurement, the nature of the 'meal', if any, and the influence of drugs (particularly narcotic analgesics) on the rate of emptying of the stomach during labour. It is no longer permissible to repeat the earlier radiological studies because of the risks of irradiation for mother and child.

The rate of emptying a watery meal from the stomach is slightly prolonged from week 34 of pregnancy (Davison et al, 1970) and the greatest delays occurred in women who complained of heartburn. Plasma motilin concentrations are reduced from week 12 of pregnancy and this could explain the slight prolongation of gastric emptying and the laxity of the gastro-oesophageal sphincter in those women who experience heartburn (Christofides et al, 1982).

Gastric emptying in patients in labour may take place at widely varying rates and is greatly influenced by the drugs administered during labour. There can be no doubt that stomach contents may be retained for many hours in the labouring woman who has received narcotic analgesics. In the days before the introduction of proper restrictions on the intake of solid food in labour and when labour might last for 48 hours, clinical experience would often confirm that food ingested 12 or more hours previously was present in the stomach at the induction of general anaesthesia. Roberts and Shirley (1976) noted that the volume of gastric contents diminished during the first 20 hours of labour and thereafter began to increase. Davison et al (1970) observed that the rate of disappearance of a saline test meal was greatly prolonged in labour. Pethidine has been found to prolong gastric emptying times to 5 hours or more in 70% of patients in labour (La Salvia and Steffen, 1950) and it is certain that the narcotic analgesics which were formerly prescribed in large doses throughout prolonged labour contributed substantially to the retention of solids and liquids in the stomach. When labour is conducted under epidural analgesia or without analgesia the gastric emptying time is only slightly prolonged (Wilson, 1978). The greatly prolonged gastric emptying times caused by the use of narcotic analgesics have been confirmed by Nimmo et al (1975). Holdsworth (1978) recorded larger volumes of gastric contents in women who had received pethidine in labour. Metoclopramide seems not to reverse the effect of narcotic analgesics, but naloxone is able to do so (Wilson, 1978). An additional factor in creating a high gastric volume in labour may be the stimulant effect on gastric secretion of the high plasma gastrin levels of pregnancy which reach their peak in labour (Attia et al, 1982). The volume and pH of gastric contents was the same at delivery and 48 hours post partum, suggesting that the risk of aspiration pneumonitis under general anaesthesia remains the same (James et al, 1984).

Although narcotic analgesics are the main cause of prolonged gastric emptying in labour and their use increases the risk of subsequent general anaesthesia, there is also a clinical impression that anxiety and stress may sometimes contribute to the delay in gastric emptying.

Gastro-oesophageal reflux. Heartburn occurs in 45–70% of pregnant women (Hart, 1978) and is usually caused by the reflux of acid gastric juice into the oesophagus (Castro, 1967). Heartburn and oesophagitis are very probably the result of a degree of incompetence of the physiological gastro-oesophageal (cardiac) sphincter. There is no true anatomical sphincter and the term 'high pressure zone' is also used. A history of heartburn should alert the obstetric anaesthetist to the probability that the gastro-oesophageal sphincter is relatively incompetent and that the likelihood of the regurgitation of stomach contents is higher than usual (Dinnick, 1967). Hiatus hernia is said to be common in pregnancy and again the symptom of heartburn should put the anaesthetist on the alert. According to Mixson and Woloshin (1956) a hiatus hernia can be detected in 27% of pregnant women who complain of heartburn. A hiatus hernia was diagnosed if the sphincter was displaced upwards into the thorax. If reflux is to cause heartburn it must be of sufficiently long standing to have exposed nerve endings in the oesophagus (Edwards, 1973). Acid reflux was demonstrated in 8 out of 10 pregnant women with heartburn and in 3 out of 10 mothers without heartburn (Hey et al, 1977). These workers demonstrated that maximum sphincter pressure is substantially reduced in the presence of heartburn. Regurgitation is commonest in the supine position (Hart, 1978).

Intragastric pressure. The pressure within the stomach is considerably increased in the last weeks of pregnancy. Spence et al (1967) recorded a mean intragastric pressure of 13.6 cmH$_2$O (1.3 kPa) in the supine position among patients at term. The mean intragastric pressure in a control series of non-pregnant patients was 7.3 cmH$_2$O (0.7 kPa). Somewhat higher values were recorded by Lind and others (1968), who noted a mean intragastric pressure of 17.2 cmH$_2$O (1.7 kPa) in pregnant women and 12.1 cmH$_2$O (1.2 kPa) in control subjects. In the series of Spence et al there was a mean further rise of 5.6 cmH$_2$O (0.5 kPa) in the lithotomy position and a mean further rise of 3.2 cmH$_2$O (0.3 kPa) in the Trendelenberg position. In a few patients with twins, hydramnios or gross obesity the intragastric pressure exceeded 40 cmH$_2$O (3.9 kPa). In early pregnancy there is a small increase in intragastric pressure. In women with heartburn at less than 20 weeks gestation the barrier pressure between stomach and oesophagus is reduced (Brock-Utne et al, 1981). Thus, even in early pregnancy, heartburn is a warning to the anaesthetist.

Regurgitation will occur when the intragastric pressure exceeds the opening pressure of the gastro-oesophageal sphincter. From the results of Lind et al (1968) it can be seen that the increase in intragastric pressure which occurs in pregnancy is accompanied by an even greater rise in sphincter opening pressure (Table 2) and that the risk of regurgitation is not enhanced. Of great significance to the anaesthetist is the observation that in pregnant

Table 2. Mean intragastric and gastro-oesophageal sphincter opening pressures* in supine women (From Lind et al, 1968)

	Controls	Term pregnancy	Term pregnancy with heartburn
Intragastric pressure	12.1 (1.2)	17.2 (1.7)	16.5 (1.6)
Sphincter opening pressure	34.8 (3.4)	44.8 (4.4)	23.8 (2.3)
Gastro-oesophageal pressure gradient	22.7 (2.2)	27.6 (2.7)	7.3 (0.7)

*Measured as cmH$_2$O with kPa shown in parentheses.

patients with heartburn the sphincter opening pressure (sphincter tone) is considerably reduced and the gastro-oesophageal pressure gradient is reduced to a mere $7.3\,cmH_2O$ (0.7 kPa). This gradient is sometimes referred to as the barrier pressure.

Metoclopramide increases the tone of the gastro-oesophageal sphincter in non-pregnant subjects (Brock-Utne et al, 1976, 1978a) but in pregnancy this action seems less consistent (Hey, 1978). Narcotic analgesics, intravenous atropine and glycopyrrolate lower the tone of the sphincter (Hall et al, 1975; Brock-Utne et al, 1976, 1978a,b; Hey et al, 1983) and these effects are reversible by metoclopramide, at least in non-pregnant subjects (Ostick and Hey, 1977). The H_2-receptor antagonists, cimetidine and ranitidine, do not alter the sphincter tone when given by mouth or intravenously (Kravitz et al, 1978; Denis et al, 1981).

It is often suggested that the fasciculations of suxamethonium may increase intragastric pressure and cause regurgitation. According to Smith et al (1978) this is not the case because suxamethonium causes an accompanying increase in sphincter tone and barrier pressure is actually increased. Pancuronium and to a lesser extent vecuronium increase sphincter tone (Hunt et al, 1984). The effect has not been studied in pregnancy.

Gastric acid secretion. There is a reduction in the quantity of hydrochloric acid secreted by the stomach during the second trimester of pregnancy, and a return to normal occurs in the last few weeks of pregnancy. Approximately 50% of women in labour have a gastric pH below 2.5 (Roberts and Shirley, 1976).

LIVER FUNCTION

The liver remains normal in size during pregnancy and its histological appearance is unaltered. The changes in liver function are in general terms not extensive, but there are alterations in plasma protein patterns and in the enzymes involved in the breakdown of certain drugs which are of interest to the anaesthetist. Hepatic blood flow is thought to be unchanged by pregnancy.

The lowering of the plasma albumin concentration and the elevation of the concentration of certain of the plasma globulin fractions which occurs in pregnancy are presumably reflections of alterations in liver metabolism. The serum bilirubin concentration is unchanged. A few women develop a reversible jaundice with increased bile viscosity and dilated bile cannaliculi. There is an increase in the concentration of some enzymes in the serum, including glutamic oxaloacetic transaminase, alkaline phosphatase and lactic dehydrogenase. The serum cholinesterase level is reduced by about 28% (Shnider, 1965; Robertson, 1966). This is insufficient to cause clinically important prolongation of suxamethonium apnoea. In gestational trophoblastic disease and after frequently repeated plasmapheresis serum cholinesterase levels may fall sharply and suxamethonium apnoea may be prolonged (Evans et al, 1980; Davies et al, 1983). The lowest cholinesterase levels in normal pregnancy are likely to occur shortly after delivery.

The rate of clearance of bromsulphthalein from the blood is frequently reduced in pregnancy (Smith et al, 1962; Brewer and Hjelte, 1965). This observation need not necessarily imply that hepatic function is impaired. Alternative explanations include a delay in the excretion of bromsulphthalein into the bile (Tindall and Beazley, 1965) and an increase in the binding of bromsulphthalein to plasma proteins which would delay the clearance of the dye from the plasma (Crawford and Hooi, 1968).

Other standard tests of liver function are not altered to any clinically important extent during normal pregnancy. Small increases in thymol turbidity and cephalin flocculation are present in about 10% of pregnant women and may be due to extrahepatic obstruction rather than to cellular damage (McNair and Jaynes, 1960). Alternatively the observations may be regarded as spurious, owing to the use of an inappropriate test.

Of interest to the anaesthetist is the observation by Crawford and Rudofsky (1966) that the ability to metabolize pethidine and certain other drugs may be reduced during pregnancy and also in women taking oral contraceptives and in the newborn. This observation was formerly attributed to an effect of oestrogens upon hepatic enzyme systems and was not confirmed by Kuhnert et al (1980). The increase in the binding capacity of the plasma proteins for drugs, which occurs during pregnancy, affects the placental transfer of drugs.

PREGNANCY, LABOUR AND THE STRESS RESPONSE

Plasma levels of adrenaline, noradrenaline and dopamine are reduced towards the end of normal pregnancy (Jones and Greiss, 1982). The concentrations of catecholamines rise progressively during painful labour, returning to normal within 20 minutes of delivery (Lederman et al, 1977). This catecholamine response is diminished when epidural analgesia is used (Falconer and Powles, 1982; Jouppila et al, 1984). Plasma cortisol levels increase during painful labour but not when pain is relieved by epidural analgesia (Maltau et al, 1979). Towards term the concentration of β-endorphin, β-lipotrophin and γ-lipotrophin increases, and there is a further increase during painful labour (Browning et al, 1983; Riss and Bieglmayer, 1984).

A picture emerges of painful labour as a stressful situation. The stress response, and presumably the stress, is largely prevented or reversed by epidural analgesia. During caesarean section under epidural or spinal anaesthesia, maternal β-endorphin levels are halved, whereas when general anaesthesia is used the β-endorphin levels increase by 50% (Datta et al, 1983). It has been postulated that the high levels of β-endorphin could explain the decrease in MAC (minimum alveolar concentration) for inhalational agents during obstetric anaesthesia (Abboud et al, 1983).

FAT AND CARBOHYDRATE METABOLISM

The pregnant woman adapts rapidly to starvation. When feeding is restricted or prohibited before surgery or during labour, there is early activation of fat metabolism. Fatty acids are utilized and glucose is thereby saved for the fetus. When nourishment is taken there is accelerated deposition in the energy depots (Dick et al, 1977).

Gluconeogenesis is decreased in pregnancy and therefore blood glucose concentrations tend to be low. Hypoglycaemia is accompanied by a large increase in ketone body formation and ketonuria is common in labour. Maternal hypoglycaemia leads to fetal hypoglycaemia and this in turn causes the fetus to draw upon its stores of glycogen.

These consequences of maternal starvation do not justify oral feeding in labour because of the possible need for general anaesthesia. Ketonuria is no longer viewed as a disaster in labour which must be prevented or treated by 'forced feeding' with intravenous sugar solutions, and the risks for the fetus and neonate of maternal hyperglycaemia are now recognized. Maternal hyperglycaemia rapidly produces the same condition in the fetus who responds by producing insulin. Delivery is followed by dangerous hypoglycaemia and acidosis (Kenepp et al, 1982; Lawrence et al, 1982). Glucose-free crystalloid solutions should be infused at caesarean section and the regimen should not cause maternal or neonatal hypoglycaemia (Thomas et al, 1984). Normoglycaemia should be the aim and a maximum glucose intake of 20 g/h has been recommended by Mendola et al (1982). Ketonuria in labour should be treated initially by infusing Hartmann's solution. The indication for glucose therapy is hypoglycaemia.

RENAL FUNCTION

Anatomical changes. Dilation of the ureters and renal pelves is present from the third month of pregnancy until term and is usually more pronounced on the right side. The cause is probably mechanical obstruction of the ureters by dilated blood vessels and the obstruction may be aggravated later in pregnancy by the enlarged uterus. A hormonal effect causing relaxation of the ureteric muscle may be an additional causal factor. Urinary stasis results from this effect and predisposes to infection. Crawford (1972) thinks that pain, especially in early labour, may originate in the dilated renal tract following upon compression by the uterus and be referred to the segmental distribution of the tenth and eleventh thoracic nerves.

Renal blood flow. Effective renal plasma flow is increased in early pregnancy, remains at a higher level until the final weeks and then falls again, even in the absence of aortocaval compression (Dunlop, 1981). Lindheimer et al (1973) observed substantial falls in renal blood flow on changing from the lateral to the supine or erect position.

Glomerular filtration rate. By week 10 or week 12 of pregnancy the glomerular filtration rate has increased by about 60% and remains at this level during the second trimester, falling again towards term. Glomerular filtration rate therefore mimics renal blood flow. Using a creatinine clearance method a glomerular filtration rate of approximately 150 ml/min is a representative value for pregnancy (Davison and Noble, 1981; Dunlop, 1981). The glomerular filtration rate is reduced in the supine, but not in the lateral, position in late pregnancy (Lindheimer et al, 1973; Chesley and Sloan, 1964). The increased glomerular filtration rate is not accompanied by an increase in the production of urea and creatinine and therefore the plasma concentration of these substances decreases.

Tubular reabsorption. The reabsorption of water and electrolytes in the renal tubules increases in proportion to the increase in the glomerular filtration rate so that the balance of salt and water is maintained.

Constituents of the urine. Glycosuria of pregnancy is associated with a lowering of the renal threshold for glucose. The glomerular filtration rate for glucose is substantially increased but tubular reabsorption is not always sufficient to cope with the increased filtration of glucose. Glycosuria may therefore occur without hyperglycaemia.

Lactose is a normal constituent of the urine in pregnancy because this sugar is not completely reabsorbed in the tubules.

THE EPIDURAL AND SUBARACHNOID SPACES

There are quite substantial pressure and volume changes in the epidural and subarachnoid spaces which have important effects upon the spread of solutions within these compartments and which significantly reduce the dose requirements of local anaesthetic drugs when epidural and subarachnoid analgesia are employed in obstetric practice with the mother in the supine position. When caval occlusion is prevented and engorgement of the epidural veins is lessened or absent, then the dose requirements of the pregnant women are similar to those of non-pregnant controls (Grundy et al, 1978).

The lumbar epidural space. The epidural veins are veins of the internal vertebral venous plexus and are part of the alternative vertebral and azygous venous system by which blood can reach the heart from the lower limbs. This venous system is important in pregnancy in compensation for the obstruction to the vena cava which is often present. In consequence the epidural veins are dilated and engorged with blood in the supine position in the final weeks of pregnancy and it is the 'space-occupying and massaging effect' of these veins which alters the response of the pregnant patient to epidural analgesia (Bromage, 1961). Because the maximum total volume of the spinal epidural space is fixed, the engorged veins act as a space-occupying lesion to reduce the volume of the extravascular portion of the space. Consequently solutions injected into the lumbar epidural space will spread more extensively when the mother is in the supine position. It is for this reason that the dose requirements for lumbar epidural analgesia are reduced by about one-third in pregnancy (Bromage, 1962). Perhaps surprisingly the spread of solutions in the epidural space is also more extensive in early pregnancy and here a non-mechanical explanation is needed. Perhaps the hyperventilation of pregnancy decreases buffering capacity and local anaesthetics remain as free salts for longer. This would allow them to remain in the epidural space for longer and therefore to spread further (Fagraeus et al, 1983). During labour there is progressive further engorgement of the epidural veins, even if caval occlusion is avoided (Galbert and Marx, 1974). Puncture of the engorged veins by an epidural catheter is common. In the sitting position the epidural veins may be distended with blood because they now lie below the level of the heart.

Studies by Harrison et al (1985), in which resin was injected into the epidural space of cadavers, suggested that the lumbar epidural space may be little more than a potential space distending after injection. These workers found that spread within the epidural space is influenced by the pressure in the subarachnoid space.

Epidural pressures. Baseline pressures, between contractions, are from 1.63 cmH$_2$O (0.16 kPa) in the lateral position in very early labour and rise to between 4 and 10 cmH$_2$O (0.4 and 1.0 kPa) by the end of the first stage. Pressures are higher in the supine position, confirming that caval occlusion further engorges the epidural veins (Galbert and Marx, 1974). Pressure in the lumbar epidural space in the non-pregnant subject is usually −1 cmH$_2$O (−0.1 kPa) (Usubiaga et al, 1967). In pregnancy the pressure is slightly positive and again becomes slightly negative a few hours after delivery (Messih, 1981). During uterine contractions the pressure in the epidural space rises by a further 2–8 cmH$_2$O (0.2–0.8 kPa) in the lateral position. The pressure increase with contractions is less marked or even absent when pain has been relieved, indicating that movement and rigidity contribute to the pressure changes observed during painful contractions (Messih, 1981). During expulsive efforts the pressure in the epidural space ranges from 20 to 60 cmH$_2$O (2.0–5.9 kPa). It is widely believed that the spread of solutions in the epidural space will be further exaggerated during contractions and that injections should be made between contractions. In the study by Sivakumaran and others (1982) spread was not thought to be influenced by injection during contractions. It is concluded that methods of identifying the lumbar epidural space which depend on the existence of a negative pressure are unsuitable for use in obstetrics. In the sitting position the cerebrospinal fluid pressure will rise in the lumbar region and the dura may bulge so that the volume of the surrounding epidural space diminishes. Dural puncture might be more likely and the spread of solutions would be more extensive in the epidural space. When a fluid is injected into the epidural space the dura is compressed, and Shah (1981) has suggested that dural compression together with escape of the fluid through the intervertebral foramina would allow rapid equilibration of epidural and cerebrospinal fluid pressures.

There appears to be no information on pressures within the sacral part of the epidural space in pregnancy and labour.

The subarachnoid space. The constituents of the cerebrospinal fluid are unaltered during pregnancy (Marx and Orkin, 1965) and therefore the modified responses to subarachnoid analgesia which occur in pregnancy are not due to alterations in the protein-binding capacity of the cerebrospinal fluid for local anaesthetic drugs. Neither are they due to changes in the specific gravity of the cerebrospinal fluid.

Cerebrospinal fluid pressures are increased by caval occlusion and by uterine contractions in labour. During pregnancy the pressure of the cerebrospinal fluid is normal in the lateral position. Baseline pressures in labour, between contractions, are $28\,cmH_2O$ ($2.7\,kPa$) in the supine position and fall to $22\,cmH_2O$ ($2.2\,kPa$) when the uterus is displaced to the left to relieve caval occlusion (Galbert and Marx, 1974). During painful contractions the cerebrospinal fluid pressure rises by 11 to $39\,cmH_2O$ ($1.1–3.8\,kPa$) above the baseline value (Marx et al, 1961; Marx et al, 1962; Galbert and Marx, 1974). Pressures are much higher in the lumbar portion of the subarachnoid space when the patient is sitting (Shah, 1981). The relief of pain results in a substantial diminution in the extent of the pressure rises which accompany uterine contractions. The small pressure rises which may be recorded even during completely painless contractions are attributed by Hopkins et al (1965) to rises in central venous and arterial pressure and to further engorgement of the epidural veins. In the second stage of labour the cerebrospinal fluid pressure may reach $70\,cmH_2O$ ($6.9\,kPa$).

It has long been recognized that the spread of local anaesthetic solutions in the cerebrospinal fluid is more extensive during pregnancy. This phenomenon is commonly attributed to the raised pressure of the cerebrospinal fluid. Hopkins and his colleagues argue that a rise in pressure does not necessarily mean that turbulence occurs and they attribute the more extensive spread of solutions in the cerebrospinal fluid to reductions in the volume of the subarachnoid space caused by pressure of the engorged epidural veins upon the dura. This view is shared by Galbert and Marx (1974). The exaggerated lumbar lordosis of pregnancy may encourage cephalad spread. The spread of local anaesthetic solutions can sometimes be rather unpredictable in pregnancy and depends also upon variables such as the nature and specific gravity of the solution, the speed of injection and the position of the patient during and after the injection.

REFERENCES

Abboud, T.K., Sarkis, F. and Hung, T.T. (1983) Effects of epidural anesthesia during labor on maternal plasma beta endorphin levels. *Anesthesiology*, **59**, 1.

Abouleish, E., Kang, Y., Uram, M., McKenzie, R. and Taylor, F. (1982) Hemodynamic changes during cesarean section under spinal analgesia using impedence cardiography. *Anesthesiology*, **57**, A397.

Andersen, G.J. and Walker, J. (1970) Effect of labour on the maternal blood–gas and acid–base status. *J. Obstet. Gynaec. Br. Commonw.*, **77**, 289.

Ang, C.K., Tan, T.H., Walters, W.A.W. and Wood, C. (1969) Postural influence on maternal capillary oxygen and carbon dioxide tension. *Br. med. J.*, **iv**, 20.

Archer, G.W. and Marx, G.F. (1974) Arterial oxygen tension during apnoea in parturient women. *Br. J. Anaesth.*, **46**, 358.

Assali, N.S., Vergon, J.M., Tada, Y. and Garber, S.T. (1952) Studies on autonomic blockade. *Am. J. Obstet. Gynec.*, **63**, 978.

Assali, N.S., Rauramo, L. and Peltonen, T. (1960) Measurement of uterine blood flow and metabolism. *Am. J. Obstet. Gynec.*, **79**, 86.

Atkins, A.J.F., Watt, J.M., Milan, P., Davies, P. and Crawford, J.S. (1981) A longitudinal study of cardiovascular dynamic changes throughout pregnancy. *Europ. J. Obstet. Gynaec. and Repr. Biol.*, **12**, 215.

Attia, R.R., Ebeid, A.M., Fischer, J.E. and Goudsouzian, N.G. (1982) Maternal, fetal and placental gastrin concentrations. *Anaesthesia*, **37**, 18.

Bader, R.A., Bader, M.E., Rose, D.J. and Braunwald, E. (1955) Hemodynamics at rest and during exercise in normal pregnancy as studied by cardiac catheterization. *J. clin. Invest.*, **34**, 1524.

Baldwin, G.R., Moorthi, D.S., Whelton, J.A. and MacDonnell, K.F. (1977) New lung functions in pregnancy. *Am. J. Obstet. Gynec.*, **127**, 235.

Bevan, D.R., Holdcroft, A., Loh, L. et al (1974) Closing volume and pregnancy. *Br. med. J.*, **i**, 13.

Bhatt, J.R. (1965) Blood volume variations during labor and the early puerperium. *Obstet. Gynec.*, **26**, 243.

Blechner, J.N., Cotter, J.R., Stenger, V.G., Hinkley, C.M. and Prystowsky, H. (1968) Oxygen, carbon dioxide and hydrogen ion concentrations in arterial blood during pregnancy. *Am. J. Obstet. Gynec.*, **100**, 1.

Blitt, C.D., Petty, W.C., Alberternst, E.E. and Wright, B.J. (1977). Correlation of plasma cholinesterase activity and duration of action of succinylcholine during pregnancy. *Anesth. Analg. curr. Res.*, **56**, 78.

Bolton, F.G. and Street, M. (1983) Changes in erythrocyte volume and shape in pregnancy. *Br. J. Obstet. Gynaec*, **89**, 1018.

Bonnar, J., Prentice, C.R.M., McNicol, G.P. and Douglas, A.S. (1970) Haemostatic mechanism in the uterine circulation during placental separation. *Br. med. J.*, **ii**, 564.

Bonnar, J., McNicol, G.P. and Douglas, A.S. (1971). Coagulation and fibrinolytic systems in pre-eclampsia. *Br. med. J.*, **ii**, 12.

Bouterline-Young, H. and Bouterline-Young, E. (1956). Alveolar carbon dioxide levels in pregnant, parturient and lactating subjects. *J. Obstet. Gynaec. Br. Emp.*, **63**, 509.

Brant, H.A. (1966) Blood loss at Caesarean section. *J. Obstet. Gynaec. Br. Commonw.*, **73**, 456.

Brewer, T.H. and Hjelte, V. (1965) Bromsulfophthalein conjugation in toxemia of late pregnancy. *Am. J. Obstet. Gynec.*, **92**, 114.

Brock-Utne, J.G., Rubin, J., Downing, J.W. et al (1976) The administration of metoclopramide with atropine. *Anaesthesia*, **31**, 1186.

Brock-Utne, J.G., Rubin, J., Welman, S. et al (1978a) The action of commonly used anti-emetics on the lower oesophageal sphincter. *Br. J. Anaesth.*, **50**, 295.

Brock-Utne, J.G., Rubin, J., Welman, S. et al (1978b) The effect of glycopyrrolate (Robinul) on the lower oesophageal sphincter. *Can. Anaesth. Soc. J.*, **25**, 144.

Brock-Utne, J.G., Dow, T.G.B., Dimopoulos, G.E. et al (1981) Gastric and lower oesophageal sphincter (LOS) pressures in early pregnancy. *Br. J. Anaesth.*, **53**, 381.

Bromage, P.R. (1961) Continuous lumbar epidural analgesia for obstetrics. *Can. med. Ass. J.*, **85**, 1136.

Bromage, P.R. (1962) Spread of analgesic solutions in the epidural space and their site of action: a statistical study. *Br. J. Anaesth.*, **34**, 161.

Browning, A.J.F., Butt, W.R., Lynch, S.S. and Crawford, J.S. (1983) Maternal and cord plasma concentrations of β-lipotrophin, β-endorphin and γ-lipotrophin at delivery: effect of analgesia. *Br. J. Obstet. Gynaec.*, **90**, 1152.

Buley, R.J.R., Downing, J.W., Brock-Utne, J.G. and Cuerden, C. (1977) Right versus lateral tilt for Caesarean section. *Br. J. Anaesth.*, **49**, 1009.

Burg, J.R., Dodek, A., Kloster, F.E. and Metcalfe, J. (1974) Alterations of systolic time intervals during pregnancy. *Circulation*, **49**, 560

Butler, N.R., Goldstein, H. and Ross, E.M. (1972) Cigarette smoking in pregnancy: its influence on birth weight and perinatal mortality. *Br. med. J.*, **ii**, 127.

Cameron, S.J., Bain, H.H. and Grant, I.W.B. (1970) Ventilatory function in pregnancy. *Scott. med. J.*, **15**, 243.

Campbell, E.J.M. and Howell, J.B.L. (1963) The sensation of breathlessness. *Br. med. Bull.*, **19**, 36.

Castro, L. de P. (1967) Reflux esophagitis as the cause of heartburn in pregnancy. *Am. J. Obstet. Gynec.*, **98**, 1.

Chesley, L.C. and Duffus, G.M. (1971) Posture and apparent plasma volume in late pregnancy. *J. Obstet. Gynaec. Br. Commonw.*, **78**, 406.

Chesley, L.C. and Sloan, D.M. (1964) The effect of posture on renal function in late pregnancy. *Am. J. Obstet. Gynec.*, **89**, 754.

Christofides, N.D., Ghatei, M.A., Bloom, S.R., Borberg, C. and Gillmer, M.D.G. (1982) Decreased plasma motilin concentration in pregnancy. *Br. med. J.*, **ii**, 1453.

Clapp, J.F. (1978) Cardiac output and uterine blood flow in the pregnant ewe. *Am. J. Obstet. Gynec.*, **130**, 419.

Colditz, R.B. and Josey, W.E. (1970) Central venous pressure in supine position during normal pregnancy. *Obstet. Gynec.*, **36**, 769.

Cole, P.V., Hawkins, L.H. and Roberts, D. (1972) Smoking during pregnancy and its effect on the fetus. *J. Obstet. Gynaec. Br. Commonw.*, **79**, 782.

Craig, D.B. and Toole, M.A. (1975) Airway closure in pregnancy. *Can. Anaesth. Soc. J.*, **22**, 665.

Crawford, J.S. (1972) *Principles and Practice of Obstetric Anaesthesia*, 3rd ed. Oxford: Blackwell.

Crawford, J.S. and Hooi, H.W.Y. (1968) Binding of bromsulphthalein by serum albumin from pregnant women, neonates and subjects on oral contraceptives. *Br. J. Anaesth.*, **40**, 723.

Crawford, J.S. and Rudofsky, S. (1966) Some alterations in the pattern of drug metabolism associated with pregnancy, oral contraceptives and the newly born. *Br. J. Anaesth.*, **38**, 446.

Crawford, J.S. and Tunstall, M.E. (1968) Notes on respiratory performance during labour. *Br. J. Anaesth.*, **40**, 612.

Crawford, J.S., Burton, M. and Davies, P. (1972) Time and lateral tilt at Caesarean section. *Br. J. Anaesth.*, **44**, 477.

Cugell, D.W., Frank, N.R., Gaensler, E.A. and Badger, T.L. (1953) Pulmonary function in pregnancy. I. Serial observations in normal women. *Am. Rev. Tuberc. pulm. Dis.*, **67**, 568.

Darmady, J.M. and Postle, A.D. (1982) Lipid metabolism in pregnancy. *Br. J. Obstet. Gynaec.*, **89**, 211.

Datta, S., Crocker, J.S. and Alper, M.H. (1977) Muscle pain following administration of suxamethonium to pregnant and non-pregnant patients undergoing laparoscopic tubal ligation. *Br. J. Anaesth.*, **49**, 625.

Datta, S., Carr, D.B., Lambert, D.H. et al (1983) Anesthesia for cesarean delivery. Relationship of maternal and fetal plasma γ-endorphins to different types of anesthesia. *Anesthesiology*, **59**, A418.

Davies, J.M., Hogg, M.I.J. and Rosen, M. (1974) Upper limits of resistance of apparatus for inhalation analgesia during labour. *Br. J. Anaesth.*, **46**, 136.

Davies, J.M., Carmichael, D. and Dymond, C. (1983) Plasma cholinesterase and trophoblastic disease. *Anaesthesia*, **38**, 1071.

Davison, J.M. and Noble, M.C. (1981) Serial changes in 24 hour creatinine clearance during normal menstrual cycles and the first trimester of pregnancy. *Br. J. Obstet Gynaec.*, **88**, 10.

Davison, J.S., Davison, M.C. and Hay, D.M. (1970) Gastric emptying time in late pregnancy and labour. *J. Obstet. Gynaec. Br. Commonw.*, **77**, 37.

Denis, P., Galmiche, J.P., Ducrotte, P. et al (1981) Effect of ranitidine on resting pressure and pentagastrin response of human lower esophageal sphincter. *Dig. Dis.*, **26**, 999.

Department of Health and Social Security (1982) *Report on Confidential Enquiries into Maternal Death in England and Wales 1976–78.* London: H.M.S.O.

Dick, W., Ahnefeld, F.W., Milewski, P. and Schoch, G. (1977) Important adaptation processes of women during pregnancy: anaesthesiologic considerations. *J. perinat. Med.*, **5**, 103.

Dinnick, O.P. (1967) Reflux reflections. *Proc. R. Soc. Med.*, **60**, 623.

Drummond, G.B., Scott, S.E.M., Lees, M.M. and Scott, D.B. (1974) Effects of posture on limb blood flow in late pregnancy. *Br. med. J.*, **iv**, 587.

Dunlop, W. (1981) Serial changes in renal haemodynamics during normal human pregnancy. *Br. J. Obstet. Gynaec.*, **88**, 1.

Eckstein, K.L. and Marx, G.F. (1974) Aortocaval compression and uterine displacement. *Anesthesiology*, **40**, 92.

Edwards, D.A.W. (1973) Symposium on gastro-oesophageal reflux and its complications. *Gut*, **14**, 233.

Evans, R.T. and Wroe, J.M. (1980) Plasma cholinesterase changes during pregnancy. Their interpretation in a case of suxamethonium-induced apnoea., *Anaesthesia*, **35**, 64.

Evans, R.T., Macdonald, R. and Robinson, A. (1980) Suxamethonium apnoea associated with plasmapheresis. *Anaesthesia*, **35**, 198.

Fadl, E.T. and Utting, J.E. (1969) A study of maternal acid–base state during labour. *Br. J. Anaesth.*, **41**, 327.

Fadl, E.T. and Utting, J.E. (1970) Acid–base disturbances in obstetrics. *Proc. R. Soc. Med.*, **63**, 77.

Fagraeus, L., Urban, B.J. and Bromage, P.R. (1983) Spread of epidural analgesia in early pregnancy. *Anesthesiology*, **58**, 184.

Falconer, A.D. and Powles, A.B. (1982) Plasma noradrenaline levels during labour. Influence of elective lumbar epidural blockade. *Anaesthesia*, **37**, 416.

Farman, J.V. and Thorpe, M.H. (1969) Compliance changes during Caesarean section. *Br. J. Anaesth*, **41**, 999.

Fisher, A. and Prys-Roberts, C. (1968) Maternal pulmonary gas exchange. *Anaesthesia*, **23**, 350.

Galbert, M.W. and Marx, G.F. (1974) Extradural pressures in the parturient patient. *Anesthesiology*, **40**, 499.

Gant, N.F., Daley, G.L., Chand, S., Whalley, P.J. and MacDonald, P.C. (1973) A study of Angiotensin II; pressor response throughout primigravid pregnancy. *J. clin. Invest.*, **52**, 2682.

Gee, J.B.L., Packer, B.S., Millen, J.E. and Robin, E.D. (1967) Pulmonary mechanics during pregnancy. *J. clin. Invest.*, **46**, 945.

Ginsburg, J. and Duncan, S. (1967) Peripheral blood flow in normal pregnancy. *Cardiovasc. Res.*, **1**, 132.

Ginsburg, J. and Duncan, S. (1969) Direct and indirect blood pressure measurements in pregnancy. *J. Obstet. Gynaec. Br. Commonw.*, **76**, 705.

Goodland, R.L. and Pommerenke, W.T. (1952) Cyclic fluctuations of the alveolar carbon dioxide tension during the normal menstrual cycle. *Fert. Steril.*, **3**, 394.

Goodland, R.L., Reynolds, J.G., McCoord, A.B. and Pommerenke, W.T. (1953) Respiratory and electrolyte effects induced by estrogen and progesterone. *Fert. Steril.*, **4**, 300.

Greiss, F.C. (1966) Pressure-flow relationships in the gravid uterine vascular bed. *Am. J. Obstet. Gynec.*, **96**, 41.

Greiss, F.C. (1972) Differential reactivity of the myometrial and placental vasculatures: adrenergic responses. *Am. J. Obstet. Gynec.*, **112**, 20.

Grundy, E.M., Zamora, A.M. and Winnie, A.P. (1978) Comparison of epidural anaesthesia in pregnant and non-pregnant women. *Anesth. Analg. curr. Res.*, **57**, 544.

Hagerdal, M., Morgan, C.W., Sumner, A.E. and Gutsche, B. (1983) Minute ventilation and oxygen consumption during labor with epidural anesthesia. *Anesthesiology*, **59**, 425.

Hall, A.W., Moasa, A.R., Clark, J., Cooley, G.R. and Skinner, D.B. (1975) The effect of premedication drugs on the lower oesophageal high pressure zone and reflux status of rhesus monkeys and man. *Gut*, **16**, 347.

Hardy, J.B. and Mellitus, E.D. (1972) Does maternal smoking during pregnancy have a long-term effect on the child? *Lancet*, **ii**, 1332.

Harlap, S. and Shiono, P.H. (1980) Alcohol, smoking and incidence of spontaneous abortion in the first and second trimester. *Lancet*, **ii**, 173.

Harrison, G.R., Parkin, I.G. and Shah, J.L. (1985) Resin injection studies of the lumbar epidural space. *Br J. Anaesth.*, **51**, 333.

Hart, D.M. (1978) Heartburn in pregnancy. *J. int. med. Res.*, **6**, Suppl. 1, 1.

Hazel, B. and Monier, D. (1971) Human serum cholinesterase: variation during pregnancy and postpartum. *Can. Anaesth. Soc. J.*, **18**, 272.

Hendricks, C.H. (1958) Hemodynamics of a uterine contraction. *Am. J. Obstet. Gynec.*, **76**, 968.

Hewlett, A.M., Hulands, G.H., Nunn, J.F. and Milledge, J.S. (1974) Functional residual capacity during anaesthesia. III. Artificial ventilation. *Br. J. Anaesth*, **46**, 95.

Hey, V.M.F. (1978) Gastro-oesophageal reflux in pregnancy: a review article. *J. int. med. Res.*, **6**, Suppl. 1, 18.

Hey, V.M.F., Cowley, D.J., Ganguli, P.C. et al (1977) Gastro-oesophageal reflux in late pregnancy. *Anaesthesia*, **32**, 372.

Hey, V.M.F., Phillips, K. and Woods, I. (1983) Pethidine, atropine, metoclopramide and the lower oesophagus. *Anaesthesia*, **38**, 650.

Holdcroft, A., Bevan, D.R., O'Sullivan, J.C. and Sykes, M.K. (1977) Airway closure and pregnancy. *Anaesthesia*, **32**, 517.

Holdsworth, J.D. (1978) Relationship between stomach contents and analgesia in labour. *Br. J. Anaesth.*, **50**, 1145.

Hopkins, E.L., Hendricks, C.H. and Cibils, L.A. (1965) Cerebrospinal fluid pressure in labor. *Am. J. Obstet. Gynec.*, **93**, 907.

Huch, A., Huch, R., Lindmark, G. and Rooth, G. (1974) Maternal hypoxaemia after pethidine. *J. Obstet. Gynaec. Br. Commonw*, **81**, 608.

Humphrey, M.D., Chang, A., Wood, E.C., Morgan, S. and Hounslow, D. (1974) A decrease in fetal pH during the second stage of labour when conducted in the dorsal position. *J. Obstet. Gynaec. Br. Commonw.*, **81**, 600

Hunt, P.C.W., Cotton, B.R. and Smith, G. (1984) Barrier pressure and muscle relaxants. Comparison of the effects of pancuronium and vecuronium on the lower oesophageal sphincter. *Anaesthesia*, **39**, 412.

Hytten, F.E. and Leitch, I. (1971) *The Physiology of Human Pregnancy*, 2nd ed. Oxford: Blackwell.

James, C.F., Gibbs, C.P. and Banner, T. (1984) Postpartum perioperative risk of aspiration pneumonia. *Anesthesiology*, **61**, 756.

Jassir, C., Yu, K.C. and Marx, G.F. (1973) Alveolar–arterial oxygen difference in parturient women with two types of uterine displacement. *Anesth. Analg. curr. Res.*, **52**, 43.

Jones, C.M. and Greiss, F.C. (1982) Effect of labor on maternal and fetal circulating catecholamines. *Am. J. Obstet. Gynec.*, **144**, 149.

Jouppila, R., Jouppila, P., Hollmen, A. and Kuikka, J. (1978a) Effect of segmental extradural analgesia on placental blood flow during normal labour. *Br. J. Anaesth.*, **50**, 563.

Jouppila, R., Jouppila, P., Kuikka, J. and Hollmen, A. (1978b) Placental blood flow during Caesarean section under lumbar extradural analgesia. *Br. J. Anaesth.*, **50**, 275.

Jouppila, R., Puolakka, J., Kauppila, A. and Vuori, J. (1984) Maternal and cord plasma noradrenaline concentrations during labour with and without segmental extradural analgesia and during Caesarian section. *Br. J. Anaesth.*, **56**, 251.

Kambam, J.R., Handtke, R.E., Brown, W.U. and Smith, B.E. (1983) Effect of pregnancy on oxygen dissociation. *Anesthesiology*, **59**, A359.

Kauppila, A., Koskinen, M., Puolakka, J., Tuimala, R. and Kuikka, J. (1980) Decreased intervillous and unchanged myometrial blood flow in supine recumbency. *Obstet. Gynec.*, **53**, 203.

Kenepp, N.B., Shelley, W.C., Gabbe, S.G. et al (1982) Fetal and neonatal hazards of maternal hydration with 5% dextrose before Caesarean section. *Lancet*, 1150.

Kerr, M.G., Scott, D.B. and Samuel, E. (1964) Studies of the inferior vena cava in pregnancy. *Br. med. J.*, **i**, 532.

Kravitz, J.J., Snape, W.J. and Cohen, S. (1978) Effects of histamine and histamine antagonists on human lower esophageal sphincter. *Gastroenterology*, **74**, 435.

Kuhnert, B.R., Kuhnert, P.M., Prochaska, A.L. and Sokol, R.J. (1980) Meperidine disposition in mother, neonate and non-pregnant females. *Clin. Pharmac. Ther.*, **27**, 486.

La Salvia, L.A. and Steffen, E.A. (1950) Delayed gastric emptying time in labor. *Am. J. Obstet. Gynec.*, **59**, 1075.

Lawrence, G.F., Brown, V., Parsons, R.J. and Cooke, I.D. (1982) Feto-maternal consequences of high-dose glucose infusion during labour. *Br. J. Obstet. Gynaec.*, **89**, 27.

Lederman, R.P., McCann, D.S. and Work, B. (1977) Endogenous plasma endorphins and norepinephrine in last-trimester pregnancy and labor. *Am. J. Obstet. Gynec.*, **129**, 5.

Lees, M.M., Scott, D.B., Kerr, M.G. and Taylor, S.H. (1967a) The circulatory effects of recumbent postural change in late pregnancy. *Clin. Sci.*, **32**, 453.

Lees, M.M., Taylor, S.H., Scott, D.B. and Kerr, M.G. (1967b) A study of cardiac output at rest throughout pregnancy. *J. Obstet. Gynaec. Br. Commonw.*, **74**, 319.

Lees, M.M., Scott, D.B. and Kerr, M.G. (1970) Haemodynamic changes associated with labour. *J. Obstet. Gynaec. Br. Commonw.*, **77**, 29.

Lehtorvita, P. and Forss, M. (1978) The acute effect of smoking on intervillous blood flow of the placenta. *Br. J. Obstet. Gynaec.*, **85**, 729.

Lind, F.J., Smith, A., McIver, D.K., Coopland, A.T. and Crispin, J.S. (1968) Heartburn in pregnancy—a manometric study. *Can. med. Ass. J.*, **98**, 571.

Lindheimer, M.D., Del Greco, F. and Ehrlich, E.N. (1973) Postural effects on Na and steroid excretion and serum renin activity during pregnancy. *J. appl. Physiol.*, **35**, 433.

Lippert, T.H., Cloeren, S.E., Fridrich, R. and Hinselmann, M. (1973) Continuous recording of uterplacental blood volume in the human. *Acta obstet. gynec. scand.*, **52**, 131.

Lucius, H., Gahlenbeck, H., Kleine, H.O., Fabel, H. and Bartles, H. (1970) Respiratory functions, buffer system and electrolyte concentrations of blood during human pregnancy. *Respiration Physiol.*, **9**, 311.

Lund, C.J. and Donovan, J.C. (1967) Blood volume during pregnancy. *Am. J. Obstet. Gynec.*, **98**, 393.

Macrae, D.J. and Palavradji, D. (1967) Maternal acid–base changes in pregnancy. *J. Obstet. Gynaec. Br. Commw.*, **74**, 11.

Maltau, J.M., Andersen, H.T. and Skrede, S. (1975) Obstetrical analgesia assessed by free fatty acid mobilization. *Acta anaesth. scand.*, **19**, 245.

Maltau, J.M., Eielsen, O.V. and Stokke, K.T. (1979) Effect of stress during labor on the concentration of cortisol and estriol in maternal plasma. *Am. J. Obstet. Gynec.*, **134**, 681.

Manning, F., Walker, D. and Feyerabend, C. (1978) The effect of nicotine on fetal breathing movements in conscious pregnant ewes. *Obstet. Gynec.*, **52**, 563.

Marx, G.F. and Greene, N.M. (1964) Maternal lactate, pyruvate and excess lactate production during labor and delivery. *Am. J. Obstet. Gynec.*, **90**, 786.

Marx, G.F. and Orkin, L.R. (1965) Cerebrospinal fluid proteins and spinal anesthesia in obstetrics. *Anesthesiology*, **26**, 340.

Marx, G.F. and Orkin, L.R. (1969) *Physiology of Obstetric Anesthesia*, p. 21. Springfield, Ill.: Charles C. Thomas.

Marx, G.F., Zemaitis, M.T. and Orkin, L.R. (1961) Cerebrospinal fluid pressures during labor and obstetrical anesthesia. *Anesthesiology*, **22**, 348.

Marx, G.F., Oka, Y. and Orkin, L.R. (1962) Cerebrospinal fluid pressures during labor. *Am. J. Obstet. Gynec.*, **84**, 213.

Marx, G.F., Murthy, P.K. and Orkin, L.R. (1970) Static compliance before and after vaginal delivery. *Br. J. Anaesth.*, **42**, 1100.

McLennan, C.E. (1943) Antecubital and femoral venous pressures in normal and toxemic pregnancy. *Am. J. Obstet. Gynec.*, **45**, 568.

McNair, R.D. and Jaynes, R.V. (1960) Alterations in liver function during normal pregnancy. *Am. J. Obstet. Gynec.*, **80**, 500.

Mendola, J., Grylack, L.J. and Scanlon, J.W. (1982) Effects of intrapartum maternal glucose infusion on the normal fetus and newborn. *Anesth. Analg. curr. Res.*, **61**, 32.

Messih, M.N.A. (1981) Epidural space pressures in the lumbar region during pregnancy. *Anaesthesia*, **36**, 775.

Metcalfe, J., Romney, S.L., Ramsey, L.H., Reid, D.E. and Burwell, C.S. (1955) Estimation of uterine blood flow in normal human pregnancy at term. *J. clin. Invest.*, **34**, 1632.

Meyer, M.B. (1978) How does maternal smoking affect birth weight and maternal weight gain? *Am. J. Obstet. Gynec.*, **131**, 888.

Miller, F.C., Petrie, R.H., Arce, J.J., Paul, R.H. and Hon, E.H. (1974) Hyperventilation during labor. *Am. J. Obstet. Gynec.*, **120**, 489.

Milne, J.A., Mills, R.J., Howie, A.D. and Pack, A.I. (1977a) Large airways function during normal pregnancy. *Br. J. Obstet. Gynaec.*, **84**, 448.

Milne, J.A., Mills, R.J., Coutts, J.R.T. et al (1977b) The effect of human pregnancy on the pulmonary transfer factor for carbon monoxide as measured by the single breath method. *Clin. Sci. Molec. Med.*, **53**, 271.

Mixson, W.J. and Woloshin, H.J. (1956) Hiatus hernia in pregnancy. *Obstet. Gynec.*, **8**, 249.

Moir, D.D. (1970) Anaesthesia for Caesarean section. *Br. J. Anaesth.*, **42**, 136.

Moir, D.D. and Amoa, A.B. (1979) Ergometrine or oxytocin? *Br. J. Anaesth.*, **51**, 113.

Moir, D.D. and Wallace, G. (1967) Blood loss at forceps delivery. *J. Obstet. Gynaec. Br. Commonw.*, **74**, 424.

Moodie, J.E. and Moir, D.D. (1976) Ergometrine, oxytocin and epidural analgesia. *Br. J. Anaesth.*, **48**, 571.

Myers, R.E., Stange, L., Joelson, I., Huzell, B. and Wussow, C. (1977) Effects upon the fetus of oxygen administration to the mother. *Acta obstet. gynec. scand.*, **56**, 195.

Newman, B. (1982) Cardiac output changes during Caesarian section. Measurement by transcutaneous aortvelography. *Anaesthesia*, **37**, 266.

Newman, B., Derrington, C. and Dore, C. (1983) Cardiac output and the recumbent position in late pregnancy. *Anaesthesia*, **34**, 332.

Nimmo, W.S., Wilson, J. and Prescott, L.F. (1975) Narcotic analgesics and delayed gastric emptying during labour. *Lancet*, **i**, 890.

Novy, M.J. and Edwards, M.J. (1967) Respiratory problems in pregnancy. *Am. J. Obstet. Gynec.*, **99**, 1024.

Ostick, D.G. and Hey, V.M.F. (1977) The action of pethidine and metoclopramide on the gastro-oesophageal sphincter in healthy volunteers. *Anaesthesia*, **32**, 101.

Ouellette, E.M., Rosett, H.L., Rosman, N.P. and Weiner, L. (1977) Adverse effects on offspring of maternal alcohol abuse during pregnancy. *New Engl. J. Med.*, **297**, 528.

Paintin, D.B. (1962) The size of the total red cell volume in pregnancy. *J. Obstet. Gynaec. Br. Commonw.*, **69**, 719.

Palahniuk, R.J., Shnider, S.M. and Eger, E.I. (1974) Pregnancy decreases the requirements for inhaled anesthetic agents. *Anesthesiology*, **41**, 82.

Parry, E., Shields, R. and Turnbull, A.C. (1970) Transit time in the small intestine in pregnancy. *J. Obstet. Gynaec. Br. Commonw.*, **77**, 900.

Pearson, J.F. and Davies, P. (1973a) The effect of continuous epidural analgesia on the acid–base status of maternal arterial blood during the first stage of labour. *J. Obstet. Gynaec. Br. Commonw.*, **80**, 218.

Pearson, J.F. and Davies, P. (1973b) The effect of continuous epidural analgesia on maternal acid–base balance and arterial lactate concentration during the second stage of labour. *J. Obstet. Gynaec. Br. Commonw.*, **80**, 225.

Pernoll, M.L., Metcalfe, J., Schlenker, T.L., Welch, J.E. and Matsumoto, J.A. (1975a) Oxygen consumption at rest and during exercise in pregnancy. *Respiration Physiol.*, **25**, 285.

Pernoll, M.L., Metcalfe, J., Kovach, P.A., Wachter, R. and Dunham, M.J. (1975b) Ventilation during rest and exercise in pregnancy and postpartum. *Respiration Physiol.*, **25**, 295.

Pirani, B.B.K., Campbell, D.M. and MacGillivray, I. (1973) Plasma volume in normal first pregnancy. *J. Obstet. Gynaec. Br. Commonw.*, **80**, 884.

Poseiro, J.J. (1967) Compression of the aorta or iliac arteries by the contracting human uterus during labor. In *Effects of Labor on Fetus and Newborn*, ed. Caldeyro-Barcia, R. New York: Pergamon Press

Pritchard, J.A. (1965) Blood volume changes during pregnancy. *Anesthesiology*, **26**, 393.

Pritchard, J.A., Wiggins, K.M. and Dickey, J.C. (1960) Blood volume changes in pregnancy and the puerperium. *Am. J. Obstet. Gynec*, **80**, 956.

Pritchard, J.A., Baldwin, R.M., Dickey, J.C. and Wiggins, K.M. (1962) Blood volume changes in pregnancy and the puerperium. *Am. J. Obstet. Gynec.*, **84**, 1271.

Prowse, C.M. and Gaensler, E.A. (1965) Respiratory and acid–base changes during pregnancy. *Anesthesiology*, **26**, 381.

Pyörälä, T. (1966) Cardiovascular response to the upright position during pregnancy. *Acta obstet. gynec. scand.*, **45**, Suppl. 5.

Quinlivan, W.L.G. and Brock, J.A. (1970) Blood volume changes and blood loss associated with labor. *Am. J. Obstet. Gynec.*, **106**, 843.

Ramanathan, S., Ghandhi, S., Arismendy, J., Chalon, J. and Turndorf, A. (1982) Oxygen transfer from mother to fetus during cesarean section under epidural anesthesia. *Anesth. Analg. curr. Res.*, **61**, 576.

Read, M.D. and Anderton, J.M. (1977) Radioisotope dilution technique for measurement of blood loss associated with lower segment Caesarean section. *Br. J. Obstet. Gynaec.*, **84**, 859.

Rekonen, A., Luotola, H., Pitkanen, M., Kuikka, J. and Pyörälä, T. (1976) Measurement of intervillous and myometrial blood flow by an intravenous ^{133}Xe method. *Br. J. Obstet. Gynaec.*, **83**, 723.

Riss, P.A. and Bieglmayer, C. (1984) Obstetric analgesia and immunoreactive endorphin peptides in maternal plasma during labor. *Gynec. Obstet. Invest.*, **17**, 127.

Roberts, R.B. and Shirley, M.A. (1976) The obstetrician's role in reducing the risk of aspiration pneumonitis. *Am. J. Obstet. Gynec.*, **124**, 611.

Robertson, G.S. (1966) Serum cholinesterase deficiency. 2. Pregnancy. *Br. J. Anaesth.*, **38**, 361.

Robertson, E.G. (1968) Increased erythrocyte fragility in association with osmotic changes in pregnancy serum. *J. Reprod. Fert.*, **16**, 323.

Romney, S.L., Reid, D.E., Metcalfe, J. and Burwell, C.S. (1955) Oxygen utilization by the human fetus in utero. *Am. J. Obstet. Gynec.*, **70**, 791.

Rubler, S., Schneebaum, R. and Hammer, N. (1973) Systolic intervals in pregnancy and the post-partum period. *Am. Heart J.*, **86**, 182.

Rush, D. (1974) Examination of the relationship between birthweight, cigarette smoking during pregnancy and maternal weight gain. *J. Obstet. Gynaec. Br. Commonw.*, **81**, 746.

Russell, I.F. and Chambers, W.A. (1981) Closing volume in normal pregnancy. *Br. J. Anaesth.*, **53**, 1043.

Scott, D.B. (1963) Inferior vena caval pressure changes during anaesthesia. *Anaesthesia*, **18**, 135.

Scott, J.S. (1968) Coagulation failure in obstetrics. *Br. med. Bull.*, **24**, 32.

Scott, J.S. (1969) Disordered blood coagulation in obstetrics. *Br. J. Hosp. Med.*, **2**, 1847.

Shah, J.L. (1981) Influence of cerebrospinal fluid on epidural pressure. *Anaesthesia*, **36**, 627.

Shnider, S.M. (1965) Serum cholinesterase activity during pregnancy, labor and the puerperium. *Anesthesiology*, **26**, 335.

Sivakumaran, C., Ramanathan, S., Chalon, J. and Turndorf, H. (1982) Uterine contractions and the spread of local anesthetics in the epidural space. *Anesth. Analg. curr. Res.*, **61**, 127.

Sjøstedt. S. (1962) Acid–base balance of arterial blood during pregnancy, at delivery and in the puerperium. *Am. J. Obstet. Gynec.*, **84**, 775.

Smith, B., Moya, F. and Shnider, S.M. (1962) Effects of anesthesia on liver function during labor. *Anesth. Analg. curr. Res.*, **41**, 24.

Smith, G., Dalling, R. and Williams, T.I.R. (1978) Gastro-oesophageal pressure gradient changes produced by induction of anaesthesia and suxamethonium. *Br. J. Anaesth.*, **50**, 1137.

Smith, N.C., Soutter, W.P., Sharp, F., McColl, J. and Ford, I. (1983) Fetal scalp blood lactate as an indication of intrapartum hypoxia. *Br. J. Obstet. Gynaec.*, **90**, 821.

Soffronoff, E.C., Kaufman, B.M. and Connaughton, J.F. (1977) Intravascular volume determinations and fetal outcome in hypertensive diseases of pregnancy. *Am. J. Obstet. Gynec.*, **127**, 4.

Spence, A.A., Moir, D.D. and Finlay, W.E.I. (1967) Observations on intragastric pressure. *Anaesthesia*, **22**, 249.

Stenger, V., Eitzman, D., Anderson, T.D. et al (1964) Observations on the placental exchange of the respiratory gases in pregnant women at Cesarean section. *Am. J. Obstet. Gynec.*, **88**, 45.

Sykes, M.K. (1975) Arterial oxygen tension in parturient women. *Br. J. Anaesth.*, **47**, 530.

Taylor, D.J. and Lind, T. (1979) Red cell mass during and after normal pregnancy. *Br. J. Obstet. Gynaec.*, **86**, 364.

Taylor, D.J., Phillips, P. and Lind, T. (1981) Puerperal haematological indices. *Br. J. Obstet. Gynaec.*, **88**, 601.

Taylor, D.J., Mallen, C. and Lind, T. (1983) Does oral iron supplementation have an erythropoietic effect? *Br. J. Obstet. Gynaec.*, **89**, 1006.

Teisner, B., Davey, M.W. and Grudzinskas, J.G. (1982) Circulating antithrombins in pregnancy. *Br. J. Obstet. Gynaec.*, **89**, 62.

Templeton, A. and Kelman, G.R. (1976) Maternal blood gases (P_{AO_2}–P_{aO_2}), physiological shunt and V_D/V_T in normal pregnancy. *Br. J. Anaesth.*, **48**, 1001.

Thind, G.S. and Bryson, T.H.L. (1983) Single dose suxamethonium and muscle pain in pregnancy. *Br. J. Anaesth.*, **55**, 743.

Thomas, P., Buckley, P. and Fox, M. (1984) Maternal and neonatal blood glucose after crystalline loading for epidural Caesarean section. *Anaesthesia*, **39**, 1240.

Thorburn, J., Drummond, M.M., Whigham, K.A. et al (1982) Blood viscosity and haematocrit factors in late pregnancy, pre-eclampsia and fetal growth retardation. *Br. J. Obstet., Gynaec.*, **89**, 117.

Tindall, V.R. and Beazley, J.M. (1965) An assessment of changes in liver function during normal pregnancy using a modified bromsulphthalein test. *J. Obstet. Gynaec. Br. Commonw.*, **72**, 717.

Toldy, M. and Scott, D.B. (1969) Blood loss during Caesarean section under general anaesthesia. *Br. J. Anaesth.*, **41**, 868.

Tyler, J.M. (1960) The effect of progesterone on the respiration of patients with emphysema and hypercapnia. *J. clin. Invest.*, **39**, 34.

Ueland, K. (1976) Maternal cardiovascular dynamics. VII. Intrapartum blood volume changes. *Am. J. Obstet. Gynec.*, **126**, 671.

Ueland, K., Gills, R.E. and Hansen, J.M. (1968) Maternal cardiovascular dynamics. *Am. J. Obstet. Gynec.*, **100**, 42.

Usubiaga, J.E., Moya, F. and Usubiaga, L.E. (1967) The effect of thoracic and abdominal pressure changes on the epidural space. *Br. J. Anaesth.*, **39**, 612.

Von Möbius, W. (1961) Atmung und Schwangerschaft. *Münch. med. Wschr.*, **103**, 1389.

Vorys, N., Ullery, J.C. and Hanusek, G.E. (1961) The cardiac output changes in various positions. *Am. J. Obstet. Gynec.*, **82**, 1312.

Wallace, G. (1967) Blood loss in obstetrics, using a haemoglobin dilution technique. *J. Obstet. Gynaec. Br. Commonw.*, **74**, 64.

Weaver, J.A., Pearson, J.F. and Rosen, M. (1977) Response to Valsalva manoeuvre before and after epidural block. *Anaesthesia*, **32**, 148.

Wiederman, J., Freund, M. and Wiederman, A. (1965) Arterial and venous pressure during uterine contractions. *Obstet. Gynec.*, **26**, 14.

Willcourt, R.J., King, J.C. and Queenen, J.T. (1983) Maternal oxygen administration and fetal transcutaneous P_{O_2}. *Am. J. Obstet. Gynec.*, **146**, 714.

Williams, C.V., Johnson, A. and Ledward, R. (1974) A comparison of central venous pressure changes in the third stage of labour following oxytocic drugs and diazepam. *J. Obstet. Gynaec. Br. Commonw.*, **81**, 596.

Wilson, J. (1978) Gastric emptying in labour, some recent findings and their clinical significance. *J. int. med. Res.*, **6**, Suppl 1, 54.

Wood, M. and Wood, A.J.J. (1981) Changes in plasma drug binding and α-acid glycoprotein in mother and newborn infant. *Clin. Pharmac. Ther.*, **29**, 522.

Zwillich, C.W., Natalino, M.R., Sutton, F.D. and Weil, J.V. (1978) Effects of progesterone on chemosensitivity in normal man. *J. clin. Invest.*, **92**, 262.

3

Pharmacology of Drugs Used in Labour

The maternal response to drugs may be somewhat modified by factors such as increased binding to plasma proteins, minor alterations in the pattern of breakdown in the liver and the alterations in cardiac output and blood volume which exist in the pregnant woman. The placental transfer of drugs and the action of drugs on the uterus are of importance to the obstetric anaesthetist and will be considered in some detail. Aspects of the pharmacology of the various drugs used in labour will be discussed.

PLACENTAL TRANSFER

The placenta rarely presents an absolute barrier to the transfer of drugs although in clinical practice the transfer of certain substances is so restricted that these substances are regarded as having no effect upon the fetus. The placental transfer of ether was recognized by John Snow in 1853 when he noted the smell of this anaesthetic agent on the breath of newborn infants. A concept of placental transfer appropriate to clinical practice is the extent of transfer after the administration of a normal therapeutic dose of a drug. This clinical concept effectively ignores, for example, the small quantities of muscle relaxant drug detectable in the fetal blood after the administration of a standard paralysing dose to the mother.

Simple diffusion is the process mainly involved in the placental transfer of most drugs and gases of interest to the anaesthetist and so the concentration gradient between maternal and fetal blood is of great importance. Placental transfer is of course a two-way process and takes place between mother and fetus or in the reverse direction depending upon the concentration gradient. The tendency is always to establish equilibrium between the two sides of the placental membrane. In the mature placenta the maternal blood in the intervillous space is separated from the fetal capillary endothelium only by a single layer of chorionic tissue and there is thus a thin and extensive surface available for the transfer process. The placental membrane is rich in lipids, so drug transfer is influenced by the lipid solubility of the drug more than by any other factor.

Other processes are involved in the placental transfer of particular substances. Proteins reach the fetus by pinocytosis, a process which involves

50

the engulfing of the protein within the microvilli of the placenta and then its disgorging into the fetal blood. Fetal blood cells may enter the maternal circulation through defects in the barrier and it is now recognized that a maternal transfusion of fetal red cells is quite a frequent occurrence, which may in certain circumstances result in the formation of antibodies by the mother. The placenta is much more than a simple filter. There are enzyme systems within the placenta which can break down certain drugs such as procaine, 2-chloroprocaine and catecholamines.

It is stressed that most studies of the placental transfer of a drug are based solely upon an estimation of the concentration in the maternal blood at the time of delivery and a simultaneous estimation of the concentration in the umbilical vein blood. An umbilical venous/maternal blood concentration ratio (U_v/M_a) is calculated. Such simple studies ignore many important factors, such as the distribution of the drug to fetal tissues, metabolism by the fetus, the extent of binding to fetal plasma proteins and the degree of ionization of the drug at the fetal pH. U_v/M_a ratios may be quite misleading and may give no accurate indications of, for example, the concentration of the drug in the fetal brain or myocardium. Fetal/maternal drug ratios of greater than unity can occur where binding in fetal plasma exceeds binding in maternal plasma. U_v/M_a ratios for diazepam may be as high as 2.0 for this reason. Conversely local anaesthetics are generally less extensively bound to fetal plasma proteins and fetal maternal ratios for bupivacaine are low. A further difficulty is the almost general ignorance of the distribution, metabolism and excretion of drugs by the infant in the first 24–48 hours of life. There is usually little indication of the total mass of drug transferred.

Gases

Oxygen. The transfer of oxygen depends mainly on the difference between the oxygen tension of the maternal blood in the intervillous space and the fetal blood in the umbilical artery. Although the maternal P_aO_2 will normally be about 100 mmHg (13.3 kPa) the Po_2 of the blood in the intervillous space varies widely in different parts of the space. A representative value for the Po_2 of the blood in the intervillous space would be 50 mmHg (6.7 kPa). The Po_2 of the fetal blood entering the placenta in the umbilical artery is about 20 mmHg (2.7 kPa) so that there is a pressure gradient of the order of 30 mmHg (4.0 kPa) to effect the transfer of oxygen. In practice the gradient varies quite widely at different times and in different sites within the placenta. The blood returning to the fetus in the umbilical vein has a Po_2 of about 30 mmHg (4.0 kPa). The value for the fetus of maternal oxygen therapy has sometimes been questioned but the present view is that increasing the maternal P_aO_2 improves fetal oxygenation, and the former belief that very high maternal oxygen tensions might be counter-productive by causing constriction of the spiral arteries of the placenta is probably invalid (Young et

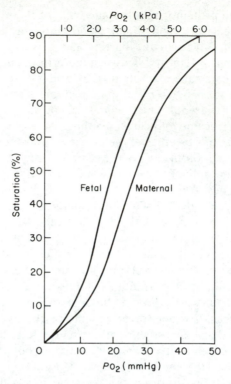

Figure 4. Oxygen dissociation curves of maternal and fetal blood at term. Typically blood in the umbilical arteries has a Po_2 of 20 mmHg (2.7 kPa) and 50% saturation and blood in the umbilical vein has a Po_2 of around 30 mmHg (4.0 kPa) and 75% saturation.

al, 1980; Ramanathan et al, 1982). Oxygen therapy is useful in fetal distress and a high F_IO_2 is appropriate during anaesthesia.

Secondary factors concerned in the placental transfer of oxygen are the functional status of the placenta, the circulation of blood through the placenta and the high haemoglobin content of the fetal blood which increases its oxygen-carrying capacity. The maternal and fetal oxygen dissociation curves are shown in Figure 4. It has been accepted that the diffusion of oxygen across the placenta is passive. There is a suggestion that active transport may occur and that there may be a specific oxygen carrier, such as cytochrome P_{450}, in the placenta (Gurtner and Burns, 1975).

The Bohr effect favours the transfer of oxygen to the fetus. As fetal blood gives up carbon dioxide it becomes more alkaline and develops a greater affinity for oxygen because of a shift to the left in its oxygen dissociation curve. At the same time this carbon dioxide has now reached the maternal blood and rendered it more acid. In consequence the oxygen dissociation curve of the maternal blood is shifted to the right and the release of oxygen to the fetus is promoted. This favourable combination of circumstances for the fetus is referred to as the double Bohr effect.

There are several analogies between the placenta and the lung and one of these concerns the consequences of inequality or mismatching of the fetal and maternal blood flows within the placenta. Just as pulmonary V/Q inequalities cause hypoxaemia so may Q_m/Q_f inequalities in the placenta cause fetal hypoxaemia (Meschia, 1978). Prostaglandin PGE_2 may have a role in correcting mismatching of the fetal and maternal placental circulations.

The placenta is itself a metabolically highly active organ. Approximately 15% of the oxygen utilized by the fetoplacental unit is accounted for by the placenta.

Carbon dioxide. The transfer of carbon dioxide from the fetus depends mainly on the pressure gradient for the gas between the blood in the umbilical artery and the maternal blood in the intervillous spaces. The fetal P_aCO_2 is thought to be about 50 mmHg (6.7 kPa). The PCO_2 of the blood in the intervillous spaces varies at different sites but probably averages about 37 mmHg (4.9 kPa). The blood which returns to the fetus in the umbilical vein has a PCO_2 of about 40 mmHg (5.3 kPa).

The high concentration of haemoglobin in the fetal blood increases its capacity for the carriage of carbon dioxide as carbaminohaemoglobin. The Haldane effect facilitates carbon dioxide transfer by two mechanisms (the double Haldane effect). First, as the maternal blood gives up oxygen it is able to carry more carbon dioxide as carbaminohaemoglobin, without a rise in PCO_2. Second, as the fetal blood takes up oxygen it releases carbon dioxide from its combination with haemoglobin without a reduction in PCO_2.

Table 3. Representative values for oxygen and carbon dioxide tensions* in maternal and fetal blood

Blood	PO_2	PCO_2
Maternal		
Arterial	100 (13.3)	30 (4.0)
Intervillous space	50 (6.7)	37 (4.9)
Fetal		
Umbilical vein	30 (4.0)	40 (5.3)
Umbilical artery	20 (2.7)	50 (6.7)

*Measured as mmHg with kPa shown in parentheses.

The foregoing is a perhaps oversimplified account of some very complex processes which are not yet fully understood. There are many apparently contradictory accounts in the literature and the values quoted for PO_2 and PCO_2 at the various sites should be regarded as broadly representative of a wide scatter of values. Representative maternal and fetal blood gas values are listed in Table 3.

Oxygen, carbon dioxide and the placental circulation. A reduction in the P_aO_2 of maternal blood appears to improve the normally rather patchy and erratic distribution of blood to different parts of the placenta (Power et al, 1967), and as flow becomes more uniform fetal oxygenation may improve.

The fear has often been expressed that abnormally high oxygen tensions in the maternal blood might cause constriction of the uteroplacental vessels and so produce fetal hypoxia and hypercapnia. This fear has sometimes made clinicians reluctant to administer oxygen in cases of fetal distress and has caused anaesthetists to hesitate to use high concentrations of oxygen at caesarean section. Recent studies do not support this concept and there appears to be no need to restrict the maternal F_IO_2 during anaesthesia (Ramanathan et al, 1982). If the fetus is hypoxaemic, then increasing the maternal P_aO_2 may be expected to facilitate the transfer of oxygen to the fetus and oxygen should be given (James et al, 1972). Greiss et al (1974) suggest that acute hyperoxia has very little effect on placental blood flow and increases in maternal P_aO_2 are usually beneficial to the fetus (Newman et al, 1967; Battaglia, 1970). Continuous transcutaneous monitoring of fetal P_{O_2} indicates that maternal oxygen therapy consistently increases fetal P_{O_2} and that fetal P_{O_2} falls when the mother moves from the lateral to the supine position (Huch et al, 1977). There is now general agreement that administration of at least 50% of oxygen at caesarean section improves the clinical and biochemical condition of the infant at birth (Rorke et al, 1968; Baraka, 1970; Moir, 1970; Marx and Mateo, 1971). Myers and others (1977) have demonstrated that fetal P_{O_2} increases 50 seconds after an increase in maternal F_IO_2. In the hypoxic fetus there is a preferential distribution of blood to the brain, heart and adrenals.

Several workers have found extreme maternal hyperventilation during general anaesthesia to be harmful to the fetus (Morishima et al, 1963; Moya et al, 1965; Motoyama et al, 1966), although Coleman (1967) failed to detect any deleterious effects. It was not clear whether the harmful effects of hyperventilation upon the fetus were due to a presumed impairment of placental blood flow due to maternal hypocapnia or to a reduction in maternal cardiac output and therefore in placental blood flow as a result of increased intrathoracic pressure (Scott et al, 1969). The question has been answered by Peng et al (1972) and by Levinson et al (1974), who have shown that maternal hypocapnia decreases the oxygen content of fetal blood by about 20% and that it is associated with fetal metabolic acidosis and low Apgar scores at birth. It was also demonstrated that intermittent positive pressure ventilation, even with normocapnia or hypercapnia, reduces uterine artery blood flow by about 25% in the absence of hypotension. It is now clear that intermittent positive pressure ventilation and hypocapnia are both independently capable of a harmful action upon the fetus. The level of P_{CO_2} necessary to produce this effect is probably 17 mmHg (2.3 kPa) or less. Spontaneous hyperventilation in painful labour can lower the P_{O_2} and base excess of fetal scalp blood (Miller et al, 1974). In the view of Baillie and others (1971) the dangers of hypocapnia may have been exaggerated. It is nevertheless recommended that extreme hyperventilation, whether spontaneous or artificial, should be avoided and normocapnia should be the aim.

Drugs

It is necessary to consider only the process of diffusion, because this is the process which is involved in the placental transfer of almost all of the drugs used for anaesthesia, analgesia and sedation.

The two principal properties of a drug which influence its placental transfer are its lipid solubility and the extent of its ionization in the blood. Most drugs do diffuse across the placental membrane. The placental barrier is rarely, if ever, absolute, although certain drugs such as the muscle relaxants cross in clinically insignificant amounts. The extent to which certain drugs, including the local anaesthetics, are bound to maternal plasma proteins is an important factor influencing placental transfer.

The following are the principal factors affecting placental transfer by diffusion:

Lipid solubility of the drug. The placental membrane contains much lipoprotein. Drugs which are soluble in lipids can therefore easily pass through the placental membrane.

Degree of ionization of the drug. The placental membrane carries an electrical charge. If an ionized drug molecule carries the same charge (positive or negative) it will be repelled but if the drug carries the opposite charge it will be retained within the placental membrane. In either circumstance the placental transfer of the ionized moiety of the drug will be almost non-existent.

Most drugs used for anaesthesia, analgesia and sedation are lipid soluble and poorly ionized in the blood and their placental transfer is almost unrestricted. The muscle relaxants on the other hand are poorly soluble in lipids, are highly ionized in the blood and their transfer is negligible.

Because it is only the unionized fraction of a partly ionized drug which can cross the placental membrane, anything which alters the degree of ionization of the drug will influence its placental transfer.

pH of maternal blood. The pH of the mother's blood can alter the degree of ionization of a drug which is partly ionized. The magnitude of this effect depends upon the ionization constant (pK_a) of the drug. The pK_a is the pH at which 50% of the drug is ionized. If the pK_a is near the pH of the blood then small changes in blood pH produce large changes in the quantity of drug ionized. Consequently the pH changes of labour may affect the placental transfer of drugs. Unfortunately a reduction in maternal blood pH facilitates the transfer of thiopentone. The progressive metabolic acidosis of painful labour is accompanied by progressive fetal infusion acidosis due to the transfer of acid substances to the fetus (Pearson and Davies, 1974). Maternal hyperventilation, common in painful labour, can cause alkalosis. A greater fraction of drug will then be present in the unionized state and available for transfer. The fetal pH is usually lower than that of the mother and therefore the degree of ionization of a drug will often vary between maternal and fetal blood.

Protein-binding. This is an important factor which may reduce the quantity of certain drugs reaching the fetus. Many drugs are bound in part to plasma proteins and the extent of this protein-binding is usually greater during pregnancy, due to alterations in the make-up of the plasma proteins. A protein-bound drug is not immediately available for placental transfer. A dynamic equilibrium exists between bound (unavailable) and unbound (available) drug so that there is a pool of bound drug from which unbound drug may be released. Protein-binding, like ionization, is influenced by blood pH. For example, protein-binding of local anaesthetics is reduced by acidosis. Protein-binding is an important factor reducing the placental transfer of bupivacaine and etidocaine. Binding is mainly to serum albumin. The concentration of serum albumin may be substantially reduced in severe pre-eclampsia, so that the proportion of unbound, transferable drug may be higher in this condition. Pregnancy is associated with the development of endogenous inhibitors of protein binding and this, together with the lower pH of the fetal blood, can cause the total quantity of drug in maternal and fetal blood to differ quite substantially.

Molecular weight of the drug. If a drug has a molecular weight above about 600 then placental transfer by diffusion does not occur. An all-or-nothing rule applies. If the molecular weight is below the critical value then placental transfer is not restricted by this property of the drug. Most drugs used in anaesthesia have a molecular weight below 600.

Maternal–fetal concentration gradient. Where a drug is capable of placental transfer by diffusion then the rate and quantity of transfer depend to a large extent upon the concentration of the drug in the maternal and fetal blood. There is a tendency to equalize the two concentrations.

The influence of the several factors concerned in placental transfer may be expressed in a formula based upon Fick's law of diffusion:

$$\frac{Q}{t} = K \frac{A(C_m - C_f)}{D}$$

where $\dfrac{Q}{t}$ = quantity transferred per unit of time

A = area of placenta available for transfer

D = thickness of placental membrane

$C_m - C_f$ = maternal–fetal concentration gradient

K = a constant for the drug, dependent upon its lipid solubility, ionization, etc.

Placental blood flow. It will be apparent that variations in placental blood flow must affect placental transfer. There is usually a reduction in uteroplacental blood flow during uterine contractions and so it has been postulated that if an intravenous injection of a drug is timed to coincide with a uterine contraction then the placental transfer of the drug may be lessened (Crawford, 1972). Intravenous injections are of course associated with extremely high, although transient, maternal–fetal concentration gradients. An interesting paradox has recently emerged. Although very light anaesthesia is usually deemed best for the fetus, there is evidence that thiopentone, nitrous oxide, relaxant anaesthesia can promote fetal acidosis because the high catecholamine levels associated with very light anaesthesia may reduce uterine artery blood flow (Palahniuk and Cumming, 1977). Maternal hypotension reduces intervillous blood flow. The pressure/flow relationship is probably simple and direct because there is no autoregulating mechanism within the placenta.

Failure to take into account all of the foregoing factors and to allow for the effects of labour, diseases of the placenta and other special circumstances may be sufficient to explain the many reported inconsistencies in the placental transfer of individual drugs and the sometimes poor correlation between measured concentrations of a drug in maternal and cord blood with the clinical condition of the infant. Some workers have measured serum concentrations and others have used whole blood and it has been unusual to acknowledge the possible influence of protein-binding and ionization.

It is worth noting that the factors which influence placental transfer are essentially the same factors which influence the transfer of substances by diffusion across the blood–brain barrier and across other biological membranes. It is therefore very unlikely that the 'ideal' analgesic or anaesthetic will be discovered. If a drug is capable of reaching its site of action within the central nervous system it must possess the very physical properties which permit its placental transfer.

The effects of drugs upon the fetus and newborn

In the final analysis it is of course the potential hazards for the fetus, or more usually for the neonate, which restrict the quantities of anaesthetic and analgesic drugs which may safely be given to the mother. The response of the fetus and neonate to drugs differs in several important ways from the response of the adult and older child. In general it may be stated that the more immature the infant, the greater will be the modification in the response to drugs. Some of the blood returning from the placenta by-passes the fetal liver in the ductus venosus and goes to the fetal brain without being first partly 'cleared' of drug in the liver. There is, however, a helpful tendency for blood from the umbilical vein to be diluted with blood from the legs and lower abdomen. The following are among the factors which make the infant more susceptible to drugs, or in a few instances, among the factors which may protect the fetus from the effects of certain drugs.

Selective uptake by fetal liver. When thiopentone is injected into the mother or into the umbilical vein, as much as 50% of the injected dose is later found in the fetal liver (Finster et al, 1972). This trapping of thiopentone by fetal liver may help to explain the apparent paradox of the awake child delivered to the anaesthetized mother. The concentration of thiopentone in the fetal liver is about 100 times greater than in the brain. More recent work has shown that the ability of the fetal liver to trap thiopentone becomes exhausted after only 2 or 3 minutes (Woods et al, 1982).

Inadequacy of liver enzyme systems. The ability of the fetus and of the newborn to metabolize most drugs is often substantially impaired owing to the inefficiency of some of the hepatic enzymes. In particular the oxidative enzymes and glucuronyl transferase are likely to be less active. Liver function may be further modified by the high concentration of oestrogens in the infant's blood (Crawford and Rudofsky, 1966), and it may be this, rather than immaturity of enzyme systems, which exaggerates and prolongs the action of drugs in the fetus and neonate. This observation was not confirmed by Kuhnert and others (1980b).

Enzyme induction. Pretreatment by the administration of enzyme-inducing agents such as phenobarbitone may activate fetal hepatic enzyme systems. Narcotic drugs may then be more rapidly metabolized and the technique has been used to protect against the development of dangerously high concentrations of unconjugated bilirubin by increasing the ability of the infant to conjugate bilirubin (Trolle, 1968). Conjugated bilirubin is less able to penetrate into the brain and so the risk of kernicterus may be reduced. Neonatal phototherapy is also used to treat severe jaundice.

Renal excretion. There may be impairment in the excretion of drugs by the kidneys.

Pulmonary excretion. The elimination of volatile anaesthetics by the lungs depends upon the establishment of adequate pulmonary ventilation at birth. Artificial ventilation may be used and the fear of volatile agents has sometimes been exaggerated. Before birth the placenta functions as a lung for the fetus.

Protein-binding, ionization and pH. The pH of fetal blood is usually lower than that of maternal blood and therefore the degree of ionization and of binding to fetal plasma proteins is usually different. The concentration of various plasma proteins is different in fetal blood and the binding capacity of these proteins is generally less. Amide-type local anaesthetics are less extensively bound to fetal plasma proteins (Tucker et al, 1970). A decrease in pH increases the ionization of amide-type local anaesthetics which are 'trapped' in the fetal circulation in greater amounts and the U_v/M concentration ratio is increased (Brown et al, 1976; Biehl et al, 1978). If fetal pH falls due to acute placental insufficiency in labour then the concentration of a basic drug such as bupivacaine may rise to dangerous levels (Kennedy et al, 1979). This concentration of a base in the acidotic fetus is known as 'ion trapping'.

Red cell binding. Some drugs such as the volatile and gaseous anaesthetics show an affinity for erythrocytes. Other drugs, such as the local anaesthetics are extensively bound to proteins and are only attached to red cells to a small extent.

Increased uptake by fetal brain. It is likely that morphine penetrates fetal nervous tissues more easily because of its low myelin content (Kupforberg and Way, 1963; Way et al, 1965). The concentration of diamorphine in fetal brain is three times greater than in maternal brain (Sanner and Woods, 1965).

Penetration of the infant's blood–brain barrier by drugs whose site of action is within the central nervous system is dependent upon the same factors which are concerned in transmission across the placental barrier. Consequently a drug whose placental transfer is free will readily reach the fetal brain. The fetal response to anaesthetics may be different. There is evidence that nitrous oxide selectively inhibits aerobic metabolism in the fetal brain, perhaps by impairing blood flow or by altering metabolism directly (Vannucci and Wolf, 1978). Hypoxic changes in the brain may be preventable by large doses of pentobarbitone in animals, but the role of such therapy is uncertain in humans (Holtzman, 1978). The administration of sedatives in labour may have a protective function when the fetus is at risk from hypoxia (Myers and Myers, 1979). Sedatives might also improve placental blood flow by relieving anxiety and reducing catecholamine levels. Animal studies suggest that etomidate may reduce the effects of hypoxia on the brain (Wauquier, 1983). There is a good deal of animal evidence which supports the concept of protection against cerebral hypoxia by barbiturates acting by reducing the rate of brain metabolism. The evidence in man is unsatisfactory and often anecdotal (Aitkenhead, 1981). Sedatives are not in clinical use for a protective action on fetal brain.

It is not surprising, in view of the large number of variables involved, that the condition of the infant at birth may sometimes be at variance with a prediction based solely upon the drugs administered during labour or on the type of anaesthesia used at delivery. Even so there is general support for the view that Apgar scores are lower and metabolic acidosis is more severe among infants born to mothers who have received a general anaesthetic in preference to a regional block (Apgar et al, 1957; Marx et al, 1969). The recent application of sensitive techniques for assessing behaviour and neurological function in neonates has demonstrated depressant effects of narcotic analgesics administered during labour (Brackbill et al, 1974; Scanlon et al, 1974). Infants whose mothers received epidural analgesia in labour did not show evidence of depression of neurological function seen in the infants whose mothers had received pethidine (Abboud et al, 1982, 1984b). Striking differences in neonatal behavioural responses have also been demonstrated following caesarean section under general anaesthesia and epidural analgesia (Palahniuk et al, 1977; Hollmen et al, 1978).

Crawford (1962) emphasized the need to eliminate the influence of obstetric factors in any attempt to evaluate the effect of an anaesthetic agent or technique on the infant. He introduced the concept of a 'clinically acceptable ideal' situation where the infant is a mature singleton, presenting by the vertex. Placental function must be satisfactory and the mother must not be in labour. These conditions can only apply at elective caesarean section. Hypotension and aorto-caval occlusion must be prevented.

Teratogenesis

There is no reason to believe that the administration of anaesthetic, analgesic or sedative drugs during labour to the mother of a mature fetus can cause any developmental abnormality. The possible risk of drug therapy of almost any type in early pregnancy is now well known. There is no evidence available to suggest that the administration of a single general anaesthetic early in pregnancy is capable of inducing a fetal abnormality in man (Pedersen and Finster, 1979; Brodsky et al, 1980), although the evidence in this field is scanty. A single exposure to halothane for 2 hours in the early days of pregnancy causes behavioural and learning abnormalities in the offspring of rats, suggestive of a teratogenic effect on the rat fetal brain (Smith et al, 1978), and perhaps these observations justify a cautious attitude to the use of anaesthetics in human pregnancy. It seems prudent to advise against a non-essential anaesthetic during pregnancy, especially in the early months. Misgivings have been expressed about a possible effect of nitrous oxide on fetal DNA synthesis. Swedish studies have revealed no association between the use of psychotropic or anti-emetic drugs in human pregnancy and fetal abnormality or death (Kullander and Kallen, 1976a,b). The short term use of such drugs for anaesthesia or premedication is not known to be harmful.

There is now a great deal of evidence that the continuous exposure to high concentrations of several volatile and gaseous anaesthetic agents for periods of 12 hours to two or three days will induce a very high incidence of abnormalities of the skeletal and nervous systems in the early developing embryos of chickens and rats (Smith et al, 1965; Fink et al, 1967; Anderson, 1968; Basford and Fink, 1968). Exposure of pregnant rats to sub-anaesthetic concentrations of halothane, methoxyflurane or nitrous oxide for 8 hours daily throughout pregnancy produced no fetal abnormalities, but retarded fetal growth (Pope et al, 1978). Litter size was reduced after daily exposure to

0.5 and 0.1% nitrous oxide throughout pregnancy (Viera et al, 1983). Chronic exposure to enflurane 200 p.p.m. did not cause abortion or fetal abnormalities in rats (Green et al, 1982) and exposure to 20 p.p.m. of halothane and enflurane had no teratogenic effect (Halsey et al, 1981). Several narcotic analgesics, including morphine, diamorphine, pethidine and methadone, were found by Geber and Schramm (1975) to substantially increase the incidence of abnormalities of the central nervous system in hamster fetuses. The children of human addicts may be at risk.

Anaesthesia during pregnancy

There is very little information on the fetal risks associated with anaesthesia during pregnancy. Brodsky and others (1980) reviewed 287 women who had been anaesthetized during the first and second trimesters. There was no increase in the incidence of fetal abnormalities, but there was an increase in the number of first trimester abortions. The survey was retrospective and the reply rate was only 70%. These features are possible sources of error. It was not possible to distinguish between the influence of anaesthesia and surgery. Pedersen and Finster (1979) also failed to find any increase in the incidence of fetal abnormalities after anaesthesia in early pregnancy.

It may be preferable to postpone non-essential surgery until after the first trimester, but there must be no question of failing to perform essential surgery. Hypoxia and hypotension could cause fetal death or brain damage if severe. The recent demonstration of the possible effect of nitrous oxide on DNA synthesis has caused some anaesthetists in the USA to avoid this agent during pregnancy. The cautious anaesthetist may select spinal or epidural anaesthesia for cervical cerclage. Folinic acid may be given if nitrous oxide is to be used.

Occupational hazards of anaesthetists in relation to pregnancy

There is now some evidence for a relationship between a high rate of spontaneous abortion and regular employment during early pregnancy among women anaesthetists and women operating theatre nurses (Askrog, 1970; Cohen et al, 1971; Knill-Jones et al, 1972; American Society of Anesthesiologists, 1974; Knill-Jones et al, 1975), and it has been suggested that the incidence of spontaneous abortion among the wives of male anaesthetists may be excessive (Askrog, 1970; Tomlin, 1979). There is also a suggestion of an abnormally high incidence of congenital abnormalities among the children of male and female anaesthetists (American Society of Anesthesiologists, 1974; Corbett et al, 1974; Tomlin, 1979). Evidence for a higher incidence of abortion among women anaesthetists is quite convincing. The evidence for a higher incidence of fetal abnormality and for hazards to the children of male anaesthetists is open to statistical criticisms.

The explanations for these presumptive relationships are unknown. The attributing of them to fetal abnormalities due to the long-term exposure to very low concentrations of anaesthetic agents in the atmosphere is at the moment speculative. Nevertheless it may seem a sensible precaution for a woman anaesthetist to avoid exposure to these agents in early pregnancy and the introduction of effective ventilation or decontamination systems for operating theatres is recommended by the Department of Health and Social Security (1976).

The placental transfer of individual drugs

It would be tedious and of little value to present an exhaustive list of drugs, accompanied by a detailed account of the placental transfer of each drug. Much of the available information is apparently contradictory and is often difficult to interpret and apply to the clinical situation due to lack of information concerning the conditions under which the information was obtained.

Information is usually confined to estimates of the fetal/maternal concentration ratio at the time of delivery. This ratio merely indicates the situation at an isolated point in time and gives little or no indication of important matters such as the total amount of drug transferred, the rate of transfer and the fate of the drug in the fetus and neonate. The effective concentration in fetal blood and tissues depends upon factors such as ionization and protein-binding and these, too, are often unknown. These comments should be kept in mind when reading the following sections concerned with individual drugs and groups of drugs.

As far as is possible the typical behaviour of the various groups of drugs will be summarized below, and where information is available on the behaviour of commonly used agents, then this will be presented.

In order to assess the effects of a drug upon the infant it is essential to eliminate obvious obstetric variables such as placental insufficiency, prematurity and postmaturity and to avoid aortocaval occlusion. Crawford (1962) has elaborated on this in relation to caesarean section and stressed that only mature infants delivered by elective section should be studied.

The volatile and gaseous anaesthetics. All the volatile and gaseous anaesthetics are able to cross biological membranes such as the blood–brain barrier and the placental barrier with ease. The process of transfer begins very shortly after administration and most agents are detectable in the cord blood within 2–3 minutes of commencing inhalation. The rate and extent of placental transfer depends upon the duration of the period of administration. Solubility coefficients of anaesthetic agents are different for maternal and fetal bloods (Gibbs et al, 1975). For example, halothane, enflurane and nitrous oxide are less soluble in fetal blood, plasma and red cells and for this and other reasons the concentration of these agents is lower in fetal than in blood thiopentone concentrations should be achieved in about 17 minutes (Dawes, 1973). The well-recognized phenomenon of the delivery of an awake baby to an anaesthetized mother is not due to any significant barrier to the placental transfer of thiopentone. It is the result of <u>dilution</u> of the drug in the fetal veins and also in part to <u>uptake by the fetal liver</u> (Finster et al, 1972), so that the quantity of thiopentone reaching the fetal brain is greatly reduced. The protective effect of liver uptake may be less than was formerly thought, because this process ceases after 2 or 3 minutes of exposure according to Woods et al (1982). The exposure of the fetal brain to thiopentone may depend more on variations in maternal distribution and elimination and on the consequences of caval occlusion than on the dose injected (Morgan et al, 1981).

Other intravenous anaesthetics. The other extremely short-acting barbiturates, including methohexitone, rapidly cross the placenta. Their behaviour resembles that of thiopentone in that peak fetal blood concentrations are reached 2 or 3 minutes after injection and, thereafter, there is an exponential decline (Marshall, 1964). Methohexitone in a dose of 1 mg/kg maternal body weight did not cause clinical depression of the neonate but a dose of 1.4 mg/kg was associated with a high percentage of low Apgar scores (Holdcroft et al, 1974). Neonatal depression is related to the dose of methohexitone, and dosage is quite critical if depression is to be avoided. Propanidid can be detected in cord blood within 4 minutes of injection (Doenicke et al, 1968). Comparison of the clinical condition of the infants at birth in series of caesarean sections revealed no significant difference between thiopentone and methohexitone (Sliom et al, 1962) and thiopentone and propanidid (Bradford and Moir, 1969). The concentration of propanidid in fetal blood is thought to be influenced by the maternal serum cholinesterase activity. Althesin certainly crosses the placenta although accurate measurements of fetal blood concentrations have not so far been made. When Althesin and thiopentone were used for the induction of anaesthesia for caesarean section there was no demonstrable difference in the condition of the infants at birth in the two groups (Downing et al, 1974). Similar comparisons have been made between thiopentone and intravenous ketamine, and clinical assessments have revealed no differences in the condition of the infants at birth (Moore et al, 1971; Peltz and Sinclair, 1973) although blood concentrations were not measured. Other studies have revealed a dose-related neonatal depression with ketamine (Eng et al, 1975b; Downing et al, 1976) as well as maternal hypertension and uterine hypercontractility (Marx et al, 1979). The placental transfer of ketamine is rapid, and metabolism of this agent is less efficient in pregnancy (Little et al, 1972).

There seem to have been no reports on the placental transfer of etomidate, but Downing and his colleagues (1979) found that etomidate caused less fetal acidosis than thiopentone and suggested that the minimal cardiovascular side-effects and rapid breakdown of etomidate made it very suitable for obstetric use.

Although agents such as Althesin and propanidid might seem attractive because of their very rapid breakdown, other factors must be taken into account. Althesin and propanidid can cause fetal metabolic acidosis due to a reduction in placental blood flow consequent upon a degree of maternal circulatory depression (Downing et al, 1974; Mahomedy et al, 1976). The side-effects and adverse reactions associated with the various agents must be considered, as well as a possible effect upon the incidence of awareness during anaesthesia. On balance, thiopentone, methohexitone and perhaps etomidate are the induction agents of first choice when given in a minimal 'sleep dose'. Althesin and propanidid are no longer in general use in the UK and thiopentone continues to be preferred by most anaesthetists.

The barbiturates. All the barbiturates readily cross the placenta. Following an intramuscular injection of sodium amytal, equilibrium is established between fetal and maternal bloods in about 30 minutes and, at this time, the concentrations in the blood of mother and infant are approximately equal (Ploman and Persson, 1957). Following an intravenous injection of quinalbarbitone or pentobarbitone the drug is detectable in the umbilical vein blood within 1 minute. Equilibrium is achieved between fetal and maternal blood in about 5 minutes and then the fetal blood concentration is approximately 70% of the concentration in maternal blood (Fealey, 1958). Other short- and medium-acting barbiturates probably behave in a similar fashion after intramuscular and intravenous injection. It has been shown that there are enzymes within the placenta which are capable of breaking down barbiturates and possibly other drugs before they can reach the fetus (Kyegombe et al, 1973) although it would appear that this process is not normally capable of preventing other than quite small quantities of barbiturates from reaching the fetus.

The barbiturates are no longer used as sedatives in normal labour because of their free placental transfer, their sometimes very prolonged action in the enzyme-deficient neonate and the lack of a specific barbiturate antagonist. Phenobarbitone when given antenatally causes enzyme induction in the fetus and can substantially reduce the incidence and severity of neonatal jaundice in the infant affected by rhesus incompatibility (Trolle, 1968; Thomas, 1976). Phenobarbitone is still sometimes prescribed for pregnant epileptics; infants of these mothers may be drowsy and unresponsive for several days after delivery.

The muscle relaxants. Happily for the anaesthetist the placental transfer of the muscle relaxants in clinical use is of such limited extent as to be of no practical importance with normal dosage. This is because these drugs are highly ionized in maternal serum and poorly soluble in lipids.

Only minute and completely insignificant quantities of D-tubocurarine (Crawford, 1956) and suxamethonium (Moya and Kvisselgaard, 1961) are present in the cord blood after the doses normally used for caesarean section, and extensive experience confirms the safety of these two drugs. Suxamethonium was detectable in clinically insignificant amounts in the serum of monkey fetuses within 10 minutes of the injection of 2.3 mg/kg body weight into the mother. This large dose was metabolized much more slowly by the relatively inactive fetal cholinesterase, and there seems a possibility of a cumulative effect from multiple large doses (Drabkova et al, 1973). If suxamethonium is used to maintain relaxation during caesarean section then a continuous infusion should be chosen.

The placental transfer of gallamine (Crawford, 1956) and alcuronium (Thomas et al, 1969a) is slightly greater than that of D-tubocurarine and suxamethonium. The fetal/maternal concentration ratio of alcuronium increases with prolongation of the induction–delivery interval at caesarean section (Ho et al, 1981). Although in practice the newborn infant seems to be unaffected by gallamine or alcuronium administered to the mother it is usual to prefer suxamethonium, pancuronium, vecuronium or atracurium for obstetric anaesthesia.

Technical problems at first prevented the estimation of the concentration of pancuronium in the blood. Spiers and Sim (1972) detected minute quantities of pancuronium in the urine of some newborn infants and Heaney (1974) has found pancuronium in the cord blood of only 2 out of 19 infants. More recently, Dailey and others (1984) measured U_v/M_a ratios averaging 0.19 for pancuronium. Clinical experience has confirmed the suitability of pancuronium for obstetric anaesthesia. The placental transfer of fazadinium is of no clinically significant extent and this non-depolarizing relaxant with a rapid onset of action was proposed as a successor to suxamethonium for inducing rapid relaxation in obstetric anaesthesia (Blogg et al, 1975). Intubation is sometimes difficult and these early hopes have not been realized. Decamethonium has been used for obstetric anaesthesia without any apparent effect upon the fetus (Lawson, 1958) but quantitative studies have not been reported.

The placental transfer of vecuronium is less extensive than the transfer of pancuronium and the duration of action of vecuronium is reduced in pregnancy (Dailey et al, 1984). U_v/M_a ratios at delivery average 0.11. Infants are clinically unaffected and, in the view of Dailey and colleagues, vecuronium may be the ideal relaxant for caesarean section. However conditions for rapid intubation are not ideal. Atracurium has been successfully used in obstetrics and its placental transfer is also clinically insignificant (Flynn et al, 1984). The fetal/maternal ratio averages 0.11 at delivery (Demetriou et al, 1982). Suxamethonium remains the best agent for rapid intubation of the trachea.

Tetrahydroaminacrine (Tacrine) has been used to prolong the action of suxamethonium in obstetric anaesthesia and has been shown to cross the placenta (Spiers, 1966). The dose requirements of suxamethonium are reduced and the drug seems not to affect the fetus (McCaul and Robinson, 1962).

In illustration of the concept that the placental barrier is never absolute it may be noted that when a regimen of curarization and intermittent positive pressure ventilation was used in the control of convulsions during pregnancy, the administration of 245 mg of D-tubocurarine in 10 hours appeared to cause neonatal paralysis (Older and Harris, 1968). The prolonged use of relaxants in the treatment of maternal tetanus has been followed by the delivery of an infant suffering from arthrogryposis (Jago, 1970). Apnoea for 6 hours after delivery was reported in the cholinesterase-deficient offspring of a cholinesterase-deficient mother (Baraka et al, 1975), confirming that 100 mg suxamethonium is followed by detectable amounts in fetal serum. Plasmapheresis is now employed in the management of rhesus-isoimmunized mothers and is followed by a reduction in plasma cholinesterase level. After repeated plasmapheresis the cholinesterase level may remain low for several weeks (Evans et al, 1980), and if the procedure is performed twice weekly then prolongation of the period of suxamethonium apnoea could occur. Plasma cholinesterase levels are also reduced in gestational trophoblastic disease (a pseudopregnancy state) and prolonged suxamethonium apnoea has been reported (Davies et al, 1983).

Narcotic analgesics. All known narcotic analgesics appear to cross the placenta in significant amounts.

The placental transfer of pethidine (meperidine) is almost unrestricted. Within 2 minutes of an intravenous injection the concentration of pethidine in the umbilical venous blood almost equals the concentration in the maternal blood. Placental transfer is of course less rapid after an intramuscular injection (Crawford and Rudofsky, 1965). The solubility of narcotic analgesics in water and lipids varies with pH and so the concentration in the fetus may be affected by the pH of its blood (Benson et al, 1976). The fetal blood concentration of pethidine may sometimes exceed that in the maternal blood (Jenkins et al, 1972). Pethidine is more extensively bound to maternal than to fetal plasma proteins (Nation, 1981). Neonatal respiratory depression is likely to be most severe if delivery takes place between 2.5 and 3.5 hours after an intramuscular injection of pethidine (Roberts and Please, 1958; Shnider and Moya, 1964) and the newborn is unlikely to suffer significant drug-induced respiratory depression if delivery occurs within 1 hour, or more than 6 hours, after an intramuscular injection. Belfrage et al (1981) confirmed that cord blood pethidine concentrations increase in the 2 or 3 hours following an intramuscular injection, and decline thereafter. The likelihood of serious depression is probably greatest if delivery occurs shortly after a single intravenous injection of pethidine. Fetal/maternal concentration ratios of pethidine increase with time. Twenty minutes after a dose the ratio is 0.6 but by 160 minutes, the ratio always exceeds 1.0. It has been widely believed that course of labour. Following an intravenous injection of diazepam the plasma concentrations in the infants at delivery 15–205 minutes later were always higher than those in the maternal blood (Gamble et al, 1977). Placental transfer is extremely rapid. After an intravenous injection diazepam can be detected in the umbilical venous blood within 30 seconds, and a maternal intravenous injection of diazepam 10 mg causes a decrease in neonatal rectal temperature (McAllister, 1980). Absorption is very unpredictable after intramuscular injection, perhaps owing to binding of the drug to muscle protein. Oral or intravenous administration results in more certain absorption.

Lorazepam behaves in a different way from diazepam. Lorazepam plasma concentrations are lower in the infant than in the mother, suggesting that protein-binding is less extensive in the fetus and neonate (McBride et al, 1979). Conjugation of lorazepam is impaired in the newborn, and the inactive glucuronide is detectable in the urine for up to seven days after birth (Whitelaw et al, 1981). The fetal/maternal concentration ratio of midazolam and its metabolite 1-hydroxymethylmidazolam is only 0.15 (Vree et al, 1984).

At the time of writing, benzodiazepine antagonists are not generally available. They can rapidly reverse even a deep coma in adults. Their half-lives are only about 2 hours, whereas the benzodiazepines have long half-lives. Repeated administration would therefore be required and these antagonists await further trials in neonates (Ashton, 1985).

Chlormethiazole has been detected in the cord blood (Duffus et al, 1969). This anticonvulsant and sedative may, like diazepam, cause neonatal hypotonia, hypothermia and apnoea in large doses.

Local anaesthetics. There is much new information on the placental transfer of local anaesthetics. Most studies are concerned solely with the fetal and neonatal blood concentrations at the time of delivery, usually under lumbar epidural analgesia. The transfer of the local anaesthetic during labour and its metabolism, distribution and excretion by the neonate have not been extensively studied. It is clear that some of the amide-type local anaesthetics reach the fetus in quantities sufficient to affect the neonate in a minor way, by reducing muscle tone (Scanlon et al, 1974), while others of this group, such as bupivacaine, need not do so (Scanlon et al, 1976). Later work by Abboud and her colleagues (1982, 1984b) has failed to detect any effect of various local anaesthetics on the fetus. The rapid hydrolysis of the ester-type drugs results in minimal or non-existent placental transfer. Procaine and 2-chloroprocaine do not affect fetal heart rate patterns in labour, whereas bupivacaine and lignocaine can produce loss of beat-to-beat variability, a phenomenon which is probably not of serious significance in this situation (Abboud et al, 1982, 1984a). Of course, regional analgesia can affect the fetus by mechanisms other than placental transfer of local anaesthetic drugs. Maternal hypoxaemia or hypotension can be disastrous for the fetus, but these problems are considered elsewhere.

The following factors influence the placental transfer of local anaesthetics and the effect of the transferred drug on the fetus:

Maternal factors:

(1) Total dose of drug. This influences the maternal–fetal concentration gradient and therefore the quantity and rate of transfer. An intravascular injection produces very high concentrations in neonatal and fetal blood.

(2) Protein-binding. Drug bound to plasma protein is unavailable for transfer. This is the principal reason for the low concentration of bupivacaine in the umbilical vein. Typical protein-binding capacities and U_v/M_a concentration ratios for amide-type local anaesthetics are shown in Table 4.

Table 4. Typical protein-binding capacities and U_v/M_a concentration ratios for amide-like local anaesthetics

	Protein-binding capacity (%)	U_v/M_a ratio
Prilocaine	55	1.0 or higher
Lignocaine	64	0.5–0.7
Mepivacaine	77	0.5–0.75
Bupivacaine	95	0.25–0.45
Etidocaine	94	0.15–0.35

(3) The ionization constant (pK_a) of the drug. Each local anaesthetic has a different pK_a. At normal maternal blood pH, 97% of procaine is ionized but only 60% of mepivacaine is in the ionized form and therefore the fraction of unionized mepivacaine available for transfer is greater.

(4) Metabolism and excretion. The ester-type agents (e.g. procaine, 2-chloroprocaine and amethocaine) are hydrolysed by serum esterases and, to a small extent, by esterases in the placenta. The amide-type drugs (e.g. lignocaine, mepivacaine and bupivacaine) are metabolized in the liver. This is a slower process and there is a tendency for these agents to accumulate in the maternal blood during continuous epidural analgesia.

(5) Injection site. Most injection sites for obstetric analgesia are vascular; absorption is therefore rapid and blood concentrations are higher.

(6) Addition of adrenaline. With drugs such as lignocaine the addition of adrenaline prolongs analgesia and reduces peak serum concentrations. With bupivacaine and etidocaine the use of adrenaline does not significantly influence duration of effect or peak serum concentrations (Reynolds et al, 1973).

(7) Placental blood flow. If this is reduced by hypotension or disease of the placenta, then transfer will be impaired. In the special case of paracervical block the local anaesthetic drug may reduce placental blood flow (Liston et al, 1973).

Fetal factors:

Less is known about the distribution and fate of local anaesthetics in the fetus although clearly these things must have an important effect on the response of the fetus and neonate to any local anaesthetic agent which reaches the fetus. To a greater or lesser extent the factors which control the maternal distribution and metabolism must apply to the infant. There are some modifying influences. The drug arriving in the umbilical vein is diluted by blood from the legs and pelvis. The amount of blood by-passing the liver in the ductus venosus is very variable and therefore uptake by the liver varies. The local anaesthetic may be less extensively bound to fetal than to maternal plasma protein so that the effective, unbound moiety may be greater (Mather et al, 1971). The reduced binding capacity of fetal plasma proteins is an important factor in the case of bupivacaine and results in approximately equal amounts of unbound bupivacaine existing in maternal and fetal plasma, although the total concentration of bupivacaine is usually much lower in the fetal plasma. Fetal hepatic enzymes may be less able to metabolize the drug. This statement probably applies to mepivacaine but not to bupivacaine (Brown et al, 1975). The breakdown of ester-type local anaesthetics by serum esterases is slower.

The fetal blood pH is lower than that of the mother and the fetal/maternal concentration ratio is thereby increased as the degree of ionization increases (Brown et al, 1976). As fetal pH falls the ionized drug is 'trapped' in the fetal blood and tissues and may reach harmful concentrations (Kennedy et al, 1979). It is unfortunate that fetal asphyxia may predispose to adverse effects of local anaesthetics on the fetal brain. Fetal hypoxia and acidosis cause more blood from the umbilical vein to by-pass the liver, go directly to the heart and so to the brain via the foramen ovale. Hypercapnia increases cerebral blood flow and these factors combine to expose the brain to more local anaesthetic.

The following information concerning individual drugs applies primarily to lumbar epidural analgesia. The doses used for subarachnoid analgesia are so small that placental transfer can be ignored.

(1) *Lignocaine (lidocaine)*. Following on an injection into the lumbar epidural space, lignocaine can be detected in the maternal blood within 3 minutes and in the blood of the umbilical vein within 12–15 minutes. The highest levels are found between 15 and 30 minutes after injection. The reported concentrations of lignocaine in fetal blood vary between 20 and 95% of the concentration in the maternal blood at the time of delivery (Beckett et al, 1965; Shnider and Way, 1968; Thomas et al, 1968; Thomas et al, 1969c; Lurie and Weiss, 1970). Accumulation has been demonstrated in the fetal blood in long labour (Lurie and Weiss, 1970; Fox et al, 1971). In practice the concentration of lignocaine in the blood of the umbilical vein is usually between 60 and 70% of the maternal venous blood concentration and the umbilical vein blood concentration is normally between 1 and 2 μg/kg. It is

therefore unlikely that serious fetal intoxication will occur if reasonable care is exercised in the conduct of epidural analgesia. Neonatal hypotonia has been attributed to the use of lignocaine for epidural analgesia (Scanlon et al, 1974). Recent studies by Abboud and her colleagues (1984a,b) indicate that lignocaine is an acceptable agent for epidural analgesia in labour and does not adversely influence Apgar scores, neurobehavioural studies, fetal heart rate patterns or uterine action. Lignocaine and bupivacaine had similar effects on infants delivered by caesarean section under epidural anaesthesia and sucking was more vigorous after 24 hours where lignocaine had been used (Klieff et al, 1984). The urine of neonates contains lignocaine and its metabolites for one to three days after delivery (Kuhnert et al, 1979). The addition of adrenaline to 1.5% lignocaine solutions had no effect on the concentrations of lignocaine in the umbilical vein blood, although it did reduce the concentration of local anaesthetic in the maternal blood (Epstein and Coakley, 1967). Fetal acidosis produces high concentrations of lignocaine in the fetal blood (Brown et al, 1976; Biehl et al, 1978) and the fetal/maternal concentration ratio may then exceed unity, owing to trapping of the now ionized lignocaine base. When continuous lumbar epidural analgesia is maintained for more than about 12 hours with lignocaine then tachyphylaxis frequently develops (Moir and Willocks, 1968) and there is then a risk of accumulation of lignocaine in maternal and fetal blood and tissues as injections are given at ever-decreasing time intervals. Loss or diminution of beat-to-beat variability of the fetal heart rate during labour has been noted during epidural analgesia with lignocaine and bupivacaine, but this was probably harmless (Boehm et al, 1975; Abboud et al, 1982). In the latter study late decelerations were more common in the absence of hypotension and this may be a reason for concern.

(2) *Prilocaine* (*propitocaine*). The local anaesthetic prilocaine is detectable in the blood of the umbilical vein 10 minutes after a lumbar epidural injection. The reported fetal/maternal ratios, like those of lignocaine, vary quite widely and may approach unity (Poppers and Finster, 1968; Hehre et al, 1969) and the concentration of prilocaine in the umbilical vein blood averages about 1.5 µg/kg. The behaviour of prilocaine is thus very like that of lignocaine.

Methaemoglobinaemia is a regular feature of prilocaine analgesia and occurs in mother and infant (Climie et al, 1967; Poppers and Mastri, 1970). The severity of methaemoglobinaemia is related to the dose of prilocaine. The conversion to methaemoglobin is due to a metabolite of prilocaine, *o*-toleridine, whose placental transfer is also extensive. Consequently prilocaine, although a very safe agent for single injections, is not recommended for continuous epidural analgesia or repeated paracervical blocks. The associated methaemoglobinaemia reduces the oxygen-carrying capacity of maternal and fetal blood. An intravenous injection of 0.2 mg/kg body weight of methylene blue will reverse methaemoglobinaemia in mother and fetus, indicating that the dye has free placental transfer. An intravenous infusion of glucose will supply methaemoglobin reductase. The urine of the neonate may become blue.

(3) *Mepivacaine*. After an epidural injection mepivacaine appears in the maternal venous blood in minutes, and peak maternal and fetal blood concentrations are attained between 30 and 40 minutes after injection (Morishima et al, 1966). Fetal/maternal concentration ratios of 0.75 were recorded when 2% mepivacaine was used for epidural analgesia. With 1% mepivacaine the ratio was 0.46 (Clark et al, 1975). The placental transfer of mepivacaine is unusually free and there is a tendency for the drug to accumulate in the fetal blood. The half-life of mepivacaine in neonatal plasma is 9 hours, a figure much greater than is seen with lignocaine (3 hours) or bupivacaine (2 hours) according to Brown et al (1975). In Morishima's study there were a number of infants whose poor condition at birth was associated with high concentrations of mepivacaine in the blood and there were also a number of toxic reactions among the mothers. Neonatal hypotonia has been attributed to mepivacaine (Scanlon et al, 1974). Mepivacaine is therefore not an agent of first choice for obstetric epidural analgesia.

(4) *Bupivacaine*. The placental transfer of this relatively long-acting local anaesthetic is significantly less than that of lignocaine, prilocaine and mepivacaine, so bupivacaine is particularly suitable for obstetric use. After an epidural injection the peak concentration of bupivacaine is reached in maternal blood in 15–30 minutes and there is then a steady decline in concentration over the next 3 hours. The concentration of bupivacaine in the blood of the umbilical vein is usually less than 30% of the concentration in the maternal venous blood, even after repeated injections (Thomas et al, 1969b; Reynolds et al, 1973). The umbilical arterial blood concentrations are lower than those in the blood of the umbilical vein (Geeronckx et al, 1974). Diminished variability of the fetal heart rate is frequently seen a few minutes after an epidural injection of bupivacaine. The effect is transient and is not thought to indicate fetal hypoxia (Abboud et al, 1982).

Binding of bupivacaine to plasma proteins is less extensive in fetal than in maternal blood (Tucker et al, 1970) and there is therefore more free drug available for distribution to fetal tissues and especially to the fetal brain. The concentration of bupivacaine in fetal tissues is probably greater than would perhaps be anticipated from the favourable fetal/maternal concentration ratio. When the fetus is hypoxic and acidotic then bupivacaine base may be 'trapped' in the acidic tissues with a resulting rise in the concentration of bupivacaine (Datta et al, 1981a). Nevertheless there is no evidence of neurobehavioural impairment in the offspring of mothers who receive bupivacaine for epidural analgesia in normal labour (Scanlon et al, 1976). Certain drugs, including pethidine, can displace bupivacaine from protein receptor sites and thus increase the potential toxicity of bupivacaine (Ghoneim and Pandya, 1974).

Epidural analgesia with bupivacaine has been associated with an increased incidence of neonatal jaundice (Friedman et al, 1978). The explanation for this association, which may not be causal, is unknown. Other factors such as oxytocin infusions, premature induction of labour and forceps delivery have also been incriminated on inconclusive evidence.

Elimination of bupivacaine by the neonate takes two days following epidural anaesthesia for caesarean section, and the principal metabolite is 2,6-pipecolylxylidine (Kuhnert et al, 1981). This slow elimination reflects the diminished ability of the neonatal liver to metabolize drugs.

In a report on a small series of patients by Reynolds and Taylor (1971) it was suggested that the addition of adrenaline to the bupivacaine solutions used for lumbar epidural block resulted in higher concentrations of bupivacaine in the fetal blood. This rather surprising finding was not confirmed in a second, larger series (Reynolds et al, 1973) and it appears that the use of adrenaline has no effect on the placental transfer of bupivacaine during lumbar epidural analgesia.

There have been reports from North America of a substantial number of maternal deaths attributable to bupivacaine toxicity and it has been suggested that bupivacaine may have a special affinity for myocardial receptors when plasma protein receptors are occupied. The pattern of death has been convulsions followed by cardiac arrest, and failure of resuscitation has been attributed by some authorities to the high concentration of bupivacaine in the heart (Albright, 1979). No such deaths have been recorded in the UK, although Thorburn and Moir (1984) have reported convulsions following a large dose of bupivacaine. Perhaps the most important safety factor may be the widespread use of incremental techniques for epidural caesarean section in the UK. These techniques are unlikely to produce toxic plasma concentrations of bupivacaine especially if the 0.5% concentration is used (Dutton et al, 1984; Thompson et al, 1985).

(5) *Procaine* and *2-chloroprocaine*. These are two local anaesthetics which are in a special category in relation to placental transfer.

Esterases in the maternal and fetal plasma rapidly break down those two agents. Placental enzymes may contribute to the process in a small way. Concentrations in fetal blood are usually very low or absent. A substantial intravenous injection of procaine at the time of delivery did allow unaltered drug to reach the fetus (Usubiaga et al, 1968). The very rapid breakdown of 2-chloroprocaine makes it a very safe, but short-acting, local anaesthetic and it has gained popularity in the USA. 2-Chloroprocaine is not marketed in the UK, although its rapid action would be useful. Maternal and cord plasma concentrations of 2-chloroprocaine are very low or even undetectable due to the breakdown of this agent by plasma cholinesterase (Kuhnert et al, 1980a). Inadvertent subarachnoid injection of a large volume of 2-chloroprocaine during attempted epidural analgesia has been followed by prolonged nerve damage (Kane, 1981) and opinion is sharply divided over the safety of this agent which is unavailable in the UK.

Mixtures of equal volumes of bupivacaine and chloroprocaine are sometimes used to obtain a rapid onset of prolonged epidural analgesia. This practice may increase the toxicity of the chloroprocaine, because amide local anaesthetics such as bupivacaine slow the rate of hydrolysis of chloroprocaine (Lalka et al, 1978). Also, the pH of the mixture is low (3.7) and repeated injections may exhaust tissue buffers, create acid conditions at the injection site and promote tachyphylaxis towards bupivacaine (Brodsky and Brock-Utne, 1978).

(6) *Etidocaine*. The placental transfer of etidocaine has been assessed in a small series of epidural blocks by Bromage et al (1974). The mean concentration of the drug in the blood of the umbilical vein at delivery was 0.16 μg/ml and was 35% of the maternal venous blood concentration. The newborn lamb can eliminate etidocaine as rapidly as the adult sheep (Pedersen et al, 1982). The authors and their colleagues recorded a high incidence of inadequate anaesthesia when using etidocaine for elective epidural caesarean section, although the rapid spread of etidocaine was a useful feature (Dutton et al, 1984).

The relatively poor placental transfer of etidocaine and bupivacaine is attributable to a high degree of binding to plasma proteins.

Adrenaline and noradrenaline. The catecholamines adrenaline and noradrenaline cross the placenta in limited amounts because they are to some extent metabolized within the placenta (Sandler et al, 1964; Morgan et al, 1972). Alterations in fetal heart rate have been associated with the administration of adrenaline to the mother but are probably the result of the effects of adrenaline on the uterine and general circulation of the mother (Beard, 1962).

Miscellaneous drugs

(1) *Atropine and hyoscine*. The placental transfer of atropine is usually unrestricted and an intravenous injection of atropine is usually followed by fetal tachycardia within 2 or 3 minutes if placental function is good (John, 1965). Hopes that this phenomenon would form the basis for an atropine test of placental function have not been substantiated (Hellman and Fillisti, 1965). The concentration of atropine in the umbilical vein is 93% of the maternal value 5 minutes after an intravenous injection (Kivalo and Saarikoski, 1977).

Hyoscine crosses the placenta and, despite its undoubted sedative action, it has been given by intravenous injection before caesarean section without apparent ill-effect upon the infant.

(2) *Neostigmine*. Although no studies appear to have been reported it is probable that neostigmine does not cross the placenta to any important extent on account of the high degree of ionization of the drug in the maternal blood. The administration of neostigmine before the delivery of the child is very unlikely.

(3) *Magnesium sulphate*. Widely used in the USA as an anticonvulsant in severe pre-eclampsia and eclampsia, magnesium sulphate increases the

magnesium content of maternal and fetal blood (Stone and Pritchard, 1970) and has caused hypotonia and hyporeflexia in the neonate. Magnesium sulphate prevents convulsions by a peripheral action at the myoneural junction and not by a central action. Its placental transfer is free and a marked diminution in the normal beat-to-beat variability of the fetal heart rate follows the intravenous administration of magnesium sulphate (Babaknia and Niebyl, 1978; Green et al, 1983).

(4) *Other therapeutic agents*. The placenta permits the passage of a vast range of drugs which may be administered during pregnancy or labour and which may exert a beneficial or a harmful effect upon the fetus. Among the drugs which cross the placenta readily are antibiotics, digoxin, frusemide, propranolol, cortisone, hydrocortisone, prednisone, prednisolone and other hormones.

Among the drugs which are known to exert a harmful effect upon the fetus and which should not normally be given to a pregnant woman are:

Tetracycline (causes discoloration of teeth, hypoplasia of enamel and possible liver damage).

Chloramphenicol (produces the 'grey infant syndrome' with hypotonia, hypothermia, inadequate ventilation and grey coloration).

Streptomycin (causes nerve deafness) and lincomycin (may cause hypotonia).

Sulphonamides (may cause neonatal jaundice and kernicterus).

Cancer chemotherapeutic agents (may cause gross fetal abnormality and death).

Dicoumarol and allied anticoagulants (may cause fetal bleeding and death). Heparin is preferred.

Antithyroid drugs (cause suppression of fetal thyroid).

Oral hypoglycaemic agents (cause fetal hypoglycaemia and perhaps are teratogenic).

H_2-receptor antagonists (cimetidine and ranitidine have free placental transfer. No known harmful effects given before anaesthesia (Howe et al, 1981; Johnston et al, 1982). Long term cimetidine may impair fetal hepatic microsomal enzymes).

Primidone and phenytoin (may cause a coagulation defect in the neonate: Mountain et al, 1970).

Phenytoin, epanutin and diphenylhydantoin (have been thought to cause hare lip and cleft palate: Shapiro et al, 1976. Congenital heart disease and various defects commoner in children of treated epileptics, American Academy of Pediatrics, 1979).

Ganglion-blocking drugs (may cause paralytic ileus in the infant).

Diazoxide (is detectable in fetal blood but has no harmful effects).

Propranolol (long-term use may cause growth retardation, bradycardia and neonatal hypoglycaemia. Intravenous use causes dangerous fetal bradycardia).

Clinical experience suggests that insulin, dextrans, methyldopa and heparin do not cross the placenta. Diabetic patients should therefore receive insulin and not oral hypoglycaemic agents and heparin should always be preferred to dicoumarol during pregnancy. Frusemide crosses the placenta and causes neonatal diuresis if given shortly before delivery.

Breast feeding and anaesthesia

There is a lack of accurate information on the excretion of anaesthetics, analgesics and sedatives in breast milk, yet it is not uncommon for a nursing mother to require anaesthesia. Most drugs reach the breast milk by simple diffusion across the mammary capillaries and the epithelium of the mammary gland. Excretion of a drug in breast milk will be influenced by its pK_a, the pH of the milk (range 6.8–7.3), the extent of drug-binding to plasma and milk proteins, lipid solubility and molecular weight. Plasma/milk concentration ratios are usually low and the total dose absorbed by the infant depends also upon the quantity of milk consumed and subsequently absorbed from the gut.

Most drugs used in anaesthesia will be excreted in the milk, but the concentration is usually low and in most cases the infant will show no clinically obvious effects (Davis, 1977). Diazepam may depress the infant (Patrick et al, 1972) and the action of morphine may be prolonged or exaggerated, owing to the deficient metabolism of this drug by glucuronyl transferase. Breast milk production may be inhibited, especially by the barbiturates. Surgical haemorrhage has occurred in an infant whose mother was receiving a coumarin derivative (Catz and Giacoia, 1972).

Early and frequent maternal contact with an active neonate is an important stimulus to lactation (Salariya et al, 1978) and regional analgesia should be used whenever possible for the mother who wishes to establish or maintain lactation. If general anaesthesia is used, the morphine should be avoided and the dose of barbiturate minimized or a non-barbiturate induction agent chosen. Inhalational agents usually have a short-lived effect and may be used (Shantha, 1977).

DRUGS ACTING ON THE UTERUS

Drugs may be administered primarily for their action on the uterus; secondary effects which are of importance to the anaesthetist are then common. Conversely there are many drugs which, although administered for other reasons, may exert a secondary action on the uterus.

The exciting advances towards the control of uterine action in labour are dealt with in chapter 4. The account which follows is concerned with the action of drugs and certain other factors on the uterine muscle. Many drugs given by anaesthetists have a secondary affect on the myometrium, and powerful drugs given by obstetricians for their effect upon the uterus have important and potentially dangerous effects upon the cardiovascular and other systems.

The uterine muscle has α- and β-adrenergic receptors and rather widely scattered cholinergic receptors. Stimulation of the α-adrenergic receptors causes an increase in resting tone and in the strength of contractions in labour. Stimulation of the β-adrenergic receptors reduces the intensity of the contractions and lowers resting tone. Adrenaline in low concentrations produces β-activity; such an effect may sometimes occur to a small extent when adrenaline is used with local anaesthetic solutions. A high concentration of adrenaline, such as would follow accidental intravascular injection, causes α-activity. Noradrenaline has α-adrenergic effects and an infusion of noradrenaline in labour produces irregular, powerful contractions and a high resting tone. Endogenous catecholamines in the frightened woman in painful labour may cause this type of incoordinate uterine action. Drugs such as methoxamine which have α-adrenergic action can produce dangerously powerful, tetanic contractions which restrict or abolish blood flow to the placenta and may kill the fetus. Cholinergic drugs increase the strength of normal contractions without altering resting tone and they may do this, at least in part, by promoting the secretion of oxytocin by the posterior pituitary.

Most drugs which act on the myometrium act also on the myocardium and blood vessel walls, often in a broadly similar way. Cardiovascular side-effects are impossible to avoid and are occasionally severe enough to limit the use of a drug. Although β-receptors have been subdivided into β_1 (in the heart) and β_2 (in the uterus), there is always an overlap in action upon these two types of receptors.

Methods of assessing the action of a drug on the contractility of the uterine muscle include the measurement of intrauterine pressures, the evaluation of the duration and intensity of contractions in Montevideo units, the recording of the effects of the drug on isolated strips of myometrium, the indirect evaluation of the adequacy of uterine contractions and retraction after delivery, by measuring blood loss, and the assessment of progress in labour either clinically or graphically. These methods are used to evaluate uterine action at various times in pregnancy and labour and are of widely varying degrees of sensitivity. In many instances one has to depend on clinical impressions of the effects of drugs upon the rate of progress in labour as the only assessment available.

Gaseous and volatile anaesthetics

Analgesic concentrations of nitrous oxide, trichloroethylene and methoxyflurane do not impede the rate of progress of normal labour.

Anaesthetic concentrations of all of the powerful volatile anaesthetics depress the contractility of the uterine muscle in rough proportion to the depth of anaesthesia. In all but the lowest concentrations, chloroform, ether, halothane, methoxyflurane, enflurane and isoflurane relax the myometrium and may cause excessive bleeding at delivery which may only be arrested by reducing the depth of anaesthesia. It is claimed that light cyclopropane anaesthesia has only a slight depressant effect on the uterine muscle (Vasicka and Kretchmer, 1961; Alfonsi and Massi, 1963) but deeper planes of cyclopropane anaesthesia will relax the uterus.

Human myometrium responds in a similar way to equipotent concentrations of halothane, enflurane and isoflurane. Depression is dose-related. Resting tension is little altered at 0.5 MAC and haemorrhage from the placental site would be unlikely. At 1.5 MAC resting tension is significantly reduced (Munson and Embro, 1977). In contrast 3% enflurane (1.75 MAC) did not depress contractility in pregnant and non-pregnant rabbits (Jones et al, 1978). The effect of halothane is probably greater on the pregnant uterus (Naftalin et al, 1977). The picture is confused by the use of animal and human uteri or strips of myometrium from pregnant or non-pregnant subjects and by the use of different perfusates with differing ionic content but it seems acceptable to use concentrations of about 0.5 MAC to supplement nitrous oxide anaesthesia.

It is seldom now that uterine relaxation is deliberately sought for the performance of intrauterine manipulations. Halothane is undoubtedly effective for this purpose but the effect upon the maternal cardiovascular system may be severe and the loss of blood may be very great.

The use of minimal concentrations of halothane, enflurane or trichloroethylene is at present popular among anaesthetists in Great Britain during obstetric anaesthesia. The object is to reduce the incidence of awareness during anaesthesia while permitting the use of high concentrations of oxygen along with nitrous oxide. Clinical experience (Crawford, 1972) and the measurement of blood loss (Moir, 1970; Galbert and Gardner, 1972; Abboud et al, 1981) suggest that methoxyflurane (0.1 or 0.2%), enflurane (0.6%) and halothane (0.5%) do not increase bleeding at caesarean section. When isolated strips of myometrium are exposed to halothane a relaxant effect is first discernible when the concentration of halothane is 0.37% (Munson et al, 1969). Serious inhibition is not observed until the concentration reaches 1.2%. The uterus which has been relaxed by halothane may not respond to oxytocic drugs.

The uterus in early pregnancy can be relaxed by halothane. Cullen et al (1970) found that halothane increased bleeding at therapeutic abortion. Isoflurane increased bleeding in similar circumstances (Dolan et al, 1972) and it is probable that the other volatile anaesthetics would have this effect in equivalent concentrations.

Intravenous anaesthetics

Thiopentone has no effect on uterine contractions in doses of up to 500 mg (Alvarez and Caldeyro-Barcia, 1954; Alfonsi and Massi, 1963) and it is probable that the other agents commonly used for the intravenous induction of anaesthesia do not directly affect the myometrium. It is possible that a reduction in uterine blood flow following a reduction in cardiac output as the result of anaesthesia would temporarily inhibit uterine contractions. Ketamine increases resting tone and the amplitude and frequency of contractions in isolated animal uteri (Jawalekar et al, 1972). The tone of the human postpartum uterus is increased by ketamine (Marx et al, 1979).

Muscle relaxants

Suxamethonium has been shown not to affect uterine contractility in vivo, by intrauterine pressure recordings (Healey, 1971; Iuppa et al, 1971). In vitro studies demonstrated that suxamethonium, gallamine and D-tubocurarine have no action on uterine muscle (Reier and Moster, 1970). The facilitation of manoeuvres such as external cephalic version by the administration of a skeletal muscle relaxant is due entirely to relaxation of the abdominal wall musculature.

Analgesics, sedatives and tranquillizers

It is now generally agreed that the narcotic analgesics, sedatives and tranquillizers do not inhibit the progress of established labour and that these drugs are very unlikely to be effective if given in the hope of abolishing established premature labour. Diazepam does not alter normal contractions in established labour in the absence of hypotension (Friedman et al, 1969). Caval occlusion tends to reduce uterine activity, presumably by reducing uterine blood flow (Caldeyro-Barcia, 1960) and this effect may be enhanced by the administration of powerful sedatives and analgesics to supine patients. Intrauterine manometry has confirmed that morphine and chlorpromazine have no inhibiting effect on the contractions of normal labour (Caldeyro-Barcia et al, 1955; Caldeyro-Barcia et al, 1958). Even bolus intravenous injections of pethidine, morphine, alphaprodine and promethazine had only minor effects on uterine contractions in established labour conducted in the lateral position (Petrie et al, 1976). Pentazocine appears not to inhibit uterine action (Filler and Filler, 1966).

When uterine action is incoordinate and labour is prolonged, painful and distressing, the administration of analgesic and sedative drugs will often be followed by a more normal type of uterine action (De Voe et al, 1969). This is of course the traditional management of prolonged labour which is summarized in the phrase 'time and morphine' and it is believed that it is the central action of these drugs in relieving pain and anxiety which results in the improvement of uterine action. One may speculate on the possibility that pain and anxiety result in high catecholamine levels in the maternal blood and that the secondary result of the exposure of the uterus to adrenaline and noradrenaline is either inhibition of contractions or an incoordinate pattern of uterine action.

Sympathomimetic drugs and antagonists and the uterus

The uterus cotains both α- and β-receptors (Miller, 1967) and these influence contraction and relaxation of the uterine muscle respectively.

α-Receptor stimulants. Agents such as noradrenaline, methoxamine and mephentermine will cause the uterus to contract, although not always in a physiological manner and the effect depends on the dose of the drug. These agents should not be used to treat hypotension.

Noradrenaline. An intravenous infusion of noradrenaline at the rate of 2–10 μg/min will result in incoordinate uterine contractions, and a higher rate of infusion may induce tetanic contractions and arterial hypertension. The violent uterine contractions may impair uteroplacental blood flow to a degree sufficient to cause fetal hypoxia which may be aggravated by spasm of the uterine arteries (Cibils et al, 1962).

Methoxamine, by its α-receptor stimulant effect, and mephentermine, by causing the release of noradrenaline, will each produce effects similar to those previously described for noradrenaline. An intravenous injection of 2–6 mg methoxamine can induce potentially dangerous hypertonic uterine contractions (Senties et al, 1970) as well as causing spasm of the uterine arteries. Severe fetal bradycardia has been reported in association with uterine hypertonus after methoxamine (Vasicka et al, 1964). Methoxamine should not be used in obstetrics.

β-Receptor stimulants. Adrenaline and the various β-receptor stimulants such as isoxuprine, orciprenaline, salbutamol and ritodrine are all capable of reducing the frequency and strength of uterine contractions. Propranolol reverses this action but may cause dangerous fetal bradycardia. The action on the uterus of the β-receptor stimulants is always accompanied by alterations in the maternal heart rate, blood pressure and stroke volume. These cardiovascular effects vary somewhat in intensity among the various drugs but β_2 effects on the uterus and β_1 effects on the heart always coexist in some degree. Plasma potassium concentration fell from 3.5 ± 0.1 to 2.7 ± 0.1 mmol/litre during salbutamol infusions but there were no electrocardiographic signs of hypokalaemia. Plasma glucose and insulin concentrations increased (Thomas et al, 1977).

(1) *Adrenaline.* When adrenaline is given by intravenous infusion at a rate of 5–20 μg/min the intensity and frequency of uterine contractions diminish and maternal tachycardia and hypertension develop (Pose et al, 1962; Zuspan et al, 1964). Signs of fetal distress may arise during an infusion of adrenaline and are probably due to a reduction in the uteroplacental blood flow (Beard, 1962). It is considered to be very unlikely that a correctly placed injection of a solution containing 1 : 200 000 adrenaline into the epidural

space, the pudendal nerve or the subcutaneous tissues would result in blood levels of adrenaline sufficient to seriously impair uterine action. Craft et al (1972) found that the rate of progress in labour was the same when plain lignocaine and lignocaine with 1 : 200 000 adrenaline were used for lumbar epidural analgesia in induced labours. Gunther and Bauman (1969) made similar observations when caudal analgesia was used in induced labours, although adrenaline did seem to delay progress in labour which had begun spontaneously. Hypotension developed in 20% of these patients and may well have contributed to the inhibition of contractions. Several β-receptor stimulants have been used in attempts to arrest premature labour and also in the hope of diminishing the intensity of hypertonic uterine contractions where it has been considered that these contractions contributed to fetal distress in labour. The apparent uterine inhibition caused by β-adrenergic compounds is the result of a chaotic fibrillation in the myometrium which prevents coordinated, powerful contractions (Schulman, 1978). In practice these agents are not always capable of abolishing established labour, particularly if the membranes have already ruptured, and the incidence of cardiovascular side-effects is often rather high.

The administration of β-adrenergic agents can create a worrying situation for the anaesthetist who is asked to anaesthetize a mother with extreme tachycardia for the urgent delivery of a distressed fetus. Propranolol will reduce the heart rate but should if possible be withheld until after delivery of the fetus because it may cause neonatal bradycardia (Knight, 1977; Schoenfeld et al, 1978). The average pulse rate during salbutamol infusion was 148 ± 4 beats/min (Thomas et al, 1977). Cardiac output usually increases substantially. β-Mimetic drugs are contraindicated in patients with heart disease and, in all patients, the heart rate should not exceed 140 beats/min. Continuous ECG monitoring is recommended. Pulmonary oedema has been reported with various β-mimetic agents, usually where corticosteroid therapy has been given to promote fetal lung maturation (Elliott et al, 1978). Hypokalaemia may complicate β-mimetic infusions. The following β-receptor stimulants have been used in clinical practice:

(2) *Isoxuprine* will reduce the frequency and intensity of oxytocin-induced contractions in labour and in early pregnancy (Hendricks et al, 1961; Hawkins, 1964) but it is doubtful if isoxuprine will completely inhibit established labour. Maternal hypertension and tachycardia are common and alterations in the fetal heart rate may occur.

(3) *Orciprenaline*. The effects of orciprenaline are similar to those of isoxuprine; maternal tachycardia, nausea and vomiting are of frequent occurrence.

(4) *Ritodrine* is also capable of diminishing the strength and frequency of contractions, although it will not always arrest established premature labour.

The incidence of cardiovascular side-effects is lower with this drug than with isoxuprine and orciprenaline (Wesselius-de Casparis et al, 1971).

(5) *Salbutamol* also causes tachycardia and occasionally nausea and vomiting, although blood pressure is usually little changed. Salbutamol is at present quite widely used for the suppression of premature labour and is occasionally given intravenously for the relief of dangerous uterine hypertonicity in labour (Liggins and Vaughan, 1973; Lunell et al, 1976). β-Adrenergic stimulators have been used to inhibit uterine activity in acute fetal distress, regardless of the aetiology (Arias, 1978). A single inhalation of salbutamol from an inhaler can produce transient uterine relaxation and has been used to facilitate obstetrical manoeuvres when uterine tone is high under epidural or spinal analgesia. There is a risk of hypotension.

α-Receptor antagonists. Most of these compounds (for example phentolamine) have no useful action upon the myometrium. Other substances, such as certain of the ergot alkaloids, possess a weak α-receptor antagonistic action on the uterus which is overwhelmed by their direct stimulant action on the uterine muscle.

β-Receptor antagonists. Propranolol has been shown to be capable of reversing the depressant effect of isoxuprine and adrenaline on the uterine muscle (Eskes et al, 1965; Barden and Stander, 1968a). When an intravenous infusion of propranolol was administered during labour the strength and frequency of contractions increased in approximately half of the patients (Barden and Stander, 1968b). It was postulated that uterine action was intensified by propranolol in those women who had high concentrations of adrenaline in their blood or who had a high level of sympathetic activity during labour. Propranolol will also reduce the tachycardia caused by β-receptor stimulants such as ritodrine and salbutamol. Unfortunately propranolol can cause severe fetal bradycardia and perhaps hypoglycaemia.

Long-term treatment with propranolol during pregnancy is said to block the responses of the mother to the haemodynamic demands of pregnancy and labour and also appears to block the fetal responses to the stress of labour (Reed et al, 1974). The incidence of infants requiring active resuscitation at birth was high in a series of infants whose mothers had received propranolol (Tunstall, 1969). Fetal growth in utero may be impaired.

Parasympathomimetic drugs and antagonists

The dominant action of acetylcholine on the uterus is muscarinic. An intravenous infusion of acetylcholine increases the strength and frequency of uterine contractions (Sala and Fisch, 1965). Acetylcholine may also stimulate the uterus indirectly by increasing the output of oxytocin from the posterior pituitary. The uterine blood flow is enhanced by acetylcholine. These effects of acetylcholine are all of very short duration and this, together with its cardiovascular effects, makes acetylcholine unsuitable for clinical use. Physostigmine enhances the effect of acetylcholine on the non-pregnant uterus but has little useful effect on the uterus during labour (Shabanah et al, 1964).

Atropine has no significant effect upon uterine contractions, even when the contractions have been induced by acetylcholine (Embrey, 1958; Sala and Fisch, 1965).

Epidural and subarachnoid block

Where epidural or subarachnoid analgesia causes hypotension then uterine contractions may cease. Restoration of an adequate uterine blood flow quickly restores uterine action (Vasicka et al, 1964). Contractions are not usually abolished unless the systolic blood pressure falls below about 80 mmHg (10.6 kPa). The injection of local anaesthetic solutions into the epidural space is sometimes followed by the abolition of uterine contractions for 10 or 15 minutes in the absence of hypotension (Vasicka and Kretchmer, 1961; Shabanah et al, 1964). The cause is probably a reduction in uterine blood flow due to caval occlusion. This inhibition is not seen when top-up injections are given in the lateral position (Schellenberg, 1977).

When labour has been incoordinate, the institution of a continuous epidural block will usually be followed by a more normal type of uterine action and an increase in the rate of dilatation of the cervix (Climie, 1964; Moir and Willocks, 1967). This improvement may be observed even when oxytocin is not administered. It is thought that the effective relief of pain by epidural analgesia reverses the adverse effects of fear, anxiety and pain on uterine action. Alternatively it is postulated that the blockade of the preganglionic sympathetic nerve fibres allows the postganglionic fibres to function more normally in the absence of impulses from higher centres.

There are reports of a slight reduction in uterine activity and prolongation of labour attributed to the addition of 1 : 200 000 adrenaline to the local anaesthetic solution (Matadial and Cibils, 1976; Jouppila et al, 1977), although no such effect was observed by Phillips and his colleagues (1977). Adrenaline offers no advantages with bupivacaine and should not be used. The first stage of labour is then unlikely to be prolonged by more than 1 hour (Potter and MacDonald, 1971). According to Studd et al (1980, 1982) epidural analgesia does not significantly influence the duration of the first stage of normal, spontaneous labour, augmented labour or induced labour.

It was the practice for many years in North America to refrain from performing an epidural block in labour until the cervix had dilated to a predetermined extent (commonly 5 or 6 cm in the primigravida). It was held that the earlier institution of epidural analgesia might inhibit uterine action. This practice is no longer justifiable, if indeed it ever was. Epidural analgesia should be given when labour is becoming painful, regardless of the dilatation of the cervix. Epidural analgesia may even be given electively on induction of labour. Oxytocin (Syntocinon) is usually given to augment labour in these circumstances.

When delivery is conducted under epidural or subarachnoid analgesia the uterus normally retracts powerfully after the delivery of the infant, and blood loss is often substantially reduced. The loss of blood at forceps deliveries and at caesarean section is approximately halved when epidural analgesia is used instead of general anaesthesia (Moir and Wallace, 1967; Moir, 1970).

Local anaesthetics. The direct action of procaine, lignocaine (lidocaine) and amethocaine (tetracaine) on the uterus has been studied using isolated strips of myometrium (McGaughey et al, 1962). In low concentrations these three local anaesthetics increased the amplitude of contractions and reduced their frequency. The resting tone between contractions was reduced. High concentrations increased the resting tone and decreased the amplitude of contractions. Cinchocaine (dibucaine) had almost no effect on isolated myometrium. It is doubtful if concentrations sufficient to produce any of these effects would be achieved within the uterus in the course of most regional blocks. The use of large doses for extensive and prolonged epidural blockade might result in concentrations approaching those used in the study (Bromage, 1967). Direct injection of various local anaesthetics into the uterine artery increased uterine tone (Greiss et al, 1976). Accidental arterial injection might occur in performing paracervical block.

Oxytocin, ergometrine and other uterine stimulants

Oxytocin is a hormone of the posterior pituitary and some of the preparations of this hormone may contain traces of vasopressin. Oxytocin increases the permeability of the myometrial cell membrane to potassium, and renders the cell more easily excitable. The relationship between oxytocin and prostaglandins in the initiation of labour is not yet fully understood. Hypertensive responses have been attributed to the presence of vasopressin. Syntocinon is a synthetic preparation of oxytocin which is now normally used in preference to the natural hormone and is of course free of vasopressin. An antidiuretic action may occur after only 15 minutes administration of a Syntocinon infusion (Abdul-Karim and Rizk, 1970). The concentration of natural oxytocin increases as labour progresses. Oxytocin is destroyed by placental oxytocinase and the concentration of this enzyme falls at the onset of labour (Ances, 1972; Gibbens and Chard, 1976).

The use of oxytocin in the first stage of labour is considered in chapter 4. It is worth noting here that oxytocin, and perhaps prostaglandins, are the only drugs capable of inducing uterine contractions which are manometrically indistinguishable from those of spontaneous onset.

Oxytocin may be given as a single intravenous injection of 5 units at delivery as an alternative to ergometrine. It is in these circumstances that the cardiovascular side-effects of oxytocin are most likely to occur. The powerful uterine contraction is likely to be accompanied by a very short-lasting but occasionally substantial reduction in arterial pressure and a small increase in central venous pressure and cardiac output which is the result of the transfer of blood from the uteroplacental circulation to the general circulation (Andersen et al, 1965; Hendricks and Brenner, 1970; Williams et al, 1974). Hypotension attributable to oxytocin has not been a feature at delivery by caesarean section under epidural analgesia when patients were well hydrated, and in the laterally tilted position (Moir and Amoa, 1979), although transient, substantial falls in arterial blood pressure were recorded under general anaesthesia by Weiss and Peak (1974). A continuous, dilute infusion of synthetic oxytocin has minimal cardiovascular effects. These actions of oxytocin make this agent preferable to ergometrine, with its hypertensive action, in cases of pre-eclampsia and in the presence of heart disease. Oxytocin and ergometrine appear to be equally effective in reducing blood loss at delivery when injected intravenously (Williams et al, 1974; Moodie and Moir, 1976; Moir and Amoa, 1979).

A further advantage of oxytocin is the avoidance of the nausea and vomiting which may occur after an intravenous injection of ergometrine in the conscious patient and especially during epidural analgesia (Milne and Murray Lawson, 1973; Moodie and Moir, 1976).

Oxytocin infusions during labour appear to be associated with an increase in the incidence and severity of neonatal jaundice. However, oxytocin is no longer considered to be a direct cause of neonatal jaundice (Lange et al, 1982); the cause may be related to the infusion of large volumes of glucose and water (Kenepp et al, 1982). This phenomenon has, probably erroneously, also been attributed to the use of epidural analgesia in labour (D'Souza et al, 1979).

Water intoxication has occurred during labour. It is the result of the infusion of large volumes of salt-free solutions such as 5% dextrose, together with the antidiuretic action of oxytocin. Convulsions, coma and death have been recorded. Both maternal and fetal hyponatraemia have been reported (Tarnow-Mordi et al, 1981). Balanced salt solutions should be preferred to solutions of dextrose in water.

Ergometrine. If ergometrine is administered during the first stage of labour it will give rise to grossly abnormal and violent contractions which will be associated with a dangerously high intrauterine pressure between contractions. These effects are likely to impair uteroplacental blood flow and cause fetal hypoxia. When ergometrine is given at delivery then a sustained hypertonicity of the uterus results and irregular contractions are superimposed.

An intravenous injection of 0.25 mg or 0.5 mg ergometrine may have important side-effects. Ergometrine has a vasoconstrictor activity which Johnstone (1972) has demonstrated by forearm plethysmography. This action, combined with the autotransfusion of blood from the uterus into the general circulation, commonly results in rises in the arterial and central venous pressures (Greenhalf and Evans, 1970; Hendricks and Brenner, 1970; Williams et al, 1974). Arterial hypertension is likely to be most severe in patients with pre-eclampsia (Baillie, 1963) and may persist for several hours. Hypertension, cerebral oedema and convulsions have been attributed to an ergot preparation given intravenously at delivery (Abouleish, 1976). Moore (1964) and Marx and Orkin (1969) stress the possibility of severe hypertension with the attendant risk of a cerebrovascular accident if a vasopressor and an oxytocic drug are given to the same patient, even after an interval of several hours. The risks of this happening would seem to be greater with ergometrine than with synthetic oxytocin on theoretical grounds. Moreover the use of vasopressors of the α-adrenergic vasoconstrictor type should be avoided in pregnancy because of their effect upon the uterus. Sinus bradycardia and nodal rhythm may be observed on the electrocardiograph after intravenous ergometrine (Baillie, 1969). Johnstone (1972) has pointed out the possibility that anaesthesia may temporarily suppress the powerful vasoconstrictor action of ergometrine and postulates that when pulmonary oedema develops shortly after obstetric anaesthesia the explanation could sometimes lie with the use of ergometrine, and that an erroneous diagnosis of Mendelson's syndrome could be made. A progressive illness together with a history of pulmonary aspiration would support a diagnosis of Mendelson's syndrome. It may be postulated that the action of ergometrine on the pulmonary vessels would aggravate aspiration pneumonitis and the administration of ergometrine might explain the high mortality rate associated with this condition in obstetric patients. The emetic effect of intravenous ergometrine has been demonstrated by Wassef et al (1974). Some cardiovascular actions of oxytocin and ergometrine are summarized in Table 5.

The potential dangers of ergometrine, especially for patients with pre-eclampsia and heart disease, deserve wider recognition and there are excellent grounds for substituting synthetic oxytocin for ergometrine. One can only speculate on the number of episodes of cardiac failure, eclampsia and cerebral haemorrhage which may have been precipitated by ergometrine. Cardiovascular side-effects are least evident after an intramuscular injection

Table 5. Some cardiovascular effects of intravenous ergometrine and oxytocin (Syntocinon) in the third stage of labour

	Ergometrine (i.v. injection)	Oxytocin (i.v. injection)	Oxytocin (i.v. infusion)
Systolic blood pressure	Considerably increased	Decreased very briefly	No change
Central venous pressure	Considerably increased	Increased moderately	Increased slightly
Peripheral resistance	Considerably increased	Decreased very briefly	Little effect

of ergometrine. An intramuscular injection of oxytocin with ergometrine (Syntometrine) will produce a uterine contraction in an average time of 2 minutes and 37 seconds, whereas an intravenous injection of ergometrine is effective in 41 seconds (Embrey, 1961).

Prostaglandins. There are at least 13 prostaglandins and they occur in a wide variety of body tissues and fluids including the lungs, the nervous system, muscle and seminal fluid. An important action of prostaglandins is their ability to induce smooth muscle to contract and, in the case of the uterine muscle, there is probably a direct stimulant action on the muscle and an indirect effect mediated through an increased output of oxytocin from the pituitary.

Prostaglandins can induce uterine contractions at any stage in pregnancy and they may be given intravenously, orally, into the uterus or intravaginally. They appear to enhance the action of oxytocin and may 'prepare' the uterus for oxytocin stimulation. The prostaglandins are still being evaluated but there is a place for these compounds in the termination of pregnancy, especially in the mid-trimester and in the induction of labour. Oral administration is attractive to the patient, although vomiting and diarrhoea occasionally occur as the result of contraction of the smooth muscle of the gastrointestinal tract. The synthetic prostaglandin Prostin appears to relax and 'ripen' the cervix and is given as a pessary to prepare the cervix for labour. Extra-amniotic administration is associated with few gastrointestinal side-effects and is currently popular.

The compounds used to stimulate uterine action are principally prostaglandins E_2 and $F_2\alpha$ (PGE_2 and $PGF_2\alpha$). These compounds are concerned in the natural onset and maintenance of labour. Among the numerous side-effects of these compounds are some of concern to the obstetric anaesthetist. When PGE_2 is injected intravenously a moderate rise in blood pressure may result and tachycardia and flushing are associated phenomena. An intravenous injection of $500\,\mu g\,PGF_2\alpha$ may cause a slight rise in blood pressure but a continuous infusion has no effect on blood pressure (Fishburne et al, 1972). The oral and intrauterine (extra-amniotic) administration of PGE_2 and $PGF_2\alpha$ do not affect blood pressure (Karim et al, 1971). For mid-trimester abortion a continuous infusion of PGE_2 or $PGF_2\alpha$ has been used and must be maintained for 48 hours or more. Extra-amniotic or intra-amniotic injections are now usually preferred. PGE_2 pessaries are extensively used to 'ripen' the cervix as an aid to the induction of labour. PGE_2 relaxes bronchial muscle and antagonizes bronchoconstrictor substances. These actions are most obvious in asthmatic subjects in whom a significant improvement in FEV_1 and peak flow rate can be measured (Cuthbert, 1969). In contrast $PGF_2\alpha$ increases the tone of bronchial muscles, especially in asthmatics, and this compound should be avoided in such patients (Fishburne et al, 1972). These opposite actions of PGE_2 and $PGF_2\alpha$ on bronchial tone have been widely accepted (Katz and Katz, 1974) but have been challenged by Mathi and others (1973), who believe that both these prostaglandins are bronchoconstrictors. Although PGE_1 is a powerful, but short-acting inhibitor of platelet aggregation (Emmons et al, 1967) its evanescent action precludes its use in the prevention and treatment of thrombosis. PGE_2 has no effect on platelet aggregation.

Spartein sulphate. Spartein sulphate has been quite extensively used to induce labour. The contractions may sometimes be tetanic or incoordinate and for this reason the drug has fallen into disuse.

Other uterine relaxants

Ethyl alcohol. An intravenous infusion of ethyl alcohol was formerly used in an attempt to inhibit premature labour. Alcohol has a direct depressant action on the myometrium and blood levels of 80–160 mg/100 ml (17.4– 34.7 mmol/litre) are required in order to achieve this effect. Such blood levels would result in the automatic conviction of a British motorist for drunken driving and some patients feel nauseated and distressed during treatment (Fuchs et al, 1967; Mantell and Liggins, 1970). Alcohol is also thought to inhibit the release of oxytocin in labour (Fuchs, 1966).

It is doubtful if ethyl alcohol, or indeed any known drug, can regularly abolish established labour, especially if the membranes have already ruptured. Alcohol is now seldom used to suppress premature labour.

Amyl nitrite. This drug was formerly administered by inhaling the contents of a crushable glass capsule. The capsule may be crushed within the rebreathing or reservoir bag of an anaesthetic apparatus.

Although amyl nitrite may sometimes briefly reduce the intensity of normal uterine contractions it has been shown to be ineffective in the treatment of tetanic contractions and constriction ring of the uterus, the conditions for which amyl nitrite was formerly advocated (Kumar et al, 1965). Amyl nitrite causes marked flushing of the skin and hypotension may result from a large dose.

The cautious introduction of halothane 2% will relax the uterus of the anaesthetized patient on the rare occasions when such a procedure seems justified.

Diazoxide. A slow intravenous injection of diazoxide is a powerful inhibitor of spontaneous and oxytocin-induced uterine contractions (Wilson et al, 1974; Caritis et al, 1979). It is difficult to judge the dose which will suppress contractions without causing hypotension. Diazoxide is not a β-adrenergic drug and may act directly on the myometrium and blood vessels; it is also a calcium antagonist.

OTHER FACTORS INFLUENCING UTERINE ACTION

Caval occlusion and posture. In the first stage of labour, contractions are more powerful when the patient lies in the lateral position (Caldeyro-Barcia, 1960) in contrast with the supine position. It is presumed that the improvement in uterine action in the lateral position is due, in part at least, to the improvement in uterine blood flow which results from the relief of pressure on the inferior vena cava. There is therefore a physiological as well as a psychological basis for an upright, semi-recumbent or lateral position during labour, although the clinical evidence for a more rapid labour is conflicting.

Alterations in pH. Experiments with isolated strips of uterine muscle demonstrate that as the environmental pH declines the strength of the contractions decreases (Mark, 1961). It is easy to imagine a situation during a prolonged labour whereby localized acidosis within the uterus and perhaps also a generalized acidosis result in a further impairment of uterine activity.

Electrolytes. The uterus, like other muscular organs, depends on a reasonably normal electrolytic environment if it is to function efficiently. Consequently the electrolyte deficiencies which may develop during prolonged labour are unlikely to be conducive to good uterine action (Hawkins and Nixon, 1957).

Calcium ions are a necessary cofactor for the functioning of smooth muscle although their precise role in myometrial function is not fully established. An intravenous injection of calcium gluconate increases uterine contractility in late pregnancy.

High concentrations of magnesium ions reduce uterine contractility and this effect may be observed when intravenous infusions of magnesium sulphate, at the rate of 0.1 g/min, are used in the treatment of pre-eclampsia (Hall et al, 1959). It is thought that magnesium ions compete with calcium ions at cellular level.

DRUGS ACTING ON THE UTEROPLACENTAL
CIRCULATION

Uteroplacental blood flow depends on alterations in cardiac output and on local and general changes in blood pressure and vascular resistance. Occlusion of the inferior vena cava by the gravid uterus in the supine position may reduce uteroplacental blood flow by obstructing the venous outflow from the uterus or by reducing cardiac output. Drugs which increase uterine contractility, particularly if the contractions are incoordinate and accompanied by hypertonicity between contractions, may reduce uterine artery blood flow. The effect of an anaesthetic or analgesic technique on uteroplacental blood flow is often of prime importance, outweighing factors such as the placental transfer of the anaesthetic agents in determining the condition of the child at birth. In clinical practice evidence of a reduction in placental blood flow is usually obtained in the form of fetal metabolic acidosis.

General anaesthesia. Measurement of uterine blood flow is technically difficult and prone to inaccuracies in the human subject. Studies based upon measurements of thermal conductivity in the myometrium in women suggest that light hexobarbitone and nitrous oxide anaesthesia does not alter uterine blood flow and that deep halothane anaesthesia substantially reduces the flow of blood, through the uterus (Nobel and Hille, 1963). Halothane and isoflurane in concentrations of up to 1.5 MAC actually improved uterine artery blood flow and fetal acidosis was absent (Palahniuk and Shnider, 1974). This interesting observation may be related to a direct action of these agents on the uterine artery. Myometrial relaxation would be expected to improve blood flow and the vasoconstrictor action of endogenous catecholamines during very light nitrous oxide anaesthesia would be avoided. The reduction in uterine blood flow with deep halothane anaesthesia is probably attributable mainly to a reduction in cardiac output. The administration of 0.5% halothane to pregnant dogs caused a 37% reduction in uterine blood flow in association with a 30% reduction in cardiac output (Einer-Jensen and Juhl, 1974).

Uterine artery blood flow has been measured in pregnant ewes and bitches by placing electromagnetic flowmeters around the uterine artery. By using this technique it was found that a single injection of thiopentone reduced uterine blood flow by 15% while the systemic arterial pressure remained steady (Wolkoff et al, 1965). A similar, transient reduction in intervillous blood flow has been observed in human mothers, using the ^{133}Xe-clearance technique (Jouppila et al, 1979). The clinical importance of this reduction is not great if the dose of thiopentone is small.

Small doses of thiopentone, methohexitone and ketamine when given for the induction of anaesthesia for caesarean section do not increase fetal metabolic acidosis and it is concluded that maternal cardiac output and uteroplacental blood flow are not seriously impaired (Levinson et al, 1973; Holdcroft et al, 1974; Buley et al, 1977). In contrast, propanidid and Althesin are associated with increased fetal metabolic acidosis, and this is indirect evidence that maternal and therefore placental circulation are impaired by these agents (Downing et al, 1974; Mahomedy et al, 1976).

Regional analgesia. In the absence of hypotension there is no alteration in uterine artery blood flow during subarchnoid analgesia, but if the systemic arterial pressure falls then uterine blood flow declines. The percentage reduction in uterine blood flow usually equals the reduction in arterial pressure although some workers have suggested that uterine vascular resistance sometimes increases in association with hypotension with a disproportionately great reduction in flow (Greiss and Crandell, 1965; Lucas et al, 1965). In the absence of hypotension uteroplacental blood flow, as measured by a ^{133}Xe method, is not significantly altered during epidural analgesia in normal labour or at caesarean section (Jouppila et al, 1978a,b). Using electromagnetic flow probes, epidural analgesia was shown not to affect uterine artery blood flow in normotensive pregnant ewes (Wallis et al, 1976).

It is not possible to lay down a 'safe' maternal arterial blood pressure which will always ensure an adequate uteroplacental blood flow. No doubt this pressure will vary from mother to mother according to the previous blood pressure. Guide lines can be obtained from the finding that signs of hypoxia appear in the fetal heart rate tracing when the systolic blood pressure remains below 60 mmHg (8.0 kPa) during spinal analgesia (Ebner et al, 1960). When mean arterial pressure remained below 70 mmHg (9.3 kPa) for more than 3 minutes during caesarean section under epidural analgesia neurobehavioural impairment was observed in the neonates (Hollmen et al, 1978). Observations by Corke and others (1982) suggest that the duration of hypotension is important and that if hypotension is corrected within 2 minutes at caesarean section under spinal anaesthesia then the infant will not be acidotic at birth.

When continuous caudal analgesia was instituted during prolonged, incoordinate labours there was a substantial improvement in the hitherto much reduced placental blood flow (Johnson and Clayton, 1955). The improvement in blood flow probably resulted from the restoration of a more normal pattern of uterine contractions following upon the provision of effective analgesia.

Vasopressor drugs. Several investigators have demonstrated by the use of electromagnetic flowmeters in animals that noradrenaline, phenylephrine, metaraminol and methoxamine have an α-adrenergic, vasoconstrictor action upon the uterine circulation and cause a substantial reduction in uterine artery blood flow (Greiss, 1963; Greiss and Van Wilkes, 1964; Shnider et al, 1968; Ralston et al, 1974). The rise in systemic arterial pressure produced by these α-adrenergic agents was accompanied by a disproportionately greater increase in uterine vascular resistance. When pregnant bitches were experimentally bled there was a reduction in uterine artery blood flow, and when the systemic arterial pressure was then raised by a vasoconstrictor drug there was a further reduction in uterine artery blood flow (Romney et al, 1963).

The dangers of hypotension for the fetus and the potential exaggeration of these risks by the use of vasoconstrictor agents are clearly established in animals and it would be wise to assume that these dangers apply to the human mother and her infant.

Vasopressor drugs which produce their pressor effect principally by a positive inotropic action upon the myocardium should be viewed in a different light from those with a mainly vasoconstrictor action. Ephedrine and to a lesser extent mephentermine are capable of increasing the systemic arterial pressure by increasing cardiac output and without causing any major reduction in uterine artery blood flow (Ralston et al, 1974). Ephedrine is also effective in preventing hypotension during caesarean section under epidural anaesthesia (Rolbin et al, 1982) and placental blood flow appears to be well maintained.

Vasopressor drugs will rarely be needed during epidural analgesia in labour if cardiac output and blood pressure are maintained by intravenous fluids and the avoidance of caval occlusion. If a vasopressor is to be administered, then, in the light of available information, the drug of choice is ephedrine. An intravenous injection of 10 mg will usually prove effective. Clinical experience indicates that ephedrine may be required in up to 30% of caesarean sections performed under epidural or spinal anaesthesia, despite preloading with 1.5 litres of crystalloid fluids.

Diazoxide. A rapid intravenous injection of a bolus of diazoxide causes maternal tachycardia and hypotension and a reduction in uterine artery blood flow. A slower infusion of the drug causes minimal cardiovascular changes and uterine artery blood flow is unaltered (Caritis et al, 1976).

GASTROINTESTINAL EFFECTS OF DRUGS USED IN LABOUR

It is widely accepted that gastric emptying times are prolonged in labour and it is probable that this is due in large measure to the administration of narcotic analgesics which reduce gastric motility and promote contraction of the pyloric sphincter. The administration of pethidine during labour increases gastric emptying time to at least 5 hours in 70% of women (LaSalvia and Steffen, 1950). Metoclopramide is capable of accelerating gastric emptying in early labour but this effect does not develop for 20 minutes after intramuscular injection (Howard and Sharp, 1973). Metoclopramide is ineffective later in labour in patients who have received narcotic analgesics (Nimmo et al, 1975). Murphy and others (1984) found that metoclopramide could sometimes be effective depending upon the time interval between the administration of metoclopramide and pethidine. Nimmo and his colleagues have confirmed that pethidine and heroin markedly delay gastric emptying by measuring the rate of absorption of paracetamol from the gut. Naloxone may prevent the delayed gastric emptying if given along with the narcotic analgesic (Wilson, 1978) but a reduction in pain relief is then likely (Girvan et al, 1976). Gastric emptying times were normal in patients in labour who had not received a narcotic analgesic, and in those who received epidural analgesia. When naloxone 1.2 mg was given intravenously after prior administration of pethidine in labour, gastric emptying was accelerated (Frame et al, 1984).

Nausea and vomiting are very common when narcotic analgesics are administered during labour. This central effect can be anticipated in up to 50% of patients given morphine or pethidine but has been found to be substantially less common after pentazocine (Mowat and Garrey, 1970; Moore and Ball, 1974). Phenothiazines, cyclizine and droperidol are helpful in preventing drug-induced nausea and vomiting and Cyclimorph (a combination of cyclizine and morphine) may be effective.

Drugs given during labour and in anaesthesia can affect the tone of the gastro-oesophageal sphincter and so alter the propensity to regurgitation. The subject has been reviewed by Hey (1978) and it is probable that narcotic analgesics, intravenous atropine and glycopyrrolate lower the sphincter tone and predispose to regurgitation (Brock-Utne et al, 1976; Hey et al, 1983). In non-pregnant subjects this action can be reversed by metoclopramide but the action of metoclopramide as a promoter of hypertonicity of the gastro-oesophageal sphincter seems less powerful in pregnancy.

Ergometrine given by intravenous injection to the conscious patient quite frequently induces retching or vomiting and this action is especially common in patients receiving epidural analgesia, even in the absence of hypotension (Moodie and Moir, 1976). A sudden, severe hypotensive episode may cause nausea or vomiting. Following on general anaesthesia for evacuation of the uterus in association with spontaneous abortion, the incidence of vomiting was uninfluenced by the administration of ergometrine or oxytocin (Deeby and Hughes, 1984). It should be remembered that nausea and vomiting are common in labour and the cause may not be apparent. The patient is not always seriously disturbed by a transient episode of sickness and treatment may be unnecessary.

DRUGS AND RESPIRATION

In most circumstances the respiratory-depressant effects of narcotic analgesics on the mother are countered by the stimulant effect of painful uterine contractions. There is usually an overall increase in minute volume during labour in women who receive pethidine, and Pearson and Davies (1973) observed a progressive decline in maternal $P_a\mathrm{CO}_2$ in women who received pethidine.

Hyperventilation is confined mainly to the period when painful contractions are present and in some women hypoventilation may occur between contractions. Continuous measurements of $P\mathrm{O}_2$ in the subcutaneous tissues have indicated that the $P\mathrm{O}_2$ usually increases in association with the hyperventilation at the time of the painful contractions. In some patients the subcutaneous $P\mathrm{O}_2$ fell to low levels between the contractions and at this time alterations in the fetal heart rate were sometimes observed (Huch et al, 1974). The patients in this series had received pethidine or a pethidine–levallorphan mixture.

That pain is the major cause of hyperventilation in labour is confirmed by the more normal ventilation seen when epidural analgesia is used (Pearson and Davies, 1973). The maternal $P_a\text{co}_2$ reflects the severity of pain and the adequacy of pain relief in labour and this is confirmation of the ineffectiveness of pethidine as an obstetric analgesic.

DRUGS AND THE LIVER

Most aspects of liver function are not altered during pregnancy, as far as can be measured by standard tests of liver function. The metabolism of pethidine and promazine is modified in pregnancy and may be incomplete. This is also the case in women taking oral contraceptives and is therefore presumed to be due to the hormonal effects of pregnancy and 'the pill' (Crawford and Rudofsky, 1966). It seems probable that the metabolism of other drugs may be modified during pregnancy.

The alterations in the plasma proteins which increase the drug-binding capacity of the plasma and the reduction in the plasma cholinesterase level in pregnancy are probably reflections of modifications in liver function. They are discussed in chapter 2.

Enflurane and probably halothane do not cause abnormal hepatic function when used in low concentrations for caesarean section in normal mothers and in mothers with severe pre-eclampsia (Crowhurst and Rosen, 1984).

CARDIOVASCULAR EFFECTS OF DRUGS USED IN LABOUR

Intramuscular injections of normal doses of analgesics, sedatives and tranquillizers rarely produce cardiovascular effects of clinical importance. Rapid intravenous injections of these agents may cause hypotension. Hypotension, if it occurs, is often postural and may be precipitated by the assumption of an upright posture or by caval occlusion in the supine position.

The sometimes considerable cardiovascular effects of intravenous injections of oxytocin and ergometrine have been considered earlier in this chapter. In summary, both drugs increase the central venous pressure and ergometrine may increase the arterial pressure whereas oxytocin briefly lowers the arterial pressure in the supine patient.

Sedatives and narcotic analgesics are often given in the hope of lowering the blood pressure in patients with pre-eclampsia. A useful hypotensive effect is seldom achieved. Effective doses of narcotic analgesics may reduce the rises in blood pressure which accompany painful contractions. Chlormethiazole is currently quite widely used in the UK as a sedative and anticonvulsant in pre-eclampsia. This drug has no hypotensive action in normal doses and the cardiac output is not reduced because any reduction in stroke volume is cancelled out by an increase in heart rate (Wilson et al, 1969).

The β-mimetic agents such as ritodrine and salbutamol can cause extreme tachycardia when given by intravenous infusion for the attempted suppression of premature labour. Pulmonary oedema is thought to result from the concomitant administration of corticosteroids. Deaths have occurred and the risks of anaesthesia are grave in these circumstances. Propranolol will reduce a dangerous maternal tachycardia but may harm the fetus. β-Mimetics should not be given to women with existing heart disease and the heart rate should not exceed 140 beats/min.

REFERENCES

Abboud, T.K., Shnider, S.M., Wright, R. et al (1981) Enflurane analgesia in obstetrics. *Anesth. Analg. curr. Res.*, **60**, 133.

Abboud, T.K., Khoo, S.S., Miller, F., Doan, T. and Hendricksen, E.H. (1982) Maternal, fetal and neonatal responses after epidural anesthesia with bupivacaine, 2-chloroprocaine and lidocaine. *Anesth. Analg. curr. Res.*, **61**, 638.

Abboud, T.K., Afrasiab, A., Sarkis, F. et al (1984a) Continuous infusion epidural anesthesia in parturients receiving bupivacaine, chloroprocaine or lidocaine. Maternal, fetal and neonatal effects. *Anesth. Analg. curr. Res.*, **63**, 421.

Abboud, T.K., David, S., Ngappala, S. et al (1984b) Maternal, fetal and neonatal effects of lidocaine with and without epinephrine for epidural anesthesia in obstetrics. *Anesth. Analg. curr. Res.*, **63**, 974.

Abdul-Karim, J.W. and Rizk, P.T. (1970) Effects of oxytocin on renal hemodynamics, water and electrolyte excretion. *Obstetl. gynec. Survey*, **25**, 805.

Abouleish, E. (1976) Postpartum hypertension and convulsion after oxytoxic drugs. *Anesth. Analg. curr. Res.*, **55**, 813.

Adamsons, K. and Joelsson, I. (1966) Effect of pharmacologic agents upon the fetus and newborn. *Am. J. Obstet. Gynec.*, **96**, 437.

Aitkenhead, A.R. (1981) Editorial. Do barbiturates protect the brain? *Br. J. Anaesth.*, **53**, 1011.

Albright, G.A. (1979) Cardiac arrest following regional anesthesia with etidocaine or bupivacaine. *Anesthesiology*, **51**, 285.

Alfonsi, P.L. and Massi, G.B. (1963) Effeti degli anestetici sulla contrattilita uterina. *Riv. Ostet. Ginec.*, **18**, 37.

Alvarez, H. and Caldeyro-Barcia, R. (1954) The normal and abnormal contractile waves of the uterus during labour. *Gynaecologia*, **138**, 190.

American Academy of Pediatrics (1979) Anticonvulsants and pregnancy. *Pediatrics*, **63**, 331.

American Society of Anesthesiologists (1974) Report of an ad hoc committee on the effect of trace anesthetics on the health of operating room personnel. Occupational disease among operating room personnel: a national study. *Anesthesiology*, **41**, 321.

Ances, I.G. (1972) Observations on the level of blood oxytocinase throughout the course of labor and delivery. *Am. J. Obstet. Gynec.*, **113**, 291.

Andersen, T.W., DePadua, C.B., Stenger, V. and Prystowsky, H. (1965) Cardiovascular effects of rapid intravenous injection of synthetic oxytocin during elective cesarean section. *Clin. Pharmac. Ther.*, **6**, 345.

Anderson, N.B. (1968) The teratogenicity of cyclopropane in the chicken. *Anesthesiology*, **29**, 113.

Apgar, V., Holaday, D.A., James, L.S., Prince, C.E. and Weisbrot, I.M. (1957) Comparison of regional and general anesthesia in obstetrics with special reference to transmission of cyclopropane across the placenta. *J. Am. med. Ass.*, **165**, 2155.

Arias, F. (1978) Intrauterine resuscitation with terbutaline: a method for the management of acute intrapartum fetal distress. *Am. J. Obstet. Gynec.*, **130**, 39.

Ashton, C.H. (1985) Editorial. Benzodiazepine overdose: are specific antagonists useful? *Br. med J.*, **290**, 805.

Askrog, V.F. (1970) Teratogenic effects of volatile anaesthetics. *3rd Europ. Anaesthesiol. Conf.*, **13**, 1.

Babaknia, A. and Niebyl, J.R. (1978) Effect of magnesium sulfate on fetal heart-rate baseline variability. *Obstet. Gynec.*, **51**, 28.

Baillie, T.W. (1963) Vasopressor activity of ergometrine maleate in anaesthetised parturient women. *Br. med. J.*, **i**, 585.

Baillie, T.W. (1969) Influence of ergometrine on the initiation of the cardiac impulse. *J. Obstet. Gynaec. Br. Commonw.*, **76**, 34.

Baillie, P., Dawes, G.S., Merlet, C.L. and Richards, R. (1971) Maternal hyperventilation and foetal hypocapnia in the sheep. *J. Physiol., Lond.*, **218**, 635.

Baraka, A. (1970) Correlation between maternal and foetal Po_2 and Pco_2 during Caesarean section. *Br. J. Anaesth.*, **42**, 434.

Baraka, A., Haroun, S., Bassili, M. and Abu-Haider, G. (1975) Response of the newborn to succinylcholine injections to homozygotic atypical mothers. *Anesthesiology*, **43**, 115.

Barden, T.P. and Stander, R.W. (1968a) Effects of adrenergic blocking agents and catecholamines in human pregnancy. *Am. J. Obstet. Gynec.*, **102**, 226.

Barden, T.P. and Stander, R.W. (1968b) Myometrial and cardiovascular effects of an adrenergic blocking drug in human pregnancy. *Am. J. Obstet. Gynec.*, **101**, 91.

Basford, A.B. and Fink, B.R. (1968) The teratogenicity of halothane in the rat. *Anesthesiology*, **29**, 1167.

Battaglia, F.C. (1970) Placental clearance and fetal oxygenation. *Pediatrics*, **45**, 563.

Beard, R.W. (1962) Response of human foetal heart and maternal circulation to adrenaline and noradrenaline. *Br. med. J.*, **i**, 443.

Beckett, A.H. and Taylor, J.F. (1967) Blood concentrations of pethidine and pentazocine in mother and infant at the time of birth. *J. Pharm. Pharmac.*, **19**, Suppl. 50.

Beckett, A.H., Boyes, R.N. and Parker, J.B.R. (1965) Determination of lignocaine in blood and urine in human subjects undergoing local analgesia procedures. *Anaesthesia*, **20**, 294.

Belfrage, P., Boreus, L.O., Hartwig, P., Irestedt, L. and Raabe, N. (1981) Neonatal depression after obstetrical analgesia with pethidine. *Acta obstet. gynec. scand.*, **60**, 43.

Benson, D.W., Kaufman, J.J. and Koski, W.S. (1976) Theoretic significance of pH dependence of narcotics and narcotic antagonists in clinical anesthesia. *Anesth. Analg. curr. Res.*, **55**, 253.

Biehl, D., Shnider, S.M., Levinson, G. and Callender, K. (1978) Placental transfer of lidocaine. *Anesthesiology*, **48**, 409.

Biehl, D.R., Tweed, A., Cote, J., Wade, J.G. and Sitar, D. (1983) Effect of halothane on cardiac output and regional flow in the fetal lamb in utero. *Anesth. Analg. curr. Res.*, **62**, 489.

Blogg, C.E., Simpson, B.R., Tyers, M.B., Martin, L.E. and Bell, J.A. (1975) Human placental transfer of AH 8165. *Anaesthesia*, **30**, 23.

Boehm, F.H., Woodruff, L.F. and Growdon, J.H. (1975) Effect of lumbar epidural anesthesia on fetal heart rate baseline variability. *Anesth. Analg. curr. Res.*, **54**, 779.

Brackbill, U., Kane, J., Manniello, R.L. and Abramson, D. (1974) Obstetric meperidine usage and assessment of neonatal status. *Anesthesiology*, **40**, 116.

Bradford, E.M.W. and Moir, D.D. (1969) Anaesthesia for caesarean section. *Br. J. Anaesth.*, **41**, 641.

Brazelton, T.B. (1970) Effect of prenatal drugs on behaviour of the neonate. *Am. J. Psychiat.*, **126**, 1261.

Brock-Utne, J.G., Rubin, J., Downing, J.W. et al (1976) The administration of metoclopramide with atropine. *Anaesthesia*, **31**, 1186.

Brodsky, J.B. and Brock-Utne, J.G. (1978) Mixing local anaesthetics. *Br. J. Anaesth.*, **50**, 1269.

Brodsky, J.B., Cohen, E.N., Brown, B.W., Wu, M.L. and Whitcher, C. (1980) Surgery during pregnancy and fetal outcome. *Am. J. Obstet. Gynec.*, **138**, 1165

Bromage, P.R. (1967) Physiology and pharmacology of epidural analgesia. *Anesthesiology*, **28**, 592.

Bromage, P.R., Datta, S. and Dunford, L.A. (1974) Etidocaine: an evaluation in epidural analgesia for obstetrics. *Can. Anaesth. Soc. J.*, **21**, 535.

Brown, W.U., Bell, G.C. and Lurie, A.O. (1975) Newborn blood levels of lidocaine and mepivacaine in the first postnatal day following maternal epidural anesthesia. *Anesthesiology*, **42**, 698.

Brown, W.U., Bell, G.C. and Alper, M.H. (1976) Acidosis, local anesthetics and the newborn. *Obstet. Gynec.*, **48**, 27.

Buley, R.J.R., Downing, J.W., Brock-Utne, J.G. and Cuerden, C. (1977) Right versus left lateral tilt for caesarean section. *Br. J. Anaesth.*, **49**, 1009.

Caldeyro-Barcia, R. (1960) Effect of position changes on the intensity and frequency of uterine contractions during labor. *Am. J. Obstet. Gynec.*, **80**, 284.

Caldeyro-Barcia, R., Alvarez, H. and Poseiro, J.J. (1955) Action of morphine on the contractility of the human uterus. *Archs int. Pharmacodyn. Ther.*, **101**, 171.

Caldeyro-Barcia, R., Poseiro, J.J., Alvarez, H. and Tost, P. (1958) The action of chlorpromazine on uterine contractility and arterial pressure in normal and toxemic pregnant women. *Am. J. Obstet. Gynec.*, **75**, 1088.

Caldwell, J. and Notarianni, L.J. (1978) Disposition of pethidine in childbirth. *Br. J. Anaesth.*, **50**, 307.

Caritis, S., Morishima, H., Stark, R.I. and James, L.S. (1976) The effect of diazoxide on uterine blood flow in pregnant sheep. *Obstet. Gynec.*, **48**, 464.

Caritis, S.N., Edelstone, D.L. and Müller-Heubach, E. (1979) Pharmacologic inhibition of preterm labor. *Am. J. Obstet. Gynec.*, **133**, 557.

Catz, C.S. and Giacoia, G.P. (1972) Drugs and breast milk. *Pediat. Clins. N. Am.*, **19**, 151.

Cibils, L.A., Pose, S.V. and Zuspan, F.P. (1962) Effect of L-norepinephrine infusion on uterine contractility and cardiovascular system. *Am. J. Obstet. Gynec.*, **84**, 307.

Clark, R.B., Jones, G.L., Barclay, D.L., Greifenstein, F.E. and McAninch, P.E. (1975) Maternal and neonatal effects of 1 per cent and 2 per cent mepivacaine for lumbar extradural analgesia. *Br. J. Anaesth.*, **47**, 1283.

Climie, C.R. (1964) The place of continuous lumbar epidural analgesia in the management of abnormally prolonged labour. *Med. J. Aust.*, **2**, 447.

Climie, C.R., McLean, S., Starmer, G.A. and Thomas, J. (1967) Methaemoglobinaemia in mother and foetus following continuous epidural analgesia with prilocaine. *Br. J. Anaesth.*, **39**, 155.

Cohen, E.N., Bellville, J.W. and Brown, B.W. (1971) Anesthesia, pregnancy and miscarriage: a study of operating room nurses and anesthetists. *Anesthesiology*, **35**, 343.

Coleman, A.J. (1967) Absence of harmful effect of maternal hypocarbia in babies delivered at caesarean section. *Lancet*, **i**, 813.

Coleman, A.J. and Downing, J.W. (1975) Enflurane anesthesia for Cesarean section. *Anesthesiology*, **43**, 354.

Corbett, T.H., Cornell, R.G., Endres, J.L. and Lieding, K. (1974) Birth defects among children of nurse anesthetists. *Anesthesiology*, **41**, 341.

Corke, B.C., Datta, S., Ostheimer, G.W. et al (1982) Spinal anaesthesia for Caesarean section. The influence of hypotension on neonatal outcome. *Anaesthesia*, **37**, 658.

Craft, J.B., Epstein, B.S.M. and Coakley, C.S. (1972) Effect of lidocaine with epinephrine versus lidocaine plain on induced labor. *Anesth. Analg. curr. Res.*, **51**, 243.

Crawford, J.S. (1956) Some aspects of obstetric anaesthesia. *Br. J. Anaesth.*, **28**, 146.

Crawford, J.S. (1962) Anaesthesia for caesarean section: proposal for evaluation with analysis of a method. *Br. J. Anaesth.*, **34**, 179.

Crawford, J.S. (1972) *Principles and Practice of Obstetric Anaesthesia*, 3rd edn. Oxford: Blackwell.

Crawford, J.S. and Rudofsky, S. (1965) Placental transmission of pethidine. *Br. J. Anaesth.*, **37**, 929.

Crawford, J.S. and Rudofsky, S. (1966) Some alterations in the pattern of drug metabolism associated with pregnancy, oral contraceptives and the newly-born. *Br. J. Anaesth.*, **38**, 446.

Cree, J.E., Meyer, J. and Hailey, D.M. (1973) Diazepam in labour: its metabolism and effect on the clinical condition and thermogenesis of the newborn. *Br. med. J.*, **iv**, 251.

Crowhurst, J.A. and Rosen, M. (1984) General anaesthesia for Caesarean section in severe pre-eclampsia. Comparison of the renal and hepatic effects of enflurane and halothane. *Br. J. Anaesth.*, **56**, 587.

Cullen, B.F., Margolis, A.J. and Eger, E.I. (1970) The effects of anesthesia and pulmonary ventilation on blood loss during elective therapeutic abortion. *Anesthesiology*, **32**, 108.

Cuthbert, M.F. (1969) Effect on airway resistance of PGE_1 given by aerosol to healthy and asthmatic volunteers. *Br. med. J.*, **iv**, 723.

Dailey, P.A., Fisher, D.M., Shnider, S.M. et al (1984) Pharmacokinetics, placental transfer and neonatal effects of vecuronium and pancuronium during cesarean section. *Anesthesiology*, **60**, 569.

Datta, S., Brown, W.U., Ostheimer, G.W. et al (1981a) Epidural anesthesia for cesarean section in diabetic parturients: maternal and neonatal acid–base status and bupivacaine concentration. *Anesth. Analg. curr. Res.*, **60**, 574.

Datta, S., Ostheimer, G.W., Naulty, J.S., Knapp, R.M. and Weiss, J.B. (1981b) General anesthesia for cesarean section. Effects of halothane on maternal and fetal acid–base and lactic acid concentration. *Anesthesiology*, **55**, A309.

Dawes, G. (1973) The distribution and action of drugs on the foetus in utero. *Br. J. Anaesth.*, **45**, Suppl. 766.

Davies, J.M., Carmichael, D. and Dymond, C. (1983) Plasma cholinesterase and trophoblastic disease. *Anaesthesia*, **38**, 1071.

Davis, J.E. (1977) Question and answer. *Anesth. Analg. curr. Res.*, **56**, 744.

Day, D.M. (1978) Nitrous oxide transfer across the placenta and condition of the newborn at delivery. *Br. J. Obstet. Gynaec*, **85**, 299.

Decanq, H.E., Bosco, J.R. and Townsend, E.H. (1965) Chlordiazepoxide in labor. *J. Pediat.*, **67**, 836.

Deeby, D. and Hughes, J.O.M. (1984) Oxytocic drug and anaesthesia. *Anaesthesia*, **39**, 764.

Demetriou, M., Depoix, J.P., Diakite, B., Fromentin, M. and Duvaldestin, P. (1982) Placental transfer of ORG NC 45 in women undergoing Caesarean section. *Br. J. Anaesth.*, **54**, 643.

Department of Health and Social Security (1976) *Pollution of Operating Departments by Anaesthetic Gases.* H.C. (76)38. London: HMSO.

De Voe, S.J., De Voe, K., Rigsby, W.C. and McDaniels, B.A. (1969) Effect of meperidine on uterine contractility. *Am. J. Obstet. Gynec.*, **105**, 1004.

Doenicke, A., Krumey, I., Kugler, J. and Klempa, J. (1968) Experimental studies of the breakdown of Epontol: determination of propanidid in human serum. *Br. J. Anaesth.*, **40**, 415.

Dolan, W.M., Eger, E.I., II and Margolis, A.J. (1972) Forane increases bleeding in therapeutic suction abortion. *Anesthesiology*, **36**, 96.

Downing, J.W., Mahomedy, M.C., Coleman, A.J., Mahomedy, Y.H. and Jeal, D.E. (1974) Anaesthetic induction for caesarean section. Althesin versus thiopentone. *Anaesthesia*, **29**, 689.

Downing, J.W., Mahomedy, N.C., Jeal, D.E. and Allen, P.J. (1976) Anaesthesia for Caesarean section with ketamine. *Anaesthesia*, **31**, 883.

Downing, J.W., Buley, R.J.R., Brock-Utne, J.G. and Houlton, P.C. (1979) Etomidate for induction of anaesthesia at Caesarean section: comparison with thiopentone. *Br. J. Anaesth.*, **51**, 135.

Drabkova, J., Crul, J.F. and Van de Kleijn, E. (1973) Placental transfer of ^{14}C labelled succinylcholine in near-term Macaca Mulatta monkeys. *Br. J. Anaesth.*, **45**, 1087.

D'Souza, S.W., Black, P., McFarlane, T. and Richards, B. (1979) The effect of oxytocin in induced labour on neonatal jaundice. *Br. J. Obstet. Gynaec.*, **86**, 133.

Duffus, G.M., Tunstall, M.E., Condie, R.G. and MacGillivray, I. (1969) Chlormethiazole in the prevention of eclampsia and the reduction of perinatal mortality. *J. Obstet. Gynaec. Br. Commonw.*, **76**, 645.

Duncan, S.L., Ginsburg, J. and Morris, N.F. (1969) Comparison of pentazocine and pethidine in normal labor. *Am. J. Obstet. Gynec.*, **105**, 197.

Dutton, D.A., Moir, D.D., Howie, H.B., Thorburn, J. and Watson, R. (1984) Choice of local anaesthetic drug for extradural Caesarean section. *Br. J. Anaesth.*, **56**, 1361.

Ebner, H., Barcohana, J. and Bartoshuk, A.K. (1960) Influence of post-spinal hypotension on the fetal electrocardiogram. *Am. J. Obstet. Gynec.*, **80**, 569.

Einer-Jensen, N. and Juhl, B. (1974) Uterine blood flow in dogs during various depths of halothane anaesthesia. *Acta anaesth. scand.*, **18**, 123.

Elliott, H.R., Abdulla, U. and Hayes, P.J. (1978) Pulmonary oedema associated with ritodrine infusion and betamethasone administration in premature labour. *Br. med. J.*, **ii**, 799.

Embrey, M.P. (1958) The effect of acetylcholine on the intact human uterus. *J. Obstet. Gynaec. Br. Emp.*, **65**, 531.

Embrey, M.P. (1961) Simultaneous intramuscular injection of oxytocin and ergometrine: a tocographic study. *Br. med. J.*, **i**, 1737.

Emmons, P.R., Hampton, J.R., Harrison, M.J.G. and Mitchell, J.R.A. (1967) Effect of prostaglandin E_1 on platelet behaviour in vitro and in vivo. *Br. med. J.*, **ii**, 468.

Eng, M., Bonica, J.J., Akamatsu, T.J. et al (1975a) Maternal and fetal responses to halothane in pregnant monkeys. *Acta anaesth. scand.*, **19**, 154.

Eng, M., Bonica, J.J., Akamatsu, T.J., Berges, P.U. and Ueland, K. (1975b) Respiratory depression in newborn monkeys at Caesarean section following ketamine administration. *Br. J. Anaesth.*, **47**, 917.

Epstein, B.S. and Coakley, C.S. (1967) Passage of lidocaine and prilocaine across the placenta. *Anesthesiology*, **28**, 246.

Erkkola, R. and Kanto, J. (1972) Diazepam and breast feeding. *Lancet*, **i**, 1235.

Eskes, T.K.A.B., Stolte, L., Seelen, J., Moed, H.D. and Vogelsang, C. (1965) Epinephrine derivatives and the activity of the human uterus. *Am. J. Obstet. Gynec.*, **92**, 871.

Evans, R.T., Macdonald, R. and Robinson, A. (1980) Suxamethonium apnoea associated with plasmapheresis. *Anaesthesia*, **35**, 198.

Fealey, J. (1958) Placental transmission of pentobarbital sodium. *Obstet. Gynec.*, **11**, 342.

Filler, W.W. and Filler, N.W. (1966) Effect of a potent non-narcotic analgesic agent (pentazocine) on uterine contractility and fetal heart rate. *Obstet. Gynec.*, **28**, 224.

Fink, B.R., Shepard, T.H. and Blandau, R.J. (1967) Teratogenic activity of nitrous oxide. *Nature, Lond.*, **214**, 146.

Finster, M., Mark, L.C., Morishima, H.O. et al (1966) Plasma thiopental concentrations in the newborn following delivery under thiopental-nitrous oxide anesthesia. *Am. J. Obstet. Gynec.*, **95**, 621.

Finster, M., Morishima, H.O., Mark, L.C. et al (1972) Tissue thiopental concentrations in the fetus and newborn. *Anesthesiology*, **36**, 155.

Fiserova-Bergerova, V. (1976) Fluoride in bone of rats anesthetized during gestation with enflurane or methoxyflurane. *Anesthesiology*, **45**, 483.

Fishburne, J.I., Brenner, W.E., Braaksma, J.T. et al (1972) Cardiovascular and respiratory responses to intravenous infusion of prostaglandin $F_2\alpha$ in the pregnant woman. *Am. J. Obstet. Gynec.*, **114**, 765.

Flynn, P.J., Frank, M. and Hughes, R. (1984) Use of atracurium in Caesarean section. *Br. J. Anaesth.*, **56**, 599.

Fox, G.S., Houle, B.L., Desjardines, P.D. and Mercier, G. (1971) Intrauterine fetal lidocaine concentrations during continuous epidural anesthesia. *Am. J. Obstet. Gynec.*, **110**, 896.

Frame, W.I., Allison, R.H., Moir, D.D. and Nimmo, W.S. (1984) Effect of naloxone on gastric emptying during labour. *Br. J. Anaesth.*, **56**, 263.

Friedman, E.A., Niswander, K.R. and Sachtleben, M.R. (1969) Effect of diazepam on labor. *Obstet. Gynec.*, **34**, 82.

Friedman, L., Lewis, P.J., Clifton, P. and Bulpitt, C. (1978) Factors influencing the incidence of neonatal jaundice. *Br. med. J.*, **i**, 1235.

Fuchs, A.R. (1966) The inhibitory effect of ethanol on the release of oxytocin during parturition in the rabbit. *J. Endocrin.*, **35**, 125.

Fuchs, F., Fuchs, A.R., Poblete, V.F. and Risk, A. (1967) Effect of alcohol on threatened premature labor. *Am. J. Obstet. Gynec.*, **99**, 627.

Galbert, M.W. and Gardner, A.E. (1972) Use of halothane in a balanced technic for cesarean section. *Anesth. Analg. curr. Res.*, **51**, 701.

Gamble, J.A.S., Moore, J., Lamki, H. and Howard, P.J. (1977) A study of plasma diazepam levels in mother and infant. *Br. J. Obstet. Gynaec.*, **84**, 588.

Geber, W.F. and Schramm, L.C. (1975) Congenital malformation of the central nervous system produced by narcotic analgesics in the hamster. *Am. J. Obstet. Gynec.*, **123**, 705.

Geeronckx, K., Vanderick, G., Van Steenberge, A.L., Bouche, R. and De Muelder, E. (1974) Bupivacaine 0.125% in epidural block analgesia during childbirth: maternal and foetal plasma concentrations. *Br. J. Anaesth.*, **46**, 937.

Ghoneim, M.M. and Pandya, H. (1974) Plasma protein binding of bupivacaine and its interaction with other drugs in man. *Br. J. Anaesth.*, **46**, 435.

Gibbens, G.L.D. and Chard, T. (1976) Observations on maternal oxytocin release during normal labor, and the effect of intravenous alcohol administration. *Am. J. Obstet. Gynec.*, **126**, 243.

Gibbs, C.P., Munson, E.S. and Tham, K. (1975) Anesthetic solubility coefficients for maternal and fetal blood. *Anesthesiology*, **43**, 100

Girvan, G.B., Moore, J. and Dundee, J.W. (1976) Pethidine compared with pethidine–naloxone administered during labour. *Br. J. Anaesth.*, **48**, 563.

Goodfriend, M.J., Shey, I.A. and Klein, M.D. (1956) Effects of maternal narcotic addiction on the newborn. *Am. J. Obstet. Gynec.*, **71**, 29.

Green, C.J., Monk, S.J., Knight, J.F. et al (1982) Chronic exposure of rats to enflurane 200 ppm: no evidence of toxicity or teratogenicity. *Br. J. Anaesth.*, **54**, 1097.

Green, K.W., Kay, T.C., Coen, R. and Rasnik, R. (1983) The effects of maternally administered magnesium sulfate on the infant. *Am. J. Obstet. Gynec.*, **146**, 29.

Greenhalf, J.O. and Evans, D.J.E. (1970) Effect of ergometrine on the central venous pressure in the third stage of labour. *J. Obstet. Gynaec. Br. Commonw.*, **77**, 1066.

Gregory, G.A., Wade, J.G., Beihl, D.R., Ong, B.Y. and Sitar, D.Y. (1983) Fetal anesthetic requirement (MAC) for halothane. *Anesth. Analg. curr. Res.*, **62**, 9.

Greiss, F.C. (1963) The uterine vascular bed. Effect of adrenergic stimulation. *Obstet. Gynec.*, **21**, 295.

Greiss, F.C. and Crandell, L. (1965) Therapy for hypotension induced by spinal anesthesia during pregnancy. *J. Am. med. Ass.*, **191**, 793.

Greiss, F.C. and Van Wilkes, D. (1964) Effects of sympathomimetic drugs and angiotensin on the uterine vascular bed. *Obstet. Gynec.*, **23**, 925.

Greiss, F.C., Anderson, S.G. and King, L.C. (1974) Uterine vascular bed: the effects of acute hyperoxia. *Am. J. Obstet. Gynec.*, **118**, 542.

Greiss, F.C., Still, J.G. and Anderson, S.G. (1976) Effects of local anesthetic agents on the uterine vasculature and myometrium. *Am. J. Obstet. Gynec.*, **124**, 889.

Gunther, R.E. and Bauman, J. (1969) Obstetrical caudal anesthesia. *Anesthesiology*, **31**, 5.

Gurtner, G. and Burns, B. (1975) Physiological evidence consistent with the presence of a specific O_2 carrier in the placenta. *J. appl. Physiol.*, **39**, 728.

Hall, D.G., McGaughey, H.S., Corey, E.L. and Thornton, W.N. (1959) The effects of magnesium therapy on the duration of labor. *Am. J. Obstet. Gynec.*, **78**, 27.

Halsey, M.J., Green, C.J., Monk, S.J. et al (1981) Maternal and paternal chronic exposure to enflurane and halothane: fetal and histological changes in the rat. *Br. J. Anaesth.*, **53**, 203.

Hawkins, D.F. (1964) Agents acting on the uterus. In *Evaluation of Drug Activities: Pharmacometrics*, ed. Laurence, D.R. and Bacharach, A.L., vol. 2, p. 665. London and New York: Academic Press.

Hawkins, D.F. and Nixon, W.C.W. (1957) Blood electrolytes in prolonged labour. *J. Obstet. Gynaec. Br. Emp.*, **64**, 641.

Healey, T.E.J. (1971) Suxamethonium and intrauterine pressure. *Br. J. Anaesth.*, **43**, 1156.

Heaney, G.A.H. (1974) Pancuronium in maternal and foetal serum. *Br. J. Anaesth.*, **46**, 282.

Hehre, F.W., Hook, W. and Hon, E.H. (1969) Continuous lumbar epidural anesthesia in obstetrics. *Anesth. Analg. curr. Res.*, **48**, 909.

Helliwell, P.J. and Hutton, A.M. (1950) Trichlorethylene anaesthesia. *Anaesthesia*, **5**, 4.

Hellman, L.M. and Fillisti, L.P. (1965) Analysis of the atropine test for placental transfer in gravidas with toxemia and diabetes. *Am. J. Obstet. Gynec.*, **91**, 797.

Hendricks, C.H. and Brenner, W.E. (1970) Cardiovascular effects of oxytocic drugs used post-partum. *Am. J. Obstet. Gynec.*, **108**, 751.

Hendricks, C.H., Cibils, L.A., Pose, S.V. and Ekes, T.K.A.B. (1961) The pharmacological control of excessive uterine activity with isoxuprine. *Am. J. Obstet. Gynec.*, **82**, 1064.

Hey, V.M.F. (1978) Gastro-oesophageal reflux in pregnancy: a review article. *J. int. med. Res.*, **6**, Suppl. 1, 18.

Hey, V.M.F., Phillips, K. and Woods, I. (1983) Pethidine, atropine, metoclopramide and the lower oesophageal sphincter. *Anaesthesia*, **38**, 650

Ho, P.C., Stephens, I.D. and Triggs, E.J. (1981) Caesarean section and placental transfer of alcuronium. *Anaesthesia and Intensive Care*, **9**, 113.

Hogg, M.I.J., Wiener, P.C., Rosen, M. and Mapleson, W.W. (1977) Urinary excretion and metabolism of pethidine and norpethidine in the newborn. *Br. J. Anaesth.*, **49**, 891.

Holdcroft, A., Robinson, M.J., Gordon, H. and Whitman, J.G. (1974) Comparison of effects of two induction doses of methohexitone on infants delivered by elective Caesarean section. *Br. med. J.*, **ii**, 472.

Hollmen, A.I., Jouppila, R., Koivisto, M. et al (1978) Neurologic activity of infants following anesthesia for cesarean section. *Anesthesiology*, **48**, 350.

Holtzman, S.D. (1978) Maternal anesthesia and fetal neuropharmacology. *Anesthesiology*, **48**, 235.

Howard, F.A. and Sharp, D.S. (1973) Effect of metoclopramide on gastric emptying during labour. *Br. med. J.*, **i**, 446.

Howe, J.P., McGowen, W.A., Moore, J., McCaughey, W. and Dundee, J.W. (1981) The placental transfer of cimetidine. *Anaesthesia*, **36**, 371.

Huch, A., Huch, R., Lindmark, G. and Rooth, G. (1974) Maternal hypoxaemia after pethidine. *J. Obstet. Gynaec. Br. Commonw.*, **81**, 608.

Huch, A., Huch, R., Schneider, H. and Rooth, G. (1977) Continuous transcutaneous monitoring of fetal oxygen tension during labour. *Br. J. Obstet. Gynaec.*, **84**, Suppl. 1, 1.

Iuppa, J.B., Smith, G.A., Colella, J.J. and Gibson, J.L. (1971) Succinylcholine effect on human myometrial activity. *Obstet. Gynec.*, **37**, 591.

Jago, R.H. (1970) Arthrogryposis following treatment of maternal tetanus with muscle relaxants: a case report. *Archs Dis. Childh.*, **45**, 277.

James, L.S., Morishima, H.O., Daniel, S.S. et al (1972) Mechanism of late deceleration of the fetal heart rate. *Am. J. Obstet. Gynec.*, **113**, 578.

Jawalekar, K.S., Jawalekar, S.R. and Mathur, V.P. (1972) Effect of ketamine on isolated murine myometrial activity. *Anesth. Analg. curr. Res.*, **51**, 685.

Jenkins, V.R., Talbert, W.M. and Dilts, P.V. (1972) Placental transfer of meperidine hydrochloride. *Obstet. Gynec.*, **39**, 254.

John, A.H. (1965) Placental transfer of atropine and the effect on the foetal heart rate. *Br. J. Anaesth.*, **37**, 57.

Johnson, G.T. and Clayton, S.G. (1955) Studies in placental action during prolonged dysfunctional labours using radioactive sodium. *J. Obstet. Gynaec. Br. Emp.*, **62**, 513.

Johnston, J.R., McCaughey, W., Moore, J. and Dundee, J.W. (1982) A field trial of cimetidine as the sole oral antacid in obstetric anaesthesia. *Anaesthesia*, **37**, 33.

Johnstone, M. (1972) The cardiovascular effects of oxytocic drugs. *Br. J. Anaesth.*, **44**, 826.

Jones, D.J., Hodgson, B.J., Stehling, L.C. and Zauder, H.L. (1978) Enflurane and uterine contractability in rabbits. *Anesth. Analg. curr. Res.*, **57**, 160.

Jouppila, P., Jouppila, R., Kaar, K. and Merila, M. (1977) Fetal heart rate patterns and uterine activity after segmental epidural analgesia. *Br. J. Obstet. Gynaec.*, **84**, 481.

Jouppila, R., Jouppila, P., Hollmen, A. and Kuikka, J. (1978a) Effect of segmental extradural analgesia on placental blood flow during normal labour. *Br. J. Anaesth.*, **50**, 563.

Jouppila, R., Jouppila, P., Kuikka, J. and Hollmen, A. (1978b) Placental blood flow during Caesarean section under lumbar extradural analgesia. *Br. J. Anaesth.*, **50**, 275.

Jouppila, P., Kuikka, J., Jouppila, R. and Hollmen, A. (1979) Effect of induction of general anaesthesia for Caesarean section on intervillous blood flow. *Acta. obstet. gynec. scand.*, **58**, 249.

Kane, R.E. (1981) Neurologic deficits following epidural or spinal anesthesia. *Anesth. Analg. curr. Res.*, **60**, 150.

Karim, S.M., Hillier, K., Somers, K. and Trussell, R.R. (1971) The effects of prostaglandins E_2 and $F_{2\alpha}$ administered by different routes on uterine activity and the cardiovascular system in pregnant and non-pregnant women. *J. Obstet. Gynaec. Br. Commonw.*, **78**, 172.

Kariniemi, V. and Ammala, P. (1981) Effects of intramuscular pethidine on fetal heart rate variability during labour. *Br. J. Obstet. Gynaec.*, **88**, 718.

Katz, R.L. and Katz, G.J. (1974) Prostaglandins—basic and clinical considerations. *Anesthesiology*, **40**, 471.

Kenepp, N.B., Shelley, W.C., Gabbe, S.G. et al (1982) Fetal and neonatal hazards of maternal hydration with 5 per cent dextrose before Caesarean section. *Lancet*, **i**, 1150.

Kennedy, R.L., Erenberg, G.A., Robillard, J.E., Merkow, A. and Turner, T. (1979) Effects of changes in maternal–fetal pH on the transplacental equilibrium of bupivacaine. *Anesthesiology*, **51**, 50.

Kivalo, I. and Saarikoski, S. (1977) Placental transmission of atropine at full-term pregnancy. *Br. J. Anaesth.*, **49**, 1017.

Klieff, M.E., James, F.M., Dewan, D.M. and Floyd, H.M. (1984) Neonatal neurobehavioral responses after epidural anesthesia for cesarean section using lidocaine and bupivacaine. *Anesth. Analg. curr. Res.*, **63**, 413.

Knight, R.J. (1977) Labour retarded by β-agonist drugs. A therapeutic problem in emergency anaesthesia. *Anaesthesia*, **32**, 639.

Knill-Jones, R.P., Rodrigues, L.V., Moir, D.D. and Spence, A.A. (1972) Anaesthetic practice and pregnancy: a controlled survey of women anaesthetists in the United Kingdom. *Lancet*, **i**, 1326.

Knill-Jones, R.P., Newman, B.J. and Spence, A.A. (1975) Anaesthetic practice and pregnancy. Controlled survey of male anaesthetists in the United Kingdom. *Lancet*, **ii**, 8070.

Koch, G. and Wandel, H. (1968) Effect of pethidine in the postnatal adjustment of respiration and acid–base balance. *Acta obstet. gynec. scand.*, **47**, 27.

Kosaka, Y., Takahashi, T. and Mark, L.C. (1969) Intravenous thiobarbiturate anesthesia for cesarean section. *Anesthesiology*, **31**, 489.

Kristianson, B., Magno, R. and Wickstrom, I. (1980) Anaesthesia for Caesarean section. VI.

Late effects on the infant of enflurane anaesthesia for Caesarean section. *Acta anaesth. scand.*, **24**, 187.

Kuhnert, B.R., Knapp, D.R., Kuhnert, P.M. and Prochaska, A.L. (1979) Maternal, fetal and neonatal metabolism of lidocaine. *Clin. Pharmac. Ther.*, **26**, 213.

Kuhnert, B.R., Kuhnert, P.M., Prochaska, A.L. and Gross, T.L. (1980a) Plasma levels of 2-chloroprocaine in obstetric patients and their neonates after epidural anesthesia. *Anesthesiology*, **53**, 21.

Kuhnert, B.R., Kuhnert, P.M., Prochaska, A.L. and Sokol, R.J. (1980b) Meperidine distribution in mother, neonate and non-pregnant females. *Clin. Pharmac. Ther.*, **27**, 486.

Kuhnert, P.M., Kuhnert, B.R., Stitts, J.M. and Gross, T.L. (1981) Use of a selected ion monitoring technique to study the disposition of bupivacaine in mother, fetus and neonate following epidural anesthesia for cesarean section. *Anesthesiology*, **55**, 611.

Kullander, S. and Kallen, B. (1976a) A prospective study of drugs in pregnancy. *Acta obstet. gynec. scand.*, **55**, 25.

Kullander, S. and Kallen, B. (1976b) A prospective study of drugs in pregnancy. II. Anti-emetic drugs. *Acta obstet. gynec. scand.*, **55**, 105.

Kumar, D., Zourlas, P.A. and Barnes, A.C. (1965) In vivo effect of amylnitrite on human pregnant uterine contractility. An objective evaluation. *Am. J. Obstet. Gynec.*, **91**, 1066.

Kunstadter, R.H., Klein, R.I., Lundeen, E.C., Witz, W. and Morrison, M. (1958) Narcotic withdrawal symptoms in newborn infants. *J. Am. med. Ass.*, **168**, 1008.

Kupforberg, H.J. and Way, E.L. (1963) Pharmacologic basis for the increased sensitivity of the newborn rat to morphine. *J. Pharmac. exp. Ther.*, **141**, 105.

Kyegombe, D., Franklin, C. and Turner, P. (1973) Drug metabolising enzymes in the human placenta, their induction and repression. *Lancet*, **i**, 405.

Lalka, D., Vicuna, N., Burrow, S.R. et al (1978) Bupivacaine and other local anaesthetics inhibit the hydrolysis of chloroprocaine by human serum. *Anesth. Analg. curr. Res.*, **57**, 534.

Lange, A.P., Westergaard, J.G., Secher, N.J. and Skovgard, I. (1982) Neonatal jaundice after labour induced or stimulated by prostaglandin E_2 or oxytocin. *Lancet*, **i**, 991.

LaSalvia, L.A. and Steffen, E.A. (1950) Delayed gastric emptying time in labor. *Am. J. Obstet. Gynec.*, **59**, 1075.

Latto, I.P. and Waldron, B.A. (1977) Anaesthesia for Caesarean section. *Br. J. Anaesth.*, **49**, 371.

Lawson, J.I. (1958) Decamethonium iodide: a reappraisal. *Br. J. Anaesth.*, **30**, 240.

Levinson, G., Shnider, S.M., Gildea, J.E. and de Lorimer, A.A. (1973) Maternal and fetal cardiovascular and acid–base changes during ketamine anaesthesia in pregnant ewes. *Br. J. Anaesth.*, **45**, 1111.

Levinson, G., Shnider, S.M. de Lorimer, A.A. and Steffenson, J.L. (1974) Effects of maternal hyperventilation on uterine blood flow and fetal oxygenation and acid–base status. *Anesthesiology*, **40**, 340.

Levy, C.J. and Owen, G. (1964) Thiopentone transmission through the placenta. *Anaesthesia*, **19**, 511.

Liggins, G.C. and Vaughan, G.S. (1973) Intravenous infusion of salbutamol in the management of premature labour. *J. Obstet. Gynaec. Br. Commonw*, **80**, 29.

Liston, W.A., Adjepon-Yamoah, K.K. and Scott, D.B. (1973) Foetal and maternal lignocaine levels after paracervical block. *Br. J. Anaesth.*, **45**, 750.

Little, B., Chang, T., Chucot, L. et al (1972) Study of ketamine as an obstetric anesthetic agent. *Am. J. Obstet. Gynec.*, **113**, 247.

Lucas, W.E., Kirschbaum, T.H. and Assali, N.S. (1965) Effects of autonomic blockade with spinal anesthesia on uterine and fetal hemodynamics and oxygen consumption in sheep. *Biologia Neonat.*, **10**, 166.

Lunell, N.O., Joelsson, I., Bjorkman, U., Lamb, P and Persson, B. (1976) The use of salbutamol in obstetrics. *Acta obstet. gynec. scand.*, **55**, 333.

Lurie, A.O. and Weiss, J.B. (1970) Blood concentration of mepivacaine and lidocaine in mother and baby after epidural anesthesia. *Am. J. Obstet. Gynec.*, **106**, 850.

Mahomedy, M.C., Downing, J.W., Jeal, D.E. and Coleman, A.J. (1976) Anaesthetic induction for Caesarean section with propanidid. *Anaesthesia*, **31**, 205.

Mandelli, M., Morselli, P.L., Nordio, S. et al (1975) Placental transfer of diazepam and its disposition in the newborn. *Clin. Pharmac. Ther.*, **17**, 564.

Mankowitz, E., Brock-Utne, J.G. and Downing, J.W. (1981) Nitrous oxide elimination by the newborn. *Anaesthesia*, **36**, 1014.

Mantell, C.D. and Liggins, G.C. (1970) The effect of ethanol on the myometrial response to oxytocin in women at term. *J. Obstet. Gynaec. Br. Commonw.*, **77**, 976.

Mark, R.F. (1961) Dependence of uterine muscle contractions on pH, with reference to prolonged labour. *J. Obstet. Gynaec. Br. Commonw.*, **68**, 584.

Mark, P.M. and Hamel, J. (1968) Librium for patients in labor. *Obstet. Gynec.*, **32**, 188.

Marshall, J.R. (1964) Human antepartum placental passage of methohexital sodium. *Obstet. Gynec.*, **23**, 589.

Marx, G.F. and Mateo, C.V. (1971) Effects of different oxygen concentrations during general anaesthesia for caesarean section. *Can. Anaesth. Soc. J.*, **18**, 587.

Marx, G.F. and Orkin, L.R. (1969) *Physiology of Obstetric Anesthesia*, p. 104. Springfield, Ill.: Charles C. Thomas.

Marx, G.F., Cosmi, E.V. and Wollman, S.B. (1969) Biochemical status and clinical condition of mother and infant at cesarean section. *Anesth. Analg. curr. Res.*, **48**, 986.

Marx, G.F., Joshi, C.W. and Orkin, L.R. (1970) Placental transmission of nitrous oxide. *Anesthesiology*, **32**, 429.

Marx, G.F., Hwang, H.S. and Chandra, P. (1979) Postpartum uterine pressures with different doses of ketamine. *Anesthesiology*, **50**, 163.

Matadial, L. and Cibils, L.A. (1976) Effects of epidural anesthesia on uterine activity and blood pressure. *Am. J. Obstet. Gynec.*, **125**

Mather, L.E., Long, G.J. and Thomas, J. (1971) Binding of bupivacaine to maternal and foetal plasma proteins. *J. Pharmac.*, **23**, 359.

Mathi, A.A., Hidqvist, P., Holmgren, A. and Svenborg, N. (1973) Bronchial hyperactivity to prostaglandin F_2 and histamine in patients with asthma. *Br. med. J.*, **i**, 193.

Matthews, A.E. (1963) Double-blind trials of promazine in labour. *Br. med. J.*, **ii**, 423.

McAllister, C.B. (1980) Placental transfer and neonatal effects of diazepam administered to women just before delivery. *Br. J. Anaesth.*, **52**, 419.

McBride, R.J., Dundee, J.W., Moore, J., Toner, W. and Howard, P. (1979) A study of the plasma concentrations of lorazepam in mothers and neonates. *Br. J. Anaesth.*, **51**, 971.

McCarthy, G.T., O'Connell, B. and Robinson, A.E. (1973) Blood levels of diazepam in infants of two mothers given large doses of diazepam during labour. *J. Obstet. Gynaec. Br. Commonw.*, **80**, 349.

McCaul, K. and Robinson, G.D. (1962) Suxamethonium 'extension' by tetrahydroaminacrine. *Br. J. Anaesth.*, **34**, 536.

McGaughey, H.S., Jr., Corey, E.L., Eastwood, D. and Thornton, W.N. (1962) Effect of synthetic anesthetics on the spontaneous motility of human uterine muscle in vitro. *Obstet. Gynec.*, **19**, 233.

McKechnie, R.B. and Converse, J.G. (1955) Placental transmission of thiopental. *Am. J. Obstet. Gynec.*, **70**, 639.

Meschia, G. (1978) Evolution of thinking in fetal respiratory physiology. *Am. J. Obstet. Gynec.*, **132**, 806.

Miller, J.W. (1967) Adrenergic receptors in the myometrium. *Ann. N.Y. Acad. Sci.*, **139**, 788.

Miller, J.R., Stoelting, V.K., Stander, P.W. and Watring, W. (1966) In vitro and in vivo responses of the uterus to halothane anesthesia. *Anesth. Analg. curr. Res.*, **45**, 583.

Miller, F.C., Petrie, R.H., Arce, J.J., Paul, R.H. and Hon, E.H. (1974) Hyperventilation during labor. *Am. J. Obstet. Gynec.*, **120**, 489.

Milne, M.K. and Murray Lawson, J.I. (1973) Epidural analgesia for caesarean section. *Br. J. Anaesth.*, **45**, 1206.

Moir, D.D. (1970) Anaesthesia for caesarean section: an evaluation of a method using low concentrations of halothane and 50 per cent oxygen. *Br. J. Anaesth.*, **42**, 136.

Moir, D.D. and Amoa, A.B. (1979) Ergometrine or oxytocin? *Br. J. Anaesth.*, **51**, 113.

Moir, D.D. and Wallace, G. (1967) Blood loss at forceps delivery. *J. Obstet. Gynaec. Br. Commonw.*, **74**, 424.

Moir, D.D. and Willocks, J. (1967) Management of inco-ordinate uterine action under continuous epidural analgesia. *Br. med. J.*, **iii**, 396.

Moir, D.D. and Willocks, J. (1968) Epidural analgesia in British obstetrics. *Br. J. Anaesth.*, **40**, 129.

Moodie, J.E. and Moir, D.D. (1976) Ergometrine, oxytocin, and epidural analgesia. *Br. J. Anaesth.*, **48**, 571.

Moore, D.C. (1964) *Anesthetic Techniques for Obstetrical Anesthesia and Analgesia*, p. 37. Springfield, Ill.: Charles C. Thomas.

Moore, J. and Ball, H.G. (1974) A sequential study of intravenous analgesic treatment during labour. *Br. J. Anaesth.*, **46**, 365.

Moore, J., McNabb, T.G. and Dundee, J.W. (1971) Preliminary report on ketamine in obstetrics. *Br. J. Anaesth.*, **43**, 779.

Moore, J., McNabb, T.G. and Glynn, J.P. (1973) The placental transfer of pentazocine and pethidine. *Br. J. Anaesth.*, **45**, Suppl. 798.

Morgan, C.D., Sandler, M. and Panigel, M. (1972) Placental transfer of catecholamines in vitro and in vivo. *Am. J. Obstet. Gynec.*, **112**, 1068.

Morgan, D.J., Blackman, G.L., Paull, J.D. and Wolf, L.J. (1981) Pharmacokinetics and plasma binding of thiopental. Studies at cesarean section. *Anesthesiology*, **54**, 474.

Morishima, H.O., Moya, F., Bossers, A. and Thorndike, V. (1963) Adverse effects on the newborn of severe maternal hyperventilation. *Anesthesiology*, **24**, 135.

Morishima, H.O., Daniel, S.S., Finster, M., Poppers, P.J. and James, L.S. (1966) Transmission of mepivacaine hydrochloride (Carbocaine) across the human placenta. *Anesthesiology*, **27**, 147.

Morrison, J.C., Todd, E.L., Lipshitz, J. et al (1982) Meperidine and normeperidine levels following meperidine administration during labor. I. Mother. *Am. J. Obstet. Gynec.*, **59**, 359.

Motoyama, E.K., Rivard, G., Acheson, F. and Cook, C.D. (1966) Adverse effect of maternal hyperventilation on the foetus. *Lancet*, **i**, 286.

Mountain, K.R., Nirsh, J. and Gallus, A.S. (1970) Neonatal coagulation defect due to anticonvulsant drug treatment in pregnancy. *Lancet*, **i**, 265.

Mowat, J. and Garrey, M.M. (1970) Comparison of pentazocine and pethidine in labour. *Br. med. J.*, **ii**, 757.

Moya, F. and Kvisselgaard, N. (1961) Placental transmission of succinylcholine. *Anesthesiology*, **22**, 1.

Moya, F., Morishima, A., Shnider, S.M. and James, L.S. (1965) Influence of maternal hyperventilation on the newborn infant. *Am. J. Obstet. Gynec.*, **91**, 76.

Munson, E.S. and Embro, W.J. (1977) Enflurane, isoflurane and halothane and isolated human uterine muscle. *Anesthesiology*, **46**, 11.

Munson, E.S., Maier, W.R. and Caton, D. (1969) Effects of halothane, cyclopropane and nitrous oxide on isolated human uterine muscle. *J. Obstet. Gynaec. Br. Commonw.*, **76**, 27.

Murphy, D.F., Nally, B., Gardiner, J. and Unwin, A. (1984) Effect of metoclopramide on gastric emptying before elective and emergency Caesarean section. *Br. J. Anaesth.*, **56**, 1113.

Myers, R.E. and Myers, S.E. (1979) Use of sedative, analgesic and anesthetic drugs during labor: bane or boon? *Am. J. Obstet. Gynec.*, **133**, 83.

Myers, R.E., Stange, L., Joelson, I., Huzell, B. and Wussow, C. (1977) Effects upon the fetus of oxygen administration to the mother. *Acta obstet. gynec. scand.*, **56**, 195.

Naftalin, N.J., McKay, D.M., Phear, W.P.C. and Goldberg, A.H. (1977) The effects of halothane on pregnant and non-pregnant human myometrium. *Anesthesiology*, **46**, 15.

Nation, R.L. (1981) Meperidine binding in maternal and fetal plasma. *Clin. Pharmac. Ther.*, **23**, 288.

Newman, W., McKinnon, L., Phillips, L., Paterson, P. and Wood, C. (1967) Oxygen transfer from mother to fetus during labor. *Am. J. Obstet. Gynec.*, **99**, 61.

Nimmo, W.S., Wilson, J. and Prescott, L.F. (1975) Narcotic analgesics and delayed gastric emptying during labour. *Lancet*, **i**, 890.

Nobel, J. and Hille, H. (1963) Durchblutungsreaktionen des Uterus in Halothan oder Barbiturat Narkose. *Anaesthetist*, **12**, 349.

Older, P.O. and Harris, J.M. (1968) Placental transfer of tubocurarine. *Br. J. Anaesth.*, **40**, 459.

Palahniuk, R.J. and Cumming, M. (1977) Foetal deterioration following thiopentone–nitrous oxide anaesthesia in the pregnant ewe. *Can. Anaesth. Soc. J.*, **24**, 361.

Palahniuk, R.J. and Shnider, S.M. (1974) Maternal and fetal cardiovascular and acid–base changes during halothane and isoflurane anesthesia in the pregnant ewe. *Anesthesiology*, **41**, 462.

Palahniuk, R.J., Scatcliffe, J., Biehl, D., Wiebe, H. and Sankaran, K. (1977) Maternal and neonatal effects of methoxyflurane, nitrous oxide and lumbar epidural anaesthesia for Caesarean section. *Can. Anaesth. Soc. J.*, **24**, 586.

Patrick, M.J., Tilstone, W.J. and Reavey, P. (1972) Diazepam and breast feeding. *Lancet*, **i**, 542.

Pearson, J.F. and Davies, P. (1973) The effect of continuous epidural analgesia on the acid–base status of maternal arterial blood during the first stage of labour. *J. Obstet. Gynaec. Br. Commonw.*, **80**, 218.

Pearson, J.F. and Davies, P. (1974) The effect of continuous lumbar epidural analgesia upon fetal acid–base status during the first stage of labour. *J. Obstet. Gynaec. Br. Commonw.*, **81**, 971.

Pedersen, H. and Finster, M. (1979) Anesthetic risk in the pregnant surgical patient. *Anesthesiology*, **51**, 439.

Pedersen, H., Morishima, H.O., Finster, M., Arthur, G.R. and Covino, B.G. (1982) Pharmacokinetics of etidocaine in fetal and neonatal lambs and adult sheep. *Anesth. Analg. curr. Res.*, **61**, 104.

Peltz, B. and Sinclair, D.M. (1973) Induction agents for caesarean section. Comparison of thiopentone and ketamine. *Anaesthesia*, **28**, 37.

Peng, A.T.C., Blancato, L.S. and Motoyama, E.K. (1972) Effect of maternal hypocapnia v. eucapnia on the foetus during caesarean section. *Br. J. Anaesth.*, **44**, 1173.

Petrie, R.H., Wu, R., Miller, F.C. et al (1976) The effect of drugs on uterine activity. *Obstet. Gynec.*, **48**, 431.

Phillips, J.C., Hochberg, C.J., Petrakis, J.K. and Van Winkle, J.D. (1977) Epidural analgesia and its effects on the 'normal' progress of labor. *Am. J. Obstet. Gynec.*, **129**, 316.

Ploman, L. and Persson, B.H. (1957) On the transfer of barbiturates to the human foetus and their accumulation in some of the vital organs. *J. Obst. Gynaec. Br. Emp.*, **64**, 706.

Pope, W.D.B., Halsey, M.J., Lansdown, A.B.G., Simmonds, A. and Bateman, P.E. (1978) Fetotoxicity in rats following chronic exposure to halothane, nitrous oxide or methoxyflurane. *Anesthesiology*, **48**, 11.

Poppers, P.J. and Finster, M. (1968) Use of prilocaine hydrochloride (Citanest) for epidural analgesia in obstetrics. *Anesthesiology*, **29**, 1134.

Poppers, P.J. and Mastri, A.R. (1970) Maternal and foetal methaemoglobinaemia caused by prilocaine. *Acta anaesth. scand.*, Suppl. **37**, 258.

Pose, S.V., Cibils, L.A. and Zuspan, F.P. (1962) Effect of L-epinephrine infusion on uterine contractility and the cardiovascular system. *Am. J. Obstet. Gynec.*, **84**, 297.

Potter, N. and MacDonald, R.D. (1971) Obstetric consequences of epidural analgesia in multiparous patients. *Lancet*, **i**, 1031.

Power, G.G., Longo, L.D., Wagner, H.N., Kuhle, D.E. and Forster, R.E. (1967) Uneven distribution of maternal and fetal placental blood flow, as demonstrated by using macro-aggregates, and its response to hypoxia. *J. clin. Invest.*, **46**, 2053.

Ralston, D.H., Shnider, S.M. and de Lorimer, A.A. (1974) Effects of equipotent ephedrine, metaraminol, mephentermine and methoxamine on uterine blood flow in the pregnant ewe. *Anesthesiology*, **40**, 354.

Ramanathan, S., Ghandhi, S., Arismendy, J., Chalon, J. and Turndorf, H. (1982). Oxygen transfer from mother to fetus during cesarean section under epidural anesthesia. *Anesth. Analg. curr. Res.*, **61**, 576.

Reed, R.L., Cheney, C.B., Fearon, R.E., Hook, R. and Hehre, F.W. (1974) Propranolol therapy throughout pregnancy: a case report. *Anesth. Analg. curr. Res.*, **53**, 214.

Refstad, S.O. and Lindbaek, E. (1980) Ventilatory depression of the newborn of women receiving pethidine or pentazocine. *Br. J. Anaesth.*, **52**, 265.

Reier, C.E. and Moster, W.G. (1970) Effects of neuromuscular blocking agents on uterine contractions in vitro. *Am. J. Obstet. Gynec.*, **108**, 610.

Reynolds, F. and Taylor, G. (1971) Plasma concentrations of bupivacaine during continuous epidural analgesia in labour: the effect of adrenaline. *Br. J. Anaesth.*, **43**, 436.

Reynolds, F., Hargrove, R.L. and Wyman, J.B. (1973) Maternal and foetal plasma concentrations of bupivacaine after epidural block. *Br. J. Anaesth.*, **45**, 1049.

Roberts, H. and Please, N.W. (1958) Respiratory minute volume in the newborn infant. *J. Obstet. Gynaec. Br. Emp.*, **65**, 33.

Rolbin, S.H., Cole, A.F.D., Hew, E.M., Pollard, A. and Virgint, S. (1982) Prophylactic intramuscular ephedrine before epidural anaesthesia for Caesarean section: efficacy and actions on the foetus and newborn. *Can. Anaesth. Soc. J.*, **29**, 148.

Romney, S.L., Gabel, P.V. and Takeda, Y. (1963) Experimental hemorrhage in late pregnancy: effects on maternal and fetal hemodynamics. *Am. J. Obstet. Gynec.*, **87**, 636.

Rorke, M.J., Davey, D.A. and Du Toit, H.J. (1968) Foetal oxygenation during caesarean section. *Anaesthesia*, **23**, 585.

Sala, N.L. and Fisch, L. (1965) Effect of acetylcholine and atropine upon uterine contracility in pregnant women. *Am. J. Obstet. Gynec.*, **91**, 1069.

Salariya, E.M., Easton, P.M. and Cater, J.I. (1978) Duration of breast feeding after early initiation of frequent feeding. *Lancet*, **ii**, 1141.

Sandler, M., Ruthven, C.R.J. and Wood, C. (1964) Metabolism of C^{14}-norepinephrine and C^{14}-epinephrine and their transmission across the human placenta. *Neuropharmacology*, **3**, 123.

Sanner, J.H. and Woods, L.A. (1965) Comparative distribution of tritium-labelled dihydromorphine between maternal and fetal rats. *J. Pharmac. exp. Ther.*, **148**, 176.

Scanlon, J.W., Brown, W.U., Weiss, J.B. and Alper, M.H. (1974) Neurobehavioral responses of newborn infants after maternal epidural anesthesia. *Anesthesiology*, **40**, 121.

Scanlon, J.W., Ostheimer, G.W., Lurie, A.O. et al (1976) Neurobehavioral responses and drug concentrations in newborns after maternal epidural anesthesia with bupivacaine. *Anesthesiology*, **45**, 400.

Schellenberg, J.C. (1977) Uterine activity during lumbar epidural analgesia with bupivacaine. *Am. J. Obstet. Gynec.*, **127**, 26.

Scher, J., Hailey, D.M. and Beard, R.W. (1972) The effect of diazepam on the fetus. *J. Obst. Gynaec. Br. Commonw.*, **79**, 635.

Schoenfeld, A., Joel-Cohen, S.J., Duparc, H. and Levy, E. (1978) Emergency obstetric anaesthesia and the use of sympathomimetic drugs. *Br. J. Anaesth.*, **50**, 969.

Schulman, H. (1978) The comparative actions of uterine inhibiting drugs. *Am. J. Obstet. Gynec.*, **130**, 684.

Scott, D.B., Lees, M.M., Davie, I.T., Slawson, K.B. and Kerr, M.G. (1969) Observations on cardiorespiratory function during caesarean section. *Br. J. Anaesth.*, **41**, 489.

Senties, G.L., Arellano, G., Casellas, F.A., Ontiveros, E. and Santos, J. (1970) Effects of some vasopressor drugs upon uterine contractility in pregnant women. *Am. J. Obstet. Gynec.*, **107**, 892.

Shabanah, E.H., Toth, A. and Maughan, G.B. (1964) The role of the autonomic nervous system in uterine contractility and blood flow. *Am. J. Obstet. Gynec.*, **89**, 841.

Shantha, T.R. (1977) Question and answer. *Anesth. Analg. curr. Res.*, **56**, 745.

Shapiro, S., Stone, D., Hartz, S.C. et al (1976) Anticonvulsants and parental epilepsy in the development of birth defects. *Lancet*, **i**, 272.

Shnider, S.M. and Moya, F. (1964) Effect of meperidine on the newborn infant. *Am. J. Obstet. Gynec.*, **89**, 1009.

Shnider, S.M. and Way, E.L. (1968) Plasma levels of lidocaine (Xylocaine) in mothers and newborn following obstetrical conduction anesthesia. *Anesthesiology*, **29**, 951.

Shnider, S.M., de Lorimer, A.A., Holl, J.W., Chapler, F.K. and Morishima, H.O. (1968) Vasopressors in obstetrics. *Am. J. Obstet. Gynec.*, **102**, 911.

Sliom, C.M., Frankel, L. and Holbrook, R.A. (1962) A comparison between methohexitone and thiopentone as induction agents for caesarean section anaesthesia. *Br. J. Anaesth.*, **34**, 316.

Smith, B.E., Gaub, M.L. and Moya, F. (1965) Teratogenic effects of anesthetic agents: nitrous oxide. *Anesth. Analg. curr. Res.*, **44**, 726.

Smith, R.F., Bowman, R.E. and Katz, J. (1978) Behavioral effects of exposure to halothane during early development in the rat. *Anesthesiology*, **49**, 319.

Spiers, I. (1966) Use of tacrine and suxamethonium in anaesthesia for caesarean section. *Br. J. Anaesth.*, **38**, 394.

Spiers, I. and Sim, W. (1972) The placental transfer of pancuronium bromide. *Br. J. Anaesth.*, **44**, 370

Stenger, V.G., Blechner, J.N. and Prystowsky, H. (1969) A study of prolongation of obstetric anesthesia. *Am. J. Obstet. Gynec.*, **103**, 901.

Stone, S.R. and Pritchard, J.A. (1970) Effect of maternally administered magnesium sulfate on the neonate. *Obstet. Gynec.*, **35**, 574.

Studd, J.W.W., Crawford, J.S., Duignan, N.M., Rowbotham, C.J.F. and Hughes, A.O. (1980) Effect of lumbar epidural analgesia upon cervimetric progress and the outcome of spontaneous labour. *Br. J. Obstet. Gynaec.*, **87**, 1015.

Studd, J.W.W., Duignan, N.M., Crawford, J.S., Rowbotham, C.J.F. and Hughes, A.O. (1982) The effect of lumbar epidural analgesia on the progress and outcome of induced labour. *J. Obstet. Gynaec.*, **2**, 230.

Tarnow-Mordi, W.O., Shaw, J.C.L., Liu, D., Gardner, D.A. and Flynn, F.V. (1981) Iatrogenic hyponatraemia of the newborn due to maternal fluid overload: a prospective study. *Br. med. J.*, **283**, 639.

Thomas, C.R. (1976) Routine phenobarbital for prevention of neonatal hyperbilirubinemia. *Obstet. Gynec.*, **47**, 304.

Thomas, J., Climie, C.R. and Mather, L.E. (1968) Placental transfer of lignocaine following lumbar epidural administration. *Br. J. Anaesth.*, **40**, 965.

Thomas, J., Climie, C.R. and Mather, L.E. (1969a) Placental transfer of alcuronium. *Br. J. Anaesth.*, **41**, 297.

Thomas, J., Climie, C.R. and Mather, L.E. (1969b) Maternal plasma levels and placental transfer of bupivacaine following epidural analgesia. *Br. J. Anaesth.*, **41**, 1035.

Thomas, J., Climie, C.R., Long, G. and Nightjoy, J.E. (1969c) Influence of adrenaline on the maternal plasma levels and placental transfer of lignocaine following lumbar epidural administration. *Br. J. Anaesth.*, **41**, 1029.

Thomas, D.J.B., Dove, A.F. and Alberti, K.G.M.M. (1977) Metabolic effects of salbutamol infusion during premature labour. *Br. J. Obstet. Gynaec.*, **84**, 479.

Thompson, E.M., Wilson, C.M., Moore, J. and McClean, E. (1985) Plasma bupivacaine levels associated with extradural anaesthesia for Caesarean section. *Anaesthesia*, **40**, 427.

Thorburn, J. and Moir, D.D. (1984) Bupivacaine toxicity in association with extradural analgesia for Caesarean section. *Br. J. Anaesth.*, **56**, 551.

Tomlin, P.J. (1979) Health problems of anaesthetists and their families in the West Midlands. *Br. med. J.*, **i**, 779.

Trolle, D. (1968) Decrease of total serum bilirubin concentration in newborn infants after phenobarbitone treatment. *Lancet*, **ii**, 705.

Tucker, G.T., Boyes, R.N., Bridenbaugh, P.O. and Moore, D.C. (1970) Binding of anilide-type local anesthetics in human plasma. II. Implications *in vivo* with special reference to transplacental distribution. *Anesthesiology*, **33**, 304.

Tunstall, M.E. (1969) The effect of propranolol on the onset of breathing at birth. *Br. J. Anaesth.*, **41**, 792.

Usubiaga, J.E., La Iuppa, M., Moya, F., Wilkinski, J.A. and Velazco, R. (1968) Passage of procaine hydrochloride and para-aminobenzoic acid across the human placenta. *Am. J. Obstet. Gynec.*, **100**, 918.

Vannucci, R.C. and Wolf, J.W. (1978) Oxidative metabolism in fetal rat brain during maternal anesthesia. *Anesthesiology*, **48**, 238.

Vasicka, A. and Kretchmer, H. (1961) Effect of conduction and inhalation anesthesia on uterine contractions. *Am. J. Obstet. Gynec.*, **82**, 600.

Vasicka, A., Hutchinson, H.T., Eng, M. and Allen, C.B. (1964) Spinal and epidural anesthesia, fetal and uterine response to acute hypo- and hypertension. *Am. J. Obstet. Gynec.*, **90**, 800.

Viera, E., Cleaton-Jones, P. and Moyes, D. (1983) Effects of low intermittent concentrations of nitrous oxide on the developing fetus. *Br. J. Anaesth.*, **55**, 67.

Vree, T.B., Reekers-Ketting, J.J., Fragen, R.J. and Arts, T.H.M. (1984) Placental transfer of midazolam and its metabolite 1-hydroxymidazolam in the pregnant ewe. *Anesth. Analg. curr. Res.*, **63**, 31.

Wallis, K.L., Shnider, S.M., Hicks, J.S. and Spivey, H.T. (1976) Epidural anesthesia in the normotensive pregnant ewe. *Anesthesiology*, **44**, 481.

Wassef, M.R., Lal, H. and Pleuvry, B.J. (1974) The cardiovascular effects of ergometrine in the experimental animal in vivo and in vitro. *Br. J. Anaesth.*, **46**, 473.

Wauquier, A. (1983) Profile of etomidate. A hypnotic, anticonvulsant and brain protective compound. *Anaesthesia*, **38**, Suppl. 26.

Way, W.L., Costley, E.C. and Way, E.L. (1965) Respiratory sensitivity of the newborn infant to meperidine and morphine. *Clin. Pharmac. Ther.*, **6**, 454.

Wearing, M.P. and Love, E.J. (1964) Effect of analgesic, amnesic and anesthetic drugs on the newborn. *Am. J. Obstet. Gynec.*, **88**, 298.

Weiss, F.R. and Peak, J. (1974) Effects of oxytocin on blood pressure during anesthesia. *Anesthesiology*, **40**, 189.

Wesselius-de Casparis, A, Thiery, M., Sian, A.Y.L. et al (1971) Results of double-blind, multi-centre study with ritodrine in premature labour. *Br. med. J.*, **iii**, 144.

Whitelaw, A.G.L., Cummings, A.J. and McFadyen, I.R. (1981) Effect of maternal lorazepam on the neonate. *Br. med. J.*, **282**, 1106.

Wiener, P.C., Hogg, M.I.J. and Rosen, M. (1977) Effects of naloxone on pethidine-induced neonatal depression. *Br. med. J.*, **ii**, 228.

Williams, C.V., Johnson, A. and Ledward, R. (1974) A comparison of central venous pressure changes in the third stage of labour following oxytocic drugs and diazepam. *J. Obstet. Gynaec. Br. Commonw.*, **81**, 596.

Wilson, J. (1978) Gastric emptying in labour: some recent findings and their clinical significance. *J. int. med. Res.*, **6**, Suppl., 54.

Wilson, J., Stephen, G.W. and Scott, D.B. (1969) A study of the cardiovascular effects of chlormethiazole. *Br. J. Anaesth.*, **41**, 840.

Wilson, K.H., Louerson, N.H., Raghoven, K.S., Fuchs, F. and Niemann, W.H. (1974) Effects of diazoxide and beta adrenergic drugs on spontaneous and induced uterine activity in the pregnant baboon. *Am. J. Obstet. Gynec.*, **118**, 499.

Wolkoff, A.S., Bawden, J.W., Flowers, C.E. and McGee, J.A. (1965) The effects of anesthesia on the newborn. *Am. J. Obstet. Gynec.*, **93**, 311.

Woods, W.A., Stanski, D.R., Curtis, J., Rosen, M. and Shnider, S. (1982) The role of the fetal liver in the distribution of thiopental from mother to fetus. *Anesthesiology*, **57**, A390.

Yeh, S.Y., Paul, R.H., Cordero, L. and Hon, E.H. (1974) A study of diazepam during labor. *Obstet. Gynec.*, **43**, 363.

Young, D.C., Popat, R., Luther, E.R., Scott, K.E. and Writer, W.D.R. (1980) Influence of maternal oxygen administration on the fetus before labor. *Am. J. Obstet. Gynec.*, **136**, 321.

Zuspan, F.P., Nelson, G.H. and Ahlquist, R.P. (1964) Epinephrine infusions in normal and toxemic pregnancy. 1. Nonesterified fatty acids and cardiovascular alterations. *Am. J. Obstet. Gynec.*, **90**, 88.

4

The Modern Management of Pregnancy and Labour

Martin J. Whittle

Fashions change relatively quickly in obstetrics and because of this some things proposed today may well be out-of-date by the time they are read. However an important, and hopefully unchanging, development has been the concept of the team approach to obstetrics. The success of this depends upon the separate members of the team understanding each others' problems, and it is with this in mind that a chapter on obstetrics appears in a book written essentially for anaesthetists. The chapter comprises two main parts: the first dealing with certain aspects of antenatal care and the second concerning the management of both normal and abnormal labour.

PREGNANCY ASSESSMENT

The first antenatal visit

The mother's first visit to the antenatal clinic is of immense importance both obstetrically and also psychologically. The obstetric aims are not only to confirm the pregnancy and establish accurately the period of gestation but also to determine the mother's general medical state. In general terms the obstetrician is seeking to establish whether or not the current pregnancy carries any particular risk factors and only when this has been done does it become possible to plan logically the subsequent care.

Calculation of gestational age. The gestational age is calculated from the first day of the last normal menstrual period (LNMP) and the estimated date of delivery (EDD) can be determined, assuming a 28-day cycle, by adding seven days to the LMP and subtracting three months (Nagaele's rule). Uterine size may be assessed by bimanual vaginal examination or, later in pregnancy, by abdominal palpation. However even with certain dates and a regular cycle the clinical estimation of the date of delivery will be wrong by at least two weeks in about 12% of cases (Persson and Kullander, 1983). However, now that routine ultrasound examinations before 20 weeks of pregnancy are more common (Campbell et al, 1984) such discrepancies tend to be minimized. Measurement of the fetal crown–rump length for up to 12 weeks (Robinson

112

and Fleming, 1975) and of biparietal diameter up to about 20 weeks (Campbell, 1969) provides an estimation of gestational age to within three to five days. Such precise dating at an early stage in the pregnancy greatly facilitates the identification and management of complications that may arise later. Thus, the diagnosis of a suspected small-for-dates fetus is virtually impossible if the gestational age is not known accurately. Similarly, the planning of an elective delivery becomes difficult if the EDD is imprecise and under these circumstances other, less satisfactory, methods of determining fetal maturity must be considered such as radiography or amniocentesis.

Apart from its use in determining gestational age early ultrasound examination is also of value in confirming the viability of the pregnancy, detecting gross fetal structural abnormalities and establishing the diagnosis of multiple pregnancy.

Assessment of medical conditions. Since pregnant women are young it is unusual for them to present for the first time in pregnancy with serious medical problems. However an examination of the cardiovascular system, for example, may reveal hypertension or occasionally cardiac bruits other than the frequently auscultated systolic 'flow' murmur of pregnancy. These women need to be investigated ideally by a physician interested in the association of medical conditions with pregnancy. Metabolic conditions such as thyroid disorders and diabetes mellitus may be seen in pregnancy and these are always best managed in conjunction with a physician, particularly diabetes, which can pose considerable difficulties. Finally a drug history is very important both from the potential risk of particular drugs to the fetus (teratogenesis) and also from the need to be aware that pregnancy may influence the metabolism of drugs and modify their effects.

When a medical or surgical problem is either suspected or, indeed, known to be present the patient should ideally be seen for investigation and advice prior to commencing the pregnancy, and although this can be difficult to arrange, prepregnancy counselling clinics are now beginning to be established.

Routine examination and investigations. As mentioned above a routine physical examination of the mother is essential at the first visit to exclude serious underlying disease but, in addition, blood must be taken for haemoglobin, blood group and rhesus status as well as syphilitic and rubella serology. In some areas of the UK a sample is also taken, when the pregnancy is about 16–18 weeks, for a serum α-fetoprotein level to aid in the detection of babies with open neural tube defects (Brock and Sutcliffe, 1972). Finally, women of 35 years or more should be offered amniocentesis to detect chromosomal abnormalities such as Down's syndrome, which becomes increasingly common as maternal age advances.

Identification of risk factors. One of the most difficult aspects of antenatal care is the reliable identification of the high risk pregnancy and, in an attempt to quantify risk, different types of scoring systems have been devised. However, although this approach has been described by groups in the USA (Creasy, 1980) and France (Kaminiski and Papiernik, 1974) to predict, for example, preterm labour it is not generally popular in the UK although the principle has been used recently with apparent success in the Sighthill Project in Edinburgh, Scotland (Boddy et al, 1980).

Table 6. Some risk factors in pregnancy

Past history	Social factors	Obstetric factors
Spontaneous abortions (×3)	Low socio-economic group	Uncertain LNMP/late booker
Previous preterm birth	Maternal age (<16 or >35 years)	Multiple pregnancy
Previous stillbirth		Polyhydramnios
Underlying medical condition	Multiparity (4 or more children)	Uterine bleeding
	Unsupported	Pre-eclampsia/hypertension
	Smokes/drinks alcohol	

Generally, high-risk groups can be identified on the basis of their past obstetric and medical history and, although some risk factors are shown in Table 6, their quantitation is difficult because of the complicated interrelations that exist between the different factors. The value of proportioning risk is that it enables a logical judgement to be made about the subsequent management of the pregnancy with regard to the frequency of antenatal visits, the need for serial biophysical and biochemical fetal evaluation and the wisdom of sharing care with the general practitioner.

Fetal evaluation

Over the last 10–15 years the fetus has come to be increasingly recognized as a patient in its own right. This has been partly because the dramatic reductions in maternal mortality, to a rate of 12 in 100 000 for 1976–1978 (Report on Confidential Enquiries into Maternal Deaths in England and Wales), have allowed the obstetrician to concentrate more on the condition of the baby. However, in addition, there is now an enhanced ability to evaluate the fetus both through biochemical techniques, which are currently less in vogue, and biophysical techniques in which major improvements have occurred in recent years.

Biochemical assessment. A major disadvantage of biochemical methods is that tests only give a 'secondhand' impression of fetal wellbeing since the placental and/or fetal products must be measured in either maternal urine or plasma. A brief description of the variety of tests available will follow:

Oestriol The estimation of this hormone illustrates the problems that are involved in biochemical assessment since the amount excreted depends on the placenta, fetus and the maternal renal function and enterohepatic circulation (Diczfalusy and Mancuso, 1969). Oestriol may be measured in either maternal urine or, in unconjugated form, in plasma and the levels obtained may be used either as a day-to-day assessment or as a screening test to detect the small-for-dates fetus. There is some evidence that daily plasma unconjugated oestriols may be of some use in identifying impending fetal demise, particularly in the diabetic (Whittle et al, 1979) but there is little to show that oestriol levels are useful as a screening test.

Human placental lactogen   This is a product of the placenta and has been shown to be of value in predicting fetal outcome in pregnancies complicated by hypertension or growth retardation (Spellacy et al, 1975). A recent report suggested that human placental lactogen may be a useful screening test for predicting the small-for-dates fetus and it performed more effectively than two other placental proteins—pregnancy specific β-glycoprotein (PSβ1) and pregnancy-associated plasma protein-A (PAPP-A) (Pledger et al, 1984).

Although other placental proteins (PSβ1, PAPP and placental protein 5) have been investigated there appears to be no real consensus as to their value either in the prediction of complications or the day-to-day evaluation of the pregnancy.

Biophysical assessment.   Non-invasive biophysical techniques, in contrast to biochemical methods, permit a direct assessment of the fetus. The two main techniques involve the evaluation of the fetal heart rate patterns and ultrasound visualization which permits both the measurement of the fetus and the observation of fetal activity.

Antepartum fetal heart rate testing (AFHRT)   Using the Doppler principle, continuous wave ultrasound can be used to determine the fetal heart rate; this has formed the basis of AFHRT. In fact detailed observations of the AFHRT were first made by Hammacher (1969) who, using phonocardiography, described the characteristic appearance of the heart rate trace. Since then a number of modifications have been made but the principle remains that the presence of accelerations in the fetal heart with movement or contractions—a reactive test—indicates a baby that is in good condition and is likely to remain so for up to seven days (Keegan and Paul, 1980). The significance of a non-reactive test is less clear so further evaluation is required under these circumstances. The test can be merely repeated within 6–12 hours or a contraction stress test performed to establish the fetal oxygen reserves (Lin et al, 1981). If fetal heart rate decelerations occur in response to contractions the test is said to be positive and this is likely to be associated with significant fetal problems in 50–60% of cases.

Ultrasound evaluation   The use of ultrasound to observe the fetus later in pregnancy (after 20 weeks) has become increasingly important as the quality of the ultrasound image improves. Three major roles for ultrasound are the evaluation of fetal growth, the detection of fetal structural abnormalities and the identification of the placental site. With respect to growth a number of different screening tests have been devised which determine the fetal head/trunk circumference ratios (Campbell and Thoms, 1977) or the product of fetal crown–rump length and trunk area (Neilson et al, 1980). These methods appear to be generally useful in detecting the small-for-dates fetus each with a sensitivity of over 80%.

However not all small-for-dates babies are necessarily at risk and an attempt at identifying those that are at risk has been made by combining information from the AFHRT with the ultrasound appearances to form a biophysical profile (Manning et al, 1985). This sort of approach is likely to prove more useful than the use of a single test of fetal wellbeing but further evaluation is clearly needed.

In general terms the purpose of all these evaluations, biochemical and biophysical, is to determine whether the baby requires to be delivered. However, fetal evaluation is still an inexact science and the greatest danger is to undertake, on the basis of abnormal antepartum tests, the inappropriate preterm delivery of a baby who subsequently develops severe respiratory problems and dies or, perhaps worse, survives with long-term handicap. The neonatal risks can be reduced by determining the state of the fetal lungs from the lung phospholipid concentration in the amniotic fluid. Although this approach is now unfashionable (Turnbull, 1983) the measurement of the lecithin/sphingomyelin ratio (Gluck et al, 1971) or the use of the lecithin/sphingomyelin ratio in combination with another lung phospholipid, phosphatidyl glycerol (Whittle et al, 1982) provide useful predictive tests which may help in the overall planning of a preterm delivery.

Maternal evaluation

Although the only hospital attendance usually necessary during pregnancy is the routine antenatal clinic it is occasionally necessary to admit the mother to hospital for closer observation and possible treatment. Complications of pregnancy such as hypertension and antepartum haemorrhage, pulmonary embolism, heart disease and diabetes are dealt with in chapter 9. However the general aim, when maternal problems arise, is to maintain the pregnancy until a gestational age is reached at which the baby, if delivered, has a high chance of survival. However, the life of the mother takes precedence over that of the baby and if her condition deteriorates the baby should be delivered regardless of gestational age.

Indications for delivery

Fetal. Delivery in the fetal interest is indicated when intrauterine existence is judged to be more dangerous than extrauterine existence. However, as it has been shown it is frequently difficult to be sure that the fetus is in jeopardy and therefore the timing of delivery is often made arbitrarily based on the obstetrician's experience and 'hunch'.

Clear indications to electively deliver the baby include the presence of severe intrauterine growth retardation, evidence of fetal hypoxia from the AFHRT and severe anaemia in association with rhesus disease. When the circumstances are less clear it may be wise to determine the extent of the risk of lung immaturity to the neonate from amniotic fluid phospholipid content. If this test suggests a low risk of respiratory distress syndrome then delivery may well be appropriate. However, if the test indicates a high risk of respiratory distress syndrome it may be necessary to reconsider delivery or, if birth seems the best option, at least prewarn the paediatric staff that a severely immature baby is to be expected.

A previously common indication for delivery was prolongation of the pregnancy beyond 40 weeks under which circumstances it was presumed that there was an increased risk of intrauterine death. However the tendency now is to leave the normal pregnancy to at least 10–14 days past the EDD. This change in practice at the Queen Mother's Hospital, for example, has resulted in a fall in induction rates from 46% in 1979 to 18% in 1984. However there has been no apparent increase in the mature stillbirth rate over this same period which suggests that the previous active induction policy was probably of little value.

Maternal indications. Delivery on maternal grounds will only usually be undertaken when the mother's life is actually or potentially in danger. Thus severe and uncontrollable hypertension is clearly an indication for delivery since it may lead to cerebrovascular accidents, heart failure or eclamptic fits. Delivery is also indicated if pregnancy is complicated by a substantial antepartum haemorrhage, although when the bleeding is the result of placenta praevia and the fetus is previable, a conservative approach may be feasible. Finally, certain maternal diseases, such as heart disease and diabetes mellitus, may indicate the need for a planned active delivery so that additional expert medical care can be scheduled to be available.

MANAGEMENT OF LABOUR

Although it can be difficult at times to establish the diagnosis of labour it is usually characterized by the onset of regular, painful uterine contractions together with a 'show' (the mucus plug released from the cervical os as it dilates) and often rupture of the membranes. In the majority of pregnancies labour starts spontaneously but occasionally induction of labour is indicated and this can be achieved in a number of ways.

Cervical priming

Prior to induction the state of the cervix can be assessed using a modified Bishop score (Table 7) (Calder et al, 1974). A low score indicates that induction of labour will be difficult and in an attempt to improve the outcome, the cervix can be 'primed' to make it more favourable. This was first attempted by giving the mother oxytocin by mouth (buccal pitocin) or starting an intravenous oxytocin infusion. More recently cervical priming has been

Table 7. Modified Bishop score (from Calder et al, 1974)

Factor	Score			
	0	1	2	3
Dilatation of cervix	<1 cm	1–2 cm	2–4 cm	>4 cm
Length of cervix	>4 cm	2–4 cm	1–2 cm	<1 cm
Consistency of cervix	Firm	Average	Soft	—
Position of cervix	Posterior	Mid; anterior	—	—
Position of head relative to ischial spines	3 cm above	2 cm above	<1 cm above	>1 cm below

achieved by using prostaglandins (Prostin E_2) placed in the vagina as tablets (Kennedy et al, 1982), intravaginally as a gel (Mackenzie and Embrey, 1977) or extra-amniotically (Calder et al, 1977). These methods all produce varying degrees of cervical 'ripening' although the problems associated with induced labour mean that the caesarean section rate may remain high in this group.

Induction of labour

The usual method for the induction of labour is membrane rupture, usually using a small plastic rod with a hook at one end (Amnihook), and intravenous oxytocin. The dose of oxytocin is slowly increased until the uterus has been stimulated to contract firmly about once every 3 minutes. The amount of oxytocin used should be titrated against the uterine activity and the progress of labour, which can be judged from the rate of cervical dilatation. Uterine activity is assessed either from a tocotransducer attached by a belt to the mother's abdomen or, more accurately, from an intrauterine catheter connected to a pressure sensitive device (Steer et al, 1978). One major advantage of oxytocin is that it has a short half-life so that the effects of overstimulation dissipate rapidly once administration ceases.

Although oxytocin remains a popular induction agent, the prostaglandins may also be of use, particularly in the multiparous mother with a favourable cervix. Prostaglandins can be administered orally so that the mother is unencumbered with intravenous lines and so can remain mobile. The disadvantages of prostaglandins are that they may produce nausea and vomiting and their action, in contrast to oxytocin, is prolonged.

Acceleration of labour

The concept of accelerating a labour was propounded by O'Driscoll in Dublin (O'Driscoll et al, 1972). When the progress of labour as assessed from cervical dilatation was slow, acceleration could be achieved by either rupturing the membranes, commencing intravenous oxytocin or both. Using this policy the vast majority of primigravidae would be delivered within 12 hours and multigravidae within 8 hours. In addition the need to use forceps was found to be markedly reduced since the mother's own powers, if suitably stimulated, were sufficient to deliver the baby.

The stages of labour

First stage of labour. The first stage of labour, which lasts from the onset of labour—often a difficult time to establish—until the cervix is fully dilated, is divided into latent and active phases. In the latent phase very little cervical dilatation occurs although subtle changes in the cervix such as softening and effacement can be detected. The duration of this phase is very variable and may well last up to 12 hours. In fact some women, particularly primigravidae, may have a very prolonged latent phase perhaps lasting a few days. During this time they may complain of intermittent painful contractions which are clearly different from the painless Braxton-Hicks' contractions experienced by virtually all pregnant women in the last trimester. In the active phase of the first stage of labour the cervix dilates rapidly (at least as fast as 1 cm) and the fetal presenting part descends through the pelvis. This phase of labour is usually said to commence when the cervix is 3–4 cm dilated so it should last no longer than 6–7 hours.

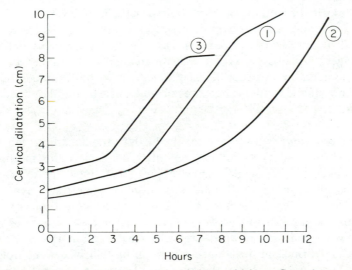

Figure 5. Partogram appearances of normal and abnormal labour. Curve 1 = normal labour; curve 2 = primary dysfunctional labour; curve 3 = secondary arrest.

The progress of the first stage is plotted on a partogram, a chart originally designed by Philpott (1972) for use in remote areas of Africa, but which is now adopted by units throughout the world. It allows cervical changes to be graphically displayed so that the arrest of progress can be readily recognized. Studd (1975) described various disorders of labour (Figure 5) which could be identified from their partogram appearances. Thus when the progress of labour was slow but steady (primary dysfunctional labour) acceleration could be achieved by rupture of intact membranes or the use of oxytocin. Conversely, rapid progress which was arrested late in the first stage (secondary arrest) was a warning of relative or absolute cephalopelvic disproportion and the chances of a safe vaginal delivery required careful re-evaluation.

Second stage of labour. This stage lasts from full dilatation of the cervix until delivery of the baby. Traditionally the second stage of labour is limited to about 2 hours in primigravidae and about an hour in multigravidae although these limits appear to have been set rather arbitrarily. However, in the absence of epidural anaesthesia there is evidence that the fetus becomes increasingly hypoxic and acidotic during delivery (Mondalou et al, 1973) partly because the prolonged expulsive efforts of the mother reduce blood flow to the placental bed, hence limiting the oxygen supply to the fetus, and partly because the mother herself becomes acidotic. However epidural anaesthesia alters considerably the pattern of the second stage probably by reducing the desire of the mother to push. This allows uterine activity alone to advance the presenting part which takes longer but is not associated with fetal acidosis and, under these circumstances, the second stage may last 3 or 4 hours (Maresh et al, 1983).

The majority of mothers manage to deliver their babies without problems although some may require an episiotomy to prevent either excessive delay in the second stage of labour or perineal lacerations. Occasionally delay in the second stage, particularly if associated with an abnormal fetal heart rate, may indicate the need for a forceps delivery which can be performed either under epidural anaesthesia if this is already established or a bilateral pudendal block if it is not.

Third stage of labour. This lasts from the birth of the baby until the delivery of the placenta and is a time of potential danger to the mother since postpartum haemorrhage can be catastrophic. To minimize the risks an active policy is adopted and in most units presently 'Syntometrine' (Syntocinon 5 units, ergometrine 0.5 mg) is given as an intramuscular injection with delivery of the anterior shoulder of the baby. Usually the placenta separates with the final expulsive contraction which delivers the baby but the Syntometrine encourages a firm and prolonged contraction which will complete the separation process and force the placenta from the upper to the lower segment of the uterus. This allows the uterine muscle to retract effectively so sealing off the placental bed and preventing haemorrhage. If the placenta only partially separates or remains in the upper segment this retraction process becomes inefficient and may lead to serious haemorrhage. Once the uterus is firmly contracted the separated placenta is removed by applying traction to the cord, the Brandt–Andrews manoeuvre.

The following complications of the third stage of labour may well demand the assistance of the anaesthetist:

Retained placenta   This is said to be retained when it remains undelivered 30 minutes after the birth of the baby. Under these circumstances the mother will require either a general or spinal anaesthetic to allow a manual removal of the placenta, unless epidural anaesthesia has been used during labour.

Atonic postpartum haemorrhage   In this circumstance the mother may lose a large volume of blood very rapidly so requiring active resuscitation with volume expanders and blood. The uterus will usually respond to massage and intravenous ergometrine (0.5 mg) but an uncontrollable haemorrhage may ultimately, but rarely, require an emergency hysterectomy.

Local birth trauma   This may also be the cause of severe haemorrhage and it will usually be necessary to anaesthetize the mother so that the vagina or cervix can be adequately explored.

Unexplained and continual haemorrhage   This may sometimes be the result of a small amniotic fluid embolus. Certainly if bleeding occurs in the presence of minor respiratory problems and slight cyanosis this diagnosis should be seriously considered and a clotting screen and blood gases determined.

Care of the mother

During labour the mother's pulse, blood pressure and temperature should be checked at regular intervals, the urine output should be charted and the presence of ketones noted. Usually oral fluids are restricted because of the concern about the delay in gastric emptying noted in mothers in labour, particularly following narcotic analgesics (Nimmo et al, 1975). Under these circumstances intravenous fluids need to be administered to prevent dehydration and ketosis if labour lasts longer than about 5 or 6 hours.

Care of the fetus

Traditionally the fetal condition in labour was assessed by the midwife auscultating the fetal heart rate for 1 minute immediately after a contraction every 15 minutes. Slowing of the heart at this time together with meconium staining of the amniotic fluid constituted the diagnosis of fetal distress.

While an abnormal heart rate and meconium still have sinister implications, the development of continuous electronic fetal heart rate monitoring by Hon (1963) and Caldeyro-Barcia et al (1966) has improved the ability to more fully assess the problem. Normally the fetal heart rate is between 120 and 160 beats/min and the baseline shows rapid changes in rate which is termed variability. This variability is the result of the physiological interplay which exists between the parasympathetic and sympathetic parts of the autonomic nervous system. This interplay may be affected not only by maternal drugs, especially the opiates, but more seriously, by fetal hypoxia. Thus, loss of variability and an elevated baseline rate, particularly if associated with other abnormalities in the heart rate and meconium in the amniotic fluid, may indicate a fetus that is becoming seriously hypoxic.

The decelerations which occur in the fetal heart rate during labour are of three types: (a) early – which occur with contractions, are of low amplitude and are probably due to head compression, (b) variable – which are very common, have a ragged appearance and are due to cord compression—a potential cause of fetal hypoxia, (c) late – which are similar in appearance to early decelerations but their timing is late in relation to contractions. Late decelerations represent the fetal response to hypoxia although only about 30% of babies showing them will be acidotic.

To be used effectively the information derived from the continuous fetal heart rate record must be matched against the clinical condition. Thus in many instances the development of late decelerations indicates a need to determine the underlying cause rather than to perform immediate caesarean section. Often such changes are the result of excessive uterine activity resulting from too much oxytocin or maternal hypotension developing either because of a supine position or conduction anaesthesia—importantly, all these factors are potentially correctible. Although normal fetal heart rate patterns give a reliable indication that the baby is well (Schifrin and Dame, 1972) abnormal patterns can be notoriously unreliable at identifying a baby in difficulties. Thus the diagnosis of fetal distress should be confirmed by assessing the fetal acid–base status using a scalp blood sample to determine pH (Beard et al, 1967) or lactate (Smith et al, 1983). A pH below 7.20 indicates severe acidosis and the need for immediate delivery.

Whether intrapartum fetal heart rate monitoring is a useful procedure remains debatable—certainly many studies suggest an increase in caesarean section rate for fetal distress (Renou et al, 1976; Havercamp et al, 1979) although the benefits in terms of improved neonatal outcome are less clear.

MANAGEMENT OF COMPLICATIONS IN LABOUR

A brief account of the abnormalities which occur in labour will be given since the anaesthetist is often involved when complications arise.

Malposition. A malposition can be defined as any position of the fetal head (vertex) in which the occiput is not anterior. Although, when labour starts, the occiput of the fetal head may be either transverse or posterior, rotation of the occiput to the anterior position usually occurs as labour proceeds. However this rotation may either never start (persistent occiput posterior position or POP) or becomes arrested with the occiput in the transverse position. Usually this arises because of inefficient uterine activity which is correctible by the administration of oxytocin. Occasionally, however, malposition indicates either a narrow pelvis or an unusually large baby in which case caesarean section is appropriate.

The partogram of a labour complicated by POP has a characteristic appearance of slow but steady progress to full dilatation. Full rotation of the head to a normal position occurs in about 50% of cases (Myerscough, 1977) although some suggest that this is less likely to occur when an epidural anaesthetic is in use (Hoult et al, 1977).

If, during the second stage of labour, a POP remains the baby may either deliver spontaneously 'face to pubes' or rotation of the head will be required either manually or with forceps. These deliveries, which require an adequate level of analgesia best produced by conduction anaesthesia, should only be performed by skilled obstetricians. Certainly rotational forceps (Keilland's model) may cause considerable trauma in untrained hands and caesarean section may, under these circumstances, be the safer option.

Malpresentation. This is defined as any presentation other than vertex.

Breech   About 2–3% of babies born at term present by the breech and, certainly over recent years, there has been an increasing tendency to perform caesarean section on the grounds that this will be safer for the baby. In fact the evidence for this is not strong and, if all preterm and congenitally abnormal babies are excluded, the perinatal mortality for breech delivery is only slightly above that for babies presenting normally. This was confirmed in a controlled trial (Collea et al, 1980) which failed to identify any obvious advantage for a breech baby to be delivered by caesarean section but identified some considerable disadvantage for the mother in terms of morbidity. The importance of a breech delivery is that it should only be conducted in carefully selected cases by a skilled obstetrician with the full support of the anaesthetist and paediatrician. The importance of good conduction anaesthesia cannot be overemphasized since it allows a slow and controlled delivery of the fetal head.

Face and brow presentation   While it is possible for a face presentation to be delivered when the fetal chin is anterior (i.e. below the symphysis) no mechanism exists when the chin is posterior. Under these latter circumstances, or when a brow presents, delivery must be by caesarean section.

Cord and compound presentations   When these presentations have been diagnosed the mother must be prepared for immediate caesarean section, providing the baby is still alive. These findings represent an obstetric emergency and there is no place for epidural anaesthesia, a formal general anaesthetic being preferred. This is because with, for example, a cord presentation (cord felt but membranes intact) the membranes may rupture at any time resulting in cord prolapse. With a compound presentation, particularly if the mother has been in labour for some time, there is a danger of uterine rupture.

MANAGEMENT OF PREMATURE LABOUR

Preterm labour is defined as labour occurring prior to 37 completed weeks of pregnancy. Two main problems arise in relation to preterm labour, the first concerning the diagnosis itself and the second concerning the decision about inhibiting labour. As mentioned above the diagnosis of labour is made in the presence of regular uterine contractions and progressive dilatation of the cervix. These criteria may also be applied to the diagnosis of preterm labour although cervical dilatation may occur relatively silently or, on occasions, excessively rapidly. At the Queen Mother's Hospital the protocol for the diagnosis of preterm labour takes account of the mother's past history so that the experience of a previous preterm delivery would lower the threshold for the diagnosis of premature labour in a subsequent pregnancy. Conversely, in the absence of a previous history, true signs of labour must be present before a diagnosis is made and 'treatment' instigated.

Table 8. Some causes of preterm labour

Recurring	Non-recurring
Cervical incompetence	Multiple pregnancy
Uterine malformation	Polyhydramnios
'Idiopathic'	Vaginal bleeding
	Intrauterine infections
	Urinary tract infections
	Intrauterine death
	Invasive procedures – amniocentesis
	– intrauterine transfusions

The causes of preterm labour are shown in Table 8 and, in general terms, can be divided into recurring and non-recurring. The recurrence risk for preterm labour depends on past history so that two previous preterm deliveries would indicate about a 30% risk (Bakketeig and Hoffman, 1981). However when conditions such as true cervical incompetence are responsible, the rate of recurrent preterm labour may be much higher.

When a pregnancy is complicated by preterm labour, in general terms, the aim should be to prevent the delivery of a premature baby who might be at serious risk of developing respiratory problems due to lung immaturity. Providing that the gestational age is accurately known it is probably reasonable to allow preterm labour to continue when the pregnancy is beyond 33 weeks since babies born after this time are unlikely to develop serious respiratory problems. However, when the pregnancy is at 33 weeks or less, or gestational age is uncertain, an attempt at tocolysis should be made.

Over recent years the aims of tocolysis have altered considerably and, whereas success was measured as the ability to continue the pregnancy to at least 37 weeks, the purpose of tocolysis is now more short-term. Thus tocolysis allows time for the pregnancy to be adequately assessed and fetal weight, presentation and normality established. If the obstetric unit is not attached to a neonatal intensive care unit tocolysis may allow the mother to be transferred, with her fetus, to a department which does have such a facility. Finally, and more contentiously, tocolysis may delay delivery for long enough to allow 48 hours of maternally administered steroids in an attempt to accelerate fetal lung maturity (Howie and Liggins, 1977).

Several groups of drugs have been used for tocolysis and they will be briefly mentioned.

β-*Sympathomimetics*. This group of drugs has been used for many years as uterine suppressants, isoxsuprine being one of the first to be used extensively (Hendricks et al, 1961). Currently, more specific β_2-agonists are available including ritodrine (Wesselius-de Casparis et al, 1971) and terbutaline (Ingemarsson, 1976).

The value of β-mimetics remains debatable and there are really no conclusive clinical trials available. However, in a review of 11 studies undertaken in the USA, Merkatz et al (1980) found a significant reduction in neonatal death for babies whose mothers received ritodrine prior to, but not after, 33 weeks.

While the efficacy of the β-mimetics remains controversial it has emerged over recent years that they may represent a potential hazard, and maternal death, usually resulting from pulmonary oedema, is now well described (Martin, 1981).

Because of the uncertain value and possible danger of the use of β-mimetics, their administration should be restricted to well-defined circumstances. However their short-term use is usually justifiable and may favourably influence the neonatal outcome.

Prostaglandin synthetase inhibitors. The use of these agents to inhibit labour was described by Zuchermann et al (1974) who administered indomethacin with apparent success. Since then a number of studies have suggested that this may be a useful method of tocolysis whic does not have the unpleasant and potentially dangerous side effects of the β-mimetics. However, effects on the fetus have been reported, the most serious of which is premature closure of the ductus arteriosus leading to pulmonary hypertension. In a review of the literature this complication developed in 20 out of 730 babies (2.7%) (Wiqvist, 1981)—probably an acceptable risk in this group of pregnancies.

Calcium antagonists. The use of this group of drugs is currently very restricted although they may ultimately be of value in tocolysis. Nifedipine has been used with apparently good effect (Andersson, 1977) but further studies are required to establish its safety and efficiency.

The use of tocolytics in preterm labour probably requires extensive re-evaluation. As mentioned, the objectives of treatment have changed considerably over recent years and now relate to a thorough evaluation of the fetus with respect to method, time and place of delivery.

Route of delivery for the preterm baby

There has been considerable debate about the optimal route for delivery of the preterm baby. However, probably the most important factor is the condition of the baby at the time of delivery (Osbourne et al, 1984), birth asphyxia having a serious impact on the baby's ultimate survival. Trauma during delivery is always a risk, particularly if the breech presents, and for this reason, many obstetricians opt to deliver the very preterm baby (less than 1500 g) by caesarean section (Howie and Patel, 1984). However, when the babies are heavier than 1500 g the advantages of a caesarean section are less obvious.

The condition of the baby throughout labour and delivery should be monitored closely so that fetal acidosis may be detected at an early stage. Analgesia during labour is best achieved by epidural anaesthesia since narcotics given to the mother may seriously depress the fetus, so exacerbating respiratory problems once the baby is born. It is essential to remember that the preterm baby will be most likely to survive if delivered carefully and in good condition to a skilled paediatrician working in a neonatal intensive care unit.

REFERENCES

Andersson, K.E. (1977) Inhibition of uterine activity by the calcium antagonist Nifedipine in preterm labour. *Proceedings of the 5th Study Group of Royal College of Obstetricians and Gynaecologists*, 101.
Bakketeig, L.S. and Hoffmann, .J. (1981) Epidemiology of preterm birth: results from a longitudinal study of births in Norway. In *Preterm Labour*, eds. Elder, M.G. and Hendricks, C.H., p. 17. London: Butterworths.
Beard, R.W., Morris, E.D. and Clayton, S.G. (1967) pH of foetal capillary blood as an indicator of the condition of the foetus. *J. Obstet. Gynaec. Br. Commonw.*, **74**, 812.
Boddy, K., Parboosingh, I.J.T. and Shepherd, W.C. (1980) *A schematic approach to prenatal care.* Edinburgh: Simpson Memorial Maternity Pavillion.
Brock, D.J.H. and Sutcliffe, R.G. (1972) Alphafetoprotein in the antenatal diagnosis of anencephaly and spina bifida. *Lancet*, ii, 197.
Calder, A.A., Embrey, M.P. and Hillier, K. (1974) Extraamniotic Prostaglandin E_2 for the induction of labour at term. *J. Obstet. Gynaec. Br. Commonw.*, **81**, 39.
Calder, A.A., Embrey, M.P. and Tait, T. (1977) Ripening of the cervix with extraamniotic prostaglandin E_2 in viscus gel before induction of labour. *Br. J. Obstet. Gynaec.*, **84**, 264.
Caldeyro-Barcia, R., Medez-Bauer, C. and Poseiro, J.J. (1966) Control of human fetal heart rate during labour. In *The Heart and Circulation in the Newborn and Infant*, ed. Cassals, D.E., New York: Grune and Stratton.
Campbell, S. (1969) The prediction of fetal maturity by ultrasonic measurement of biparietal diameter. *J. Obstet. Gynaec. Br. Commonw.*, **76**, 603.

Campbell, S. and Thoms, A. (1977) Ultrasound measurement of the fetal head to abdomen circumference ratio in the assessment of growth retardation. *Br. J. Obstet. Gynaec.*, **84**, 165.
Campbell, S., Whittle, M.J. and Trickey, N. (1984) *Report of the RCOG Working Party on Routine Ultrasound Examination in Pregnancy*. Royal College of Obstetricians and Gynaecologists.
Collea, J.V., Chein, C. and Quilligan, E.J. (1980) The randomized management of term frank breech presentation. A study of 208 cases. *Am. J. Obstet. Gynec.*, **137**, 235.
Creasy, R.K. (1980) System for predicting spontaneous preterm birth. *Obstet. Gynec.*, **55**, 695.
Diczfalusy, E. and Mancuso, S. (1969) Oestrogen metabolism in pregnancy. In *Foetus & Placenta*, eds. Klopper, A. and Diczfalusy, E., p. 191. Oxford: Blackwell.
Gluck, L., Kulovich, M.M., Borer, R.C. et al (1971) Diagnosis of RDS by amniocentesis. *Am. J. Obstet. Gynec.*, **109**, 440.
Hammacher, K. (1969) The clinical significance of cardiotocography. In *Perinatal Medicine*, eds. Huntingford, P.S., Huter, E.A. and Saling, E., 80. New York: Academic Press.
Haverkamp, A.D., Orleans, M., Langendoerfer, S. et al (1979) A controlled trial of the differential effects of intrapartum monitoring. *Am. J. Obstet. Gynec.*, **134**, 399.
Hendricks, C.H., Cibils, L.A., Pose, S.V. and Eskes, T.K.A.B. (1961) The pharmacological control of excessive uterine activity with isoxsuprine. *Am. J. Obstet. Gynec.*, **82**, 1064.
Hon, E.H. (1963) The classification of fetal heart rate. I. A working classification. *Obstet. Gynec.*, **22**, 137.
Hoult, I.J., MacLennan, A.H. and Carrie, L.E.S. (1977) Lumbar epidural analgesia in labour: relation to fetal malposition and instrumental delivery. *Br. med. J.*, **i**, 14.
Howie, R.N. and Liggins, G.C. (1977) Clinical trial of antepartum betamethasone therapy for the prevention of RDS in the preterm infant. In eds. Anderson, A. et al, *Pre-term Labour*, 281. 5th Study Group of Royal College of Obstetricians and Gynaecologists.
Howie, P.W. and Patel, N.B. (1984) Obstetric management of preterm labour. *Clinics Obstet. Gynec.*, **11**, 373.
Ingemarsson, I. (1976) Effect of terbutaline on premature labour: a double blind placebo controlled study. *Am. J. Obstet. Gynec.*, **125**, 520.
Kaminiski, M. and Papiernik, E. (1974) Multifactorial study of the risk of prematurity at 32 weeks of gestation. Comparison between an empirical prediction and a discriminant analysis. *Journal of Perinatal Medicine*, **2**, 37.
Keegan, K.A. and Paul, R.H. (1980) Antepartum fetal heart rate testing IV. The nonstress test as a primary approach. *Am. J. Obstet. Gynec.*, **136**, 75.
Kennedy, J.H., Gordon-Wright, A.P., Stewart, P., Calder, A.A. and Elder, M.G. (1982) Induction of labour with a stable based prostaglandin E_2 vaginal tablet. *Europ. J. Obstet. Gynec. Reproduct. Biol.*, **14**, 203.
Lin, C., Devoe, L.D., River, P. and Moawad, A.H. (1981) Oxytocin challenge test and intrauterine growth retardation. *Am. J. Obstet. Gynec.*, **140**, 282.
Mackenzie, I.Z. and Embrey, M.P. (1977) Cervical ripening with intravaginal prostaglandin E_2 gel. *Br. med. J.*, **2**, 1381.
Manning, F.A., Morrison, I., Lange, I.R., Harman, C.R. and Chamberlain, P.F. (1985) Fetal assessment based on fetal biophysical profile scoring: experience in 12 620 referred high risk pregnancies. *Am. J. Obstet. Gynec.*, **151**, 343.
Maresh, M., Choong, K-H. and Beard, R.W. (1983) Delayed pushing with lumbar epidural analgesia in labour. *Br. J. Obstet. Gynaec.*, **90**, 623.
Martin, A.J. (1981) Severe unwanted effects associated with β-mimetics when used in the treatment of preterm labour; causes; incidence and preventive measures. *Br. J. clin. Pract.*, **35**, 325.
Merkatz, I.R., Peter, J.B. and Barden, T.P. (1980) Ritodrine a betamimetic agent for use in preterm labour. *Obstet. Gynec.*, **56**, 7.
Mondalou, H., Yeh, S.Y., Hon, E.H. and Forsythe, E. (1973) Fetal and neonatal biochemistry and Apgar scores. *Am. J. Obstet. Gynec.*, **117**, 942.
Myerscough, P.R. (1977) Occipito-posterior positions: transverse arrest. In Munro Kerr's *Operative Obstetrics*, 64. London: Baillière Tindall.
Neilson, J.P., Whitfield, C.R. and Aitchison, T.C. (1980) Screening for the small-for-dates fetus: a two stage ultrasound examination schedule. *Br. med. J.*, **1**, 1203.
Nimmo, W.S., Wilson, J. and Prescott, L.F. (1975) Narcotic analgesics and delayed gastric emptying during labour. *Lancet*, **i**, 890.

O'Driscoll, K., Jackson, R.J.A. and Gallagher, J.T. (1972) Prevention of prolonged labour. *Br. med. J.*, **ii**, 477.
Osbourne, G.K., Patel, N.B. and Howat, R.C.L. (1984) A comparison of the outcome of low birth weight pregnancy in Glasgow and Dundee. *Hlth. Bull.*, **42** (2), 68.
Persson, P.H. and Kullander, S. (1983) Longterm experience of general ultrasound screening in pregnancy. *Am. J. Obstet. Gynec.*, **146**, 942.
Philpott, R.H. (1972) Graphic records in labour. *Br. med. J.*, **iv**, 163.
Pledger, D.R., Belfield, A., Calder, A.A. and Wallace, A.M. (1984) The predictive value of three pregnancy-associated proteins in the detection of the light-for-dates baby. *Br. J. Obstet. Gynaec.*, **91**, 870.
Renou, P., Chang, A., Anderson, I. and Wood, C. (1976) A controlled trial of fetal intensive care. *Am. J. Obstet. Gynec.*, **126**, 470.
Report on Confidential Enquiries into Maternal Deaths in England and Wales, 1976–78. London: HMSO.
Robinson, H. and Fleming, J.E.E. (1975) A critical evaluation of sonar 'crown–rump length' measurements. *Br. J. Obstet. Gynaec.*, **82**, 702.
Schifrin, B.S. and Dame, L. (1972) Fetal heart rate patterns prediction of Apgar scores. *J. Am. med. Ass.*, **219**, 1322.
Smith, N.C., Soutter, W.P., Sharp, F. and McColl, J. (1983) Fetal scalp blood lactate as an indication of intrapartum hypoxia. *Br. J. Obstet. Gynaec.*, **90**, 821.
Spellacy, W.N., Buhi, W.C. and Birk, S.A. (1975) The effectiveness of human placental lactogen as an adjunct in decreasing perinatal deaths. *Am. J. Obstet. Gynec.*, **121**, 835.
Steer, P.J., Carter, M.C., Gordon, A.J. and Beard, R.W. (1978) The use of catheter-tip pressure transducers for the measurement of intrauterine pressure in labour. *Br. J. Obstet. Gynaec.*, **85**, 561.
Studd, J. (1975) The partographic control of labour. *Clinics Obstet. Gynec.*, 140.
Turnbull, A.C. (1983) The lecithin/sphingomyelin ratio in decline. *Br. J. Obstet. Gynaec.*, **90**, 993.
Wesselius-de Casparis, A., Thiery, M., Yo le Sian, A. et al (1971) Results of a double blind multicenter study with ritodrine in premature labour. *Br. med. J.*, **iii**, 144.
Whittle, M.J., Anderson, D., Lowensohn, R.J. et al (1979) Estriol in pregnancy. VI. Experience with unconjugated plasma estriol assays and antepartum fetal heart rate testing in diabetic pregnancies. *Am. J. Obstet. Gynec.*, **135**, 764.
Whittle, M.J., Wilson, A.I., Whitfield, C.R., Paton, R. and Logan, R.W. (1982) Amniotic fluid PG and the L/S ratio in the assessment of fetal lung maturity. *Br. J. Obstet. Gynaec.*, **89**, 727.
Wiqvist, N. (1981) Preterm labour: other drug possibilities including drugs not to use. In *Preterm Labour*, eds. Elder, M.G. and Hendricks, C.H., 148. London: Butterworths.
Zuchermann, H., Reiss, U. and Rubinstein, I. (1974) Inhibition of human premature labour by indomethacin. *Obstet. Gynec.*, **44**, 787.

5

Pain Relief in Labour—Systemic and Inhalational Analgesia

SYSTEMIC ANALGESIA

It will be assumed that the reader has a knowledge of the general pharmacology of the commonly used analgesics, sedatives and tranquillizers. Some special aspects of pharmacology in obstetrics are considered in chapter 3. The present account is concerned with practical aspects of the use of drugs in the management of pain and anxiety in labour.

Despite the increasing use of epidural analgesia most British women have to depend on narcotic analgesics for the relief of pain in the first stage of labour. Analgesic drugs are commonly supplemented by inhalational analgesia towards the end of the first stage and in the second stage of labour. This is because the administration of analgesia is in most cases carried out by midwives who use the fairly simple and safe techniques approved by the National Boards for Nursing, Midwifery and Health Visiting. The effectiveness of these techniques has often proved disappointing in the opinion of the person who matters most, the patient. In one study on the efficiency of Entonox and intramuscular pethidine more than 75% of a large series of mothers said that they had obtained little or no relief from pethidine. Only 2% of these women had felt no pain and had been given no analgesic (Holdcroft and Morgan, 1974). Only 60% of a series of primigravidae who received liberal and frequent doses of narcotic analgesics on demand and inhalational analgesia later in labour were satisfied with the pain relief provided (Beazley et al, 1967).

Despite the often poor results of narcotic analgesia in labour it will be necessary for some years to direct efforts towards improving these results while at the same time making more effective techniques such as epidural analgesia available to more women. There is an unfulfilled need for a simple, safe and effective method of obstetric analgesia, suitable for use by midwives and junior obstetricians without special training in anaesthesia.

The relief of pain in labour by pharmacological means entails a compromise between the provision of effective analgesia and the avoidance of all risks to mother and child. The greatest restriction on the administration of powerful narcotic analgesics is that imposed by the free placental transfer of all drugs of this category and the resultant possibility of causing neonatal respiratory depression. Although the narcotic antagonists have improved the treatment of this type of respiratory depression it is preferable that the

129

condition should not arise. A further restriction upon the administration of depressant drugs to the mother is imposed by the impaired ability of the fetus and newborn to metabolize these drugs. The neonate may require three or four days to metabolize certain barbiturates. Pethidine given by intramuscular injection in the first stage of labour is associated with a mild, progressive maternal and fetal metabolic acidosis, and it is thought that this acidosis reflects the inadequacy of the pain relief obtained, because it does not occur with epidural analgesia (Pearson and Davies, 1973, 1974). More and more women have come to resent the drowsiness and disorientation frequently caused by narcotic analgesics and would prefer to participate actively in labour, even if this entails enduring some pain.

It is worth recalling that the ideal analgesic for use in labour does not exist because all analgesics, sedatives and tranquillizers cross the placental barrier. This unfortunate circumstance is explained by the need for these drugs to cross the blood–brain barrier to reach their site of action in the nervous system. The properties of the two biological barriers are similar with regard to the passage of drugs.

Drug-induced respiratory depression in the newborn is most likely to occur when delivery takes place about 3 hours after the intramuscular injection of pethidine to the mother (Roberts and Please, 1958; Shnider and Moya, 1964) and carbon dioxide retention is detectable at birth in infants whose mothers received pethidine up to 5 hours before delivery (Koch and

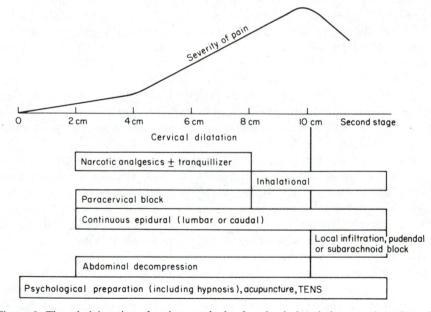

Figure 6. The administration of various methods of analgesia in relation to pain and cervical dilatation. Pain, rather than cervical dilatation, is the primary indication for analgesia. The effect of narcotic analgesia may persist until delivery (TENS = transcutaneous electrical nerve stimulation).

Wandel, 1968). After an intramuscular injection the levels of pethidine in the fetal blood average 77% of the maternal blood concentration (Apgar et al, 1952). An intravenous injection of pethidine results in extremely rapid placental transfer of the drug. Within 2 minutes the levels in maternal and fetal bloods are almost equal (Crawford and Rudofsky, 1965). The depressant effects of pethidine on the neonate may have sometimes been overemphasized and they can be reversed by naloxone.

It is now clear that pethidine depresses neurobehavioural responses in the newborn for up to 48 hours and that sucking, feeding and mother and infant interrelationships are all adversely affected, even in infants born with high Apgar scores (Brackbill et al, 1974; Corke, 1977; Wiener et al, 1977; Hodgkinson and Husain, 1982).

It is likely that the behaviour of all the narcotic analgesics is broadly similar to that just described for pethidine. Claims for the greater safety for the infant of one drug over another are often based mainly on the enthusiasm of the claimant. Equi-analgesic doses of the different narcotic analgesics have roughly equal respiratory depressant effects (Bonica, 1967). There is, however, evidence that the placental transfer of pentazocine is somewhat less than that of pethidine (Beckett and Taylor, 1967) and the clinical impression that morphine is particularly prone to depress neonatal respiration may be substantiated by the greater ability of morphine to penetrate the central nervous system of the infant (Way et al, 1965).

The indication for the administration of an analgesic drug in labour is pain. This statement of the obvious is not always acted upon. There are those who will not prescribe an analgesic for a woman in painful labour because the cervix is not dilated to some predetermined extent for fear that labour may be inhibited. This practice is condemned and rests on no sound basis. Analgesic drugs do not inhibit established uterine contractions and indeed they may improve the efficiency of incoordinate contractions. Only a very small minority of women experience no pain in labour and it is wrong to assume that the rather stoical 'good patient' does not need pain relief. The patient must be the judge of the severity of her pain and the effectiveness of the analgesic. The anaesthetist who is perhaps most familiar with postoperative pain should bear in mind that while that pain tends progressively to diminish, the pain of labour tends to increase as labour advances. Pain is often most severe towards the end of the first stage. A linear analogue is probably the most effective way of evaluating pain and pain relief in clinical studies. The patient marks on a 10 cm line the severity of her pain, graded from 'no pain at all' to 'as much as she can possibly imagine' (Revill et al, 1976) (Figure 6). The pain of labour can be extremely severe. In the view of Euripides a woman suffers more in childbirth than a soldier in the front rank of infantry in two hard battles. Melzack and his colleagues (1981) reported that the mean pain score of women in labour exceeded that of any painful pathological condition. This was also true of women who had attended classes in psychoprophylaxis and who experienced 30% less pain than unprepared women.

O'Driscoll (1975) has emphasized that good, personal care given continuously throughout labour by the obstetrician and midwife can reduce the need for analgesia because it reduces the emotional stress of fear and loneliness. He advocates the acceleration of established labour by oxytocin but is against the induction of labour, other than on medical grounds. If vaginal delivery has not taken place within 12 hours of the onset of labour, then caesarean section is performed. By all these means O'Driscoll claims to have substantially reduced the need for analgesic drugs.

There is a minority of women who will claim that pain is a necessary or even desired aspect of the experience of childbirth (Morgan et al, 1984). Doubtless the duration and severity of acceptable pain would vary with the individual. It is worthwhile to list some unphysiological and sometimes harmful effects of painful labour. These include:

Maternal and fetal acidosis
Raised catecholamine levels
Raised cortisol levels
Arterial hypertension
Increased oxygen requirements
Hyperventilation and hypocapnia
Decreased intervillous blood flow
Abnormal uterine action and prolonged labour

The concentration of endogenous opioids increases during painful labour suggesting that nature attempts to relieve this pain. While not seeking to impose any particular method of analgesia on a woman in normal labour there is a good case to be made for the physical and psychological value of pain relief, and no woman should hesitate to accept measures designed for the relief of pain. The woman who has had a pain-free labour is likely to be in a state of mind conducive to bonding with her newborn child.

Some individual analgesics

It is not proposed to detail the individual pharmacology of a long list of drugs. It will rarely be necessary to look beyond a short list of well established agents with which the user should be completely familiar. The advantages of one drug over another will often be related to the side-effects of the two drugs upon the mother, whether useful or unwanted, or the claimed but not always substantiated difference in the depressant effect of the drugs upon the newborn. One may accept the emetic sequelae and probably greater depressant effect of morphine because of its ability to relieve pain and anxiety in the anxious patient or one may choose pentazocine for its lower incidence of nausea and vomiting.

Pethidine. Pethidine remains the standard analgesic drug for obstetrics in Great Britain and its use by midwives is authorized by the National Boards for Nursing, Midwifery and Health Visiting. Midwives must comply with the Misuse of Drugs Regulations, 1973.

It is advocated that the first dose of pethidine should be 100 mg by intramuscular injection in the hope that this will relieve pain to a satisfactory extent. An intramuscular injection of 150 mg pethidine gave useful but incomplete relief of pain to 50–60% of mothers (Grant et al, 1970) and 50 to 100 mg pethidine was helpful to 40% of women in labour (Moore et al, 1970). Although perhaps slightly more effective, the 150 mg dose is more likely to cause unpleasant side-effects in the mother. Analgesia may be maintained by subsequent injections of 100 mg at intervals of approximately 3 hours. In this way the faith of the patient in her attendants and in the drug may not be lost. The first dose should be given when pain is becoming noticeable and not when it is already severe and becoming more severe. In view of the depressant effects of pethidine on the neonate and the relative ineffectiveness of pethidine as an analgesic in labour, it is unwise to give more than one or two intramuscular injections in labour unless there is no alternative form of analgesia available. Where possible, the need for a second dose of analgesic drug is an indication for epidural analgesia.

Nausea and vomiting occur in about half of the patients who receive pethidine in labour (Moore et al, 1970; Mowat and Garrey, 1970; Moore and Ball, 1974). Other maternal side-effects are uncommon after intramuscular injection although some hypoxia between contractions has been demonstrated (Huch et al, 1974). Some women will experience drowsiness, disorientation and loss of self-control which will cause them to resent the administration of pethidine. This resentment may be aggravated by failure to obtain adequate pain relief.

The placental transfer of pethidine is extensive, the fetal blood levels averaging 70% of those in the maternal blood (Apgar et al, 1952) and neonatal respiratory depression is likely to be greatest between 3 and 3.5 hours after injection. The depressant effect of pethidine on neurobehavioural functions and feeding in the neonate persists for 48 hours (Brackbill et al, 1974; Wiener et al, 1977). Naloxone reverses this effect and intramuscular injections may be repeated every 6 or 8 hours.

Pethidine and morphine, even in low doses, reduce the extent of beat-to-beat variability in the fetal heart rate in labour (Petrie et al, 1978). Fetal heart rate variability is an important indicator of fetal wellbeing and therefore the influence of drugs is of practical significance.

The relative inefficiency of pethidine as an analgesic in labour has been demonstrated by Holdcroft and Morgan (1974). In what may be a unique, randomized controlled trial of analgesia in labour, pethidine and Entonox were significantly less effective than epidural analgesia, and the incidence of feelings of deprivation was unaffected by the method of pain relief (Robinson et al, 1980a). The incidence of postpartum perineal discomfort was similar in the two groups. The forceps delivery rate was higher in those who received epidural analgesia with 0.5% bupivacaine, a concentration which is associated with more frequent instrumental deliveries (Thorburn and Moir, 1981). A weaker concentration of bupivacaine might well have reduced the forceps delivery rate. Poor analgesia is quite often associated with unwanted drowsiness and an unpleasant dissociated state (O'Driscoll and Stronge, 1973). Loss of self-control without effective relief of pain is a complaint of some articulate mothers. Uterine action is not inhibited and may be enhanced. Nalorphine, levallorphan and naloxone are antagonists.

Pentazocine. The use of pentazocine as an alternative to pethidine is accepted and this drug has been approved by the National Board for Nursing, Midwifery and Health Visiting for England and Wales. The advantages claimed for pentazocine are a much lower incidence of nausea and vomiting (Moore et al, 1970; Mowat and Garrey, 1970; Moore and Ball, 1974), a less extensive placental transfer (Beckett and Taylor, 1967) and the absence of liability to produce addiction. The condition of the infant at birth may be no better after pentazocine than after pethidine (Duncan et al, 1969). According to Filler et al (1967) pentazocine does not inhibit uterine contractions and does not alter the fetal heart rate even when given intravenously. Pentazocine 40 mg is claimed to be as effective as 100 mg pethidine; better results may be obtained from 60 mg pentazocine. The Misuse of Drugs Regulations do not apply to pentazocine. Hallucinations are an occasional unwelcome side-effect.

There is a suggestion that the respiratory depressant action of pentazocine may be limited. When the drug was given in doses of 40 mg/70 kg body weight, respiratory depression was maximal and higher doses did not increase the depressant action (Ominsky et al, 1969). The concept of a maximal depressant dose was also substantiated by Refstad and Lindbaeck (1980) who found that neonatal respiratory depression reached a plateau level after 60 mg/kg maternal weight. It is postulated that pentazocine at first combines with agonist receptors producing analgesia and depressant effects and that higher doses subsequently combine with antagonist receptors. Nalaxone is an effective antagonist. Methylphenidate (Ritalin) has some antagonistic action but is no longer marketed. Nalorphine and levallorphan are ineffective. Pentazocine is not extensively used in obstetrics, despite some earlier enthusiasm.

Meptazinol. This new analgesic has been promoted as offering relief of pain with little or no respiratory depression. Such a claim arouses a healthy scepticism and a sense of 'déja vu'. Nevertheless early experiences seem quite encouraging. Meptazinol was found by Jordan and others (1979) to cause less respiratory depression than pentazocine or morphine. A double-blind, randomized trial of intramuscular pethidine and meptazinol in 360 women in labour indicated that meptazinol gave superior analgesia in the first hour after injection and that thereafter the pain relief was similar (Nicholas and Robson, 1982). The duration of analgesia was similar, as was the incidence of nausea and vomiting. Neonatal assessments were inconclusive although there were more high 1-minute Apgar scores after meptazinol. Further trials are required.

Morphine. Because of its ability to relieve anxiety and pain, morphine retains a place in the management of prolonged labour by traditional means and is still prescribed for the anxious primigravida in early labour. Unfortunately morphine seems to have a particular propensity towards depressing neonatal respiration, perhaps because of its greater ability to penetrate the infant's brain (Way et al, 1965) and it is customary to restrict the administration of morphine to occasions when delivery is not anticipated within the ensuing 5 hours. Nalorphine, levallorphan and naloxone are antagonists. The modern, active management of labour has greatly reduced the need for morphine.

Heroin (diamorphine). Heroin retains a small place in British obstetrics because of its outstanding ability to relieve anxiety in the terrified and weeping patient. A dose of 5 mg induces marked euphoria without also producing drowsiness. The narcotic antagonists are effective. Heroin has been found to be the most effective of the narcotic analgesics (Beazley et al, 1967) but it is not recommended for routine use.

Other analgesics. The only advantage of any of the narcotic analgesics over the standard drugs such as pethidine, morphine and pentazocine may be in the incidence of maternal side-effects in relation to their analgesic action. It is unlikely that equianalgesic doses produce more or less neonatal respiratory depression. Oxymorphone probably causes less vomiting than the parent morphine. Methadone and alphaprodine have not been shown to have any clear advantages in labour. Dihydrocodeine (DF 118) in doses of 30–60 mg is said to cause less vomiting and less respiratory depression than equivalent doses of morphine and pethidine. The analgesic potency of dihydrocodeine is rather less than that of morphine and pethidine, and larger doses of dihydrocodeine may cause profound hypotension.

Intravenous analgesia

Single intravenous injections of pethidine are liable to produce vomiting and hypotension in the mother and are associated with extremely rapid and extensive placental transfer (Crawford and Rudofsky, 1965; Moore and Ball, 1974). Single intravenous injections of pentazocine are rather less severe in their effects, but are not without danger (Moore and Ball, 1974). The infant may be adversely affected by the direct depressant effect of the analgesic drug upon its brain or by the reduction in placental blood flow which may result from maternal hypotension. It may be possible to reduce the rate of placental transfer of drug by giving the intravenous injection during a uterine contraction when the uteroplacental blood flow is diminished. The intravenous administration, over a 10-minute period of up to 50 mg pethidine diluted in 10 ml of water for injection, is occasionally justified if pain is very severe, inhalational analgesia is inadequate and epidural analgesia is unavailable.

It is considered that continuous dilute infusion of a narcotic analgesic is likely to be safer and perhaps more effective than a single intravenous injection. A continuous drip of 100 mg or 200 mg of pethidine in 500 ml of a suitable fluid was advocated by Jeffcoate et al in 1952. An infusion of pethidine 175 mg, promethazine 100 mg, scopolamine 0.6 mg and levallorphan 2 mg has been used but the incidence of over-sedation was unacceptably high (Zarou et al, 1967). An ingenious drip clamp which allows the patient to control her own pethidine dosage has been described (Scott, 1970). The use of electronic drip rate counters and motor driven syringes should improve the control over dosage with continuous intravenous techniques. Continuous intravenous analgesia has a place in obstetric practice if more effective alternatives to intermittent intramuscular injections are unavailable or are contraindicated. Encouraging results have been claimed for patient-controlled intermittent intravenous injections of pethidine. Doses of 15–25 mg at intervals of at least 10 minutes can give complete or considerable relief to 73% of mothers, and the duration of the injection can be prolonged to 3 or 4 minutes to reduce maternal–fetal concentration gradients (Evans et al, 1976; Rosen, 1979). In a subsequent randomized, controlled trial self-administered pethidine 0.25 mg/kg at intervals of 10 minutes or more was not significantly more effective than intramuscular pethidine, although maternal ratings favoured the intravenous route (Robinson et al, 1980b). The total dose requirements were lower with the intravenous technique. The apparatus is available as the Cardiff Palliator and it has been successfully used in a general practitioner unit (Harper et al, 1983).

The narcotic antagonists

The limitations imposed by the depressant action of the narcotic analgesics have been lessened, although not abolished, by the introduction of the narcotic antagonists. The availability of an effective antagonist will often influence the choice of drug for use in labour. The established antagonists nalorphine and levallorphan and the recently introduced naloxone are compounds in clinical use. Naloxone is the preferred agent.

Nalorphine and levallorphan. These *N*-allyl derivatives of the narcotic analgesics morphine and levorphanol are capable of reversing the already existing depressant effects of the various opioid analgesics (but not of pentazocine). The antagonistic action of a single injection may be quite short-lived and the dose ratio of agonist to antagonist is critical. The antagonist itself may depress respiration when given in excess or when given to a patient whose respiratory depression is due to a cause other than the prior administration of an opioid drug. For these reasons and because of the difficulty of predicting the occurrence of neonatal respiratory depression with any accuracy, the prophylactic administration of the antagonist to the mother shortly before delivery as formerly advocated is not advised. A narcotic antagonist should be given to the newborn infant who demonstrates respiratory depression which is considered likely to be caused by a narcotic analgesic given during labour. Nalorphine and levallorphan are no longer recommended because they can produce respiratory depression when given in inappropriate circumstances.

Naloxone. This *N*-allyl derivative of oxymorphone differs significantly from nalorphine and levallorphan in having absolutely no morphine-like action when given alone (Jasinski and Martin, 1967; Jasinski et al, 1967). A second important attribute of naloxone is its ability to antagonize the narcotic effects of pentazocine as well as those of the various opioid drugs. Payne (1973) views the use of pentazocine, with its restricted potential for respiratory depression, and naloxone, with its safe antagonism of pentazocine (and other narcotics), as offering a greater degree of safety in obstetric practice than has hitherto been achieved and naloxone is now the narcotic antagonist of choice.

The following suggested doses of the three narcotic antagonists will antagonize approximately 100 mg pethidine or the equivalent dose of other analgesics. Only naloxone is effective against pentazocine.

	Mother	*Newborn*
Levallorphan	0.5–1 mg	0.05–0.1 mg
Nalorphine	5–10 mg	0.25–0.5 mg
Naloxone	0.4 mg	0.04 mg

It may be necessary to attempt to titrate the dose of the antagonist against that of the agonist. Neonatal injections are most effectively made into the umbilical vein although this procedure is not without risk. Intramuscular injections may result in inadequate absorption of the drug. The short action of naloxone suggests that an intravenous injection of 0.04 mg may usefully be accompanied by an intramuscular injection of 0.2 mg in order to prolong the effect.

When naloxone is given intramuscularly to the neonate in the relatively very large dose of 0.2 mg, the depressant effects of intrapartum pethidine on behavioural patterns and in particular on the establishment of feeding are prevented (Wiener et al, 1977, 1979).

Narcotic and antagonist mixtures (Pethilorfan). The mixture of 100 mg pethidine and 1.25 mg levallorphan in 2 ml of solvent (Pethilorfan) was quite extensively used in obstetrics and is still approved by the National Board for

Nursing, Midwifery and Health Visiting for England and Wales. It has been claimed that Pethilorfan can give analgesia without respiratory depression. Unfortunately this claim does not stand up to close inspection (Clark et al, 1968). The effect of narcotic and antagonist mixtures seems to depend upon the proportions of the two drugs in the mixture. In the case of pethidine and levallorphan mixtures an excess of antagonist enhances depression; an excess of pethidine does result in some reduction in the depressant effect of the mixture. A balanced mixture of pethidine and levallorphan produces the same degree of respiratory depression as that dose of pethidine would if given alone (Rouge et al, 1969). In healthy volunteers the respiratory depression of Pethilorfan was slightly greater than that of pethidine alone (Campbell et al, 1965). It is also widely held that the analgesic action of Pethilorfan is less than that of pethidine (Baker, 1957; Bullough, 1959; Hamilton et al, 1967). The continued use of Pethilorfan can no longer be justified on any rational basis.

Although naloxone is free of inherent depressant action, pethidine-naloxone mixtures have proved disappointing. A mixture of pethidine 100 mg and naloxone 0.4 mg given intramuscularly in labour gave less pain relief than pethidine 100 mg, and the incidence of side-effects was little different (Girvan et al, 1976).

Endogenous opioids. These natural analgesics are polypeptides and include the enkephalins and the endorphins. The concentration of endorphins increases during labour and seems to be a natural attempt at pain relief. This may suggest that pain is not a phenomenon which should be preserved. The presence of endorphins in the placenta and in cord blood suggests a role in the relief of fetal pain during delivery. β-Endorphin levels are lower in women who receive pethidine during labour and are highest in those who receive nitrous oxide (Thomas and Fletcher, 1983). Does nitrous oxide owe its analgesic action to the release of endorphins?

Sedatives and tranquillizers

The decision to give a sedative, hypnotic or tranquillizer drug to a woman in labour should be preceded by a consideration of the needs of that patient. The administration of any depressant drug in labour carries a statistically increased risk of causing depression in the newborn (Shnider and Moya, 1964) and therefore the giving of a sedative or tranquillizer routinely to every patient is difficult to justify. (There are of course no effective specific antidotes to these drugs presently available and their action may be greatly prolonged in the fetus and the newborn.) Antagonists to the benzodiazepines have been developed, but are not yet freely available. Their duration of action is considerably shorter than that of the benzodiazepines (Ashton, 1985).

Among the reasons for giving a sedative, hypnotic or tranquillizer are:

To allay fear and anxiety.
To promote sleep in early labour.
To provide amnesia.
To treat hypertension.
To prevent convulsions.
To obtain an antiemetic effect.

Fear and anxiety. Those who administer a tranquillizer such as promazine or promethazine routinely in labour would argue that all women are anxious or afraid during childbirth. There is evidence that the fetuses of primates (rhesus monkeys) subjected to a psychological stress may then develop acidosis and bradycardia, indicating that intervillous blood flow diminished, perhaps as the result of uterine artery constriction induced by catecholamines (Morishima et al, 1978). Anxiety is best relieved by antenatal preparation, the presence of a sympathetic attendant and the promise of adequate analgesia. If these criteria can be met, then anxiolytic drugs will often be unnecessary. It is, of course, usually unwise to give a sedative drug without providing relief for coexisting pain and most of the narcotic analgesics have a sedative as well as a pain-relieving action.

Sleep. In early or premonitory labour it may occasionally be desirable to prescribe a hypnotic drug when labour is not to be stimulated with oxytocin and especially at night. A non-barbiturate hypnotic will be safer for the child whose hepatic enzymes will be inefficient in breaking down barbiturates and barbiturates should no longer be prescribed in normal labour.

Amnesia. Several of the drugs which may be prescribed in labour will promote amnesia in a proportion of recipients. The obsolete technique of twilight sleep was based on the production of total amnesia for the events of an often long and painful labour by the injection of a single dose of morphine and hyoscine, followed by later injections of hyoscine only. Certainly the memory of a long and painful labour has in the past caused women to avoid all further pregnancies (Jeffcoate et al, 1952) but the idea that pain is of no importance if it is not consciously remembered is no longer acceptable. The modern aim is to have a mother who is free from pain, free of fear and fully involved in the events concerning the birth of a wished-for child.

Hypertension. Sedatives and tranquillizers are now seldom used in the treatment of hypertension in pregnancy. This is principally because the effectiveness of these drugs in controlling hypertension is slight and the depressant effect upon the fetus is unwelcome. The value of prolonged bed rest for moderate hypertension is doubtful. The treatment of hypertension is discussed in chapter 9.

Anticonvulsants. Certain sedatives have an accepted place in the prevention and treatment of eclampsia because of their anticonvulsant action. The barbiturates have been largely replaced by chlormethiazole, phenytoin and diazepam in the modern management of severe pre-eclampsia. Rectal bromethol has joined the ranks of obsolete treatments. The management of pre-eclampsia is considered in chapter 9.

Antiemetic action. The phenothiazines such as promethazine, trifluoperazine, perphenazine and prochlorperazine, the butyrophenones droperidol and haloperidol, and the antihistamine cyclizine are helpful in the prevention and treatment of the nausea and vomiting which may occur in as many as 50% of women who receive narcotic analgesics in labour (Moore and Ball, 1974). Not all sickness in labour is due to the administration of drugs. The cause is often obscure and antiemetic drugs are not always indicated.

Some individual sedatives and tranquillizers

Familiarity with the general properties and actions of these groups of drugs is assumed and, as with the narcotic analgesics, a small number of familiar drugs will be adequate for almost all purposes. It is proposed to concentrate on the uses of the various categories of drugs in labour. The placental transfer and the influence of these drugs on uterine action are discussed in some detail in chapter 3. It may be recalled that all of these drugs can be expected to cross the placenta and that they do not inhibit the uterine contractions of established labour.

Current opinion mainly holds that sedatives and tranquillizers are not indicated in normal labour. 'Normal labour' is of course sometimes accelerated and artificially shortened so that fear and anxiety are lessened, and the element of loneliness is usually minimized by the presence of the father and a sympathetic attendant. The knowledge that labour will not be permitted to last for more than perhaps 12 hours can be of enormous encouragement to an anxious woman in pain (O'Driscoll and Stronge, 1973).

Chloral hydrate. Chloral hydrate, triclofos (Tricloryl) and dichloralphenazone (Welldorm) are converted into trichlorethanol after absorption from the gut and it is trichloroethanol which is responsible for the mild, safe sedative and hypnotic action of these three drugs. Chloral hydrate is only obtainable in liquid form (syrup of chloral) and is now seldom used because it has an unpleasant taste and is a gastric irritant. Triclofos and dichloralphenazone tablets are preferred. Welldorm tablets contain 1.3 g dichloralphenazone and 0.65 g chloral hydrate. These drugs may be prescribed by midwives on their own initiative and are then used as a simple oral sedative in early labour. They are a safe alternative to the barbiturates for use in labour.

Chlormethiazole (Heminevrin) has been given by mouth in the form of 500 mg capsules as a simple, safe sedative in labour. The anticonvulsant properties of chlormethiazole have been known to psychiatrists for some time for the treatment of delirious and confused states. It is in the management of severe pre-eclampsia that chlormethiazole finds its principal application in obstetrics. Chlormethiazole is then used as an 0.8% solution by intravenous infusion, solely as a sedative and anticonvulsant. The drug possesses no analgesic action and hypotension does not occur in normal dosage (Wilson et al, 1969).

The barbiturates. The administration of a short- or medium-acting barbiturate as a sedative or hypnotic in labour can now rarely be justified. This is because of the protracted action of this group of drugs on the newborn. Placental transfer is free and uterine action is not inhibited when labour is established. If a sedative or hypnotic is required in labour there are now many safer agents available. A choice might be made from nitrazepam, triclofos, dichloralphenazone, one of the phenothiazine derivatives, diazepam or lorazepam.

In the past the barbiturates had been liberally prescribed for patients with pre-eclampsia both before and during labour. This practice is now happily abandoned. The effectiveness of barbiturates in the treatment of pre-eclampsia is perhaps no greater than the effectiveness of rest in bed. Hypertension is usually not effectively controlled and the cumulative depressant effect upon the fetus may be considerable. The barbiturates have often been prescribed for their anticonvulsant action, especially during labour in patients with severe pre-eclampsia. Chlormethiazole and diazepam should be preferred for this purpose. A barbiturate may be administered after delivery. Midwives are not authorized to prescribe barbiturates.

Diazepam (Valium) Early reports on the use of diazepam as a sedative in labour were favourable and it was said to reduce the requirement for pethidine and to do no harm to the infant (Bepko et al, 1965; Nisbet et al, 1967). Later reports were in conflict over the efficacy of diazepam in labour. According to Niswander (1969) and to Flowers et al (1969) when intermittent injections of pethidine and diazepam are given during labour the pethidine requirement is much lower than is the case when the injections consist of pethidine and a placebo. In the study carried out by Elder and Crossley (1969) pethidine and diazepam injections were no more effective than injections of pethidine and a placebo, the pethidine requirements were not reduced and amnesia was not a feature. Lee (1968) also found diazepam to be of no value.

In a double-blind trial diazepam was found to improve the mothers' opinion of the pain-relieving qualities of pethidine but the dose requirements of pethidine were unaltered (Davies and Rosen, 1977). It is probable that 5–10 mg diazepam does exert a tranquillizing effect but that pethidine analgesia is not potentiated. Intramuscular injections are slowly and erratically absorbed and intravenous administration is preferable (Gamble et al, 1975; Sturdee, 1976). Uncertain absorption from muscle may explain the divergent experiences with diazepam.

As experience with diazepam has increased, several potentially serious risks for the newborn have been recognized which may do more than any debate about its effectiveness as a sedative to diminish the use of diazepam in labour. Concentrations of diazepam in fetal blood and tissues often substantially exceed the maternal concentrations because the drug is extensively bound to fetal proteins. Hypotonia, lethargy, respiratory depression and apnoea have all been observed in the neonate after the administration of diazepam in labour (McCarthy et al, 1973) and these effects may all result from poor muscle tone. Neonatal hypothermia has been reported (Owen and Irani, 1972) and this too may be due to hypotonia or the cause may lie in a central action of diazepam on the heat-regulating mechanism. During labour there may be a loss of the normal beat-to-beat variations in fetal heart rate (Scher et al, 1972) and this may indicate a loss of adaptability of the circulatory system. It has been suggested that the sodium benzoate in which diazepam is dissolved may uncouple bilirubin from albumin (Adoni et al, 1973) although this may not occur in vivo because benzyl benzoate is readily broken down in the liver. The elimination of bilirubin may be impaired by diazepam because both the drug and the pigment are conjugated with glucuronic acid before excretion (Erkkola and Kanto, 1972). Raised levels, particularly of unconjugated bilirubin, could result in kernicterus in the newborn.

It is likely that these potentially hazardous effects are dose-related and it is probably safe to use diazepam if the dose in labour is restricted to 30 mg. In view of the numerous other sedatives and tranquillizers available it seems inadvisable to use diazepam routinely although its use as an anticonvulsant by infusion or by intermittent intravenous injection in severe pre-eclampsia is warranted. Intravenous diazepam is given by some obstetricians before artificial rupture of the membranes. While often effective in calming the anxious patient there is a risk of overdose with depression of reflexes and loss of consciousness, and close supervision of the patient is necessary.

Midazolam (Hypnovel). This agent has a shorter half-life than diazepam and has not been extensively studied in obstetrics. The placental transfer of midazolam is rather restricted and fetal/maternal ratios average 0.15 (Vree et al, 1984). The amnesic effect of midazolam exceeds that of diazepam, but amnesia is rarely required in modern obstetric practice.

Nitrazepam (Mogadon). Although nitrazepam, like diazepam, is a benzodiazepine derivative there have been no reports of any special hazards for the newborn with nitrazepam. The low toxicity of nitrazepam makes it a suitable sedative or hypnotic for administration by mouth in early labour if this is required.

Lorazepam (Ativan). When a 2 mg tablet of lorazepam was given early in labour the analgesic action of subsequently administered pethidine was enhanced (McAuley et al, 1982). The incidence of amnesia was increased and there was an insignificant rise in the number of infants with signs of respiratory depression.

Chlordiazepoxide (Librium), a benzodiazepine derivative, has been found to be of little value as a tranquillizer in labour (Mark and Hamel, 1968). An intravenous infusion of chlordiazepoxide has been successfully used in the control of severe pre-eclampsia and eclampsia (Lean et al, 1968a,b).

The phenothiazine derivatives have several properties which may be useful in labour. They have been widely prescribed for their sedative and anxiolytic properties and they may be administered for their antiemetic and antihistaminic actions. They have been used in the management of pre-eclampsia and eclampsia. The near-routine use of tranquillizers has decreased in recent years.

Promazine (Sparine) and promethazine (Phenergan) were commonly used along with pethidine to enhance sedation and, it is sometimes claimed, to reduce the requirements for pethidine. MacVicar and Murray (1960) claimed that a mixture of 50 mg pethidine with 50 mg promazine was superior to 100 mg pethidine alone and Matthews (1963) could distinguish between promazine and a placebo given in labour. The effectiveness of promazine has been disputed by McQuitty (1967) but most clinicians would agree that the drug has a calming and perhaps a 'pethidine-sparing' action. It is well known that under experimental conditions promazine was shown to have an analgesic action and to potentiate the analgesic effect of pethidine, and that promethazine actually had an antianalgesic action (Moore and Dundee, 1961a,b; Dundee and Moore, 1962). The relevance of these observations on artificial pain to the pain of labour may be questioned but they may constitute grounds for preferring promazine to promethazine.

The extent to which anxiety may exaggerate pain is well-known and it may be that the clinically often apparent 'analgesic' action of the phenothiazine derivatives and of other sedatives is sometimes the result of their anxiolytic properties rather than a true analgesic effect. The phenothiazine derivatives cross the placenta and it therefore seems unwise to prescribe them routinely for all women in labour. Ideally anxiety should be prevented by antenatal preparation and the presence of sympathetic attendants and an understanding husband or partner. In practice it may be necessary to attempt to allay anxiety by the use of drugs, promazine is then a suitable choice. The National Board for Nursing, Midwifery and Health Visiting for England and Wales has authorized the prescribing of promazine by midwives.

Where an antiemetic action is required a phenothiazine derivative with a piperazine side-chain may be used and a choice may be made from perphenazine (Fentazin), prochlorperazine (Stemetil, Compazine) and trifluoperazine (Stelazine). Promethazine was as effective as metoclopramide in preventing nausea and vomiting when pethidine was given during labour, but the analgesic effect of pethidine was reduced by promethazine (Vella et al, 1985).

Hypotension is uncommon after the intramuscular injection of the commonly used phenothiazine derivatives although mixtures of one or two phenothiazine derivatives with pethidine have been used in the treatment of severe pre-eclampsia and eclampsia.

INHALATIONAL ANALGESIA

Inhalational analgesia in the UK is administered very largely by midwives and therefore the agents and the apparatus used are almost always those approved by the National Board for Nursing, Midwifery and Health Visiting. The following account is therefore concerned mainly with inhalational analgesia as used by midwives. It is necessary that anaesthetists should be familiar with the techniques available to midwives and with the regulations concerning the use of these methods. The anaesthetist must of course concern himself with any drugs administered to his patients and anaesthetists have often been involved in the design of apparatus and in efforts to improve the efficacy of all forms of analgesia. The instruction of midwives in the methods of pain relief in labour is regarded by the National Board for Nursing, Midwifery and Health Visiting as a duty of the anaesthetist and it is recommended that student midwives should receive four lectures from an anaesthetist.

Approval was withdrawn for the use of trichloroethylene (Trilene) by British midwives in 1984 and in that year methoxyflurane (Penthrane) became unavailable. In practice, therefore, the only agent currently available for use by midwives in the UK is Entonox.

Nitrous oxide

Nitrous oxide is now always administered with oxygen and mainly in the form of premixed gases from the Entonox apparatus. The Entonox apparatus is approved for use by midwives in all parts of the UK. The Lucy Baldwin apparatus has been approved for unsupervised use by midwives in Northern Ireland only. The approval for the use of nitrous oxide and air mixtures by midwives was withdrawn in 1970.

Apparatus for nitrous oxide analgesia

The Lucy Baldwin apparatus was developed as an intermittent flow apparatus for the self-administration of nitrous oxide and oxygen in the hope that it would prove suitable for use by midwives as a safer and more powerful alternative to the gas and air apparatus. The apparatus has only been fully approved for use by midwives in Northern Ireland.

The two gases are not premixed but are supplied from separate cylinders and mixed in a mixing chamber. The oxygen content of the mixture is normally variable between 30% and 50%. Pure oxygen may also be delivered and, after unlocking a safety lock, a mixture containing 20% oxygen in nitrous oxide may be obtained for use only by a doctor. The apparatus is a modified Walton Five apparatus and is named after the Countess Baldwin of Bewdley, founder of the Anaesthetics Appeal Fund of the National Birthday Trust. The Lucy Baldwin apparatus is acceptably accurate at the high minute volumes which are usual in women in painful labour (McAneny and Doughty, 1963; Moir and Bissett, 1965) but at minute volumes below 5 litres, the oxygen percentage actually delivered may be significantly lower than is indicated by the dial setting (Cole et al, 1970). A safety device permits the entrainment of room air if the supply of either gas fails.

The Entonox apparatus. The familiar Entonox apparatus is approved by the National Board for Nursing, Midwifery and Health Visiting.

The apparatus was developed by Tunstall (1961) from demand valves used in underwater swimming. There is a cylinder of premixed nitrous oxide and oxygen, present in equal proportions and evenly mixed. There is also a head comprising a pressure-reducing valve, a demand valve and a cylinder contents gauge. A non-interchangeable pin-index system is used to prevent the administration of the wrong gas. The Entonox apparatus is compact and robust and generally of sound design. The resistance of the valves to breathing, although variable, is always acceptably low at any flow rates likely to be required in labour (Davies et al, 1974a,b). The resistance of the apparatus falls well below the calculated upper limits of acceptable resistance to laminar flow of 0.26 cmH$_2$O/litre/min (0.05 kPa/litre/min) (Hogg et al, 1974). This low resistance makes breathing feel easy even at high flow rates and is important in making the apparatus acceptable to the patient. The Entonox apparatus, with additions, has formed the basis of readily portable equipment for the administration of general anaesthesia in domiciliary obstetrics (Davidson et al, 1970; Whitford et al, 1973) and obstetric and accident flying squads.

The gas mixture supplied by the Entonox apparatus is normally sufficiently constant for clinical purposes and the only recognized hazard is associated with excessive cooling of the cylinder. Cooling to below $-7°C$ causes separation of the two gases. The heavier nitrous oxide then gravitates to the lowermost part of the cylinder. If the cylinder is then used the emergent gas mixture will at first consist mostly of oxygen until, when the cylinder is almost empty, the issuing gas will be almost pure nitrous oxide (Gale et al, 1964). It has been suggested that the separation may be less complete if the cylinder is horizontal.

Temperatures of $-7°C$ or lower may be anticipated on perhaps 10 or 20 nights of the year in many parts of the British Isles and they occur regularly in parts of North America and Scandinavia. No satisfactory device has yet been produced to give warning that cooling has occurred and reliance must therefore be placed mainly upon the avoidance of exposure to cold.

A subcommittee of the Medical Research Council on Nitrous Oxide/Oxygen Analgesia in Midwifery has made precise recommendations on the handling and storing of premixed gas cylinders (Cole et al, 1970). Because of their importance certain recommendations are quoted in detail:

500-litre cylinders (These are small cylinders intended for domiciliary use).

(1) If a cylinder of premixed oxygen and nitrous oxide has been exposed to cold the two gases may separate. Observation of the following procedure will ensure safety at any time of the year. The gases may be remixed by warming the cylinder to a safe temperature and then agitating the contents by inverting the cylinder three times. A safe temperature is achieved by keeping the cylinder either in the delivery room or in a room above 10°C (50°F) for at least 2 hours before use, or by placing it in warm water at body temperature for 5 minutes. Hot water should not be used and care should be taken not to allow water into the valve.

(2) The following warning label should be indelibly attached to all 500-litre cylinders: '*Do not store in the open. Always protect from cold. Immediately before use ensure that the cylinder has been adequately warmed and then invert it completely three times. Never use grease or oil on the valve.*'

The responsibility for the safe handling and storage of the 500-litre cylinders rests with the user.

2000-litre and 5000-litre cylinders (cylinders for hospital use).

(1) On receipt, the cylinders should be date-marked and, before use, stored in a horizontal position for 24 hours in an area maintained at a temperature above 10°C (50°F) but not exceeding 45°C (113°F).

(2) During delivery from the storage area to the final destination point in the hospital the cylinder must not be exposed to a freezing temperature for more than 10 minutes.

The responsibility for the safe storage and handling of these larger cylinders is placed upon the hospital authority. The manufacturer is specifically excluded from responsibility. Cooling may occur during transportation to the hospital and this is the reason for requiring storage for 24 hours in a warm atmosphere before use. When used in a piped gas system with multiple outlets there is the possibility that a high rate of usage might cause cooling in the master cylinder and it is suggested that some form of flow restriction should be employed. In practice this possibility is now virtually eliminated by the limitation of flow to a maximum of 300 litres/min in pipeline installations (McGregor et al, 1972).

Cylinder requirements. The average volume of gas used in a home confinement has been found to be about 500 litres. This figure of course may vary widely but it is recommended that a midwife should take two 500-litre cylinders to the house.

The technique of nitrous oxide analgesia

Expectant mothers should be instructed in the techniques of inhalational analgesia during pregnancy and most hospitals offer this instruction to women who attend the antenatal clinic. It is important that complete pain relief from inhalational analgesia should not be promised to all patients. Practical demonstration of the apparatus used should reduce the common fear of the mask and encourage correct use of the equipment. The UK Joint Council for Nursing, Midwifery and Health Visiting advises that pregnant women should inhale Entonox only when in labour and that neither patients nor midwives should inhale Entonox while receiving or giving antenatal instruction. It may be possible to modify the Entonox apparatus to allow the inhalation of air or oxygen for instructional purposes. It is with regrettable frequency that one sees a patient breathing air because the face mask is not in proper contact with her face. Objection to the rubber face mask is common and a more acceptable improvement is a disposable mouth-piece in the form of a tube which is held between the teeth (Dolan and Rosen, 1975). The device is recommended and has been approved, in 1985, by the Joint Council for Nursing, Midwifery and Health Visiting.

The basis for effective intermittent inhalational analgesia with nitrous oxide is that some 45 seconds are necessary for the attainment of a near-maximal analgesic effect. This was stressed from practical experience by Minnitt in 1933 and has been calculated on theoretical grounds by Waud and Waud (1970). It is therefore necessary that the inhalation of nitrous oxide should begin about 45 seconds before pain is experienced. In the first stage of labour it is recommended that the initial painless phase of the uterine

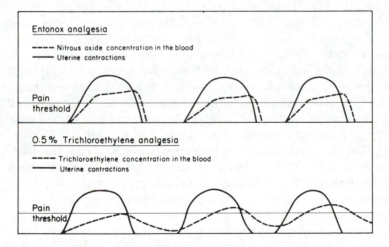

Figure 7. Entonox analgesia. A diagrammatic representation of the analgesic action of Entonox and trichloroethylene. Note that nitrous oxide very rapidly reaches analgesic concentrations in the blood and that the concentration falls rapidly between contractions. In contrast, the trichloroethylene concentration rises slowly, does not fall to zero between contractions and tends to accumulate in blood and tissues.

contractions be used to permit the build-up of an analgesic concentration of nitrous oxide. The inhalation is, of course, continued during the painful phase of the contraction (see Figure 7). Analgesia will not be satisfactory if inhalation is not begun until pain is present. This technique is based upon the fact that nitrous oxide is a relatively insoluble gas whose uptake and excretion are very rapid. Deep and relatively slow breathing should be encouraged in preference to the shallow and rapid respiratory pattern which some women adopt. Extreme hyperventilation may be harmful to the fetus (Morishima et al, 1963; Moya et al, 1965) and maternal tetany may occur. Analgesia wears off rapidly when the inhalation of nitrous oxide ceases, and the same pattern of administration must be repeated with each contraction. In the expulsive phase of the second stage of labour it will be necessary to encourage the patient to take two or three deep inhalations of the gas before each expulsive effort. The patient may breathe in and out from the mask during the crowning of the head. Inhalational analgesia may be helpful during vaginal examination, delivery of the placenta and other procedures which may be associated with discomfort. Nitrous oxide analgesia is not suitable by itself for forceps delivery, perineal suture and manual removal of the placenta, although it may be helpful during forceps or breech delivery under pudendal nerve block. Artificial rupture of the membranes causes pain to about 25% of mothers (Caseby, 1974) and the inhalation of nitrous oxide will then be helpful.

The inhalation of 50% nitrous oxide in oxygen for 5 minutes did not depress the laryngeal closure reflex (Cleaton-Jones, 1976), although the continuous inhalation of this mixture for 30 minutes did permit the entry of a radio-opaque dye into the trachea and bronchi of 2 out of 10 volunteers (Rubin et al, 1977). It seems unlikely that Entonox would depress laryngeal reflexes when inhaled intermittently, although the possibility cannot be excluded in mothers who have received narcotic and sedative drugs.

Nitrous oxide, unlike trichloroethylene and methoxyflurane, does not accumulate in the maternal and fetal tissues and there need be no restriction on the time over which it is used in labour. Although it is at present customary to restrict the administration of nitrous oxide to the second stage and the late part of the first stage of labour, it would be perfectly safe, and in some cases helpful, to use nitrous oxide analgesia for the greater part of the entire labour. The National Board for Nursing, Midwifery and Health Visiting impose no limit on the duration of Entonox analgesia. The inhalation of 50% oxygen may be beneficial to the fetus, especially if the fetus is hypoxic; Philips and Macdonald (1971) found evidence to support this contention.

The effectiveness of nitrous oxide analgesia. There is now a willingness to admit that nitrous oxide analgesia is often imperfect, and to accept that the explanation may lie with the agent and not always with the patient or the technique of administration. This more honest approach may be in part related to the wider availability of more effective analgesic methods such as epidural analgesia.

Nitrous oxide alone was twice as effective as pethidine alone in Holdcroft and Morgan's series (1974) where it was found that 22.4% of patients claimed satisfactory relief of pain from intramuscular injections of 100 mg or 150 mg pethidine, and 46.2% of women assessed analgesia with Entonox only as satisfactory. The earlier administration of pethidine did not alter the effectiveness of Entonox analgesia. Almost half (47.7%) of the patients claimed no pain relief from pethidine and 30% found Entonox analgesia completely ineffective. There is close agreement between Holdcroft and Morgan's findings and the results of the Medical Research Council's Subcommittee (Cole et al, 1970). These are summarized here:

Analgesia	MRC (1970)	Holdcroft and Morgan (1974)
Satisfactory	54%	46%
Slight	16%	18%
None	30%	30%

The administration of a 70:30 nitrous oxide/oxygen mixture was only marginally more effective than a 50:50 mixture (Cole et al, 1970). Analgesia was then satisfactory in 59%, slight in 16% and absent in 25%. The administration of 70% nitrous oxide was associated with a slight increase in the incidence of unconsciousness and lack of cooperation. In the study of Beazley et al (1967) the picture was similar. Despite the liberal administration of narcotic analgesics and inhalational agents, 40% of the patients regarded analgesia as unsatisfactory. Beazley's patients were primigravidae but Holdcroft and Morgan found that the effectiveness of pethidine and Entonox analgesia was uninfluenced by parity. The highest success rate with Entonox was that of Rosen et al (1969) who reported that 72% of mothers claimed considerable or complete pain relief. There is the intriguing possibility that nitrous oxide exerts its analgesic action by the release of endogenous opioids since the concentration of β-endorphin is increased when Entonox is inhaled (Thomas and Fletcher, 1983).

It is possible that continuous nitrous oxide analgesia might be more effective than the usual intermittent administration which is critically dependent upon correct timing for its success. Latto et al (1973) have measured nitrous oxide concentrations in arterial blood during intermittent Entonox inhalations, and they suggest that the continuous inhalation of 20–25% of nitrous oxide would give equivalent and sustained arterial blood concentrations. Fetal and maternal arterial blood concentrations of nitrous oxide would be expected to be in full equilibrium after about 40 minutes of commencing inhalations (Blechner et al, 1969; Marx et al, 1970). Arthurs and Rosen (1979) report improved pain relief in labour from the continuous inhalation of 5 litres of Entonox by nasal catheter, augmented by the inhalation of Entonox by mouth-piece during contractions. Mean end tidal nitrous oxide concentrations were 14.8% (1.9% with intermittent inhalations alone). The nasal catheter was accepted initially by 85% of mothers, but only

56% retained it until delivery; this may be the major difficulty with a potentially valuable technique. Maternal drowsiness, nausea and vomiting may be more common. In a later extended field trial 70% of mothers retained the nasal catheter until delivery (Arthurs and Rosen, 1981). The usual reason for rejection of the catheter was watering of the eyes. The improvement in analgesia in the field trial was small and was less than in the earlier local trial. The technique has been approved for use by midwives but is not extensively used.

An old technique has been revived by Levack and Tunstall (1984) who combined Entonox with up to 0.5% of trichloroethylene administered from an Oxford Miniature Vaporizer connected in series with the Entonox demand valve. This has been valuable where labour has suddenly become painful and delivery is imminent. The technique is not approved for use by midwives and there is a possibility of depression of consciousness, airway obstruction or pulmonary aspiration.

Trichloroethylene and methoxyflurane

In 1984 approval was withdrawn for the use of the Emotril Automatic and Tecota Mark 6 inhalers for the administration of trichloroethylene (Trilene) by British midwives. While this decision may be regretted it recognized that trichloroethylene had been used rarely, if ever, in many British hospitals for some years. The manufacture of trichloroethylene continues. The manufacture of methoxyflurane (Penthrane) is understood to have ceased, although the Cardiff inhaler has not been withdrawn from authorized use by midwives. The British Standards Institution no longer undertakes the annual testing of the Emotril Automatic, Tecota Mark 6 and Cardiff inhalers. The effect of all these factors is that trichloroethylene and methoxyflurane are unavailable for use by midwives in the UK. The techniques, the apparatus and the regulations governing the use of trichloroethylene and methoxyflurane by midwives need therefore no longer be described. There may be a limited use for trichloroethylene outwith the UK and the relevant information is to be found in the earlier editions of this book. Limited experience by one of the authors (Moir) suggests that the advantages of trichloroethylene in the form of low cost, high boiling point and simple apparatus may be outweighed in some third world countries by ignorance and distrust of the technique on the part of women in labour.

Enflurane and isoflurane   There has been some interest in the use of these two agents for pain relief in labour. Abboud et al (1981) thought that enflurane and nitrous oxide were equipotent and McGuinness and Rosen (1984) reported that a small series of volunteer mothers got better pain relief from 1% enflurane than Entonox. Drowsiness was more marked with enflurane. These observations are perhaps rather surprising because enflurane is not especially noted for its analgesic properties. It is also rather remarkable that the interest in enflurane should coincide with the near demise of two established effective inhalation agents, trichloroethylene and methoxyflurane. Enflurane does not impair renal function and serum inorganic fluoride concentrations are not raised (Abboud et al, 1981).

In a small preliminary series McLeod et al (1985) found that 0.75% isoflurane gave superior analgesia to 50% of nitrous oxide but drowsiness, unpleasant odour and high cost were potential drawbacks.

ANALGESIA AND THE NATIONAL BOARDS FOR NURSING, MIDWIFERY AND HEALTH VISITING

The anaesthetist who practises in association with midwives should be aware of the drugs which midwives are authorized to administer and the conditions which must be complied with when the various drugs are used. The right to administer certain powerful drugs on her own responsibility is one of the special privileges of the midwife.

The National Board for Nursing, Midwifery and Health Visiting has declared that: 'A practising midwife must not on her own responsibility use any drug, including an analgesic, unless in the course of her training whether before or after enrolment she has been thoroughly instructed in its use and is familiar with its dosage and methods of administration or application.' The student midwife is required to attend four lectures on analgesia, anaesthesia and resuscitation given by an anaesthetist and these topics are included in the examination for qualification as a State Certified Midwife.

When she has complied with the foregoing provisions the midwife is permitted to administer, on her own responsibility, the following drugs. The National Board for Nursing, Midwifery and Health Visiting lists the drugs which a midwife may prescribe but do not state the dose to be used. The doses listed below are those generally administered:

Sedatives and hypnotics
Chloral hydrate 1–2 g
Syrup of chloral 0.6–2 g
Triclofos (Tricloryl) tablets 0.5–1 g
Triclofos (Tricloryl) syrup 0.5–1 g (5–10 ml)
Dichloralphenazone (Welldorm) tablets (each contains chloral hydrate 0.65 g and phenazone 1.3 g)
Promazine 25–50 mg

Analgesics
Pethidine up to 200 mg (doses of 100 mg usually recommended)
Pethilorfan (pethidine 100 mg with levallorphan 1.25 mg in 2 ml)
Pentazocine 40–60 mg usually recommended.

The midwife who prescribes pethidine or Pethilorfan must comply with the Misuse of Drugs Act, 1973 (formerly Dangerous Drugs Act) and in particular she must maintain a register and must keep the drug in a locked receptacle. Pethidine is usually supplied to a domiciliary midwife by her employing authority who will normally recommend the maximum dose to be administered. Pentazocine is, of course, exempt from the provisions of the Misuse of Drugs Act.

Midwives are authorized to administer on their own responsibility Entonox from the Entonox apparatus. The midwife must use only an approved apparatus and must not administer an inhalational analgesic unless:

(1) She has either before or after enrolment received, at an institution approved by the Board for the purpose, special instruction in the essentials of obstetric analgesia and satisfied the institution or the Board that she is thoroughly proficient in the use of the apparatus.

(2) The patient has at some time during her pregnancy been examined by a registered medical practitioner who has signed a certificate that he finds no contraindications to the administration of analgesia by a midwife and if any illness which required medical attention subsequently developed during the pregnancy, the midwife obtained confirmation from a medical practitioner that the certificate remained valid (Central Midwives Board for England and Wales, 1955). In Scotland the ruling is that the patient has been examined 'within one month before her confinement'. The authors can envisage few, if any, contraindications to the use of Entonox other than maternal rejection of this form of pain relief.

Midwives are permitted to infiltrate the perineum with a local anaesthetic solution and to perform an episiotomy. The National Board for England and Wales has recommended the use of 10 ml of a 0.5% solution or 5 ml of a 1% solution of lignocaine or similar agent.

Midwives in England and Wales are permitted to administer 'top-up' injections through an epidural catheter (see page 265). Midwives in certain Scottish hospitals were authorized to give 'top-ups' in 1978.

The Central Midwives Board has from time to time authorized individual midwives or groups of midwives in specified hospitals to administer drugs which are not normally approved for use by midwives. This procedure may be used for clinical trials of a new drug.

PSYCHOLOGICAL PREPARATION FOR LABOUR

A brief account of the various approaches to the preparation of the patient for labour and delivery is appropriate because many of the women with whom the anaesthetist comes into contact will have been exposed to some form of psychological and educational preparation. Almost all hospitals offer instruction on a voluntary basis to the patients who attend the antenatal clinic and the instruction is usually given by the midwife or a physiotherapist.

Obstetricians and anaesthetists are often now involved in these instructional classes and fathers-to-be as well as mothers-to-be often attend. Classes should be small and informal. A lecture is inappropriate. Questions should be encouraged and answered with absolute honesty. The analgesic techniques available in the hospital should be simply described and no one technique should be unduly favoured. The efficacy of each technique should be stated and perfect analgesia should not be promised.

The great importance of avoiding the fear which arises from ignorance and from loneliness in labour has been rightly stressed by O'Driscoll (1975). No woman should be left alone in labour and wherever appropriate the father should be present. There is evidence that maternal psychological stress can reduce intervillous blood flow causing fetal bradycardia and acidosis. The presumptive mechanism is uterine artery constriction as the result of increased catecholamine concentrations (Morishima et al, 1978).

The instruction normally includes an explanation of the processes of labour and delivery. Often a method of mental and physical preparation for labour is also taught and this is intended to abolish or reduce the pain of labour. There is usually a description of the methods of pain relief used in the hospital and a demonstration of apparatus for inhalational analgesia. Sometimes a mother will attend classes offering preparation for labour which are not held under the auspices of the hospital and she may express strong and unorthodox views on the management of her labour.

The acquisition of factual information about childbirth is certainly valuable and will often dispel irrational fears which stem from ignorance. It is the various specific regimens of mental and physical preparation for 'painless childbirth' which arouse controversy. There is no single technique of preparation and of pain relief in labour which is applicable to every woman. Some women can gain much emotional satisfaction from a chosen method, even if pain is not completely relieved. The first duty of the medical attendants is to ensure the safety of mother and child. Extravagant claims for fetal and neonatal well-being have been made for certain regimens and are without scientific basis. A range of methods should be available, the patient's wishes should be respected and the choice should be arrived at by the patient, the obstetrician and the anaesthetist, in consultation and after evaluation of any obstetric problems.

Alternative positions. There is much support for the view that the dorsal or 'stranded whale' position is unnatural and unphysiological, predisposing to caval occlusion, supine hypotension and inefficient uterine action. The first stage of labour may be shortened in the upright position (Mendez-Bauer et al, 1975) although others have failed to confirm this claim (McManus and Calder, 1978; Williams et al, 1980). It would be expected that the lateral position would improve uterine blood flow and thereby improve uterine action and this has been demonstrated by Caldeyro-Barcia et al (1960). A squatting position has been thought to expedite delivery (Dunn, 1976) but this was not confirmed by Calder (1982).

While the avoidance of the dorsal position seems entirely beneficial, certain other positions may be a mixed blessing for the anaesthetist, obstetrician and midwife. Birthing chairs allow a squatting position but may make access difficult and vulvar oedema soon develops. The Borning and the Rockett beds allow mobility and access in most positions. There is a theoretical risk of severe hypotension if epidural analgesia is used in an upright position. There is reason to think that more efficient labour may be less painful labour.

Michel Odent of Pithiviers is a powerful advocate of the adoption of the posture of the mother's choice and he encourages delivery in a squatting position. Odent uses no analgesics and pain is undoubtedly present. Fetal monitoring is impossible in some positions unless radiotelemetry is used and this is a disadvantage. Not all claims made for the benefits of alternative positions have been substantiated by objective measurements. Nevertheless the wish to adopt a chosen position should be accepted within the bounds of maternal and fetal safety.

Natural childbirth. In 1935 Dr Grantly Dick-Read introduced the technique of natural childbirth. This was based on the sometimes erroneous belief that women of primitive tribes experienced no pain in labour and that civilized women could create a state of mind in which labour would be painless. Too much was expected of natural childbirth and deep-seated feelings of failure were sometimes engendered in patients who experienced pain despite having followed Dick-Read's precepts. A modified method of natural childbirth is taught by the physiotherapist Helen Heardman and her followers. This regimen includes exercises designed to bring about relaxation and therefore to prevent or relieve pains in labour.

The Leboyer method of 'birth without violence' has some attractive features such as immediate skin-to-skin contact between mother and newborn and the use of gentleness. Other aspects such as delivery in a darkened room have obvious dangers and are rarely implemented.

Psychoprophylaxis. This method originated in Russia and was developed by Lamaze and by Vellay in France in the 1950s. The basis of psychoprophylaxis is the Pavlovian conditioned reflex. It is held that most women have been conditioned into believing that the uterine contractions of labour are painful. It is therefore necessary that the patient be first deconditioned and then reconditioned to believe that contractions are not painful. Exercises are taught and these include breathing patterns for use during contractions. Patients are not taught to expect complete absence of pain and are told that conventional analgesia will be available if necessary. Patients will often retain self-control during a painful contraction. The use of psychoprophylaxis does not appear to influence the physical character of the labour, although the diminished use of regional nerve block may increase the number of spontaneous deliveries (Scott and Rose, 1976; Charles et al, 1978).

Charles and his colleagues (1978) claim a reduction in the need for analgesia and anaesthesia in mothers who had taken training in psycho-prophylaxis and comment that the level of pain is reduced, although rarely abolished, and the level of enjoyment is increased. The lack of scientifically controlled studies with random allocation and the elimination of observer prejudice is stressed by Beck and Hall (1978). The feasibility of a properly controlled trial in this context is doubtful. The study by Melzack et al (1981) used pain scoring and therefore merits attention. Pain was often very severe and was reduced by 30% on average in mothers who received instruction in psychoprophylaxis. Comparisons between mothers and neonates delivered with conventional methods, with psychoprophylaxis or with the Leboyer method have shown no important differences in the condition of the infants at birth or in their subsequent development (Scott and Rose, 1976; Hughey et al, 1978; Nelson et al, 1980).

The whole question of psychological preparation for childbirth is highly emotive and objective evaluation is difficult. Many anaesthetists will be inclined, by training and perhaps by nature, to favour pharmacological and conduction analgesia. The various psychological regimens, if not always effective, are of course free from respiratory and cardiovascular depressant actions. The provision of accurate factual information about labour is always beneficial. The various relaxation and breathing exercises will not guarantee a painless labour and it is a serious mistake to allow the patient to believe that she has failed in some way if she experiences pain. Enthusiasm on the part of teacher and pupil is necessary but extremes of enthusiasm may require to be curbed.

There is probably a relationship between fear, tension and pain. Fear may stem from ignorance and so the provision of information is important. It is postulated that fear may create muscular tension which in turn causes pain. Relaxation and breathing exercises may reduce muscular tension and it is probable that these exercises may also act as a type of distraction therapy. Some teachers seem to induce a state akin to hypnosis by talking in a slow soothing voice and suggesting relaxation and peaceful thoughts.

Birthing rooms. These are intended to provide a home-like atmosphere with rapid access to hospital facilities in emergency. The woman's husband or partner and existing older children are sometimes present during labour. Birthing rooms are a North American concept and have found limited acceptance in the UK. Perhaps birthing rooms have stronger attractions in North America where transfer to a 'mini-operating theatre' has been usual for the delivery, and the need for these rooms is perhaps less in Great Britain where normal labour and delivery are usually managed in the same room. The range of procedures to be carried out in the birthing room should be clearly defined and not all hospitals permit forceps delivery and epidural analgesia. A benefit of the institution of a birthing room may be a revision of attitudes of staff towards the wishes of women for the conduct of their labours.

Hypnosis. The advantages of successful hypnosis for mother and child are readily apparent in the avoidance of the side-effects of pharmacological analgesia. Unfortunately the applicability of hypnosis is limited. Only about 25% of obstetric patients can be hypnotized to a depth at which the appreciation of pain is abolished or substantially reduced (Moya and James, 1960; Wahl, 1962). Even among women selected as being suitable subjects for hypnosis the quality of analgesia is frequently unsatisfactory. In Moya and James' series pain was satisfactorily relieved in only 23% of women, in Gross and Posner's (1963) series analgesia was satisfactory in 41% and in Davidson's (1962) series pain relief was satisfactory in 59%. Women should not expect complete relief of pain. Antenatal hypnosis can do much to relieve anxiety and fear of labour and can be valuable for women with unnatural fears.

The need for the hypnotist to be present during labour is a major objection to the wider use of hypnosis. Patients have been taught self-hypnosis for use in labour but the failure rate is high in a busy labour ward. If hypnosis is to be used it is essential that all staff have understanding of the technique and behave in an appropriate manner towards the hypnotized patient. While the application of hypnosis in labour is in practice rather restricted, there may well be a few patients for whom it is the method of choice. These women should have realistic expectations of the method. Hypnosis should not be used in patients who are psychiatrically disturbed.

White sound (audio analgesia). White sound is a mixture of sounds of many frequencies and is analogous to the colour white which is composed of many colours. White sound is rather like the sound of rushing water. The patient wears earphones and the sound intensity is increased during painful contractions. Soothing music may be transmitted between contractions and the patient may control the volume of the white sound. The technique is a form of distraction therapy, is harmless and has been used in obstetrics and dentistry. Although probably helpful, pain relief is incomplete. Analgesic drugs should also be given and the effectiveness of these drugs is said to be enhanced, although the dose requirement was unaltered (Burt and Korn, 1964; Barbe and Sattenspiel, 1965).

Abdominal decompression. Abdominal decompression was introduced as a method of pain relief in labour by the South African Heyns in 1955 (Heyns, 1959). The patient's chest, abdomen and thighs are sealed within a rigid plastic shell or a light plastic bag. A powerful negative pressure is created within the shell or Heyn's bag by an electrically-operated suction apparatus, such as a vacuum cleaner motor. Usually the patient controls the negative pressure by placing her finger over a hole in the tubing. Decompression is used with each contraction in labour.

Abdominal decompression is said to lessen pain and to accelerate labour. It is held that the negative pressure relaxes the muscles of the abdominal wall so that the uterus assumes a more spherical shape which is conducive to a more efficient type of uterine contraction. The effectiveness of the method seems rather uncertain (Scott and Louden, 1960; Shulman and Birnbaum, 1966; Castellanos et al, 1968). There are undoubtedly patients who have obtained worthwhile relief, and faith of the patient and her attendants in the method is important for success. There is probably also an element of distraction in this technique.

Experiences with abdominal decompression in the Queen Mother's Hospital were unhappy and the method was abandoned. Patients were often terrified by the apparatus and by the loud noise of the electric motor and some women begged in tears to have the apparatus removed. Sometimes a feeling of constriction is experienced around the chest and, especially with the plastic shells, the suction may cause liquor amnii to drain in a rather unpleasant manner. The restricted access for examination and monitoring is a disadvantage.

It has been suggested that abdominal decompression increases utero-placental blood flow and improves fetal oxygenation and reduces acidosis. This claim has not been substantiated by fetal blood gas analyses (Newman and Wood, 1967). The sensational claim that regular abdominal decompression during pregnancy improves the intelligence of the infant still awaits verification in a controlled trial. The infants about whom this claim was made were the offspring of volunteer white South African mothers and comparisons with the bulk of the population are unlikely to be valid.

Acupuncture. Acupuncture is part of a whole system of medicine and not just a technique of analgesia. Acupuncture has been in use in China and other South East Asian countries for 5000 years and includes a concept of Chi energy flowing through 12 channels or meridians linking internal organs. Disease and stress are believed to upset the balance of energy flow and proper balance can be restored by acupuncture. Even if some concepts are viewed with scepticism, acupuncture might be explained by the release of natural endorphins and enkephalins or by the 'gate' theory of pain control. It is quite widely accepted that acupuncture can reduce the perception of pain and even produce partial or complete anaesthesia for surgical operations.

There appears to have been only one reported use of acupuncture during labour by Western physicians (Wallis et al, 1974) and these writers state that acupuncture has, perhaps surprisingly, not been recorded in the Chinese literature as a method of analgesia in labour.

In the experience of Wallis and his colleagues and in the opinion of their volunteer patients, acupuncture was unable to relieve the pain of labour and delivery in 19 out of 21 patients. The time requirements and the need for trained personnel and patient education would restrict the applicability of acupuncture, even if it were an effective technique.

Transcutaneous electrical nerve stimulation (TENS). The technique, which is, like acupuncture, explained by the 'gate' theory of pain control of Melzack and Wall (1965), involves the application of a variable electrical stimulus to the skin at the site of pain or to the area on either side of the spine at the level of T11–L1 nerve roots. Currents vary from 0–40 mA at a frequency of 40–150 Hz. There is 'great' or 'considerable' relief of pain in 20–24% of mothers and about 60% get slight benefit (Robson, 1979; Stewart, 1979). The method is said to be most helpful for backache. Analgesia is not immediate and may not develop for up to 40 minutes. The high frequency current may close the 'gate' in the spinal cord whereas the low frequency current may promote the release of endorphins and so account for the delayed action. Analgesia is partially reversed by naloxone, an observation which supports the endogenous opioid theory. Perineal pain at delivery is usually unrelieved. The technique is harmless to mother and infant but not very effective.

TENS can reduce the requirement for pethidine (Jones, 1980) but mothers should not expect complete analgesia. TENS is less effective if given after epidural analgesia, an unlikely sequence in labour (Davies, 1982). In a study by Cushieri et al (1985) TENS did not relieve pain after abdominal surgery.

Low intensity currents of 8–10 mA at a frequency of 750–1000 Hz have been passed through electrodes applied to the frontal and mastoid regions by Russian workers, who claim that most women get relief of pain in labour and that incoordinate uterine action becomes more normal (Persianinov, 1975). Such claims await substantiation.

REFERENCES

Abboud, T.K., Shnider, S.M., Wright, R.H. et al (1981) Enflurane analgesia in obstetrics. *Anesth. Analg. curr. Res.*, **60**, 133.
Adoni, A., Kapitulnik, J., Kaufman, N.A., Ron, M. and Blondheim, S.H. (1973) Effect of maternal administration of diazepam on bilirubin-binding capacity of cord blood serum. *Am. J. Obstet. Gynec.*, **115**, 577.
Apgar, V., Burnes, J.J., Brodie, B.B. and Papper, E.M. (1952) Transmission of meperidine across the human placenta. *Am. J. Obstet. Gynec.*, **64**, 1368.
Arthurs, G.J. and Rosen, M. (1979) Self-administered intermittent nitrous oxide analgesia for labour. *Anaesthesia*, **34**, 301.
Arthurs, G.J. and Rosen, M. (1981) Acceptability of continuous nasal nitrous oxide during labour. Field trial in six maternity hospitals. *Anaesthesia*, **36**, 384.
Ashton, C.H. (1985) Editorial. Benzodiazepines: are specific antagonists useful? *Br. med. J.*, **290**, 805.
Baker, F.J. (1957) Pethidine and nalorphine in labour. *Anaesthesia*, **12**, 282.
Barbe, D.P. and Sattenspiel, E. (1965) Audioanalgesia in labor and delivery. *Obstet. Gynec.*, **25**, 683.
Beazley, J.M., Leaver, E.P., Morewood, J.H.M. and Bircumshaw, J. (1967) Relief of pain in labour. *Lancet*, **i**, 1033.
Beck, N.C. and Hall, D. (1978) Natural childbirth: a review and analysis. *Obstet. Gynec.*, **52**, 371.

Beckett, A.H. and Taylor, J.F. (1967) Blood concentrations of pethidine and pentazocine in mother and infant at the time of birth. *J. Pharm. Pharmac.*, **19**, Suppl. 50.

Bepko, F., Lowe, E. and Waxman, B. (1965) Relief of the emotional factor in labor with parenterally administered diazepam. *Obstet. Gynec.*, **26**, 852.

Blechner, J.N., Makowski, E.L., Cotter, J.R., Meschia, G. and Barron, D.H. (1969) Nitrous oxide transfer from mother to fetus in sheep and goats. *Am. J. Obstet. Gynec.*, **105**, 368.

Bonica, J.J. (1967) *Principles and Practice of Obstetric Analgesia and Anaesthesia*, vol. I, p. 245. Oxford: Blackwell.

Brackbill, Y., Kane, J., Manniello, R.S. and Abramson, D. (1974) Obstetric meperidine usage and assessment of neonatal status. *Anesthesiology*, **40**, 116.

Bullough, J. (1959) Use of pre-mixed pethidine and antagonists in obstetrical analgesia. *Br. med. J.*, **ii**, 859.

Burt, R.K. and Korn, G.W. (1964) Audioanalgesia in obstetrics. *Am. J. Obstet. Gynec.*, **88**, 361.

Calder, A.A. (1982) Posture during labour and delivery. *Mat. Child Health*, **7**, 475.

Caldeyro-Barcia, R., Guerra, L., Cibils, L.A. et al (1960) Effect of position changes on the intensity and frequency of uterine contractions during labor. *Am. J. Obstet. Gynec.*, **80**, 284.

Campbell, D., Masson, A.H.B. and Norris, W. (1965) The clinical evaluation of narcotic and sedative drugs. 2. A re-evaluation of pethidine and Pethilorfan. *Br. J. Anaesth.*, **37**, 199.

Caseby, N. (1974) Epidural analgesia for the surgical induction of labour. *Br. J. Anaesth.*, **46**, 747.

Castellanos, R., Aguero, O. and de Soto, E. (1968) Abdominal decompression. *Am. J. Obstet. Gynec.*, **100**, 924.

Charles, A.G., Norr, K.L., Block, C.R., Meyering, S. and Meyers, E. (1978) Obstetric and psychological effects of psychoprophylactic preparation for childbirth. *Am. J. Obstet. Gynec.*, **131**, 44.

Clark, R.B., Cooper, J.O., Stephens, S.R. and Brown, W.E. (1968) Neonatal acid–base studies. *Obstet. Gynec.*, **33**, 30.

Cleaton-Jones, P. (1976) The laryngeal closure reflex and nitrous oxide–oxygen analgesia. *Anesthesiology*, **45**, 569.

Cole, P.V., Crawford, J.S., Doughty, A.G. et al (1970) Specifications and recommendations for nitrous oxide/oxygen apparatus to be used in obstetric analgesia. *Anaesthesia*, **25**, 317.

Corke, B.C. (1977) Neurobehavioural responses of the newborn: the effect of different forms of maternal analgesia. *Anaesthesia*, **32**, 539.

Crawford, J.S. and Rudofsky, S. (1965) Placental transmission of pethidine. *Br. J. Anaesth.*, **37**, 929.

Cushieri, R.J., Morran, C.G. and McArdle, C.S. (1985) Transcutaneous electrical stimulation for postoperative pain. *Annals Roy. Coll. Surg. Engl.*, **67**, 127.

Davidson, J.A. (1962) Assessment of the value of hypnosis in pregnancy and labour. *Br. med. J.*, **ii**, 951.

Davidson, J.A., Beddard, J.B., Bennett, J.A. and Whiteford, J.H.W. (1970) A new technique for domiciliary flying squad anaesthesia. *Br. J. Anaesth.*, **42**, 565.

Davies, J.R. (1982) Ineffective transcutaneous nerve stimulation following epidural anaesthesia. *Anaesthesia*, **37**, 453.

Davies, J.M. and Rosen, M. (1977) Intramuscular diazepam in labour. A double-blind trial in multiparae. *Br. J. Anaesth.*, **49**, 601.

Davies, J.M., Hogg, M.I.J. and Rosen, M. (1974a) Upper limits of resistance of apparatus for inhalation analgesia during labour. *Br. J. Anaesth.*, **46**, 136.

Davies, J.M., Hogg, M.I.J. and Rosen, M. (1974b) The resistance of Entonox valves. *Br. J. Anaesth.*, **46**, 145.

Dolan, P.F. and Rosen, M. (1975) Inhalational analgesia in labour: facemask or mouth piece? *Lancet*, **ii**, 1030.

Duncan, S.L., Ginsburg, J. and Morris, N.F. (1969) Comparison of pentazocine and pethidine in normal labour. *Am. J. Obstet. Gynec.*, **105**, 197.

Dundee, J.W. and Moore, J. (1962) The phenothiazines. *Br. J. Anaesth.*, **34**, 247.

Dunn, P.M. (1976) Obstetric delivery today: for better or for worse? *Lancet*, **i**, 790.

Elder, M.G. and Crossley, J. (1969) A double blind trial of diazepam in labour. *J. Obstet. Gynaec. Br. Commonw.*, **76**, 264.

Erkkola, R. and Kanto, J. (1972) Diazepam and breast feeding. *Lancet*, **i**, 1235.

Evans, J.M., Rosen, M., McCarthy, J.P. and Hogg, M.I.J. (1976) Apparatus for patient-controlled administration of intravenous narcotics during labour. *Lancet*, **i**, 17.

Filler, W.W., Hall, W.C. and Filler, N.W. (1967) Analgesia in obstetrics: the effect of analgesia on uterine contractility and fetal heart rate. *Am. J. Obstet. Gynec.*, **98**, 832.

Flowers, C.E., Rudolph, A.J. and Desmond, M.M. (1969) Diazepam (Valium) as an adjunct in obstetric analgesia. *Obstet. Gynec.*, **34**, 68.

Gale, C.W., Tunstall, M.E. and Wilton-Davies, C.C. (1964) Pre-mixed gas and oxygen for midwives. *Br. med. J.*, **i**, 732.

Gamble, J.A.S., Dundee, J.W. and Assaf, R.A.E. (1975) Plasma diazepam levels after single dose oral and intramuscular administration. *Anaesthesia*, **30**, 164.

Girvan, C.B., Moore, J. and Dundee, J.W. (1976) Pethidine compared with pethidine–naloxone administered during labour. *Br. J. Anaesth.*, **48**, 563.

Grant, A.M., Holt, E.M. and Noble, A.D. (1970) A comparison between pethidine and phenazocine (Narphen) for relief of pain in labour. *J. Obstet. Gynaec. Br. Commonw.*, **77**, 824.

Gross, H.N. and Posner, N.A. (1963) Evaluation of hypnosis for obstetric delivery. *Am. J. Obstet. Gynec.*, **87**, 912.

Hamilton, R.C., Dundee, J.W., Clarke, R.S.J., Loan, W.B. and Morrison, J.D. (1967) Alterations in response to somatic pain associated with anaesthesia. XVIII. Studies with some opiate antagonists. *Br. J. Anaesth.*, **39**, 490.

Harper, N.J.N., Thomson, J. and Brayshaw, S.A. (1983) Experience with self-administered pethidine with special reference to the general practitioner obstetric unit. *Anaesthesia*, **38**, 52.

Heyns, O.S. (1959) Abdominal decompression in the first stage of labour. *J. Obstet. Gynaec. Br. Emp.*, **66**, 220.

Hodgkinson, R. and Husain, F.J. (1982) The duration of effect of maternally administered meperidine on neonatal neurobehavior. *Anesthesiology*, **56**, 51.

Hogg, M.I.J., Davies, J.M., Mapleson, W.W. and Rosen, M. (1974) Proposed upper limit of respiratory resistance for inhalation apparatus used in labour. *Br. J. Anaesth.*, **46**, 149.

Holdcroft, A. and Morgan, M. (1974) An assessment of the analgesic effect in labour of pethidine and 50 per cent nitrous oxide in oxygen (Entonox). *J. Obstet. Gynaec. Br. Commonw.*, **81**, 603.

Huch, A., Huch, R., Lindmark, G. and Rooth, G. (1974) Maternal hypoxaemia after pethidine. *J. Obstet. Gynaec. Br. Commonw.*, **81**, 608.

Hughey, M.J., McElin, T.W. and Young, T. (1978) Maternal and fetal outcome of Lamaze-prepared patients. *Obstet. Gynec.*, **51**, 643.

Jasinski, D.R. and Martin, W.R. (1967) Evaluation of a new photographic method for assessing pupil diameters. *Clin. Pharmac. Ther.*, **8**, 271.

Jasinski, D.R., Martin, W.R. and Haertzen, C.A. (1967) The human pharmacology and abuse potential of N-allylnoroxymorphone (naloxone). *J. Pharmac. exp. Ther.*, **157**, 420.

Jeffcoate, T.N.A., Baker, K. and Martin, R.H. (1952) Inefficient uterine action. *Surgery Gynec. Obstet.*, **95**, 257.

Jones, C.M.H.M. (1980) Transcutaneous nerve stimulation in labour. *Anaesthesia*, **35**, 372.

Jordan, C., Lehane, J.R., Robson, P.J. and Jones, J.G. (1979) A comparison of the respiratory effects of meptazinol, pentazocine and morphine. *Br. J. Anaesth.*, **51**, 497.

Koch, G. and Wandel, H. (1968) Effect of pethidine on the postnatal adjustment of respiration and acid–base balance. *Acta obstet. gynec. scand.*, **47**, 27.

Latto, I.P., Molloy, M.J. and Rosen, M. (1973) Arterial concentrations of nitrous oxide during intermittent patient-controlled inhalation of 50% nitrous oxide in oxygen (Entonox) during the first stage of labour. *Br. J. Anaesth.*, **45**, 1029.

Lean, T.H., Ratnam, S.S. and Sivasamboo, R. (1968a) Use of chlordiazepoxide in patients with severe pregnancy toxaemia. *J. Obstet. Gynaec. Br. Commonw.*, **75**, 853.

Lean, T.H., Ratnam, S.S. and Sivasamboo, R. (1968b) Use of benzodiazepines in the management of eclampsia. *J. Obstet. Gynaec. Br. Commonw.*, **75**, 856.

Lee, D.T. (1968) The effects of diazepam (Valium) on labor. *Can. med. Ass. J.*, **98**, 446.

Levack, I.D. and Tunstall, M.E. (1984) Systems modification in obstetric analgesia. *Anaesthesia*, **39**, 183.

MacVicar, J. and Murray, M.H. (1960) Clinical evaluation of promazine as an adjuvant to predelivery sedation. *Br. med. J.*, **i**, 595.

Mark, P.M. and Hamel, J. (1968) Librium for patients in labor. *Obstet. Gynec.*, **32**, 188.

Marx, G.F., Joshi, C.W. and Orkin, L.R. (1970) Placental transmission of nitrous oxide. *Anesthesiology*, **32**, 429.

Matthews, A.E.B. (1963) Double-blind trials of promazine in labour. *Br. med. J.*, **ii**, 423.

McAneny, T.M. and Doughty, A.G. (1963) Self-administered nitrous oxide/oxygen analgesia in obstetrics. *Anaesthesia*, **18**, 488.

McCarthy, G.T., O'Connell, B. and Robinson, A.E. (1973) Blood levels of diazepam in infants of two mothers given large doses of diazepam during labour. *J. Obstet. Gynaec. Br. Commonw.*, **80**, 349.

McAuley, D.M., O'Neill, M.P. and Moore, J. (1982) Lorazepam premedication for labour. *Br. J. Obstet. Gynaec.*, **89**, 149.

McGregor, W.G., Bracken, A. and Fair, J.A. (1972) Piped pre-mixed 50% nitrous oxide and 50% oxygen mixture (Entonox). *Anaesthesia*, **27**, 14.

McGuiness, C. and Rosen, M. (1984) Enflurane as an analgesic in labour. *Anaesthesia*, **39**, 24.

McLeod, D.D., Ramayya, G.P. and Tunstall, M.E. (1985) Self-administered isoflurane in labour. *Anaesthesia*, **40**, 424.

McManus, T.J. and Calder, A.A. (1978) Upright posture and the efficiency of labour. *Lancet*, **i**, 72.

McQuitty, F.M. (1967) Relief of pain in labour. *J. Obstet. Gynaec. Br. Commonw.*, **74**, 925.

Melzack, R. and Wall, P.D. (1965) Pain mechanism: a new theory. *Science, N.Y.*, **150**, 971.

Melzack, R., Taenzer, P., Feldman, P. and Kinch, R.A. (1981) Labour is still painful after prepared childbirth training. *Can. med. Assoc. J.*, **125**, 357.

Mendez-Bauer, C., Arroyo, J., Ramos, C.G. et al (1975) Effect of standing position on spontaneous uterine contracting and other aspects of labor. *J. Perinat. Med.*, **3**, 89.

Moir, D.D. and Bissett, W.I.K. (1965) An assessment of nitrous oxide apparatus used for obstetric analgesia. *J. Obstet. Gynaec. Br. Commonw.*, **72**, 265.

Moore, J. and Ball, H.G. (1974) A sequential study of intravenous analgesic treatment during labour. *Br. J. Anaesth.*, **46**, 365.

Moore, J. and Dundee, J.W. (1961a) Alterations in response to somatic pain associated with anaesthesia. V. The effect of promethazine. *Br. J. Anaesth.*, **77**, 830.

Moore, J. and Dundee, J.W. (1961b) Alterations in response to somatic pain associated with anaesthesia. VII. The effect of nine phenothiazine derivatives. *Br. J. Anaesth.*, **33**, 422.

Moore, J., Carson, R.M. and Hunter, R.J. (1970) A comparison of the effects of pentazocine and pethidine administered during labour. *J. Obstet. Gynaec. Br. Commonw.*, **77**, 830.

Morgan, B.M., Bulpitt, C.J., Clifton, P. and Lewis, P.J. (1984) The consumers' attitude to obstetric care. *Br. J. Obstet. Gynaec.*, **91**, 624.

Morishima, H., Moya, F., Bossers, A. and Thorndike, V. (1963) Adverse effects on the newborn of severe maternal hyperventilation. *Anesthesiology*, **24**, 135.

Morishima, H., Pederson, H. and Finster, M. (1978) Influence of maternal psychological stress on the fetus. *Am. J. Obstet. Gynec.*, **131**, 286.

Mowat, J. and Garrey, M.M. (1970) Comparison of pentazocine and pethidine in labour. *Br. med. J.*, **ii**, 757.

Moya, F. and James, L.S. (1960) Medical hypnosis for obstetrics. *J. Am. med. Ass.*, **174**, 2026.

Moya, F., Morishima, H., Shnider, S.M. and James, L.S. (1965) Influence of maternal hyperventilation on the newborn infant. *Am. J. Obstet. Gynec.*, **91**, 76.

Nelson, M.N., Enkin, M.W., Saigal, S. et al (1980) Randomised clinical trial of Leboyer approach to childbirth. *New Engl. J. Med.*, **302**, 655.

Newman, J.W. and Wood, E.C. (1967) Abdominal decompression and foetal blood gases. *Br. med. J.*, **iii**, 368.

Nicholas, A.D.G. and Robson, P.J. (1982) Double-blind comparison of meptazinol and pethidine in labour. *Br. J. Obstet. Gynaec.*, **89**, 318.

Nisbet, R., Boulas, S.H. and Kantor, H.I. (1967) Diazepam (Valium) during labor. *Obstet. Gynec.*, **29**, 726.

Niswander, K.R. (1969) Effect of diazepam on meperidine requirements of patients in labor. *Obstet. Gynec.*, **34**, 62.

O'Driscoll, K. (1975) An obstetrician's view of pain. *Br. J. Anaesth.*, **47**, 1053.

O'Driscoll, K. and Stronge, M. (1973) Active management of labour. *Br. med. J.*, **iii**, 590.

Ominsky, A.J., Kallos, T. and Smith, T.C. (1969) Respiratory depression by opioid antagonists and its complete reversal by a new opioid antagonist. *Proc. Am. Soc. Anesthesiologists*, October (Cited by Payne, 1973).

Owen, J.R. and Irani, S.F. (1972) The effect of diazepam administered to mothers during labour on temperature regulation of the neonate. *Archs Dis. Childh.*, **47**, 107.

Oyama, T., Matsuki, A., Taneichi, T., Ling, N. and Guillemin, R. (1980) β-endorphin in obstetric analgesia. *Am. J. Obstet. Gynec.*, **137**, 613.

Payne, J.P. (1973) Narcotic antagonists and their use in obstetrics. *Br. J. Anaesth.*, **45**, Suppl. 794.

Pearson, J.F. and Davies, P. (1973) The effect of continuous epidural analgesia on the acid–base status of maternal arterial blood during the first stage of labour. *J. Obstet. Gynaec. Br. Commonw.*, **80**, 218.

Pearson, J.F. and Davies, P. (1974) The effect of continuous lumbar epidural analgesia upon fetal acid–base status during the first stage of labour. *J. Obstet. Gynaec. Br. Commonw.*, **81**, 971.

Persianinov, L.S. (1975) The use of electro-analgesia in obstetrics and gynecology. *Acta obstet. gynec. scand.*, **54**, 373.

Petrie, R.H., Yeh, S., Murata, Y. et al (1978) The effect of drugs on fetal heart rate variability. *Am. J. Obstet. Gynec.*, **130**, 294.

Philips, T.J. and Macdonald, R.R. (1971) Comparative effects of pethidine, trichloroethylene and Entonox on fetal and neonatal acid–base and Po_2. *Br. med. J.*, **iii**, 558.

Refstad, S.O. and Lindbaek, E. (1980) Ventilatory depression of the newborn of women receiving pethidine or pentazocine. *Br. J. Anaesth.*, **52**, 265.

Revill, S.I., Robinson, J.O., Rosen, M. and Hogg, M.I.J. (1976) The reliability of a linear analogue for evaluating pain. *Anaesthesia*, **31**, 1191.

Roberts, H. and Please, N.W. (1958) Respiratory minute volume in the newborn infant. *J. Obstet. Gynaec. Br. Emp.*, **65**, 33.

Robinson, J.O., Rosen, M., Evans, J.M. et al (1980a) Maternal opinion about analgesia for labour. A controlled trial between epidural block and intramuscular pethidine combined with inhalation. *Anaesthesia*, **35**, 1173.

Robinson, J.O., Rosen, M., Evans, J.M. et al (1980b) Self-administered intravenous and intramuscular pethidine. A controlled trial in labour. *Anaesthesia*, **35**, 763.

Robson, J.E. (1979) Transcutaneous nerve stimulation for pain relief in labour. *Anaesthesia*, **34**, 357.

Rosen, M. (1979) Systemic and inhalational analgesia. *Br. J. Anaesth.*, **51**, 118.

Rosen, M., Mushin, W.W., Jones, P. and Jones, E.V. (1969) Field trial of methoxyflurane, nitrous oxide and trichloroethylene in obstetric analgesia. *Br. med. J.*, **iii**, 263.

Rouge, J.C., Banner, M.P. and Smith, T.C. (1969) Interactions of levallorphan and meperidine. *Clin. Pharmac. Ther.*, **10**, 643.

Rubin, J., Brock-Utne, J.G., Greenberg, M., Bortz, J. and Downing, J.W. (1977) Laryngeal incompetence during experimental 'relative analgesia' using 50 per cent nitrous oxide in oxygen. *Br. J. Anaesth.*, **49**, 1005.

Scher, J., Hailey, D.M. and Beard, R.W. (1972) The effect of diazepam on the fetus. *J. Obstet. Gynaec. Br. Commonw.*, **79**, 635.

Scott, J.S. (1970) Obstetric analgesia. A consideration of labor pain and a patient-controlled technique for its relief with meperidine. *Am. J. Obstet. Gynec.*, **106**, 959.

Scott, D.B. and Louden, J.D.O. (1960) A method of abdominal decompression in labour. *Lancet*, **i**, 1181.

Scott, J.R. and Rose, N.B. (1976) Effect of psychoprophylaxis (Lamaze preparation) on labor and delivery in primipara. *New Engl. J. Med.*, **294**, 1205.

Shnider, S.M. and Moya, F. (1964) Effect of meperidine on the newborn infant. *Am. J. Obstet. Gynec.*, **89**, 1009.

Shulman, H. and Birnbaum, S.J. (1966) Evaluation of abdominal decompression during first stage of labor. *Am. J. Obstet. Gynec.*, **95**, 421.

Stewart, P. (1979) Transcutaneous nerve stimulation as a method of analgesia in labour. *Anaesthesia*, **34**, 361.

Sturdee, D.W. (1976) Diazepam: routes of administration and rates of absorption. *Br. J. Anaesth.*, **48**, 1091.

Thomas, T.A. and Fletcher, J.E. (1983) Endogenous opioids. *Europ. J. Obstet. Gynaec. Reproduct. Biol.*, **15**, 353.

Thorburn, J. and Moir, D.D. (1981) Extradural analgesia. The influence of volume and concentration on the mode of delivery, analgesic efficacy and motor block. *Br. J. Anaesth.*, **53**, 933.

Tunstall, M.E. (1961) Use of a fixed nitrous oxide and oxygen mixture from one cylinder. *Lancet*, **ii**, 964.

Vella, L., Houlton, P. and Reynolds, F. (1985) Comparison of the antiemetics metoclopramide and promethazine in labour. *Br. med. J.*, **290**, 1173.

Vree, T.B., Reekers-Ketting, J.J., Fragen, R.J. and Arts, T.H.M. (1984) Placental transfer of midazolam and its metabolite 1-hydroxymethylmidazolam in the pregnant ewe. *Anesth. Analg. curr. Res.*, **63**, 31.

Wahl, C.W. (1962) Contraindications and limitations of hypnosis in obstetric analgesia. *Am. J. Obstet. Gynec.*, **84**, 1969.

Wallis, L., Shnider, S.M., Palahniuk, R.J. and Spivey, H.T. (1974) An evaluation of acupuncture analgesia in obstetrics. *Anesthesiology*, **41**, 596.

Waud, B.E. and Waud, D.R. (1970) Calculated kinetics of distribution of nitrous oxide and methoxyflurane during intermittent administration in obstetrics. *Anesthesiology*, **32**, 306.

Way, W.L., Costley, E.C. and Way, E.L. (1965) Respiratory sensitivity of the newborn infant to meperidine and morphine. *Clin. Pharmac. Ther.*, **6**, 454.

Whitford, J.H., Cory, C.E. and Beddard, J.B. (1973) A clinical trial of apparatus for domiciliary midwifery. *Br. J. Anaesth.*, **45**, 1153.

Wiener, P.C., Hogg, M.I.J. and Rosen, M. (1977) Effects of naloxone on pethidine-induced neonatal depression. *Br. med. J.*, **ii**, 228.

Wiener, P.C., Hogg, M.I.J. and Rosen, M. (1979) Neonatal respiration, feeding and neurobehavioural state. *Anaesthesia*, **34**, 996.

Williams, R.M., Thom, M.H. and Studd, J.W.W. (1980) A study of the benefits and acceptability of ambulation in spontaneous labour. *Br. J. Obstet. Gynaec.*, **87**, 122.

Wilson, J., Stephen, G.W. and Scott, D.B. (1969) A study of the cardiovascular effects of chlormethiazole. *Br. J. Anaesth.*, **41**, 840.

Zarou, D.M., Eposito, J.M. and Zarou, G.S. (1967) Continuous intravenous analgesia in labor. *Am. J. Obstet. Gynec.*, **97**, 1101.

6

General Anaesthesia

It is now possible to describe a single basic technique of anaesthesia which, with only minor modifications, makes the best and safest use of the presently available drugs and skills and which may be used for almost every obstetric operation currently performed in the UK. The inhalational or intravenous anaesthetic of brief duration, administered without intubation of the trachea to provide oblivion at the moment of delivery, has no place in British practice, although it has been widely used in North America.

It is thought probable that the standardization of obstetric general anaesthesia which has occurred over the past 25 years in the UK should enhance the safety of this always hazardous branch of anaesthetic practice. Unfortunately this statement cannot be fully substantiated in terms of maternal mortality, as will be discussed below, although it may be correct in relation to perinatal mortality. Nevertheless familiarity with and confidence in a technique are likely to increase its safety, particularly when used by the junior anaesthetists who still administer many obstetric anaesthetics without immediate supervision and assistance. The technique of general anaesthesia used, with a few minor variations, by almost all British anaesthetists for operative deliveries owes much to the work of the late Hamer Hodges of Portsmouth in demonstrating the harmful effects upon the fetus of the older techniques which relied heavily upon the powerful volatile and gaseous anaesthetics (Hodges et al, 1959; Hodges and Tunstall, 1961).

Most obstetric anaesthetics are emergency procedures. Even when the procedure is planned and the patient is not in labour, special problems always exist. Among these are the raised maternal intragastric pressure, the acidity of the gastric contents, the probability of caval occlusion if the supine position is employed and the possibility of endangering the fetus from the transplacental passage of drugs or as the result of maternal hypoxaemia or hypotension.

The influence of anaesthesia upon the fetus and neonate has been clarified by detailed studies of the various intravenous induction agents, aortocaval compression and varying inspired oxygen concentrations at elective caesarean section. These variables are of potential importance when the fetus is premature, placental function is inadequate or acute hypoxia has developed in labour. Nevertheless all infants delivered by caesarean section under light endotracheal anaesthesia are likely to show depression of various behavioural reflexes for up to 48 hours (Palahniuk et al, 1977; Hodgkinson et al, 1978; Hollmen et al, 1978), and the time to sustained respiration may be prolonged.

164

For these and other reasons there is a swing towards epidural analgesia for caesarean section.

Deaths associated with anaesthesia

From 1964 to 1978 in England and Wales the number of deaths associated with anaesthesia for every 100 true (direct) maternal deaths was as follows:

1964–6	1967–9	1970–2	1973–5	1976–8
8.7	10.9	10.4	13.2	13.2

The absolute number of deaths attributable to complications of anaesthesia fell from 50 (in 1967–1969) to 30 (in 1976–1978). The deaths associated with anaesthesia for every 100 000 maternities fell from 2.03 (in 1967–1969) to 1.61 (in 1973–1975) and rose slightly to 1.72 (in 1976–1978) (Department of Health and Social Security, 1969, 1972, 1975, 1979, 1982). These figures should be viewed against an increase in the number of caesarean sections performed (from 25 940 in 1963 to 45 114 in 1978). The mortality rate per caesarean section is then seen to fall from 1 per 3848 sections in 1963 to 1 per 5013 sections in 1978. The great majority of deaths from anaesthesia are connected with anaesthesia for emergency caesarean section.

During the years 1967–1969 just over half of the deaths associated with anaesthesia were due to the entry of stomach contents into the lungs. In 1976–1978, 14 out of 30 anaesthetic deaths were due to this cause. These deaths were almost all due to aspiration pneumonitis (Mendelson's syndrome) rather than to acute obstructive asphyxia and many of these mothers had received magnesium trisilicate. Difficulty with intubation of the trachea resulted in 16 deaths in 1976–1978 and this was a substantial increase from the 7 deaths from this cause in 1973–1975. Intubation difficulties caused death from aspiration pneumonitis or from acute hypoxia. It is evident that aspiration pneumonitis and the consequences of difficult or failed intubation account for the substantial majority of maternal deaths associated with anaesthesia and that regional analgesia rarely causes death (Hunter and Moir, 1983).

Assessors in anaesthesia have been appointed in England and Wales and in Scotland and this has already improved the accuracy with which the contribution of anaesthesia to a particular maternal death is evaluated.

Between 1972 and 1975, 7 out of 50 true maternal deaths in Scotland were due to general anaesthesia and no deaths due to regional analgesia. Mendelson's syndrome and hypoxic cardiac arrest caused these deaths and difficult or failed intubation was a major factor in four cases (Scottish Home and Health Department, 1978). Complications of intubation caused 17% of deaths in Harrison's (1978) large series of 240 000 anaesthetics. In Ireland in 1978 anaesthesia contributed to 16.6% of true (direct) maternal deaths (Maternal Mortality Committee, I.M.A., 1980).

It is difficult to ascertain the percentage of maternal deaths in the USA attributable to anaesthesia. Death rates vary widely in different regions and there is no national enquiry comparable to those in the UK. The term 'maternal death' is sometimes taken to exclude deaths due to medical causes during pregnancy and the puerperium, so comparisons between the UK and the USA are difficult. Bonica (1967) calculates that about 10% of maternal deaths between 1957 and 1967 in the USA were the result of anaesthesia. The principal cause of these deaths was aspiration of stomach contents (30%) and the second most frequent cause of death was 'spinal shock'. Baggish and Hooper (1974) agree that the aspiration of acid is a major cause of obstetric anaesthetic deaths in the USA and estimate that 2% of all maternal deaths are due to that cause, and Roberts and Shirley (1976) considered that there had been an anaesthetic error in 8% of 950 maternal deaths in the USA.

It is certain that aspiration of stomach contents into the lungs is a leading cause of death in association with obstetric anaesthesia on both sides of the Atlantic. Aspiration more commonly results in delayed death from pneumonitis rather than instant asphyxiation from the aspiration of solid food particles. The precise mortality rate among obstetric patients who aspirate stomach contents is uncertain. Crawford and Oppit (1976) estimated that at least 25% of mothers who aspirate acid material die, and Hutchison and Newson (1975) recorded a 10% mortality rate among obstetric and surgical patients who aspirated and a 33% mortality rate among those who developed a severe pulmonary acid aspiration syndrome.

The administration of obstetric anaesthesia by inexperienced anaesthetists has been a factor in several fatal catastrophes and there is a suggestion that senior anaesthetists with a special interest in obstetric anaesthesia can achieve a better safety record (Breheny and McCarthy, 1982). The importance of general anaesthesia as a cause of maternal death is confirmed by the experience at Queen Charlotte's Maternity Hospital where anaesthesia was the leading cause of death between 1958 and 1978 (Morgan, 1980). Training and experience in obstetric anaesthesia and analgesia are essential parts of general professional training in the UK and in the USA over 90% of residents have a rotation, usually of two months duration, to obstetric anaesthesia (Millar and Plumer, 1982). It is hoped that these and other measures will reduce maternal mortality.

There is of course only one certain way of avoiding pulmonary aspiration during general anaesthesia and that is the substitution of an appropriate form of regional analgesia. Morgan et al (1983) suggested that, even in the hands of junior anaesthetists, the complications of epidural anaesthesia for caesarean section are likely to be less serious and more easily treatable than the complications of general anaesthesia. For a variety of reasons general anaesthesia is likely to remain in use, at least for caesarean section, in the foreseeable future. In 1984 general anaesthesia was used for 35% of emergency and 19% of elective caesarean sections in the Queen Mother's Hospital. General anaesthesia was used for 28% of all caesarean sections, a figure which does not reach Davis's (1982) theoretical minimum of 16%, nor the remarkable figure of 3.5% achieved by Sosis and Bodner (1983).

The importance of replacing a 'flying squad' attitude to obstetric anaesthesia with anticipation and preparation by a resident anaesthetist has been stressed by Morgan (1980) and should enable most patients to come to anaesthesia in a safer condition. There will then often be time to allow the induction of regional analgesia.

The contribution of anaesthesia to fetal and neonatal mortality is unknown but the hazards of hypoxia and hypotension are obvious and will be even greater if the infant is already at risk because of immaturity, placental insufficiency or maternal disease.

The requirements of obstetric anaesthesia

The requirements of the ideal obstetric anaesthetic have been listed (Moir, 1974). An obstetric anaesthetic should, in so far as is possible:

(1) Avoid the aspiration of stomach contents into the lungs.

(2) Avoid neonatal respiratory depression.

(3) Avoid hypoxia and provide the optimal Po_2 for fetal oxygenation.

(4) Avoid hypotension (including supine hypotension) and maintain uteroplacental blood flow.

(5) Avoid uterine atony and consequent haemorrhage.

(6) Avoid extreme maternal hyperventilation.

(7) Provide satisfactory operating conditions, including relaxation of the abdominal or pelvic floor muscles and, in a few special circumstances, permit relaxation of the uterus.

(8) Ensure unconsciousness throughout any general anaesthetic.

(9) Comply with the mother's wish to be awake or unconscious at the delivery.

The prevention of pulmonary aspiration of stomach contents

The methods used in order to reduce the risk of pulmonary aspiration occurring and to minimize the harmful consequences of aspiration, should it occur despite preventive measures, are as follows:

(1) The use of a suitable dietary regimen in labour.

(2) The administration of oral alkalis and an H_2-receptor antagonist.

(3) The use of physical or pharmacological methods intended to empty the stomach and prevent regurgitation.

(4) The presence of an anaesthetist skilled in obstetric anaesthesia and in tracheal intubation at every anaesthetic.

(5) The use of regional rather than general anaesthesia whenever possible.

Diet in labour. No patient in established labour should ever receive solid food. Oral intake should be restricted to sips of water or sucking of an ice cube. Impressed by an increase in the number of caesarean sections performed for fetal distress which could not have been predicted before labour and in the number of anaesthetics given for manual removal of the placenta, it was decided 12 years ago in the Queen Mother's Hospital, Glasgow, to give no food and no drink to any patient in established labour. This policy may seem less harsh when viewed against a situation in which many women receive an intravenous infusion of water and electrolytes and where labour rarely lasts longer than 12 hours and frequently lasts for only 6 or 8 hours. The good physical condition of the patients and the rarity of ketoacidosis are impressive and it is likely that the risks of anaesthesia are decreased by this policy. The avoidance or restriction of oral intake is of course directed towards the avoidance of asphyxial death from vomiting or regurgitation of stomach contents. Such deaths are now less common, at least in the UK and in the USA, where deaths from Mendelson's syndrome now outnumber acute asphyxial deaths. The principal cause of a large volume of gastric contents is prolonged labour and the often associated administration of narcotic analgesic drugs. Labour is today regarded as prolonged when it exceeds 10 hours in duration.

Reduction of gastric acidity

Mendelson's syndrome or the acid aspiration syndrome is unlikely to be severe unless the pH of the aspirated gastric juice is below 2.5 and the volume exceeds 0.4 ml/kg body weight (Roberts and Shirley, 1974). This observation is based upon animal experiments, but is usually assumed to be valid for pregnant women.

According to Taylor and Prys-Davies (1966), Peskett (1973) and Roberts and Shirley (1974), from 43 to 55% of women in labour have a gastric pH below 2.5, while 71% of pregnant women who were not in labour were found to have a gastric pH below 2.5 (Johnson et al, 1982a,b). At least three factors influence the development of a potentially fatal aspiration pneumonitis. A minimum volume of 0.4 ml/kg must be inhaled. This is about 28 ml for a 70 kg woman. The pH of the material is relevant. Mendelson (1946) showed that 0.1 M hydrochloric acid could produce a fatal pneumonitis, and Lewis et al (1971) observed that no patients survived who aspirated gastric contents whose pH was below 1.7 and all survived if the pH of the gastric juice exceeded 2.4. The presence of food particles makes gastric juice more irritant, whatever the pH, and Schwartz et al (1980) noted that gastric contents at pH 5.9 which contained many food particles were as irritant as pure hydrochloric acid at pH 1.8. Awe et al (1966) observed that severe pneumonitis occurred if large quantities of food particles were present and the pH was above 2.5. One can also join with Scott (1978) in speculating on the possibility that muscle relaxants and IPPV may worsen the prognosis after aspiration by forcing the irritant material into the bronchioles and alveoli.

Johnstone (1972) has postulated that the profound and prolonged vasocon-strictor action of ergometrine may cause pulmonary hypertension which aggravates the chemical pneumonitis. Preventive measures are certainly indicated and may be directed towards (a) pH control, (b) reduction of gastric juice volume, and (c) the avoidance of solid food. To these measures might be added the avoidance of ergometrine and the delaying of IPPV until after the application of tracheal suction in a case of aspiration. The most effective preventive measure is of course the substitution of regional for general anaesthesia whenever possible.

Particulate alkalis. Mendelson (1946) and Dinnick (1957) suggested that alkalis be given to women in labour and the proposal was eventually implemented by Taylor and Prys-Davies in 1966. The practice soon became widespread in the UK, was later adopted in North America and elsewhere, and has only been challenged since 1979 when Gibbs and others demonstrated that particulate alkalis could cause lung damage. In 1982 the Belfast workers reported on the use of H_2-receptor antagonists for the control of gastric pH. Throughout the 1970s deaths occurred among mothers who had received the recommended regimen of 15 ml of magnesium trisilicate mixture (British Pharmaceutical Codex) every 2 hours during labour with a final dose of 30 ml before anaesthesia. During the years 1973–1978 in England, Wales and Scotland 48% of pregnant women who died of aspiration pneumonitis following anaesthesia had received an alkali, usually in the form of magnesium trisilicate (Department of Health and Social Security, 1979, 1982; Scottish Home and Health Department, 1978) and case reports of death after magnesium trisilicate and magnesium and aluminium hydroxide mixture have been published (Whittington et al, 1979; Bond et al, 1979).

There is a failure to attain or to maintain a 'safe' pH of 2.5 or higher in 1–8% of mothers (Peskett, 1973; Crawford and Potter, 1984). If a pH of 3.0 or higher is chosen as being 'safe' then the failure rate may reach 20% with the magnesium trisilicate regimen (White et al, 1976). The factors which can cause the failure of magnesium trisilicate, and probably of other particulate alkalis to raise gastric pH, are now well documented as a result of the work of Holdsworth et al (1980). These factors include:

The alkali was not given or was refused by the woman.
The dose was inadequate in time or quantity.
The alkali was vomited up.
The magnesium trisilicate mixture was not freshly prepared in the hospital pharmacy.
Mixing with stomach contents was incomplete.
Food particles were present and increased the irritant properties of gastric juice.
The particulate alkali acted as a lung irritant.

Incomplete mixing of magnesium trisilicate with the stomach contents is an important cause of failure and is attributable to the viscous and particulate nature of this alkali which tends to coat the gastric mucosa or to form a separate layer (Holdsworth et al, 1980). There is also the possibility of two separate gastric sacs forming on either side of the vertebral column so that the alkali may enter one sac only. Crawford and Potter (1984) have shown that commercial preparations of magnesium trisilicate are less effective than freshly prepared mixtures. The preparation used should be the BPC mixture because its sodium bicarbonate content is necessary for a rapid pH change. Aluminium hydroxide is less effective than magnesium trisilicate (Taylor and Prys-Davies, 1966). Proprietary mixtures of aluminium and magnesium hydroxides have been used in the USA in preference to magnesium trisilicate.

A disturbing aspect of the use of particulate alkalis for the prevention of aspiration is the possibility that the alkalis themselves might be a cause of fatal pneumonitis if aspirated. There is undoubted evidence that a mixture of aluminium and magnesium hydroxides can cause death when inhaled by animals and that surviving animals develop multiple granulomatous lesions in the lungs, each of which is centred on the particles of alkali (Gibbs et al, 1979). Human fatality is thought to have been caused entirely or mainly by the inhalation of this mixture of aluminium and magnesium hydroxide (Bond et al, 1979). The mixture of hydroxides, perhaps not surprisingly, does not prevent the irritant effect of inhaled food particles (Gibbs et al, 1980). Similar experiments have not been performed using magnesium trisilicate but the comparable particulate nature of this alkali makes the possibility of comparable results quite strong. Human fatality has not been directly blamed upon the inhalation of magnesium trisilicate, but here again this is a possible explanation for at least some of the maternal deaths which have occurred following its use. It is this possibility which has caused the authors and many other anaesthetists to abandon the administration of all particulate alkalis in labour and before anaesthesia. Crawford and Potter (1984) continue to advocate the use of magnesium trisilicate throughout labour. If this regimen is begun it should be maintained until delivery because cessation of alkali therapy might cause rebound secretion of excess acid.

There are two alternatives to particulate alkalis for the elevation of gastric pH before anaesthesia. They are the administration of a clear, saline-type alkali and the administration of an H_2-receptor antagonist. The subject has been reviewed elsewhere (Moir, 1983).

Clear alkalis. Clear alkalis which have been used and in some measure evaluated include 0.3 M sodium citrate, sodium bicarbonate 8.4% and the proprietory preparations Bicitra and Alka-Seltzer Effervescent. These all have a rapid action although the duration of action is usually short. Most of the published information concerns 0.3 M sodium citrate. If 30 ml of this solution is given then there will be a rapid increase in gastric pH in almost all patients (Foulkes and Jenning, 1981; Gibbs et al, 1982). It is important that the 0.3 M concentration is used and the volume is at least 30 ml. Larger volumes prolong the action by only a small extent in vivo (O'Sullivan and Bullingham, 1984). A 'safe' pH may not be maintained for more than 40 minutes, although the mean duration of action as measured by radiotelemetry is 85 minutes (O'Sullivan and Bullingham, 1985). Sodium citrate does not cause serious pneumonitis in experimental animals (Gibbs et al, 1981) and it mixes well with gastric contents (Holdsworth et al, 1980). Sodium bicarbonate is also rapidly effective (Thompson et al, 1984) but the administration of 20 ml of an 8.4% solution liberates 509 cm^3 of carbon dioxide in contact with acid and this could cause a dangerous increase in intragastric pressure. Bicitra (Gibbs and Banner, 1984) is effective and Alka Seltzer Effervescent, while effective (Chen et al, 1984), might also cause gaseous distension of the stomach. The clear antacids are generally effective in producing a rapid but rather short-lived increase in gastric pH. They are normally given a few minutes before the induction of anaesthesia and their repeated administration during labour is inappropriate and unnecessary. The short action of these alkalis might result in a low gastric pH at emergence from anaesthesia.

H$_2$-receptor antagonists. Great interest is now being shown in the use of the agents cimetidine and ranitidine in obstetric anaesthesia and many anaesthetists now use these drugs. The H$_2$-receptor antagonists inhibit the secretion of hydrochloric acid but do not neutralize acid which is already within the stomach. The volume of gastric juice is reduced and this is a useful secondary effect. Elevation of gastric pH must await emptying of the stomach by physiological, pharmacological or mechanical means unless an alkali is also administered. If no alkali is given then elevation of gastric pH to above 2.5 takes 1 or 2 hours. If gastric emptying time is prolonged by the administration of narcotic analgesics in labour then several hours may be needed for the pH to change. Narcotic analgesics also delay pH change by slowing the absorption of ranitidine.

Cimetidine and ranitidine are very effective when given before elective caesarean section and their use is strongly recommended in this situation. It is important to adhere to a regimen which ensures adequate dosage and provides sufficient time for elevation of gastric pH to take place. Hodgkinson et al (1983) gave cimetidine 300 mg by mouth in the evening before elective caesarean section and cimetidine 300 mg by intramuscular injection on the morning of operation and gastric pH was above 2.5 in all patients in a substantial series. In a smaller series Johnston and colleagues (1982) found cimetidine 400 mg to be effective if given 90–150 minutes before anaesthesia. Cimetidine has been associated with central nervous system side-effects (Williams, 1983) and interference with hepatic microsomal enzyme systems which may inhibit the metabolism of lignocaine (Hodgkinson, 1984). The placental transfer of cimetidine is extensive but there have been no observed adverse effects on large numbers of neonates, and neonatal gastric acidity is normal (Ostheimer et al, 1982; McAuley et al, 1984). Ranitidine 150 mg by mouth on the evening before operation and again in the morning is also totally effective and gastric volumes are reduced (McAuley et al, 1983; O'Sullivan et al, 1985). Ranitidine is preferred because it does not affect hepatic enzymes and has a longer duration of action than cimetidine. If caesarean section is not performed within 5 hours of the morning dose of ranitidine then a further dose should be given by mouth or by intramuscular injection.

It is in the prevention of aspiration pneumonitis in association with emergency caesarean section in labour that opinions vary most widely and it is in these circumstances that the risk of death is greatest (Department of Health and Social Security, 1975, 1979, 1982). The traditional approach is based upon the 2-hourly administration of magnesium trisilicate 15 ml to all women in labour, with a final dose of 30 ml given shortly before anaesthesia. This regimen continues to be advocated by Crawford and Potter (1984). Deaths have occurred when this regimen has been used and the possible mechanisms of failure have been discussed above. An alternative policy is the 6-hourly administration of ranitidine 150 mg by mouth to all women in labour (McAuley et al, 1984). This regimen is very effective in maintaining a 'safe' pH but it is expensive and involves medication of large numbers of mothers and unborn infants. There is no evidence that the practice is harmful. It can be calculated that 127 000 women and fetuses must be treated in the hope of preventing one death from aspiration pneumonitis. In the Queen Mother's Hospital, Glasgow, only 3% of women in labour receive general anaesthesia because regional analgesia is extensively used for labour and for operative delivery. It is therefore not our practice to give routine prophylaxis to all women in labour. Only those women who are to be delivered, or seem likely to be delivered by caesarean section, are treated. Such women receive cimetidine 200 mg by intramuscular injection whenever caesarean section is decided upon or seems a probability (ranitidine 50 mg would be an acceptable alternative). In addition 30 ml of 0.3 M sodium citrate is given by mouth within 5 minutes of the induction of general anaesthesia. In a series of 100 consecutive, unselected women who had emergency caesarean section under general anaesthesia this combined approach produced a gastric pH above 2.5 in all cases (Thorburn and Moir, to be published). This regimen combines the rapid but short action of sodium citrate with the delayed but prolonged action of an H_2-receptor antagonist and is thought to be both safe and effective. A combination of ranitidine and sodium citrate or sodium bicarbonate is also effective (Thompson et al, 1984).

Only time and vast experience together with accurate collection of statistical data will tell whether these new approaches will prove superior to the particulate alkalis in preventing maternal deaths. It cannot be overemphasized that the control of gastric acidity is but one of many measures which should be used for the prevention of aspiration pneumonitis. The use of alkalis and H_2-receptor antagonists does not lessen the importance of dietary restriction, cricoid pressure, gastric emptying and the use of regional analgesia whenever possible.

Emptying the stomach. Although the dietary regimen described should result in a substantial reduction in the volume of the gastric contents in most instances, it is never justifiable to assume that any woman in labour has an empty stomach. Gastric emptying is frequently delayed in labour and this is usually the result of the administration of narcotic analgesics (LaSalvia and Steffen, 1950; Nimmo et al, 1975). The largest volumes of gastric contents are found in women who have received narcotic analgesics during labour. The smallest volumes occur where epidural analgesia has been used (Holdsworth, 1978a). Prolonged labour may be associated with gastrointestinal distension by fluid and gas and the anaesthetic risks may then be compared to those of intestinal obstruction. Fortunately such cases are now rare.

It is the author's opinion that deliberate emptying of the stomach is now seldom indicated before an obstetric anaesthetic in a properly organized labour ward. In the completely unprepared patient who presents with a prolapsed cord or some other condition demanding immediate anaesthesia the risks of attempts to empty the stomach may be great for the fetus and may well not be justified if a balanced view is taken of the whole problem. It should scarcely be necessary to point out that neither the stomach tube nor apomorphine can ensure a completely empty stomach. Efforts to empty the stomach are justifiable where it is considered that the intragastric pressure is particularly high and the risk of regurgitation is therefore greatest. The mean intragastric pressure in patients at term, in the supine position, was 13.6 cmH$_2$O (1.3 kPa), a pressure which was nearly twice the value found in non-pregnant subjects (Spence et al, 1967). An even higher mean intragastric pressure of 17.2 cmH$_2$O (1.7 kPa) in pregnancy was recorded by Lind et al (1968). Mothers with multiple pregnancy, gross obesity and hydramnios had very high intragastric pressures (Spence et al, 1967).

If a stomach tube is used it is advised that it should be removed or withdrawn until its tip lies within the oesophagus, just before the induction of anaesthesia and after gastric suction. It is believed that the presence of an intragastric tube may render the gastro-oesophageal sphincter incompetent, allowing the regurgitation of liquid stomach contents alongside the tube.

Apomorphine was introduced by Holmes in 1956 as a way of emptying the stomach before anaesthesia and this method is advocated by Holdsworth (1978b) although it is probably not extensively practised. A 3 mg ampoule of apomorphine is diluted to 10 ml with water. The concentration is now 0.3 mg apomorphine per ml. The patient sits up, holding a receiver for the vomitus while the apomorphine solution is slowly injected into a vein until vomiting occurs. The injection is stopped when retching begins, and when the vomiting has ceased an intravenous injection of atropine 1.0 mg is given through the intravenous needle or cannula. Salivation is often profuse. The proponents of this pharmacological gastric emptying claim that it upsets the patient less than the passage of a stomach tube, but confirm that neither apomorphine nor a stomach tube guarantees an empty stomach (Holdsworth et al, 1974). These workers failed to detect any harmful effect of apomorphine on the neonate. Holdsworth (1978b) found that 75% of stomach contents are vomited. At the time of writing apomorphine is not sold as a solution for injection and must be prepared by the hospital pharmacist (Burns, 1982).

Although Nimmo et al (1975) found that metoclopramide did not counteract the delaying effect of pethidine on gastric emptying when given along with pethidine, Murphy et al (1984) showed that an intravenous injection of metoclopramide 10 mg was effective when given at least 1 hour before the narcotic. It is concluded that intravenous metoclopramide can accelerate gastric emptying when no narcotic analgesic is administered or when given at least 1 hour before the narcotic. Metoclopramide increases the tone of the gastro-oesophageal sphincter (high pressure zone) and this is a useful action, but acceleration of gastric emptying should not be relied upon if pethidine has been given. The volume of gastric juice is reduced by cimetidine and ranitidine and is of course increased by oral alkalis.

The volume and pH of gastric contents were unchanged for up to 45 hours after delivery. All standard precautions should therefore be taken when anaesthetizing women in the early puerperium (James, 1984). It is not possible to state when the risks become those of a non-pregnant female.

Regurgitation and the gastro-oesophageal sphincter. Reference has already been made to the increase in intragastric pressure associated with pregnancy. Fortunately the increased pressure is, in most patients, well compensated for by a concomitant increase in the tone of the gastro-oesophageal sphincter. The gradient between the intragastric pressure and the sphincter pressure was $27.6 \, \text{cmH}_2\text{O}$ (5.0 kPa) on average (Lind et al, 1968), a value somewhat higher than that observed in non-pregnant women. It is of course this pressure difference which constitutes the barrier pressure and which resists the reflux of stomach contents into the oesophagus.

In one important group of pregnant women the pressure gradient between the stomach and the gastro-oesophageal sphincter is much lower. In a considerable number of patients who suffer from heartburn during pregnancy the intragastric pressure is elevated to the extent usually associated with pregnancy but the sphincter pressure is not increased. In these women the barrier pressure averaged only $7.3 \, \text{cmH}_2\text{O}$ (1.4 kPa). In consequence it appears that the normal pregnant woman may actually be rather less prone to regurgitate gastric contents, despite her high intragastric pressure. The risk of regurgitation is however abnormally high in patients with heartburn where sphincter tone is low, and in patients with obesity, multiple pregnancy and hydramnios who may have very high intragastric pressure.

There is another mechanism which may operate in favour of reducing the predisposition to regurgitation. Alkalinization of the stomach contents increases the tone of the gastro-oesophageal sphincter (Castell and Harris,

1970; Higgs et al, 1974). This may result from the release of gastrin in response to the rise in pH, although this explanation is not accepted by all authorities.

The fasciculations often associated with an intravenous injection of suxamethonium may, in a small number of patients, produce a sharp rise in intragastric pressure which is of very short duration (Andersen, 1962; Roe, 1962) although no such rises were observed by Spence et al (1967) using a less responsive technique of manometry. The fear that suxamethonium might cause regurgitation has been shown to be unfounded by Smith et al (1978) who demonstrated a compensatory increase in the tone of the gastro-oesophageal sphincter when suxamethonium is administered.

The action of drugs on the gastro-oesophageal sphincter in pregnancy has not been fully elucidated. Metoclopramide increases sphincter tone in non-pregnant subjects by 29 cmH$_2$O (2.8 kPa) but its action seems less certain in pregnancy (Brock-Utne et al, 1976; Hey and Ostick, 1978). Intravenous atropine and glycopyrrolate reduce sphincter tone in pregnant and non-pregnant subjects (Brock-Utne et al, 1976; Brock-Utne et al, 1978; Dow et al, 1978). Intravenous atropine is now given only if a second dose of suxamethonium is required. An intravenous injection of metoclopramide 10 mg will maintain sphincter tone if given with atropine (Brock-Utne et al, 1976). Intravenous pethidine, morphine and diazepam relax the gastro-oesophageal sphincter (Hall et al, 1975) and should be avoided. There are therefore fairly good grounds for giving metoclopramide 10 mg intravenously before induction of anaesthesia, more in the hope of raising the tone of the gastro-oesophageal sphincter and preventing regurgitation than in the hope of increasing the rate of gastric emptying, and the drug itself appears to be harmless.

Cricoid pressure (Sellick (1961) is now extensively used to prevent the emergence of any regurgitated material from the oesophagus into the pharynx. Sellick's manoeuvre has been found to be capable of preventing this disastrous occurrence when the intragastric pressure ranged from 50 to 94 cmH$_2$O, mean 74 cmH$_2$O (9–17 kPa, mean 13.4 kPa). A pressure of up to 64 N is required in order to occlude the oesophagus in some subjects and, in practice, an adequate pressure is not always applied (Howells et al, 1983). When correctly used Sellick's manoeuvre should be able to cope with the great majority of intragastric pressures likely to be encountered in pregnancy. The highest intragastric pressures were observed in pregnant women in the lithotomy position, when 7 out of 31 patients had values between 40 and 60 cmH$_2$O (7.2 and 10.9 kPa) (Spence et al, 1967) and whenever possible anaesthesia should not be induced in this position. If regurgitation occurs when Sellick's manoeuvre is allegedly being performed it is most likely to be due to incorrect application of cricoid pressure. Rosen (1981) has emphasized the value of cricoid pressure and stressed the need for skilled assistance for the anaesthetist at the induction of anaesthesia. Unfortunately, incorrect application of cricoid pressure can make intubation difficult or impossible,

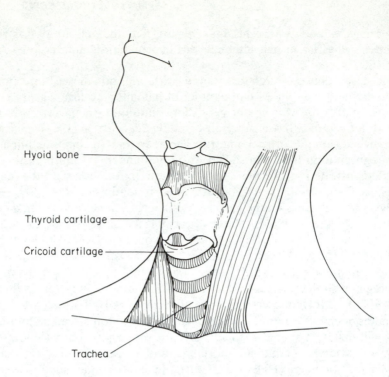

Hyoid bone

Thyroid cartilage

Cricoid cartilage

Trachea

Figure 8. The position of the cricoid cartilage in relation to the thyroid cartilage and the trachea.

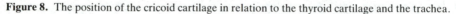

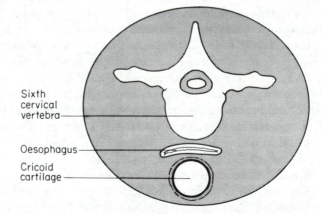

Sixth
cervical
vertebra

Oesophagus

Cricoid
cartilage

Figure 9. Diagrammatic cross-section of the neck at the level of the cricoid cartilage to show how the oesophagus can be compressed between the cricoid cartilage and the body of the sixth cervical vertebra.

while perhaps failing to prevent regurgitation. Considerable force is needed in order to prevent regurgitation and adequate pressure was applied in only half of the patients in one series (Howells et al, 1983; Wraight et al, 1983). Absence of an experienced assistant has caused maternal deaths and is an administrative failure on the part of the hospital authority or the consultant anaesthetists.

'Silent' regurgitation was detected in 20% of patients anaesthetized with nitrous oxide, a muscle relaxant and a narcotic analgesic, in whom the trachea was intubated (Turndorf et al, 1974). These patients were not pregnant and 'silent' regurgitation meant the presence of gastric juice in the oesophagus although not necessarily in the pharynx.

Premedication

It is probably impossible to administer an effective sedative premedication to an obstetric patient without producing some depressant action on the infant at birth. The patient who is in labour may have received sedatives and narcotic analgesics during labour and some of these patients will not fear anaesthesia and operative delivery but will welcome the ending of pain and distress and the birth of the baby.

The main problem arises with patients for elective caesarean section. These patients will be naturally anxious for their own and their infant's wellbeing. The authors administer no sedative premedication before elective caesarean section and prefer to rely on explanation and reassurance for the relief of anxiety. Most women willingly agree to forego sedatives and narcotic analgesics in the best interests of the infant. If the mother is very anxious then a shorter acting benzodiazepine, such as temazepam or midazolam, is unlikely to cause serious neonatal depression.

Intravenous atropine is avoided as it relaxes the gastro-oesophageal sphincter. An intramuscular injection of atropine or hyoscine is not given because salivation is rarely troublesome with modern techniques of anaesthesia, unless precipitated by neostigmine. The intravenous injection of atropine may be replaced by an injection of hyoscine 0.6 mg in the hope of reducing the incidence of awareness during anaesthesia. This measure alone may slightly reduce but does not eliminate this distressing occurrence. Latto and Wainwright (1972) state that anterograde amnesia does not appear for 20 minutes after the intravenous injection of hyoscine and that therefore the injection should be given well before the induction of anaesthesia. They attribute the amnesia obtained mainly to the use of methoxyflurane. Intravenous atropine reduces the tone of the gastro-oesophageal sphincter, predisposing to regurgitation, and may be accompanied by an intravenous injection of metoclopramide 10 mg to prevent this action (Brock-Utne et al, 1976). An intravenous injection of the anticholinergic agent glycopyrrolate (0.3 mg) may be substituted for atropine but this drug also relaxes the gastro-oesophageal sphincter (Brock-Utne et al, 1978). Glycopyrrolate reduces gastric acidity but the reduction is not always adequate as the sole alkalinizing measure (Baraka et al, 1977). Glycopyrrolate and atropine have similar effects on maternal heart rate when given intravenously and do not cause fetal tachycardia when given shortly before the induction of anaesthesia in a dose of atropine 0.01 mg/kg and glycopyrrolate 0.005 mg/kg (Abboud et al, 1983).

The administration of metoclopramide 10 mg intravenously is of uncertain value. It does not reduce the volume of gastric content at elective caesarean section (Cohen et al, 1984) and its probable value would lie in reducing the risk of regurgitation by its action on the gastro-oesophageal sphincter (Brock-Utne et al, 1976).

Immediate preparations for anaesthesia

Most of the preparations listed under this heading are part of any sound anaesthetic practice and need not be elaborated upon. A few are peculiar to obstetric anaesthesia. The following are essential preliminaries which should be omitted in only the most acute emergencies:

The identity of the patient. This should be checked by verbal enquiry and against the identity band on the wrist.

Antacid. The anaesthetist should satisfy himself that an antacid has been given. If this is not the case then a dose of 30 ml 0.3 M sodium citrate should be given before inducing anaesthesia. Ideally oral ranitidine 150 mg should have been given from 2 to 6 hours earlier. Alternatively an intramuscular injection of ranitidine 50 mg or cimetidine 300 mg is acceptable.

Stomach tube. If a stomach tube is in place it is recommended that this be aspirated and then withdrawn. It is thought that if the tube is left in position then the gastro-oesophageal sphincter may be rendered incompetent and that Sellick's manoeuvre may be ineffective.

Pulse and blood pressure. The pulse and blood pressure should be checked before inducing anaesthesia. Supine hypotension should be prevented by the use of a lateral or laterally tilted position. Hypotension due to caval occlusion is often associated with bradycardia (Lees et al, 1967). The use of an automatic blood pressure recorder is recommended.

ECG monitoring. Continuous electrocardiographic monitoring is advised in all cases as a safety precaution.

Intravenous infusion. An intravenous infusion of normal saline or a balanced salt solution should be set up before every caesarean section. A central venous pressure line may be useful, for example in antepartum haemorrhage and in the presence of serious heart disease. When the patient has been deprived of oral fluids, during labour or overnight before elective caesarean section, she may be dehydrated and hypovolaemic. It is therefore a good practice to administer 0.5 litre or 1.0 litre of crystalloid fluid intravenously before the induction of anaesthesia.

Blood for transfusion. As a matter of routine there should be two units of compatible blood for every patient undergoing caesarean section and this blood should be within the operating suite. The anticipation of the possibility of an operative delivery during labour should ensure that this recommendation is implemented at the great majority of caesarean sections. Slow progress in labour, fetal distress, previous caesarean section and indeed almost any variation from normality should indicate a request to the laboratory for the cross-matching of blood. 'Screened' group O negative blood may be kept for use in emergencies and this blood is probably safer than blood which has been cross-matched by an emergency method. Experience indicates that only between 5 and 10% of women actually receive a blood transfusion at caesarean section. This does not remove the need to have blood readily available for all patients. Reisner (1983) cites a cross-match/transfusion rate of between 17:1 and 64:1 and advocates a 'type and screen' policy whereby all patients for caesarean section are grouped and screened for antibodies. If antibodies are detected then blood is cross-matched. If there are no antibodies then serum is retained and a rapid cross-match is done if blood is required. Such a policy could be satisfactory in most situations with the important proviso that blood will always be available within 15 minutes of request.

Purely from the standpoint of volume crystalloid solutions may suffice. Dextran of mean molecular weight 70 000 (Macrodex) is an effective blood substitute, at least in volumes of up to 1 litre (Vickers et al, 1969). However blood losses of up to 2.5 litres may occur at caesarean section (Brant, 1966; Wallace, 1967; Toldy and Scott, 1969) and at forceps delivery under general anaesthesia losses of up to 1.5 litres are not rare (Moir and Wallace, 1967). Although blood transfusion is now usually given only to the 5 or 10% or so of women who lose substantially over 1 litre of blood at section, this is no justification for the unavailability of compatible blood for transfusion.

Blood warming. A safe and efficient apparatus for the warming of blood should be available and should be used for transfusions whose volume exceeds 500 ml. An apparatus employing a coil of tubing within a water bath or electrically warmed compartment is probably the safest type although the need to transfuse under pressure is a disadvantage if any but the lowest flow rates are required.

Blood filtration. A blood filter should be used for all transfusions of more than 500 ml in order to prevent microemboli reaching the lungs.

Assistance for the anaesthetist. It is essential that the anaesthetist should have the undivided attention of an assistant who is capable of performing cricoid pressure and who is reasonably familiar with anaesthetic techniques. It may be helpful to mark the point of cricoid pressure on the skin with a ball-point pen. Failure to provide the anaesthetist with a trained assistant has caused the deaths of several women.

Equipment and drugs. Within the normal full range of anaesthetic equipment, including a ventilator and cardiac monitor, certain items are of particular importance to the obstetric anaesthetist. Among these are an efficient suction apparatus, with a reserve foot-operated apparatus for use in emergencies, a selection of cuffed endotracheal tubes of size ranging from 5.0 to 9.0 mm, two laryngoscopes and a stilette to facilitate intubation. It has been the practice in the Queen Mother's Hospital, Glasgow, for 20 years to keep trays of carefully labelled anaesthetic drugs in a refrigerator in the anaesthetic room for immediate use. Also instantly available are endotracheal tubes, with connections attached, and an infusion of Ringer lactate solution. The various items which might be required in order to deal with a difficult or failed intubation must be immediately to hand and are discussed below.

An operating table capable of both head-down and lateral tilt is preferred for caesarean section. For operative vaginal delivery a modern obstetric bed is essential. Steel's obstetric table has been most effective in the writer's experience and a head-down tilt can be effected by pressure with the foot, leaving the hands free. The Oxford Labour Ward Bed is also suitable. Unfortunately neither of these beds has a lateral tilt mechanism. Lateral tilt frightens some patients in labour and would create difficulties in manufacture (Steel, 1977, personal communication). In the absence of a laterally tilting bed or table the uterus must be displaced from the vena cava by the insertion of a folded towel or a specially made wedge under the right buttock. An effective and inexpensive wedge can be made by inflating with air a 3 litre plastic bag of the type used for bladder irrigation. Inflation is easily performed by attaching a sphygmomanometer bulb to a length of infusion tubing (Carrie, 1982). The use of a mechanical device to displace the uterus to the left is popular in some North American centres.

Position of the patient. No patient who is in the later weeks of pregnancy should ever lie in the unmodified supine position before or during the induction of anaesthesia. A laterally tilted position is essential in these circumstances and must be maintained until delivery of the infant. The evidence for improved fetal oxygenation in the absence of caval occlusion is totally convincing (Ansari et al, 1970; Goodlin, 1971; Crawford et al, 1972; Downing et al, 1974a) and it is recommended that patients should be transported to theatre in the left lateral position (Crawford et al, 1973). This 'journey tilt' was found to reduce maternal metabolic acidosis. Patients transported in the supine position and then anaesthetized in the tilted position developed a greater metabolic acidosis prior to delivery than those transported and anaesthetized in the tilted position. Caval occlusion was thought to cause acid metabolites to accumulate in the legs, only to be released when a lateral tilt was introduced. The degree of lateral tilt necessary for the avoidance of caval occlusion is quite small. Ten degrees of tilt is more than sufficient and a tilt to the left is probably more effective than a tilt to the right (Drummond et al, 1974; Buley et al, 1977; Newman et al, 1983). Maternal as well as fetal oxygenation is improved by lateral tilting (Downing et al, 1974a). There is probably a small minority of patients for whom a tilt to the right is more effective.

Anaesthesia should not be induced while the patient is in the lithotomy position. If it is not possible, as for example during breech delivery, to place the patient in the supine, laterally tilted position then the legs should be removed from the lithotomy supports and held by two assistants. By this means the increase in intragastric pressure which occurs in the full lithotomy position will be minimized (Spence et al, 1967) and the patient may be quickly turned on her side if she should vomit. Regional analgesia is preferred for breech delivery. The use of general anaesthesia is a dangerous anachronism. The head-up position is not recommended because it will not prevent regurgitation, intubation is rather difficult with a steep head-up tilt, and cardiac output and cerebral blood flow may be compromised in poor risk patients.

The induction of anaesthesia

When the foregoing preliminaries have been completed the induction of anaesthesia may proceed.

Preoxygenation should be carried out by the administration of oxygen at a flow rate of 8 litres/min for a full 3 minutes. The Magill (Mapleson A), Bain or other non-rebreathing circuit should be preferred in order to encourage the washout of nitrogen from the alveoli. Archer and Marx (1974) have observed that when preoxygenation for 4 minutes was followed by apnoea of duration 1 minute the reduction in arterial Po_2 during apnoea was substantially greater in pregnant women at term than in non-pregnant controls. The mean reduction in Po_2 during apnoea was 139 mmHg (18.5 kPa) in the pregnant subjects and 58 mmHg (7.7 kPa) in the controls. Although Po_2 did not fall to hypoxic levels in any of the patients in 1 minute of apnoea it is likely that the pregnant woman will be less tolerant of a prolonged or difficult intubation than her non-pregnant sister. Archer and Marx attributed their observations to the higher metabolic requirements of pregnancy. Sykes (1975) has suggested alternative (or perhaps additional) explanations including the reduced FRC and increased closing volumes of pregnancy. A rapid alternative method of preoxygenation involves the inhalation of oxygen during three maximal inspirations and is effective in extremely urgent situations (Drummond and Park, 1984).

Preoxygenation can usefully be supervised by the anaesthetist's assistant and during this 3 minute period the anaesthetist can recheck drugs and equipment. Metoclopramide 10 mg may be injected.

The placental transfer of the currently used intravenous induction agents is discussed in chapter 3. Thiopentone 3.0–3.5 mg/kg body weight remains the induction agent of choice. The placental transfer and fetal distribution of thiopentone are such that if delivery of the infant takes place not less than 3–5 minutes after an injection and the dose is restricted to the recommended quantity, then neonatal depression due to the induction agent is unlikely (Morgan et al, 1981).

Inhalational agents are now hardly ever used for the induction of anaesthesia for obstetric surgery in the UK, although they have been extensively used for the production of unconsciousness at the moment of birth in the USA and Canada. If an inhalational induction is to be carried out in a patient in whom intravenous induction is considered to be too hazardous or impossible, then cyclopropane is in the writer's experience satisfactory. When skilfully administered, induction with cyclopropane is very swift and if the agent is used solely as a substitute for the intravenous agent and the technique of anaesthesia is otherwise unaltered, then the depressant effect on the infant and on myometrial contractility should be negligible (Kristoffersen, 1979).

Cricoid pressure should be applied by an assistant at the induction of anaesthesia. Some authorities advocate the performance of Sellick's manoeuvre before the injection of the induction agent. Because this has sometimes resulted in unwelcome and potentially dangerous movement by the patient it is suggested that cricoid pressure be applied at the moment when consciousness is lost. Fatal aspiration has occurred despite cricoid pressure (Whittington et al, 1979) and these authors advocate attempts to empty the stomach as well as cricoid pressure. Correctly applied cricoid pressure is highly effective and failure suggests faulty technique. Accurate application should not make intubation more difficult unless the mother's neck is flexed. Flexion can be countered by upward pressure of the assistant's free hand which is placed behind the patient's neck. The assistant should avoid lateral displacement of the larynx.

The injection of the induction agent is followed immediately by the intravenous injection of suxamethonium. It is strongly recommended that 100 mg or 1.5 mg/kg body weight of suxamethonium be given to ensure optimal conditions for intubation. Pretreatment with a small dose of a non-depolarizing muscle relaxant is strongly condemned. So-called 'self-taming' is ineffective, dangerous and unnecessary. Fasciculations and after-pains are not prevented, significant myoneural blockade is produced and intubation is made more difficult (Masey et al, 1983). In a minority of patients 3 mg of D-tubocurarine will cause dyspnoea, reduce maximum ventilation and predispose to aspiration (Bruce et al, 1984). After-pains are, in any case, uncommon in pregnancy (Thind and Bryson, 1983). When the jaw muscles are fully relaxed the trachea is intubated with a cuffed tube and the cuff is inflated forthwith. A tube of 8.5 mm or at the most 9.0 mm diameter is preferred in order to reduce the likelihood of failure to intubate. A selection of tubes ranging down to 5.0 mm diameter should be to hand in case of difficulty. It is a most important feature of this technique that no attempt should be made to inflate the lungs by face mask before intubation of the trachea. If preoxygenation has been conscientiously performed then arterial hypoxaemia will not occur until apnoea has lasted for at least 1 minute and very probably for substantially longer (Archer and Marx, 1974). Although intubation should be performed as swiftly and smoothly as possible in order to minimize the risk of regurgitation, speculation upon the data of Archer and Marx suggests that preoxygenation for at least 3 minutes may allow the period of apnoea to extend well beyond 60 seconds without hypoxia. Marx and Mateo (1971) observed maternal P_aO_2 values of below 100 mmHg (13.3 kPa) following difficult intubation even after preoxygenation and in these patients the onset of neonatal respiration was delayed.

The hypertensive response to intubation. The hypertensive response to intubation could, in theory, provoke intracranial bleeding and death in mothers with existing hypertensive disease. The intravenous administration of hydralazine 0.4 mg/kg 10 minutes before anaesthesia should prevent a serious rise in arterial blood pressure (Davies et al, 1981). A more rapid response may be obtained with sodium nitroprusside (Stoelting, 1979) or nitroglycerine which has the advantage of a very short duration of action should excessive hypotension result, with attendant placental insufficiency (Hood et al, 1983). Topical anaesthesia of the larynx is ineffective and predisposes to the aspiration of stomach contents. Deep anaesthesia with powerful volatile agents is probably effective in preventing the hypertensive response to intubation but cannot be generally recommended for obstetric patients. The choice of muscle relaxant influences the hypertensive response. The response is marked with pancuronium and absent with alcuronium (Cummings et al, 1983) but alcuronium is not suitable for rapid intubation in the obstetric patient.

Failed or difficult intubation

Failed intubation, difficult intubation and misplacement of the endotracheal tube together constitute the leading cause of maternal death in association with anaesthesia. The number of deaths from this cause now exceeds the number due to inhalation of stomach contents (Department of Health and Social Security, 1982; Scottish Home and Health Department, 1978). Death usually results from hypoxia or from associated regurgitation and aspiration of gastric contents. The effect of hypoxia may be aggravated by hypotension as a result of aortocaval occlusion.

Failed intubation occurs in at least 1 in every 300 obstetric general anaesthetics. This estimate is based upon experience in the Queen Mother's

Hospital, Glasgow, St James's University Hospital, Leeds, and Queen Charlotte's Maternity Hospital, London. The complication is therefore apparently commoner in obstetric anaesthesia than in other branches of anaesthesia. Factors which predispose to difficult or failed intubation include:

Short thick neck
Prominent incisor teeth
Narrow atlanto-occipital gap, inhibiting extension of the head (Nichol and Zuck, 1983)
Abnormalities of the cervical spine
Unusually deep inferior ramus of the mandible
Arthritis of the temporomandibular and laryngeal joints
Trismus
Laryngeal oedema in pre-eclampsia (Brock-Utne et al, 1977), fluid overload (Dobb, 1978) and raised venous pressure in prolonged labour (Mackenzie, 1978)

In clinical practice it is not always easy to predict difficult or impossible intubation. It is essential that every anaesthetist should have a plan of action for use when faced with failure to intubate the trachea. The failed intubation drill which is set out below is based on the drill described by Tunstall in 1976. The individual anaesthetist may wish to make minor modifications to accord with her or his own skills and with the clinical situation. The value of preoxygenation before every obstetric anaesthetic cannot be overemphasized and will prevent or delay the development of serious hypoxia in a crisis.

A failed intubation drill

(1) The anaesthetist must be willing to accept failure after two or three attempts which will probably involve the use of mechanical aids such as an introducer, a laryngoscope with a polio blade, a modified polio blade (Jellicoe and Harris, 1984) or a prism. A tube of small diameter should have been tried. Anyone can fail to intubate and it is no disgrace. Deaths have occurred due to too frequent and prolonged attempts at intubation, sometimes by a succession of anaesthetists of ascending seniority and where common sense seems to have been in inverse proportion to their seniority. There must be no attitude of 'I will intubate this patient even if it kills her' and acceptance of failure is the first and most vital step in the drill.

(2) Cricoid pressure is maintained. Correctly applied cricoid pressure does not make intubation more difficult. Incorrect application may displace the larynx to one side.

(3) An oropharyngeal airway is inserted.

(4) The lungs are ventilated with oxygen by bag and mask until spontaneous ventilation returns. If this is difficult then a nasopharyngeal tube may be helpful.

(5) If assistance is available then the mother is turned onto her left side, while maintaining cricoid pressure.

(6) A suction catheter is inserted into the mouth and left in position.

A decision must now be made in conjunction with the obstetrician as to the time of delivery.

If delivery is not urgent then the mother should be allowed to regain consciousness. This should happen quickly if the recommended technique of induction with thiopentone and suxamethonium has been used and a long-acting non-depolarizing relaxant has not been administered. The operation can be performed later under epidural or spinal anaesthesia. The use of these techniques entails a very small additional risk if an abnormally high block should result in a patient who cannot be intubated. This risk must be accepted. It is sometimes suggested that spinal anaesthesia is safer because an 'accidental spinal' will not occur but Russell (1985) has reported very high blocks with respiratory impairment when using plain bupivacaine for caesarean section. Spinal anaesthesia has a failure rate of 4–8% and hypotension may be sudden and severe. Epidural anaesthesia seems, on balance, the method of choice and a cautious incremental technique should be used in order to minimize the risk of a dangerously high block.

If immediate delivery is essential then general anaesthesia should be continued using a powerful volatile agent delivered by face mask to a spontaneously breathing mother. Anaesthesia should be maintained at a moderate depth in order to permit surgical access and to prevent active vomiting. The risk of myometrial hypotonia is recognized. Rapid delivery is important. Although it is possible to perform caesarean section in the left lateral position, it may be expedient to return the patient to the supine laterally inclined position. At the end of the operation the mother should be placed in the lateral, head-down position in anticipation of vomiting. An alternative approach involves the use of infiltration analgesia of the abdominal wall. Conditions are rarely perfect but this must be accepted in the interest of safety. A technique is described on page 316 and obstetricians should be able to carry out this technique.

The foregoing plan will deal safely with most cases of failed intubation, but it assumes that an adequate airway can be maintained and that the lungs can be ventilated without intubation of the trachea. In the rare situation in which these essentials are impossible then the situation is indeed grave. An airway may be created by puncture of the trachea or cricothyroid membrane. A formal tracheostomy will be inappropriate and a wide-bore intravenous cannula or the point of an intravenous infusion set should be used. A mini-tracheostomy set has recently become available for this purpose. These devices should be immediately available in every obstetric theatre along with suitable connectors to enable oxygen and anaesthetic gases to be administered. Excessive pressure within the airways must be prevented and an expiratory valve must be included in the circuit. High frequency transtracheal jet ventilation can be performed but the authors know of a maternal death from displacement of the tracheal cannula into the tissues. An alternative to a simplified tracheostomy in cases where obstruction is not due to laryngeal oedema or blockage is the insertion of an oesophagogastric tube airway (oesophageal obturator airway) as described by Don Michael et al in 1968 and used successfully by Tunstall and Geddes in 1984. This device has a blind distal end and perforations in the pharyngeal portion to permit the exit of oxygen. The proximal end passes through a face mask which has an oxygen inlet. The tube is passed blindly into the oesophagus and will sometimes relieve upper airway obstruction when other means fail. The lungs can be ventilated with oxygen (Merrifield and King, 1981) and inhalational anaesthesia administered. This device should be available in the obstetric theatre.

Inadvertent intubation of the oesophagus may be the outcome of repeated attempts at tracheal intubation. The anaesthetist is understandably anxious to believe that his tube is in the trachea at last and may be encouraged in this belief by the absence of cyanosis when a proper preoxygenation procedure has been undertaken. Several deaths have occurred in these circumstances and cardiac arrest may occur at about the time of delivery of the infant. Howells and Riethmuller (1980) agree that the diagnosis of oesophageal intubation can sometimes be difficult and point out that 'wheezing' and spurious chest movements may occur.

Fazadinium has minimal placental transfer and has been proposed as a substitute for suxamethonium for obstetric use (Blogg et al, 1975). The conditions for intubation are too often dangerously unsatisfactory (Young et al, 1975; Corall et al, 1977), and despite the advantages of absence of fasciculations and hyperkalaemia, the use of fazadinium for intubation is not recommended. Neither atracurium (Gergis et al, 1983) nor vecuronium (Scott and Goat, 1982; Stirt et al, 1984) can equal suxamethonium for rapid and easy intubation. Vecuronium is suitable for the maintenance of relaxation after intubation and appears to offer cardiovascular stability. The duration of action of vecuronium is shorter in pregnancy according to Dailey et al (1984). The placental transfer of atracurium is quite extensive and it appears not to be a primary choice for routine obstetric use (Frank et al, 1983). The placental transfer of suxamethonium is clinically insignificant except where cholinesterase activity is inadequate (Finster and Marx, 1976), maternal apnoea is not prolonged (Blitt et al, 1977) and the incidence of 'after-pains' is only 20% after a suxamethonium infusion in pregnancy (Datta et al, 1977). Following a single injection of 100 mg suxamethonium 'after pains' are experienced by only 7.5% of mothers (Thind and Bryson, 1983).

Suxamethonium remains the relaxant of choice for intubation in obstetric anaesthesia, despite other drawbacks. The oft-repeated claim that the fasciculations of suxamethonium might cause regurgitation of stomach contents has been proved false by Smith et al (1978) by their demonstration that any rise in intragastric pressure is negated by an increase in pressure at the lower oesophageal sphincter.

The maintenance of anaesthesia

There are certain problems and requirements which are peculiar to obstetric anaesthesia. Most of these requirements are in the fetal interest and so are only relevant up until delivery of the infant. The problems and requirements are perhaps greatest at caesarean section and it is at elective caesarean section that the influence of anaesthesia upon the condition of the infant, for good or bad, is most apparent. In recent years the influence of several factors, sometimes previously unsuspected, upon the condition of the infant at birth has been demonstrated. Unfortunately, despite quite intensive publicity there are anaesthetists who have not yet absorbed this information into their practice. The placental transfer of drugs is now better understood and the influence of maternal P_aO$_2$ and P_aCO$_2$ upon the fetus has been clarified. The major influence of caval occlusion for harm is so easily prevented, yet one hears of hospitals where caesarean sections are performed in the supine position without lateral tilt.

Drug-induced neonatal respiratory depression. There are of course many causes of neonatal asphyxia and respiratory depression and many of these causes are unrelated to anaesthesia. It is in the 'clinically acceptable, ideal case' for elective caesarean section that adverse effects of drugs, if any, may be demonstrated in the newborn (Crawford, 1962).

Dose-related depression of the Apgar score and delay in establishing respiration at birth have been recorded with methohexitone, ketamine and Althesin (Downing et al, 1973; Holdcroft et al, 1974; Downing et al, 1976), but this may be anticipated with excessive doses of any intravenous induction agent. Depression of the infant in the first minutes of life is unlikely to be of serious extent if a minimal 'sleep dose' of one of the intravenous agents is used. Fetal metabolic acidosis is probably greater after Althesin and propanidid than after thiopentone, methohexitone, ketamine or etomidate (Levinson et al, 1973; Downing et al, 1974b; Downing et al, 1979). This suggests that there is some impairment of placental blood flow with Althesin and propanidid due perhaps to a reduction in maternal cardiac output. The circulation is well maintained under light thiopentone and etomidate anaesthesia (Morgan et al, 1975; Chamberlain et al, 1977).

Although the careful use of minimal doses of most induction agents is unlikely to cause serious drug-induced depression or metabolic acidosis in the mature fetus with good placental function delivered by elective caesarean section, the small differences between the various agents could be important when the fetus is at risk. Induction of anaesthesia with thiopentone can cause a transient reduction in intervillous blood flow, even in the absence of hypotension (Jouppila et al, 1979). Unless prolonged this is unlikely to harm a healthy fetus. Factors such as unpleasant or even dangerous reactions and the avoidance of awareness during surgery must also influence the choice of induction agent, and in the writer's view, the choice lies between thiopentone, methohexitone and etomidate. Thiopentone is preferred, but a case can be made for etomidate, which appears to cause even less fetal metabolic acidosis than thiopentone (Downing et al, 1979). Downing and his colleagues injected 0.3 mg/kg etomidate and 1 mg/kg suxamethonium from the same syringe and minimized pain and movement. The dose of any induction agent should ideally be based upon the mother's weight and a dose of 3.0–3.5 mg/kg thiopentone is appropriate.

Nitrous oxide is used as the principal agent for the maintenance of unconsciousness in nearly all current techniques of anaesthesia for caesarean section. The mean concentration of nitrous oxide in the fetal blood was 79% of the maternal blood concentration when delivery took place between 2 and 19 minutes after commencing the administration of the gas (Marx et al, 1970). The range was wide, varying from 55 to 91%. There was a tendency for the fetal concentration to rise as administration was prolonged and this tendency was also noted by others (Stenger et al, 1967; Stenger et al, 1969). The observation that prolonged nitrous oxide anaesthesia resulted in an increased incidence of neonatal asphyxia (Crawford, 1962) was probably the result of caval occlusion in the supine position. Mankowitz et al (1981) have shown that the administration of nitrous oxide to the mother does not cause diffusion hypoxia in the neonate.

When caesarean section is performed with a maternal F_IO_2 of up to 66% and caval occlusion is prevented, then the fetus is unlikely to be rendered acidotic if the time from induction of anaesthesia to incision of the uterus does not exceed 30 minutes (Crawford et al, 1972; Crawford et al, 1976). However, Palahniuk and Cumming (1977) observed a progressive fetal acidosis attributed to vasoconstriction in the uteroplacental circulation in the pregnant ewe in the lateral position, anaesthetized with thiopentone and 70% of nitrous oxide. It was suggested that this fetal deterioration was due to the increased output of catecholamines which is known to occur under light nitrous oxide anaesthesia (Smith et al, 1970) and to the use of a rather low F_IO_2 (30%). The transient reduction in intervillous blood flow which follows an injection of thiopentone does not usually cause fetal acidosis (Jouppila et al, 1979). Adrenaline is known to constrict the uterine arteries in pregnant ewes (Rosenfeld et al, 1976). In contrast, deeper anaesthesia with 1.0 and 1.5 MAC of halothane, methoxyflurane and isoflurane was associated with slight increases in uterine artery blood flow under otherwise similar circumstances (Palahniuk and Shnider, 1974; Smith et al, 1975) and these studies provide further evidence in favour of a high maternal F_IO_2 and the use of a volatile agent as part of the technique of anaesthesia. A higher fetal Po_2 and a lesser degree of metabolic acidosis has been recorded in human infants delivered by caesarean section using methoxyflurane with 99% oxygen instead of unsupplemented 70% nitrous oxide (Palahniuk et al, 1977) and there is reason to think that ultra-light anaesthesia may not be best for the fetus. Even 0.5% halothane when used as a supplement to nitrous oxide may improve placental blood flow and reduce fetal acidosis (Datta et al, 1981).

Until 1969, when Wilson and Turner drew attention to the high incidence of awareness when nitrous oxide was used in concentrations of up to 75% in oxygen for caesarean section it was unusual to supplement nitrous oxide with intravenous or inhalational agents during anaesthesia for caesarean section. In order to reduce the incidence of awareness during obstetric anaesthesia it is now a common practice to add a low concentration of a volatile agent to the nitrous oxide and oxygen mixture. It is also accepted practice to administer 50%, or even 66%, of oxygen in order to achieve maximal or near-maximal oxygenation of the umbilical venous blood.

Halothane 0.5% (Moir, 1970; Galbert and Gardner, 1972; Skovstedt et al, 1973; Kangas et al, 1976), methoxyflurane 0.1 and 0.2% (Crawford, 1971a; Wilson, 1971; Crawford et al, 1976), trichloroethylene 0.2% (Crawford et al, 1985) and enflurane (Downing et al, 1979; Warren et al, 1983) have all been used. The relative effectiveness of these agents is difficult to evaluate because various concentrations of nitrous oxide have been used. The incidence of awareness with various concentrations of methoxyflurane and trichloro-ethylene given with 33–66% of oxygen varies from 1 to 10%. Experiences with 0.5% halothane and 50% nitrous oxide have been substantially better. This mixture has now been used for over 3000 caesarean sections in the Queen Mother's Hospital and awareness has been reported in under 1%. Latto and Waldron (1977) calculate that 0.2% halothane should suffice, but vaporizers capable of delivering this concentration accurately are rarely available. There is no doubt that when the powerful volatile and gaseous anaesthetics are used as the sole or principal agents for obstetric anaesthesia then the infant is more likely to be depressed at birth (Apgar et al, 1957; Hodges et al, 1959). These techniques are now rarely used. The use of very low concentrations of halothane, enflurane and methoxyflurane to ensure unconsciousness is not associated with any clinically detectable increase in the incidence of neonatal asphyxia and, as discussed above, may actually reduce fetal metabolic acidosis. In one series the Apgar scores of the infants were actually higher when halothane 0.5% was used (Moir, 1970), an observation then attributed to concomitant administration of a high percentage of oxygen (Galbert and Gardner, 1972) but perhaps due also to an increase in placental blood flow as a result of the addition of halothane (Datta et al, 1981). The concentration of halothane in the fetal blood is likely to be about 35% of the concentration in the maternal blood and the fetal blood methoxyflurane concentration is likely to lie between 48% and 70% of the maternal blood concentration (Siker et al, 1968; Clark et al, 1970; Latto and Waldron, 1977). When 0.1% methoxyflurane was administered during caesarean section the concentration in the umbilical vein had reached between 50% and 70% of the concentration in the maternal arterial blood after 15 minutes (Latto and Wainwright, 1972).

It is recommended that nitrous oxide and oxygen anaesthesia be supplemented by either 0.6% enflurane, 0.2% trichloroethylene or 0.5% halothane to ensure that awareness is unlikely to occur. The reduction in uterine artery blood flow associated with unsupplemented nitrous oxide anaesthesia may be prevented. These concentrations should not normally be exceeded. Higher concentrations may result in neonatal respiratory depression, maternal cardiovascular depression and uterine hypotonia. The use of intravenous narcotic analgesics is contraindicated before delivery due to their very rapid placental transfer. They may usefully be given after the delivery, especially during elective caesarean section, where the mother has received no preoperative analgesic drug.

Oxygen concentration. In an important publication in 1968, Rorke et al reported that as the maternal P_aO_2 increased towards 300 mmHg (39.9 kPa) the PO_2 of the fetal blood also increased and that further increases in maternal P_aO_2 were not accompanied by further increases in fetal PO_2. The patients were undergoing elective, repeat caesarean section and were in the 'clinically acceptable ideal' category of Crawford (1962). The patients received 33%, 66% or 100% of oxygen and fetal oxygenation and Apgar scores were best when 66% of oxygen was administered throughout the period before delivery. This important observation has been confirmed clinically and biochemically by others (Baraka, 1970; Moir, 1970; Marx and Mateo, 1971; Fox and Houle, 1971) although the failure to obtain further improvement in fetal oxygenation with inspired oxygen concentrations in excess of 66% was not always observed. The former view that maternal hyperoxia might cause constriction of the spiral arteries of the placenta is now regarded as suspect and there is no sound basis for limitation of the maternal F_IO_2.

It is clear that the oxygen percentage in the inspired gas mixture should be sufficient to produce an oxygen tension of about 300 mmHg (39.9 kPa) in the maternal arterial blood and that in the pregnant woman at term this is likely to require the use of a mixture containing at least 60% of oxygen. If a 40:60 or even a 50:50 mixture of nitrous oxide and oxygen is used without supplement and without sedative premedication then the incidence of awareness is likely to be high. It is therefore recommended that this gas mixture be supplemented with a minimal concentration of a volatile agent in the manner described above.

Palahniuk and his colleagues (1977) recorded the highest fetal oxygen tensions when giving 99% of oxygen during caesarean section, and Palahniuk and Cumming (1977) comment that there may be a trend towards the exclusion of nitrous oxide and the reliance upon a volatile agent given with about 100% of oxygen. This comment fails to allow for the probable depressant effect of the necessary concentration of volatile agent on the myometrium and the consequent risk of haemorrhage. Direct estimation of PO_2 in the monkey fetus in utero indicates that fetal PO_2 increases some 50 seconds after an increase in maternal F_IO_2 and decreases if placental blood flow is reduced (Myers et al, 1977).

Hyperventilation. There have been those who practised deliberate hyperventilation, sometimes of extreme degree, in the hope of further depressing consciousness during nitrous oxide and oxygen anaesthesia. At first sight this practice might seem to offer advantages in obstetrics as a way of diminishing the requirements for pharmacological anaesthesia although it is not necessarily effective (Wilson and Turner, 1969). There is now a great deal of evidence which indicates that maternal hyperventilation may be harmful to the fetus. Rather extreme hyperventilation is probably necessary to produce this effect. Moya et al (1965) observed that when the maternal Pco_2 was reduced to 17 mmHg (2.3 kPa) or lower, then the fetus developed a metabolic and respiratory acidosis. In most circumstances it is difficult to lower the Pco_2 to such levels, but it should be remembered that the P_aco_2 during pregnancy averages 30 or 31 mmHg (4.0 or 4.1 kPa) (Bouterline-Young and Bouterline-Young, 1956) and that in painful labour the maternal P_aco_2 is likely to average about 25 mmHg (3.3 kPa) and may be as low as 10 or 15 mmHg (1.3 or 2.0 kPa) (Sjøstedt, 1962; Fisher and Prys-Roberts, 1968; Andersen and Walker, 1970).

For some time it had been uncertain whether the harmful effects of hyperventilation on the fetus were due to a reduction in uteroplacental blood flow as the direct result of the low maternal P_aco_2 or were due to a reduction in uteroplacental blood flow following upon a decrease in cardiac output caused by high inflation pressures during IPPV. This question is discussed on page 54 but it now appears that both of these mechanisms may operate concurrently (Levinson et al, 1974).

It is concluded that hyperventilation should be avoided during obstetric anaesthesia. Normocapnia should be sought and in pregnancy this implies a P_aco_2 of about 30 mmHg (4.0 kPa). Burger and others (1983) suggest that optimal fetal pH is obtained when maternal pulmonary ventilation is performed at 100 ml/kg/min. Measurement of end-tidal Pco_2 will of course permit precise control of maternal P_aco_2.

The addition of carbon dioxide to the inspired gas mixture in the hope of increasing placental blood flow is probably ineffective and the high fetal Pco_2 which might result from this practice may prove harmful to the infant (Ivankovic et al, 1970; Hollmen and Jagerhorn, 1972).

Awareness during anaesthesia. The problem of awareness during obstetric anaesthesia has already been referred to on several occasions and this is an indication of the many ways in which the need to avoid this disturbing occurrence influences anaesthetic technique.

The extent of the problem was highlighted by Wilson and Turner (1969) when they reported that 8 or 9% of patients anaesthetized for caesarean section with thiopentone, nitrous oxide and a muscle relaxant had undoubted factual recall of events which had occurred during anaesthesia. Auditory recall was common and memory of pain was variable, due presumably to the analgesic properties of nitrous oxide. Nitrous oxide was used in concentrations of 50–75% in oxygen and hyperventilation was sometimes employed but neither the varying percentages of nitrous oxide nor the use of hyperventilation seemed to influence the occurrence of awareness. In addition to true awareness (factual recall) Wilson and Turner recorded a history of unpleasant and distressing dreams in 17% of their patients. Unpleasant dreams are thought to be related to the phenomenon of awareness and are often regarded as a lesser form of awareness.

Until these alarming figures were published, although most anaesthetists knew of the possibility of awareness during caesarean section, few had suspected that it might occur in 9% of patients. The initial response to Wilson and Turner's (1969) paper was the use of diazepam (Turner and Wilson, 1969) and hyoscine (Crawford, 1971a) for their sedative and amnesic properties. Unfortunately diazepam did not alter the incidence of awareness and substantially increased the percentage of patients who had unpleasant dreams during anaesthesia. When hyoscine was used instead of atropine as premedication there was a reduction in the incidence of awareness to between 2 and 4% and the incidence of unpleasant dreams was 5%. Clearly neither hyoscine nor diazepam can reduce the occurrence of awareness to acceptable levels although hyoscine is probably of value as part of a technique of anaesthesia (Crawford, 1971a). The use of narcotic analgesics is contraindicated until after the delivery of the infant.

Happily it was found that awareness was abolished in a series of 250 patients who were anaesthetized for caesarean section and who received a 50:50 mixture of nitrous oxide and oxygen supplemented with 0.5% halothane throughout the procedure (Moir, 1970). Anaesthesia had been induced with 200–250 mg thiopentone and a muscle relaxant was administered. Since this original publication, this technique has been used for over 3000 caesarean sections and the incidence of factual recall has been under 1%.

The reported incidence of awareness (factual recall and unpleasant dreams) in representative series of caesarean sections of reasonable size is as

Table 9. The reported incidence of awareness in representative series of caesarean sections

Nitrous oxide (%)	Supplement (%)	Awareness (%)	Reference
50–75	None	26	Wilson and Turner, 1969
50	None	17	Warren et al, 1983
67	None	21	Famewo, 1976
50	Halothane 0.5	<1	Moir, 1970 and later
50	Halothane 0.5	Nil	Warren et al, 1983
40	Halothane 0.5	Nil	Galbert and Gardner, 1972
33	Halothane 0.2	10	Crawford et al, 1985
33	Halothane 0.5	Nil	Crawford et al, 1985
33	Trichloroethylene 0.2	9.6	Crawford et al, 1985
33	Trichloroethylene 0.3	0.8	Crawford et al, 1985
50	Enflurane 0.6	Nil	Coleman and Downing, 1975
50	Enflurance 1.0	Nil	Warren et al, 1983
50	Isoflurane 0.75	Nil	Warren et al, 1983
Nil	Cyclopropane 7.5–25	2.5	Kristoffersen, 1979

shown in Table 9. The induction agent was thiopentone and intravenous supplements were avoided. In Kristoffersen's (1979) series anaesthesia was induced with cyclopropane.

An incidence of factual recall greater than about 1% is considered unacceptable, especially as there are now indications that very light, unsupplemented nitrous oxide anaesthesia may actually be undesirable because it may reduce placental blood flow and so promote fetal metabolic acidosis (Palahniuk and Cumming, 1977). Volatile agents in concentrations of 1.0–1.5 MAC do not reduce placental blood flow and may actually increase it (Palahniuk and Shnider, 1974; Smith et al, 1975). The anaesthetist must strive for optimal fetal oxygenation while maintaining unconsciousness and he should not be unduly afraid of the frequently over-emphasized risks of neonatal depression. One may speculate that awareness during caesarean section would act as a powerful stress and that the resulting production of catecholamines would impair uteroplacental blood flow, thus resulting in fetal acidosis.

Inspection of the awareness incidence listed above suggests that a nitrous oxide concentration below 50% increases the chance of awareness and that if less than this concentration is to be used in the fetal interest, then a higher concentration of volatile supplement will be required. The duration of anaesthesia and particularly of the induction–delivery (I-D) interval probably affects the chance of awareness, because it is during this time that very light anaesthesia has usually been sought. Tunstall (1979) recommends the use of 66% of nitrous oxide for 3 minutes after intubation for the reduction of awareness. A higher F_IO_2 is used thereafter. The short-term use of a higher percentage of nitrous oxide has a secondary benefit in accelerating the uptake of halothane by virtue of the second gas effect (Tunstall and Hawksworth, 1981) and seems to offer a practical technique for reducing the risk of awareness in the early minutes of anaesthesia when thiopentone levels are falling rapidly.

From experiences with 50% of nitrous oxide supplemented by 0.2 or 0.65% of halothane, Latto and Waldron (1977) estimated that 0.57 MAC was insufficient and 0.89 MAC was excessive for the prevention of awareness. The average MAC awake is 0.58 (Stoelting et al, 1970). Using nitrous oxide 50% with 0.5% halothane the predicted MAC values are 0.6 after 3 minutes and 0.8 after 10 minutes (Tunstall and Hawksworth, 1981) and these values are in the range required for the avoidance of awareness. This calculation is supported by an incidence of factual recall of under 1% in over 3000 caesarean sections where anaesthesia was maintained with 50% of nitrous oxide and 0.5% of halothane in the Queen Mother's Hospital. It should be remembered that the MAC for halothane is reduced by 16% in pregnancy (Strout and Nahrwold, 1981).

As has been stated, there may be a trend towards a very high F_IO_2 and a higher concentration of a volatile agent, with perhaps complete avoidance of nitrous oxide. The principal objection to such techniques must be the risk of uterine haemorrhage and a clinical compromise may be struck in the shape of the writers' preferred mixture of 50% nitrous oxide and 0.5% halothane which does not increase bleeding (Moir, 1970); 0.6% enflurane and 0.75% isoflurane also proved effective with 50% nitrous oxide (Coleman and Downing, 1975; Downing et al, 1979; Warren et al, 1983). The association between enflurane and excitation of the central nervous system suggests that it should be avoided in pre-eclampsia. The problem of awareness must be faced, for it is a terrifying experience and one which some patients find difficult to communicate, but may yet harm the attitude of the patient for all time towards anaesthesia. There is the possibility that such severe emotional stress might cause fetal hypoxia as a result of constriction of the uterine arteries (Morishima et al, 1978).

Tunstall (1979) has described the ingenious isolated forearm technique for the detection of awareness during anaesthesia. An arterial tourniquet prevents the entry of muscle relaxant to one forearm. The patient is then able to make prearranged hand signals to indicate awareness or pain. Tunstall (1980) has used this technique on a woman who wished to be awake but free of pain, although most anaesthetists would prefer regional anaesthesia for such a patient. The isolated forearm technique has shown that mothers may quite frequently be conscious during 'anaesthesia' and yet fail to recollect the events which occurred. In Tunstall's (1979) experience this occurred in 60% of mothers.

For some patients awareness while paralysed can be a terrifying experience. In the words of Claude Bernard they become 'sensitive beings locked in immobile bodies ... the torture which the imagination of the poets has invented can be found produced in nature by the action of the American poison'. Elimination of awareness is the aim but its complete achievement would mean the use of unnecessarily deep anaesthesia in the great majority of cases and a very low incidence of awareness may have to be accepted (Blacher, 1984).

Time. Speculation suggests several mechanisms whereby the passage of time might influence the condition of the infant at birth.

A very short I-D interval might result in the birth of the child at a time when the concentration of thiopentone or other induction agent in its blood is high (Morgan et al, 1981) and the infant might then suffer from drug-induced respiratory depression.

A prolonged I-D interval might result in the accumulation of nitrous oxide (Stenger et al, 1969) or volatile anaesthetic agent in the fetus. If the patient is in the supine position, without lateral tilt, then concealed or revealed caval occlusion is probable. Even if revealed caval occlusion (supine hypotension) does not arise it is likely that placental circulation may be impaired in the supine position and that the impairment may be exaggerated with the prolongation of the I-D interval. Failure to allow for the effect of caval occlusion probably accounts for much of the conflict of opinion about the influence of time on the condition of the infant in earlier studies.

If the delivery of the child is prolonged or difficult, whether at caesarean section or at operative vaginal delivery, it seems possible that this may cause asphyxia at birth. The consequences of partial separation of the placenta, cord compression and trauma are likely to be greater if delivery is prolonged. Aspiration of liquor amnii is more likely if respiratory efforts take place during a difficult delivery.

From the observations of Crawford and colleagues (1976) it appears that, with certain important provisos, the I-D interval is of no clinical importance in the production of fetal acidosis if that interval does not exceed 25 minutes. The provisos are (a) that caval occlusion is prevented by lateral tilt, (b) that a high F_IO_2 is used (66% in Crawford's series), (c) that a volatile supplement is used along with nitrous oxide, and (d) that anaesthetic accidents are avoided which might cause hypotension or hypoxia. If the nitrous oxide percentage is high (70%) and a volatile agent is omitted, then progressive fetal metabolic acidosis may develop due perhaps to constriction of the uterine arteries by endogenous adrenaline released under light nitrous oxide anaesthesia (Palahniuk and Cumming, 1977). If caval occlusion is permitted, then fetal metabolic acidosis is also likely to increase with the prolongation of the I-D interval (Crawford et al, 1972) and time and tilt are interconnected in the production of fetal acidosis. Perhaps the optimal I-D interval lies between 10 and 20 minutes if the above provisos are adhered to. This interval would allow the fetal blood concentrations of the intravenous induction agent to fall and would be well within the safe interval of 25 minutes.

The time between incision of the myometrium and delivery of the child (the U-D interval) influences the condition of the infant, even where the anaesthetic technique complies with the criteria above (Crawford et al, 1976). As the U-D interval increases, the extent of the fetal metabolic acidosis increases (Crawford et al, 1973; Crawford et al, 1976; Downing et al, 1976). If the U-D interval exceeds 90 seconds, then fetal asphyxia becomes probable. The U-D interval is often prolonged when the infant presents by the breech and in this situation the child is more likely to show signs of hypoxia when general anaesthesia is used. Epidural anaesthesia is better for abdominal breech delivery (Crawford and Davies, 1982). The explanation for this phenomenon lies less in anaesthetic than in obstetric factors such as partial placental separation, impaired placental blood flow and fetal breathing before a difficult delivery is completed. Handling the uterus may cause reflex constriction of myometrial vessels supplying the placental site. Obstetric expertise is clearly important for the delivery of the child.

Time is also of importance when delivery is spontaneous and caval occlusion is not prevented. Wood et al (1973) found that shortening of the second stage of labour reduced the biochemical evidence of neonatal asphyxia when delivery was conducted in the dorsal position. Humphrey et al (1974) demonstrated that fetal pH decreased progressively during the second stage when delivery was conducted in the dorsal position. When the dorsal position with leftward tilt was used the decline in fetal pH no longer occurred. It would be reasonable to assume that prolongation of forceps delivery and vaginal breech delivery when conducted in the dorsal position might produce biochemical evidence of asphyxia in the baby. Conversely it is considered acceptable to allow prolongation of the second stage when the fetal condition is known to be satisfactory, caval occlusion is avoided and descent of the presenting part of the fetus is anticipated.

Lateral tilt. It will now be apparent that time and tilt are interrelated phenomena in their effects on the fetus. The far-reaching effects of caval occlusion in the supine position in later pregnancy are reviewed in chapter 2 and it will be recalled that complete blockage of the inferior vena cava occurs in the majority of unanaesthetized women at term.

For the anaesthetist the most important consequence of caval occlusion is a reduction in maternal cardiac output by up to 50% if there is accompanying bradycardia (Scott et al, 1969). Among the results of this reduction in cardiac output is a probable diminution in uteroplacental blood flow. The fall in cardiac output is likely to be even greater if the patient is under the influence of general anaesthesia or an epidural or subarachnoid block. It is emphasized that a normal blood pressure in the arm must not be taken as signifying that all is well with the uterine and placental circulation (Crawford et al, 1972). It is possible and even probable that the reduction in cardiac output has elicited a compensatory increase in peripheral resistance. Constriction of the uterine arteries may therefore well form part of the response to caval occlusion. Caval occlusion may be 'revealed' in the small percentage of patients in whom overt supine hypotension develops and this is usually accompanied by bradycardia. Much more often caval occlusion is 'concealed' and in this situation the absence of readily observable signs in the mother may lead to the erroneous conclusion that all is well with the infant in utero. An additional mechanism by which caval occlusion may impair uteroplacental circulation is by obstruction of the venous outflow from the uterus.

A relationship between caval occlusion in the supine position and biochemical evidence of birth asphyxia during caesarean section was suggested by the work of Ansari et al (1970) and Goodlin (1971) and has been more firmly established by Crawford et al (1972, 1973) and Downing et al (1974a). Fetal acidosis is significantly reduced when elective caesarean section is performed in the lateral tilt position. The condition of mother and child is further improved if a lateral position has been adopted during the 30 minutes before the induction (Crawford et al, 1973). This is the so-called 'journey tilt'. The improvement in fetal Po_2 observed by Ansari et al (1970) in the tilt position was much greater where spinal anaesthesia was used but was also observed with general anaesthesia. Maternal and umbilical vein Po_2 values were significantly higher in the tilt position in Downing's (1974a) series, so that mother as well as infant benefits from the avoidance of aortocaval occlusion. Comparable observations of equally great importance have been made with respect to vertex deliveries. According to Humphrey et al (1974) there is an average fall of 0.26 of a pH unit in the fetal blood after 30 minutes in the second stage of labour when the mother is in the dorsal position. By the simple expedient of elevating the right buttock the fetal acidosis could be prevented.

It is possible to make certain recommendations about the preferred position of the mother from the point of view of fetal and maternal wellbeing:

(1) If possible the patient should be in the full lateral or lateral tilt position for 30 minutes before the induction of general or epidural anaesthesia. Anaesthesia should be induced and maintained in the tilt position, at least until delivery of the infant. A tilt to the left is usually preferred, although a very few women may fare better with a tilt to the right.

(2) Patients in labour should whenever possible assume a lateral or tilted position. If labour is managed under epidural analgesia it is essential that the supine position be avoided.

(3) If the dorsal or lithotomy position is used for any vaginal delivery a lateral tilt should be employed. Elevation of the right buttock on a towel or wedge should suffice.

It now seems probable that some of the 'unexplained' cases of neonatal asphyxia at elective caesarean section have resulted from the use of the supine position. It may also be that the infant who unexpectedly suffers from asphyxia after a spontaneous delivery in the dorsal position may have paid the price for failure to prevent caval occlusion. Perhaps a return to the lateral position for delivery is indicated. Any position seems preferable to the unmodified supine 'stranded whale' position. If caval occlusion can exert such an important effect on the condition of the full-term normal infant at birth, how much more may it jeopardize the infant delivered prematurely or in emergency circumstances?

Because caval occlusion is such a dominant factor in determining the biochemical and clinical incidence of asphyxia neonatorum any studies designed to assess the influence of any other factor on the occurrence of asphyxia should be performed on patients in the tilted position. In the past most studies on the influence of time, hyperventilation, maternal oxygenation and various anaesthetic agents have been carried out with the mothers in the supine position and some doubt must therefore arise concerning the validity of some of the conclusions of these investigations. It should also be emphasized that with careful, modern light general anaesthesia the infant is usually born without evidence of serious asphyxia. Nevertheless a proportion of infants delivered by elective caesarean section show unexpected asphyxia and the explanation is not always obvious. It is in these cases that caval occlusion, hyperventilation, suboptimal maternal oxygenation and delay in delivery may provide the explanation. Laryngeal inhibition from over-vigorous pharyngeal suction is a further explanation of 'unexplained' asphyxia neonatorum (see chapter 10). Very light, unsupplemented nitrous oxide anaesthesia may result in diminished placental blood flow. The stress response to surgical stimuli is not prevented by light anaesthesia (Namba et al, 1980). Catecholamine levels increase and uteroplacental blood flow may be diminished as a result of constriction of the uterine arteries. The consequence of this will be fetal hypoxia and acidosis (Palahniuk and Cumming, 1977). Epidural anaesthesia blocks painful stimuli and intervillous blood flow is not reduced (Jouppila et al, 1978).

The choice of muscle relaxant. For intubation of the trachea suxamethonium in a dose of 100 mg or 1.5 mg/kg body weight is at present the relaxant of choice. The fasciculations of suxamethonium are often minimal or even absent in pregnancy and they do not increase the risk of regurgitation of stomach contents (Smith et al, 1978). None of the non-depolarizing muscle relaxants can produce the rapid and complete relaxation needed for safe intubation in the obstetric patient.

For the maintenance of relaxation after intubation, any of the currently used muscle relaxants is acceptable. It is customary to avoid using gallamine because the placental transfer of this drug is somewhat greater than that of the other relaxants, although unlikely to be sufficient to affect the infant at birth (Crawford, 1956). The placental transfer of alcuronium also occurs to a rather greater extent (Thomas et al, 1969) and this drug, too, is not a relaxant of first choice for obstetric anaesthesia. The choice may be based upon properties of the remaining muscle relaxants which are unrelated to their placental transfer. Pancuronium and vecuronium are suitable because of their clinically negligible placental transfer. In hypertensive patients D-tubo-curarine is preferred for its tendency to lower blood pressure. In normotensive patients undergoing caesarean section the incidence of unwanted hypotension is greater with D-tubocurarine than with pancuronium (Neeld et al, 1974). A suxamethonium drip (1 mg/ml) may be used. Intermittent injections of suxamethonium are appropriate for only very short periods of time and may be conveniently used for examination under anaesthesia in cases of antepartum haemorrhage. An intravenous injection of atropine 1.0 mg should be given before using suxamethonium by either of these techniques. Tetrahydroaminacrine (Tacrine) has been successfully used to prolong the action of intermittent injections of suxamethonium during caesarean section (Spiers, 1966). Tetrahydroaminacrine crosses the placenta.

It should be noted that the skeletal muscle relaxants have no action upon the uterine muscle (Reier and Moster, 1970; Healey, 1971; Iuppa et al, 1971). The clinical impression that oxytocin (Syntocinon) when given by infusion during labour prolonged the action of suxamethonium (Hodges et al, 1959) has not been substantiated by further human and animal observations (Keil, 1962; Ichiyanagi et al, 1963). The incidence of suxamethonium after-pains has been found to be lower in pregnancy (Crawford, 1971b; Datta et al, 1977; Thind and Bryson, 1983).

The delivery of the infant and placental separation

The delivery of the infant, the subsequent separation of the placenta and the injection of an oxytocic drug are frequently associated with sudden and far-reaching effects upon the cardiovascular system. The more important changes are:

External blood loss.
Expulsion of blood from the uterine into the general circulation.
The relief of caval occlusion.
The effects of oxytocin and ergometrine on the circulation.

Consequently alterations in central venous pressure, cardiac output, arterial pressure and peripheral resistance are all likely to be observable at delivery and for some time thereafter. The final state of the circulation after delivery will depend upon the algebraic sum of these various changes. The cardiovascular changes of pregnancy, labour and delivery are discussed in some detail in chapter 2 and the circulatory effects of ergometrine and oxytocin (Syntocinon) are considered in chapter 3. They may be summarized as follows:

External blood loss at caesarean section under general anaesthesia averages 700–1000 ml and may be as great as 2.5 litres. Blood loss at forceps delivery under thiopentone, nitrous oxide, muscle relaxant anaesthesia averages over 500 ml and may reach 1.5 litres or more.

Retraction of the uterus after delivery is accompanied by the expulsion of blood from the uterine into the general circulation. The volume of blood involved in this process is not known with certainty but may be about 500 ml. Thus 'autotransfusion' helps in compensating for the external loss of blood. It may even over-compensate and result in a relative increase in circulating blood volume if external bleeding has been slight. This increase in blood volume could embarrass the circulation in a patient suffering from serious heart disease. This relative hypervolaemia could be aggravated by the vasoconstrictor action of ergometrine.

Where caval occlusion has been permitted to occur in the supine position, the emptying of the uterus should abolish or diminish the obstruction to venous return with a consequent increase in cardiac output. Even if a lateral tilt has been used there is often a substantial increase in cardiac output after delivery of the child by caesarean section, suggesting that caval compression has not been entirely prevented in these cases (Newman, 1982).

Delivery of the infant is usually accompanied by a substantial fall in central venous pressure (CVP). Placental separation by itself causes little alteration in CVP. The rises in CVP which may occur in the third stage are closely related to the oxytocic drug and its route of administration. An intravenous injection of 0.5 mg ergometrine causes a rise of about 5 cmH$_2$O (0.5 kPa) in CVP, which persists for 30–60 minutes. An intramuscular injection of 1 ml Syntometrine (ergometrine 0.5 mg and Syntocinon 5 units) causes changes which are only slightly less extensive. In contrast an intravenous injection of 10 units oxytocin (Syntocinon) produces a rise of only 1 or 2 cmH$_2$O (0.1 or 0.2 kPa) in CVP and this small effect persists for less than 30 minutes. Blood loss appears to be equally well controlled by ergometrine or Syntocinon given by intravenous injection.

An intravenous injection of ergometrine will sometimes cause an appreciable rise in arterial pressure due to the α-adrenergic stimulant action of this drug. This hypertensive effect is probably most frequently seen in patients with pre-eclampsia and possibly in patients who have previously received a vasopressor drug. Ergometrine may cause constriction of the pulmonary vessels (Johnstone, 1972). This could mimic the clinical picture of aspiration pneumonitis during or after anaesthesia and could render actual aspiration even more serious. It can be conjectured that the use of ergometrine contributes to the apparent high mortality rate for aspiration pneumonitis in the obstetric patient. Ergometrine may have caused bronchospasm during caesarean section although such an event must be extremely rare. An intravenous injection of Syntocinon produces a transient vasodilatation. The natural hormone oxytocin is no longer used in obstetric practice and the hypertensive action which was sometimes observed with this substance was attributable to the presence of vasopressin.

Among the practical conclusions which may be drawn from the foregoing summary is that the obstetric patient is probably quite well protected against blood loss at delivery by her pre-existing increase in blood volume and by the movement of blood from the uterine to the general circulation after delivery. It is therefore the writers' practice not to transfuse blood during caesarean section unless the blood loss exceeds 1.2–1.5 litres, or unless (and this rarely happens) there are alterations in the vital signs. This certainly does not mean that compatible blood need not be available for every patient undergoing caesarean. When blood loss reaches 1.5 litres there may be a sudden deterioration in the condition of the patient demanding transfusion. Each patient for caesarean section receives 1 litre of a balanced salt solution.

The second practical conclusion is that the effects of intravenous ergometrine upon arterial and central venous pressure are greater and potentially more harmful than those of Syntocinon. In addition, it is concluded that Syntocinon should be the routine oxytocic agent and should certainly be preferred for patients with pre-eclampsia, essential hypertension and heart disease and for those who have received a vasopressor drug during labour. A bolus intravenous injection of 5 units oxytocin (Syntocinon) is followed by an intravenous infusion of 10 or 20 units in 500 ml of fluid.

Immediately after delivery by caesarean section there is an improvement in total lung compliance of about 20% (Farman and Thorpe, 1969) and this results in an increase in tidal volume where a pressure-cycled ventilator is in use and may call for an increase in gas flows or a reduction of inflation pressure.

The postdelivery phase

When the infant and the placenta have been delivered and uterine bleeding has been controlled then obstetric operations present few further special problems to the anaesthetist. It is necessary to avoid causing uterine relaxation by restricting the administration of powerful volatile and gaseous anaesthetics. It is therefore suggested that the concentration of halothane should not exceed 0.5% and the concentration of other volatile agents should be kept to equivalent values. Blood loss is not increased when 0.65% enflurane is used (Abboud et al, 1981). The proportion of nitrous oxide may usefully be increased to 70% in the expectation that the risk of awareness may be diminished.

An intravenous injection of narcotic analgesic after delivery may further reduce the possibility of the occurrence of awareness. If an elective caesarean section is being performed the administration of an analgesic drug will be helpful in alleviating the postoperative pain which will often develop rapidly where no opiate premedication has been given. The use of methoxyflurane or trichloroethylene during anaesthesia should supply a measure of postoperative analgesia.

Buprenorphine 0.6 mg has been found to provide 7–8 hours of analgesia after caesarean section. Although the decrease in diastolic blood pressure was greater than that produced by morphine 15 mg, no serious side-effects were observed (Downing et al, 1977).

Epidural opiates have been successfully used to give prolonged analgesia, even after general anaesthesia. The attractions of epidural analgesia without cardiovascular side-effects are obvious. Breast feeding may be more easily established and the mother may be ambulant. Pruritus may be common and the rare but potentially catastrophic complication of delayed respiratory failure demands careful observation for many hours.

REFERENCES

Abboud, T.K., Shnider, S.M., Wright, R.G. et al (1981) Enflurane analgesia in obstetrics. *Anesth. Analg. curr. Res.*, **60**, 133.

Abboud, T.K., Raya, J., Sadri, S. et al (1983) Fetal and maternal cardiovascular effects of atropine and glycopyrrolate. *Anesth. Analg. curr. Res.*, **62**, 426.

Andersen, N. (1962) Changes in intragastric pressure following the administration of suxamethonium. *Br. J. Anaesth.*, **34**, 363.

Andersen, G.J. and Walker, J. (1970) Effect of labour on the maternal blood–gas and acid–base status. *J. Obstet. Gynaec. Br. Commonw.*, **77**, 289.

Ansari, I., Wallace, G., Clemetson, C.A.B., Mallikarjuneswara, V.R. and Clemetson, C.D.M. (1970) Tilt caesarean section. *J. Obstet. Gynaec. Br. Commonw.*, **77**, 713.

Apgar, V., Holaday, D.A., James, L.S., Prince, C.E. and Weisbrot, I.M. (1957) Comparison of regional and general anesthesia in obstetrics. *J. Am. med. Ass.*, **165**, 2155.

Archer, G.W. and Marx, G.F. (1974) Arterial oxygen tension during apnoea in parturient women. *Br. J. Anaesth.*, **46**, 358.

Awe, W.C., Fletcher, W.S. and Jacob, S.W. (1966) The pathophysiology of aspiration pneumonitis. *Surgery*, **60**, 232.

Baggish, M.S. and Hooper, S. (1974) Aspiration as a cause of maternal death. *Obstet. Gynec.*, **43**, 327.

Baraka, A. (1970) Correlation between maternal and foetal Po_2 and Pco_2 during caesarean section. *Br. J. Anaesth.*, **42**, 434.

Baraka, A., Saab, M., Salem, M.R. and Winnie, A.P. (1977) Control of gastric acidity by glycopyrrolate premedication in the parturient. *Anesth. Analg. curr. Res.*, **56**, 642.

Blacher, R.S. (1984) Editorial. Awareness during surgery. *Anesthesiology*, **61**, 1.

Blitt, C.D., Petty, W.C., Alberternst, E.E. and Wright, B.J. (1977) Correlation of plasma cholinesterase activity and duration of action of succinylcholine during pregnancy. *Anesth. Analg. curr. Res.*, **56**, 78.

Blogg, C.E., Simpson, B.R., Tyers, M.B., Martin, L.E. and Bell, J.A. (1975) Human placental transfer of AH 8165. *Anaesthesia*, **30**, 23.

Bond, V.K., Stoelting, R.K. and Gupta, C.D. (1979) Pulmonary aspiration syndrome after inhalation of gastric fluid containing antacids. *Anesthesiology*, **51**, 452.

Bonica, J.J. (1967) *Principles and Practice of Obstetric Analgesia and Anesthesia*, vol. 1, p. 751. Oxford: Blackwell.

Bouterline-Young, H. and Bouterline-Young, E. (1956) Alveolar carbon-dioxide levels in pregnant, parturient and lactating subjects. *J. Obstet. Gynaec. Br. Emp.*, **63**, 509.

Boys, J.E. (1983) Failed intubation in obstetric anaesthesia. A case report. *Br. J. Anaesth.*, **55**, 187.

Brant, H.A. (1966) Blood loss at caesarean section. *J. Obstet. Gynaec. Br. Commonw.*, **73**, 456.

Breheny, F. and McCarthy, J. (1982) Maternal mortality. A review of maternal death over twenty years at the National Maternity Hospital, Dublin. *Anaesthesia*, **37**, 561.

Brock-Utne, J.G., Rubin, J., Downing, J.W. et al (1976) The administration of metoclopramide with atropine. *Anaesthesia*, **31**, 1186.

Brock-Utne, J.G., Downing, J.W. and Seedat, F. (1977) Laryngeal oedema associated with pre-eclamptic toxaemia. *Anaesthesia*, **32**, 556.

Brock-Utne, J.G., Rubin, J., Welman, S. et al (1978) The effect of glycopyrrolate (Robinul) on the lower oesophageal sphincter. *Can. Anaesth. Soc. J.*, **25**, 144.

Bruce, D.L., Downs, J.B., Kulkarni, P.S. and Capan, L.M. (1984) Precurarization inhibits maximal ventilatory effort. *Anesthesiology*, **61**, 618.

Buley, R.J.R., Downing, J.W., Brock-Utne, J.G. and Cuerden, C. (1977) Right versus left lateral tilt for Caesarean section. *Br. J. Anaesth.*, **49**, 1009.

Burger, G.A., Datta, S., Chantigian, R.A. et al (1983) Optimal ventilation in general anesthesia for cesarean delivery. *Anesthesiology*, **59**, A420.

Burns, T.H.S. (1982) Apomorphine in obstetric anaesthesia. *Anaesthesia*, **37**, 346.

Carrie, L.E.S. (1982) An inflatable obstetric 'wedge'. *Anaesthesia*, **37**, 745.

Castell, D.O. and Harris, L.D. (1970) Hormonal control of gastro-esophageal sphincter strength. *New Engl. J. Med.*, **282**, 886.

Chamberlain, J.H., Seed, R.G.F.L. and Chung, D.C.W. (1977) Effect of thiopentone on myocardial function. *Br. J. Anaesth.*, **49**, 865.

Chen, C.I., Toung, T.J.R., Haupt, H.M., Hutchies, G.M. and Cameron, J.L. (1984) Evaluation of Alka-Seltzer Effervescent in gastric acid neutralization. *Anesth. Analg. curr. Res.*, **63**, 325.

Clark, R.B., Cooper, J.O., Brown, W.E. and Greifenstein, F.E. (1970) The effect of methoxyflurane on the foetus. *Br. J. Anaesth.*, **42**, 286.

Cohen, S.E., Jasson, J., Talafre, M.-L., Chauvelot-Moachin, L. and Barrier, G. (1984) Does metoclopramide decrease the volume of gastric contents in patients undergoing cesarean section? *Anesthesiology*, **61**, 604.

Coleman, A.J. and Downing, J.W. (1975) Enflurane anesthesia for cesarean section. *Anesthesiology*, **43**, 354.

Corall, I.M., Ward, M.E., Page, J. and Strunin, L. (1977) Conditions for tracheal intubation following fazadinium and pancuronium. *Br. J. Anaesth*, **49**, 615.

Crawford, J.S. (1956) Some aspects of obstetric anaesthesia. *Br. J. Anaesth.*, **28**, 146.

Crawford, J.S. (1962) Anaesthesia for caesarean section: a proposed method for evaluation with analysis of a technique. *Br. J. Anaesth.*, **34**, 179.

Crawford, J.S. (1971a) Awareness during operative obstetrics under general anaesthesia. *Br. J. Anaesth.*, **43**, 179.

Crawford, J.S. (1971b) Suxamethonium muscle pains and pregnancy. *Br. J. Anaesth.*, **43**, 677.

Crawford, J.S. (1980) Bronchospasm following ergometrine. *Anaesthesia*, **35**, 397.

Crawford, J.S. and Davies, P. (1982) Status of neonates delivered by elective Caesarean section. *Br. J. Anaesth.*, **54**, 1015.

Crawford, J.S. and Oppit, L.J. (1976) A survey of anaesthetic service to obstetrics in the Birmingham Hospital Region. *Anaesthesia*, **31**, 56.

Crawford, J.S. and Potter, S.R. (1984) Magnesium trisilicate mixture B.P.. Its physical characteristics and effectiveness as a prophylactic. *Anaesthesia*, **39**, 535.

Crawford, J.S., Burton, M. and Davies, P. (1972) Time and lateral tilt at caesarean section. *Br. J. Anaesth.*, **44**, 477.

Crawford, J.S., Burton, M. and Davies, P. (1973) Anaesthesia for caesarean section: further refinements of a technique. *Br. J. Anaesth.*, **45**, 726.

Crawford, J.S., James, F.M., Davies, P. and Crawley, M. (1976) A further study of general anaesthesia for Caesarean section. *Br. J. Anaesth.*, **48**, 661.

Crawford, J.S., Lewis, M. and Davies, P. (1985) Maternal and neonatal responses related to the volatile agent used to maintain anaesthesia at Caesarean section. *Br. J. Anaesth.*, **57**, 482.

Cummings, M.F., Russell, W.J. and Frewin, D.B. (1983) Effects of pancuronium and alcuronium on the changes in arterial pressure and plasma catecholamine concentrations during tracheal intubation. *Br. J. Anaesth.*, **55**, 619.

Dailey, P.A., Fisher, D.M., Shnider, S.M. et al (1984) Pharmacokinetics, placental transfer and neonatal effects of vecuronium and pancuronium during cesarean section. *Anesthesiology*, **60**, 569.

Datta, S., Crocker, J.S. and Alper, M.H. (1977) Muscle pain following administration of suxamethonium to pregnant and non-pregnant patients undergoing laparoscopic tubal ligation. *Br. J. Anaesth.*, **49**, 625.

Datta, S., Ostheimer, G.W., Naulty, J.S., Knapp, R.M. and Weiss, J.B. (1981) General anesthesia for cesarean section. Effects of halothane on maternal and fetal acid base and lactic acid concentration. *Anesthesiology*, **55**, A309.

Davies, M.J., Cronin, K.D. and Cowie, R.W. (1981) The prevention of hypertension at intubation. *Anaesthesia*, **36**, 147.

Davis, A.G. (1982) Anaesthesia for Caesarean section. The potential for regional block. *Anaesthesia*, **37**, 748.

Department of Health and Social Security (1969) *Report on Confidential Enquiries into Maternal Deaths in England and Wales 1964–66*. London: H.M.S.O.

Department of Health and Social Security (1972) *Report on Confidential Enquiries into Maternal Deaths in England and Wales 1967–69*. London: H.M.S.O.

Department of Health and Social Security (1975) *Report on Confidential Enquiries into Maternal Deaths in England and Wales 1970–72*. London: H.M.S.O.

Department of Health and Social Security (1979) *Report on Confidential Enquiries into Maternal Deaths in England and Wales 1973–75*. London: H.M.S.O.

Department of Health and Social Security (1982) *Report on Confidential Enquiries into Maternal Deaths in England and Wales 1976–78*. London: H.M.S.O.

Dinnick, O.P. (1957) Reflux reflections. *Proc. R. Soc. Med.*, **60**, 623.

Dobb, G. (1978) Laryngeal oedema complicating obstetric anaesthesia. *Anaesthesia*, **33**, 839.

Don Michael, T.A., Lambert, E.H. and Mehran, A. (1968) 'Mouth to lung airway' for cardiac resuscitation. *Lancet*, **ii**, 1329.

Dow, T.G.B., Brock-Utne, J.G., Rubin, J. et al (1978) The effect of atropine on the lower esophageal sphincter in late pregnancy. *Obstet. Gynec.*, **51**, 426.

Downing, J.W., Coleman, A.J. and Meer, F.M. (1973) An intravenous method of anaesthesia for caesarean section. III. Althesin. *Br. J. Anaesth.*, **45**, 381.

Downing, J.W., Coleman, A.J., Mahomedy, M.C., Jeal, D.E. and Mahomedy, Y.H. (1974a) Lateral table tilt for caesarean section. *Anaesthesia*, **29**, 696.

Downing, J.W., Mahomedy, M.C., Coleman, A.J., Mahomedy, Y.H. and Jeal, D.E. (1974b) Anaesthetic induction for Caesarean section. Althesin versus thiopentone. *Anaesthesia*, **29**, 689.

Downing, J.W., Mahomedy, M.C., Jeal, D.E. and Allen, P.J. (1976) Anaesthesia for Caesarean section with ketamine. *Anaesthesia*, **31**, 883.

Downing, J.W., Leary, W.P. and White E.S. (1977) Buprenorphine: a new potent long-acting synthetic analgesic. Comparison with morphine. *Br. J. Anaesth.*, **49**, 251.

Downing, J.W., Buley, R.J.R., Brock-Utne, J.G. and Houlton, P.C. (1979) Etomidate for induction of anaesthesia at Caesarean section: a comparison with thiopentone. *Br. J. Anaesth.*, **51**, 135.

Drummond, G.B. and Park, G.R. (1984) Arterial oxygen saturation before intubation of the trachea. An assessment of oxygenation techniques. *Br. J. Anaesth.*, **56**, 987.

Drummond, G.B., Scott, S.E.M., Lees, M.M. and Scott, D.B. (1974) Effects of posture on limb blood flow in late pregnancy. *Br. med. J.*, **iv**, 587.

Evans, R.T. and Wroe, J.M. (1980) Plasma cholinesterase changes during pregnancy. *Anaesthesia*, **35**, 651.

Famewo, C.E. (1976) Awareness and dreams during general anaesthesia for Caesarean section: a study of incidence. *Can. Anaesth. Soc. J.*, **23**, 636.

Farman, J.V. and Thorpe, M.H. (1969) Compliance changes during caesarean section. *Br. J. Anaesth.*, **41**, 999.

Finster, M. and Marx, G.F. (1976) Neonatal distribution of succinylcholine. *Anesthesiology*, **44**, 89.

Fisher, A. and Prys-Roberts, C. (1968) Maternal pulmonary gas exchange. A study during normal labour and extradural blockade. *Anaesthesia*, **23**, 350.

Foulkes, E. and Jenning, L.C. (1981) A comparative evaluation of cimetidine and sodium citrate to decrease gastric acidity and effectiveness at induction of anaesthesia. *Canad. Anaesth. Soc. J.*, **28**, 29.

Fox, G.S. and Houle, G.L. (1971) Acid–base studies in elective caesarean section during epidural and general anaesthesia. *Can. Anaesth. Soc. J.*, **18**, 60.

Frank, M., Flynn, P.J. and Hughes, R. (1983) Atracurium in obstetric anaesthesia. *Br. J. Anaesth.*, **55**, 113 S.

Galbert, M.W. and Gardner, A.E. (1972) Use of halothane in a balanced technic for cesarean section. *Anesth. Analg. curr. Res.*, **51**, 701.

Gergis, S.D., Sokoll, M.D., Mehta, M., Kenmotsu, O. and Rudd, G.D. (1983) Intubation conditions after atracurium and suxamethonium. *Br. J. Anaesth.*, **55**, 835.

Gibbs, C.P. and Banner, T.C. (1984) Effectiveness of Bicitra as a preoperative antacid. *Anesthesiology*, **61**, 97.

Gibbs, C.P., Schwartz, D.J., Wynne, J.W., Hood, C.I. and Kuck, E.J. (1979) Antacid pulmonary aspiration in the dog. *Anesthesiology*, **51**, 380.

Gibbs, C.P., Kuck, E.J., Hood, C.I. and Ruiz, B.C. (1980) Antacid plus foodstuff aspiration in the dog. *Anesthesiology*, **53**, S307.

Gibbs, C.P., Spohr, L. and Schmidt, D. (1981) In vitro and in vivo evaluation of sodium citrate as an antacid. *Anesthesiology*, **55**, A311.

Gibbs, C.P., Spohr, L. and Schmidt, D. (1982) The effectiveness of sodium citrate as an antacid. *Anesthesiology*, **57**, 44.

Goodlin, R.C. (1971) Aortocaval compression during cesarean section. *Obstet. Gynec.*, **37**, 702.

Hall, A.W., Moosa, A.R., Clark, J., Cooley, G.R. and Skinner, D.B. (1975) The effects of premedication drugs on the lower oesophageal high pressure zone and reflux status of rhesus monkeys and man. *Gut.*, **16**, 347.

Harrison, G.C. (1978) Death attributable to anaesthesia: a 10-year survey (1967–1976). *Br. J. Anaesth.*, **50**, 1041.

Healey, T.E.J. (1971) Suxamethonium and intrauterine pressure. *Br. J. Anaesth.*, **43**, 1156.

Hey, V.M.F. and Ostick, D.G. (1978) Metoclopramide and the gastro-oesophageal sphincter in pregnant women with heartburn. *Anaesthesia*, **33**, 462.

Higgs, R.H., Smyth, R.D. and Castell, D.O. (1974) Gastric alkalinization. Effect on lower esophageal sphincter pressure and serum gastrin. *New Engl. J. Med.*, **291**, 486.

Hodges, R.J.H. and Tunstall, M.E. (1961) Choice of anaesthesia and its influence on perinatal mortality in caesarean section. *Br. J. Anaesth.*, **33**, 572.

Hodges, R.J.H., Bennett, J.R., Tunstall, M.E. and Knight, R.F. (1959) General anaesthesia for operative obstetrics. *Br. J. Anaesth.*, **31**, 152.

Hodgkinson, R. (1984) Potential interactions between cimetidine and local anesthetics. *Anesthesiology*, **60**, 508.

Hodgkinson, R., Bhatt, H., Kim, S.S., Grewal, G. and Marx, G.F. (1978) Neonatal neurobehavioral tests following cesarean section under general and spinal anesthesia. *Am. J. Obstet. Gynec.*, **132**, 670.

Hodgkinson, R., Glassenberg, R., Joyce, T.H. et al (1983) Comparison of cimetidine (Tagamet) with antacid for safety and effectiveness in reducing gastric acidity before elective cesarean section. *Anesthesiology*, **59**, 86.

Holdcroft, A., Robinson, M.J., Gordon, H. and Whitwam, J.G. (1974) Comparison of effect of two induction doses of methohexitone on infants delivered by elective Caesarean section. *Br. med. J.*, **ii**, 472.

Holdsworth, J.D. (1978a) Relationship between stomach contents and analgesia in labour. *Br. J. Anaesth.*, **50**, 1145.

Holdsworth, J.D. (1978b) The place of apomorphine prior to obstetric anaesthesia. *J. int. med. Res.*, **6**, Suppl. 1, 26.

Holdsworth, J.D., Furness, R.M.B. and Roulston, R.G. (1974) A comparison of apomorphine and stomach tubes for emptying the stomach before general anaesthesia in obstetrics. *Br. J. Anaesth.*, **46**, 526.

Holdsworth, J.D., Johnson, K., Mascall, G., Roulston, G. and Tomlinson, P.A. (1980) Mixing of antacids with stomach contents. Another approach to the prevention of acid aspiration (Mendelson's) syndrome. *Anaesthesia*, **35**, 641.

Hollmen, A. and Jagerhorn, M. (1972) Does increased maternal $P_a co_2$ during general anaesthesia for Caesarean section improve foetal acid–base parameters? *Acta anaesth. scand.*, **16**, 221.

Hollmen, A., Jouppila, R., Koivisto, M. et al (1978) Neurologic activity of infants following anesthesia for cesarean section. *Anesthesiology*, **48**, 350.

Holmes, J.A. (1956) Prevention of inhaled vomit during obstetric anaesthesia. *J. Obstet. Gynaec. Br. Commonw.*, **63**, 239.

Hood, D.D., Dewan, D.M., James, F.M. III, Bogard, T.D. and Floyd, H.M. (1983) The use of nitroglycerin in preventing the hypertensive response to tracheal intubation in severe pre-eclamptics. *Anesthesiology*, **59**, A423.

Howells, T.H. and Riethmuller, R.J. (1980) Signs of endotracheal intubation. *Anaesthesia*, **35**, 984.

Howells, T.H., Chamney, A.R., Wraight, W.J. and Simons, R.S. (1983) The application of cricoid pressure. An assessment and a survey of its practice. *Anaesthesia*, **38**, 457.

Humphrey, M.D., Chang, A., Wood, E.C., Morgan, S. and Hounslow, D. (1974) A decrease in fetal pH during the second stage of labour when conducted in the dorsal position. *J. Obstet. Gynaec. Br. Commonw.*, **81**, 600.

Hunter, A.R. and Moir, D.D. (1983) Editorial. Confidential Enquiry into Maternal Deaths. *Br. J. Anaesth.*, **55**, 367.

Hutchison, B.R. and Newson, A.J. (1975) Pre-operative neutralisation of gastric acidity. *Anaesth. intensive Care*, **3**, 198.

Ichiyanagi, K., Ito, Y. and Aoki, E. (1963) Effects of oxytocin on the response to suxamethonium and D-tubocurarine in man. *Br. J. Anaesth.*, **35**, 611.

Iuppa, J.B., Smith, G.A., Colella, J.J. and Gibson, J.L. (1971) Succinylcholine effect on human myometrial activity. *Obstet. Gynec.*, **37**, 591.

Ivankovic, A.D., Elam, J.O. and Huffman, J. (1970) Effect of maternal hypercarbia on the newborn infant. *Am. J. Obstet. Gynec.*, **107**, 939.

James, C.F., Gibbs, C.P. and Banner, T. (1984) Postpartum perioperative risk of aspiration pneumonia. *Anesthesiology*, **61**, 756.

Jellicoe, J.A. and Harris, N.R. (1984) A modification of a standard laryngoscope for difficult tracheal intubation in obstetric cases. *Anaesthesia*, **39**, 800.

Johnston, J.R., McCaughey, W., Moore, J. and Dundee, J.W. (1982a) Cimetidine as an oral antacid before elective Caesarean section. *Anaesthesia*, **37**, 26.

Johnston, J.R., McCaughey, W., Moore, J. and Dundee, J.W. (1982b) A field trial of cimetidine in obstetric anaesthesia. *Anaesthesia*, **37**, 33.

Johnstone, M. (1972) The cardiovascular effects of oxytocic drugs. *Br. J. Anaesth.*, **44**, 826.

Jouppila, R., Jouppila, P., Kuikka, J. and Hollmen, A. (1978) Placental blood flow during Caesarean section under lumbar extradural analgesia. *Br. J. Anaesth.*, **50**, 275.

Jouppila, P., Kuikka, J., Jouppila, R. and Hollmen, A. (1979) Effect of induction of general anaesthesia for Caesarean section on intervillous blood flow. *Acta obstet. gynec. scand.*, **58**, 249.

Kangas, L., Erkkola, R., Kanto, J. and Mansikka, M. (1976) Halothane anaesthesia in Caesarean section. *Acta anaesth. scand.*, **20**, 189.

Keil, A. McL. (1962) Effects of oxytocin on the response to suxamethonium in rabbits, sheep and pigs. *Br. J. Anaesth.*, **34**, 306.

Kristoffersen, M.B. (1979) Cyclopropane and Caesarean section. *Br. J. Anaesth.*, **51**, 227.

Lahiri, S.K., Thomas, T.A. and Hodgson, R.M.H. (1973) Single-dose antacid therapy for the prevention of Mendelson's syndrome. *Br. J. Anaesth.*, **45**, 1143.

LaSalvia, L.A. and Steffen, E.A. (1950) Delayed gastric emptying time in labor. *Am. J. Obstet. Gynec.*, **59**, 1075.

Latto, I.P. and Wainwright, A.C. (1972) Anaesthesia for caesarean section: analysis of blood concentration of methoxyflurane using 0.1 per cent methoxyflurane and 40 per cent oxygen. *Br. J. Anaesth.*, **44**, 1050.

Latto, I.P. and Waldron, B.A. (1977) Anaesthesia for Caesarean section. *Br. J. Anaesth.*, **49**, 371.

Lees, M.M., Taylor, S.H., Scott, D.B. and Kerr, M.G. (1967) A study of cardiac output at rest throughout pregnancy. *J. Obstet. Gynaec. Br. Commonw.*, **74**, 319.

Levinson, G., Shnider, S.M., Gildea, J.E. and de Lorimier, A.A. (1973) Maternal and foetal cardiovascular and acid–base changes during ketamine anaesthesia in pregnant ewes. *Br. J. Anaesth.*, **45**, 1111.

Levinson, G., Shnider, S.M., de Lorimier, A. and Steffenson, J.L. (1974) Effects of maternal hyperventilation on uterine blood flow and fetal oxygenation and acid–base status. *Anesthesiology*, **40**, 340.

Lewis, R.T., Burgess, J.H. and Hampson, L.G. (1971) Cardio-respiratory studies in critical illness: changes in aspiration pneumonitis. *Arch. Surg.*, **103**, 335.

Lind, F.J., Smith, A.M., McIver, D.K., Coopland, A.T. and Crispin, J.S. (1968) Heartburn in pregnancy, a manometric study. *Can. med. Ass. J.*, **98**, 571.

Mackenzie, A.I. (1978) Layngeal oedema complicating obstetric anaesthesia. *Anaesthesia*, **33**, 271.

Mankowitz, E., Brock-Utne, J.G. and Downing, J.W. (1981) Nitrous oxide elimination by the newborn. *Anaesthesia*, **36**, 1014.

Marx, G.F. and Mateo, C.V. (1971) Effects of different oxygen concentrations during general anaesthesia for elective caesarean section. *Can. Anaesth. Soc. J.*, **18**, 587.

Marx, G.F., Joshi, C.W. and Orkin, L.R. (1970) Placental transmission of nitrous oxide. *Anesthesiology*, **32**, 429.

Masey, S.A., Glazebrook, C.W. and Goat, V. (1983) Suxamethonium. A new look at pretreatment. *Br. J. Anaesth.*, **55**, 729.

Maternal Mortality Committee (1980) I.M.A. Maternal Mortality Report, 1978. *Irish med. J.*, **73**, 148.

McAuley, D.M., Moore, J., McCaughey, W., Donnelly, D.B. and Dundee, J.W. (1983) Ranitidine as an antacid before elective Caesarean section. *Anaesthesia*, **38**, 108.

McAuley, D.M., Moore, J., Dundee, J.W. and McCaughey, W. (1984) Oral ranitidine in labour. *Anaesthesia*, **39**, 433.

Mendelson, C.L. (1946) The aspiration of stomach contents into the lungs during obstetric anesthesia. *Am. J. Obstet. Gynec.*, **52**, 191.

Merrifield, A.J. and King, S.J. (1981) The oesophageal obturator airway. A study of cadaver lung ventilation through obturator airways and tracheal tubes. *Anaesthesia*, **36**, 672.

Millar, W.L. and Plumer, M.H. (1982) Obstetric anesthesia teaching in U.S. anesthesia residencies. *Anesthesiology*, **57**, A431.

Moir, D.D. (1970) Anaesthesia for caesarean section. An evaluation of a method using low concentrations of halothane and 50 per cent of oxygen. *Br. J. Anaesth.*, **42**, 136.

Moir, D.D. (1974) Drugs used during labour. In *Obstetric Therapeutics*, ed. Hawkins, D.F., p. 429. London: Baillière Tindall.

Moir, D.D. (1983) Editorial. Cimetidine, antacids and pulmonary aspiration. *Anesthesiology*, **59**, 81.

Moir, D.D. and Wallace, G. (1967) Blood loss at forceps delivery. *J. Obstet. Gynaec. Br. Commonw.*, **74**, 424.

Morgan, B.M. (1980) Maternal death. A review of maternal deaths at one hospital from 1958 to 1978. *Anaesthesia*, **35**, 344.

Morgan, M., Lumley, J. and Whitwam, J.G. (1975) Etomidate, a new water soluble non-barbiturate intravenous induction agent. *Lancet*, **i**, 955.

Morgan, D.J., Blackman, G.L., Paull, J.D. and Wolf, L.H. (1981) Pharmacokinetics and plasma binding of thiopental. Studies at cesarean section. *Anesthesiology*, **54**, 474.

Morgan, B.M., Aulakh, J.M., Barker, J.P., Goroszeniuk, T. and Trojanowski, A. (1983) Anaesthesia for Caesarean section. A medical audit of junior anaesthetic staff practice. *Br. J. Anaesth.*, **55**, 885.

Morishima, H.O., Pedersen, H. and Finster, M. (1978) Influence of maternal psychological stress on the fetus. *Am. J. Obstet. Gynec.*, **131**, 286.

Moya, F., Morishima, H., Shnider, S.M. and James, L.S. (1965) Influence of maternal hyperventilation on the newborn infant. *Am. J. Obstet. Gynec.*, **91**, 76.

Murphy, D.F., Nally, B., Gardiner, J. and Unwin, A. (1984) Effect of metoclopramide on gastric emptying before elective and emergency Caesarean section. *Br. J. Anaesth.*, **56**, 1113.

Myers, R.E., Strange, L., Joelson, I., Huzell, B. and Wussow, C. (1977) Effects upon the fetus of oxygen administration to the mother. *Acta obstet. gynec. scand.*, **56**, 195.

Namba, Y., Smith, J.B., Fox, G.S. and Challis, J.R.G. (1980) Plasma cortisol concentrations during Caesarean section. *Br. J. Anaesth.*, **52**, 1027.

Neeld, J.B., Seabrook, P.D., Chastain, G.M. and Frederickson, E.L. (1974) A clinical comparison of pancuronium and tubocurarine for cesarean section. *Anesth. Analg. curr. Res.*, **53**, 7.

Newman, B. (1982) Cardiac output changes during Caesarean section. Measurement by transcutaneous aortvelography. *Anaesthesia*, **37**, 270.

Newman, B., Derrington, C. and Dore, C. (1983) Cardiac output and the recumbent position in late pregnancy. *Anaesthesia*, **34**, 332.

Nichol, H.C. and Zuck, D. (1983) Difficult laryngoscopy. The 'anterior' larynx and the atlanto-occipital gap. *Br. J. Anaesth.*, **55**, 141.

Nimmo, W.S., Wilson, J. and Prescott, L.F. (1975) Narcotic analgesics and delayed gastric emptying in labour. *Lancet*, **i**, 890.

Ostheimer, G.W., Morrison, J.A. and Lavoie, C. (1982) The effect of cimetidine on mother, newborn and neonatal behavior. *Anesthesiology*, **57**, A405.

O'Sullivan, G.M. and Bullingham, R.E.S. (1984) Does twice the volume of antacid have twice the effect in pregnant women at term? *Anesth. Analg. curr. Res.*, **63**, 752.

O'Sullivan, G.M. and Bullingham, R.E.S. (1985) Non-invasive assessment by radiotelemetry of antacid effect during labor. *Anesth. Analg. curr. Res.*, **65**, 95.

O'Sullivan, G.M., Sear, J.W., Bullingham, R.E.S. and Carrie, L.E.S. (1985) The effect of magnesium trisilicate mixture, metoclopramide and ranitidine on gastric pH, volume and serum gastrin. *Anaesthesia*, **40**, 246.

Palahniuk, R.J. and Cumming, M. (1977) Foetal deterioration following thiopentone–nitrous oxide anaesthesia in the pregnant ewe. *Can. Anaesth. Soc. J.*, **24**, 361.

Palahniuk, R.J. and Shnider, S.M. (1974) Maternal and fetal cardiovascular and acid–base changes during halothane and isoflurane anesthesia in the pregnant ewe. *Anesthesiology*, **41**, 462.

Palahniuk, R.J., Scatliff, J., Biehl, D., Wiebe, H. and Sankaran, K. (1977) Maternal and neonatal effects of methoxyflurane, nitrous oxide and lumbar epidural anaesthesia for Caesarean section. *Can. Anaesth. Soc. J.*, **24**, 586.

Peskett, W.G.H. (1973) Antacids before obstetric anaesthesia. A clinical evaluation of the effectiveness of mist. magnesium trisilicate B.P.C. *Anaesthesia*, **28**, 509.

Reier, C.E. and Moster, W.G. (1970) Effect of neuromuscular blocking agents on uterine contractions in vitro. *Am. J. Obstet. Gynec.*, **108**, 610.

Reisner, L.S. (1983) Type and screen for cesarean section: a prudent alternative. *Anesthesiology*, **58**, 476.

Roberts, R.B. and Shirley, M.A. (1974) Reducing the risk of acid aspiration during cesarean section. *Anesth. Analg. curr. Res.*, **53**, 859.

Roberts, R.B. and Shirley, M.A. (1976) The obstetrician's role in reducing the risk of aspiration pneumonitis. *Am. J. Obstet. Gynec.*, **124**, 611.

Roe, R.B. (1962) The effect of suxamethonium on intragastric pressure. *Anaesthesia*, **17**, 179.

Rorke, M.J., Davey, D.A. and Du Toit, H.J. (1968) Foetal oxygenation during caesarean section. *Anaesthesia*, **23**, 585.

Rosen, M. (1981) Editorial. Deaths associated with anaesthesia for obstetrics. *Anaesthesia*, **36**, 145.

Rosenfeld, C.R., Barton, M.D. and Neschea, G. (1976) Effects of epinephrine on distribution of blood flow in the pregnant ewe. *Am. J. Obstet. Gynec.*, **124**, 156.

Russell, I.F. (1985) Inadvertent total spinal for Caesarean section. *Anaesthesia*, **40**, 199.

Schwartz, D.J., Wynne, J.W., Gibbs, C.P., Hood, C.I. and Kuck, E.J. (1980) The pulmonary consequences of aspiration of gastric contents at pH values greater than 2.5. *Am. Rev. Resp. Dis.*, **121**, 119.

Scott, D.B. (1978) Editorial. Mendelson's syndrome. *Br. J. Anaesth.*, **50**, 977.

Scott, R.P.F. and Goat, V. (1982) Atracurium: its speed of onset. A comparison with suxamethonium. *Br. J. Anaesth.*, **54**, 909.

Scott, D.B., Lees, M.M., Davie, I.T., Slawson, K.B. and Kerr, M.G. (1969) Observations on cardiorespiratory function during caesarean section. *Br. J. Anaesth.*, **41**, 489.

Scottish Home and Health Department (1978) A Report on an Enquiry into Maternal Deaths in Scotland, 1972–75. Edinburgh: H.M.S.O.

Scottish Home and Health Department (1985) *A Report on an Enquiry into Maternal Deaths in Scotland, 1976–80*. Edinburgh: H.M.S.O.

Sellick, R.A. (1961) Cricoid pressure to control regurgitation of stomach contents during induction of anaesthesia: preliminary communication. *Lancet*, **ii**, 404.

Siker, E.S., Wolfson, B., Dubnansky, J. and Fitting, G.M. (1968) Placental transfer of methoxyflurane. *Br. J. Anaesth.*, **40**, 588.

Sjøstedt, S. (1962) Acid–base balance of arterial blood during pregnancy, at delivery and in the puerperium. *Am. J. Obstet. Gynec.*, **84**, 775.

Skovstedt, P., Misfeldt, B.B., Mogensen, J.V. and Brockner, J. (1973) Effects of anaesthesia on blood loss at Caesarean section. *Acta anaesth. scand.*, **17**, 153.

Smith, N.T. et al (1970) The cardiovascular and sympathomimetic responses to the addition of nitrous oxide to halothane in man. *Anesthesiology*, **32**, 410.

Smith, J.B., Manning, F.A. and Palahniuk, R.J. (1975) Maternal and foetal effects of methoxyflurane anaesthesia in the pregnant ewe. *Can. Anaesth. Soc. J.*, **22**, 449.

Smith, G., Dalling, R. and Williams, T.I.R. (1978) Gastro-oesophageal pressure gradient changes produced by induction of anaesthesia and suxamethonium. *Br. J. Anaesth.*, **50**, 1137.

Sosis, W. and Bodner, A. (1983) Is general anaesthesia becoming obsolete for Caesarean section? *Anaesthesia*, **38**, 702.

Spence, A.A., Moir, D.D. and Finlay, W.E.I. (1967) Observations on intragastric pressure. *Anaesthesia*, **22**, 249.

Spiers, I. (1966) Use of tacrine and suxamethonium in anaesthesia for caesarean section. *Br. J. Anaesth.*, **38**, 394.

Stenger, V.G. et al (1967) Observations on pentothal, nitrous oxide and succinylcholine anesthesia at cesarean section. *Am. J. Obstet. Gynec.*, **99**, 690.

Stenger, V.G., Blechner, J.N. and Prystowsky, H. (1969) A study of prolongation of obstetric anesthesia. *Am. J. Obstet. Gynec.*, **103**, 901.

Stirt, J.A., Katz, R.L., Schehl, D.L. and Lee, C. (1984) Atracurium for intubation in man. A clinical and electromyographic study. *Anaesthesia*, **39**, 1214.

Stoelting, R.K. (1979) Attenuation of blood pressure response to laryngoscopy and intubation with sodium nitroprusside. *Anesth. Analg. curr. Res.*, **58**, 116.

Stoelting, R.K., Longnecker, D.E. and Eger, E.I., II. (1970) Minimum alveolar concentrations in man on awakening from methoxyflurane, halothane, ether and fluroxene anesthesia: M.A.C. awake. *Anesthesiology*, **33**, 5.

Strout, C.D. and Nahrwold, M.L. (1981) Halothane requirement during pregnancy and lactation in rats. *Anesthesiology*, **55**, 322.

Sykes, M.K. (1975) Arterial oxygen tension in parturient women. *Br. J. Anaesth.*, **47**, 530.

Taylor, G. and Prys-Davies, J. (1966) Prophylactic use of antacids in the prevention of the acid-pulmonary-aspiration syndrome (Mendelson's syndrome). *Lancet*, **i**, 288.

Thind, G.S. and Bryson, T.H.L. (1983) Single dose suxamethonium and muscle pain in pregnancy. *Br. J. Anaesth.*, **55**, 743.

Thomas, J., Climie, C.R. and Mather, L.E. (1969) Placental transfer of alcuronium. *Br. J. Anaesth.*, **41**, 297.

Thompson, E.M., Loughran, P.G., McAuley, D.M., Wilson, C.M. and Moore, J. (1984) Combined treatment with ranitidine and saline antacids prior to obstetric anaesthesia. *Anaesthesia*, **39**, 1086.

Toldy, M. and Scott, D.B. (1969) Blood loss during caesarean section under general anaesthesia. *Br. J. Anaesth.*, **41**, 868.

Tunstall, M.E. (1976) Failed intubation drill. *Anaesthesia*, **31**, 850.

Tunstall, M.E. (1979) The reduction of amnesic wakefulness during Caesarean section. *Anaesthesia*, **34**, 316.

Tunstall, M.E. (1980) On being aware by request. *Br. J. Anaesth.*, **52**, 1049.

Tunstall, M.E. and Geddes, C. (1984) 'Failed intubation' in obstetric anaesthesia. An indication for the use of the 'Esophageal Gastric Tube Airway'. *Br. J. Anaesth.*, **56**, 659.

Tunstall, M.E. and Hawksworth, G.M. (1981) Halothane uptake and nitrous oxide concentration. Arterial halothane levels during Caesarean section. *Anaesthesia*, **36**, 177.

Turndorf, H., Rodis, I.D. and Clark, T.S. (1974) 'Silent' regurgitation during general anesthesia. *Anesth. Analg. curr. Res.*, **53**, 700.

Turner, D.J. and Wilson, J. (1969) Effect of diazepam on awareness during caesarean section under general anaesthesia. *Br. med. J.*, **ii**, 736.

Vickers, M.D., Heath, M.L. and Dunlap, D. (1969) A comparison of Macrodex and stored blood as replacement for blood loss during planned surgery. I. Blood volume maintenance. *Br. J. Anaesth.*, **41**, 677.

Wallace, G. (1967) Blood loss in obstetrics using a haemoglobin dilution technique. *J. Obstet. Gynaec. Br. Commonw.*, **74**, 64.

Warren, T.M., Datta, S., Ostheimer, G.W. et al (1983) Comparison of the maternal and neonatal effects of halothane, enflurane and isoflurane for cesarean delivery. *Anesth. Analg. curr. Res.*, **62**, 516.

White, W.D., Clark, J.M. and Stanley-Jones, G.H.M. (1976) The efficacy of antacid therapy. *Br. J. Anaesth.*, **48**, 1117.

Whittington, R.M., Robinson, J.S. and Thompson, J.M. (1979) Fatal aspiration (Mendelson's) syndrome despite antacids and cricoid pressure. *Lancet*, **ii**, 228.

Williams, J.C. (1983) H$_2$-receptor antagonists in anaesthesia. *Can. Anaesth. Soc. J.*, **30**, 264.

Wilson, J. (1971) Awareness during operative obstetrics under general anaesthesia. *Br. J. Anaesth.*, **43**, 723.

Wilson, J. and Turner, D.J. (1969) Awareness during caesarean section under general anaesthesia. *Br. med. J.*, **i**, 280.

Wood, C., Ng, K.H., Hounslow, D. and Benning, H. (1973) Time—an important variable in normal delivery. *J. Obstet. Gynaec. Br. Commonw.*, **80**, 295.

Wraight, W.J., Chamney, A.R. and Howells, T.H. (1983) The determination of an effective cricoid pressure. *Anaesthesia*, **34**, 461.

Young, H.S.A., Clarke, R.S.J. and Dundee, J.W. (1975) Intubating conditions with AH8165 and suxamethonium. *Anaesthesia*, **30**, 30.

7

Regional Analgesia in Obstetrics

The superior quality of the pain relief obtainable with regional analgesia in comparison with narcotic analgesic drugs is indisputable (Beazley et al, 1967; Crawford, 1972a; Holdcroft and Morgan, 1974; Moir et al, 1974). For operative vaginal deliveries the advantages and safety of regional analgesia over general anaesthesia are well-recognized. Where technique is impeccable, subarachnoid and epidural analgesia have certain advantages over general anaesthesia for caesarean section. An obstetric anaesthesia service which does not make epidural analgesia available is an incomplete service.

The introduction of continuous caudal analgesia by Hingson and Edwards in the USA in 1942 was an important landmark in the history of obstetrics and of anaesthesia. Belated, but nevertheless welcome, has been the development of services for obstetric epidural analgesia in many centres in the UK since about 1968. The provision of continuous epidural analgesia for patients in labour is the most important contribution which anaesthetists can make to the relief of pain in childbirth and is moreover a professional activity capable of giving a great deal of satisfaction to the anaesthetist as well as to his patients. There are of course potential dangers inherent in regional analgesic techniques just as in other forms of anaesthesia and analgesia and it is essential that the anaesthetist who practises regional analgesia in obstetrics should possess a sound knowledge of the relevant anatomy, physiology and pharmacology and be aware of the effects of epidural analgesia and other techniques on the mother and her infant in labour.

The techniques and indications for epidural analgesia are constantly changing in detail and are being adapted by various anaesthetists to meet the circumstances in which they practise. In a survey of London teaching hospitals with a 24-hour epidural service Doughty (1978) noted that the proportion of patients receiving continuous lumbar epidural analgesia for pain relief in labour, varied from 5% to 60%. Despite the clearly superior pain relief offered by epidural analgesia, Robinson et al (1980), in a study of patients who selected their method of pain relief in labour (either epidural or intramuscular pethidine) during the antenatal period, found that a similar proportion selecting each method were satisfied, and 66% would choose the same method again. This is contrasted by the results of a survey by Morgan et al (1982) who observed that patients apparently related disappointment following childbirth to the duration of labour and to the increased number of forceps deliveries which occurred in those who received epidural analgesia, despite the effective pain relief. It is clear that the proportion of patients receiving epidural analgesia in labour is related to the complex interplay of the beliefs and aspirations of the mother, the midwives and the obstetricians and not simply to the efficacy of the method of analgesia.

ANATOMICAL CONSIDERATIONS

The uterus and the lower birth canal possess a sensory and a motor nerve supply.

Sensory pathways. The now classic description of the nerve supply of the birth canal was given by Cleland in 1933 and, with minor modifications, this description is accepted today. Controversy exists mainly over the sensory function, if any, of the pelvic parasympathetic nerves (nervi erigentes).

The uterus. All parts of the uterus, including the cervix, share a common sensory pathway. The afferent nerve fibres from the uterus travel with the sympathetic nerves but are themselves A delta and C afferent fibres (Bonica, 1979). Emerging from the uterus on each side of the cervix, the sensory fibres pass laterally in the paracervical tissues, traversing the uterine and cervical plexus (Frankenhauser's plexus) and lying in the base of the broad ligament. The fibres then pass centrally through the inferior, middle and superior hypogastric plexuses to enter the lumbar and lower thoracic parts of the sympathetic chain of ganglia. The central connection from the sympathetic chain is by the white rami communicantes of the eleventh and twelfth thoracic nerves, the posterior roots of these nerves and the spinal cord. The first lumbar nerves effect an additional central connection in many women (Doughty, 1972). The sensory innervation of the uterus is of course bilateral and so paracervical blocks and paravertebral blocks must be performed bilaterally for the relief of uterine pain (see Figure 10).

The concept of an additional sensory nerve supply from the cervix with fibres travelling to the sacral portion of the spinal cord with the pelvic parasympathetics (S2, S3 and S4) is no longer accepted by all who have considered the question (Doughty, 1972; Bonica, 1979). Nevertheless the existence of such a nerve supply would provide a ready explanation for the severe backache of certain labours which is not always relieved by an epidural injection which blocks T11 and T12 segments and relieves the abdominal component of the pain (Moir and Willocks, 1967). Bonica (1979) states that the usual explanation for backache lies in the fact that the cutaneous branches of the posterior divisions of T10 to L1 nerves supply skin 8–10 cm caudal to their point of origin. The first lumbar nerve supplies skin over the middle of the sacrum. Bonica accepts that the severe backache which may accompany an occipitoposterior position or dystocia may require a block of the lumbar and sacral segments, but suggests that the pain originates in intrapelvic structures other than the uterus. The afferent fibres in the pelvic

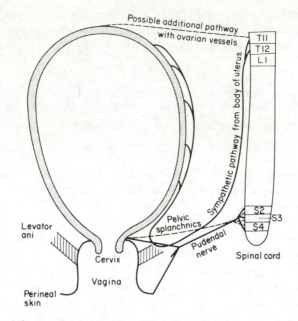

Figure 10. The pathways of pain in labour. The pain of uterine contractions enters the spinal cord at segments T11, T12 and L1. The pain of the second stage is also transmitted by the pudendal nerve to cord segments S2, S3 and S4. In a few patients uterine pain fibres may accompany the ovarian vessels. The role of the pelvic splanchnic nerves (n. erigentes) is uncertain but they have been thought to transmit painful sensations originating in the cervix and which are felt as backache.

parasympathetics are involved in Ferguson's reflex, whereby stimulation of these fibres increases uterine activity in animals and perhaps in man.

In a proportion of patients sensory fibres from the uterus accompany the ovarian vessels to enter the spinal cord directly at the eleventh and twelfth thoracic segments or perhaps at a higher level. It is possible that these fibres could be excluded from an otherwise successful epidural or subarachnoid block.

The lower birth canal. The principal sensory nerve of the vagina, vulva and perineum is the pudendal nerve (S2, S3 and S4) and it supplies these areas through its three terminal branches (the haemorrhoidal and perineal nerves and the dorsal nerve of the clitoris). The fourth sacral nerve is the motor nerve to the levator ani muscle. Small areas of perineal and vulval skin receive a sensory supply from the ileo-inguinal, genitofemoral and posterior femoral cutaneous nerves and the cutaneous branches of the second, third and fourth sacral nerves. A small area of the vaginal vault is supplied through the pelvic parasympathetics.

Motor pathways. There is debate also about the precise motor innervation of the uterus and about the roles of these nerves in the initiation and maintenance of labour. Certainly an intact motor innervation is not essential for the onset of labour and for its continuance in the human species. Patients with motor lesions at high levels in the spinal cord are capable of normal uterine activity although incapable of expulsive efforts in the second stage of labour. It is now agreed that even a high epidural block does not abolish the contractions of established labour unless severe hypotension results.

Sympathetic and parasympathetic nerves are involved in the motor innervation of the uterus. Preganglionic parasympathetics (nervi erigentes) arise from S2, S3 and S4 spinal segments and accompany the uterine artery to the uterus. The synapse between pre- and postganglionic fibres takes place in the paracervical tissues very close to the uterus. Consequently the postganglionic fibres are not interrupted by any regional block.

Preganglionic sympathetic fibres originate in a portion of the spinal cord which includes the fifth thoracic to the second lumbar segments. These fibres then synapse, according to their level of origin in the coeliac, aortic, inferior mesenteric or hypogastric plexuses or in the lumbar sympathetic chain. Finally these various motor fibres unite to form the hypogastric nerves and these, together with the pelvic parasympathetics, enter the pelvic (Frankenhauser's) plexus.

A subarachnoid or epidural block will interrupt the preganglionic sympathetic fibres and leave the postganglionic sympathetic fibres intact. Although uterine action in established normal labour is unaffected by epidural analgesia in that the rate of progress in labour is unaltered, there is commonly a brief inhibition of contractions after an epidural injection. It is thought that this transient inhibition may result from the interruption of the preganglionic sympathetic nerves and that uterine activity returns under the control of the postganglionic fibres. Similarly the more normal pattern of uterine action which frequently develops after the institution of epidural analgesia in patients with incoordinate uterine action could be due to the removal of adverse influences from higher centres by interruption of the preganglionic sympathetic fibres.

The nature of pain in labour. The reason why uterine contractions are usually painful in labour is not known with certainty. Dilatation of the cervix is the usual explanation preferred. Manual dilatation of the cervix mimics labour pains.

Uterine pain is felt mainly, but not exclusively, within the cutaneous distribution of the first lumbar and eleventh and twelfth thoracic nerves. Pains in the first stage of labour are thus felt mainly in the lower abdomen, the groins and the lower lumbar and sacral region. If pain is severe than it is frequently felt in areas supplied by adjacent nerves. The A delta and C afferent fibres which carry painful sensations from the uterus terminate mainly in lamina V of the dorsal horn and synapse there with cells (second sensory neurons) which also receive afferents from areas of skin supplied by the same cord segments (Wall, 1967). This anatomical arrangement provides a basis for the referred pain of uterine contractions. Backache is often the most distressing feature of unusually painful labour and seems to occur with particular severity in association with occipitoposterior positions and incoordinate uterine action.

In the second stage of labour and during delivery the descent of the presenting part produces pain in the distribution of the pudendal nerve within the perineum and vulva. The pain of uterine contractions continues to be experienced in the abdomen and back. Commonly pain is less severe in the second stage of labour, perhaps because delivery is imminent and the patient is now actively involved. The fully dilated cervix is no longer a source of pain. The most painful time in many labours occurs towards the end of the first stage. Pain in labour tends to become worse with time, unlike postoperative pain, and the intensity of pain is certainly influenced by emotional and environmental factors. A prolonged labour produces fear in the mother for the safety of her child, even when pain has been relieved by epidural block. Fear and pain cause the woman to secrete catecholamines which may promote incoordinate uterine action and thereby further prolong labour and increase pain and anxiety.

Doughty (1972), from extensive observation of women in labour, states that 70% of patients experience hypogastric pain and that 20% suffer backache during labour. He believes that backache may be a personal characteristic of some women and is not necessarily related to an occipitoposterior position or an incoordinate labour. A particularly distressing phenomenon is rectal pain, usually occurring when labour is well advanced and not always relieved by epidural block. Doughty and also Holdcroft and Morgan (1974) agree that very few women (perhaps 2% only) have a naturally painless labour.

A LIST OF TECHNIQUES OF REGIONAL ANALGESIA

A consideration of the foregoing anatomical details leads to the following conclusions:

All the undernoted techniques can be used to relieve the pain of uterine contractions in the first stage of labour (Moir, 1971). All these techniques have been used for this purpose at some time although with varying degrees of success and appropriateness.

Paracervical block (uterosacral block)—bilateral.
Paravertebral block of the eleventh and twelfth thoracic nerves—bilateral.
Paravertebral block of the second lumbar sympathetic ganglion—bilateral.
Lumbar epidural block.
Caudal block.
Subarachnoid block.
Subcutaneous infiltration of groins and back (areas of referred pain).

The following techniques will relieve the pain experienced in the lower birth canal during the second stage of labour and delivery:

Infiltration of the perineum and vulva.
Pudendal nerve blocks—bilateral.
Lumbar epidural block.
Caudal block.
Subarachnoid block.

There are only three techniques capable of relieving pain of uterine contractions and of the second stage of labour and delivery:

Lumbar epidural block.
Caudal block.
Subarachnoid block.

The sites at which pain may be blocked are indicated in Figure 11.

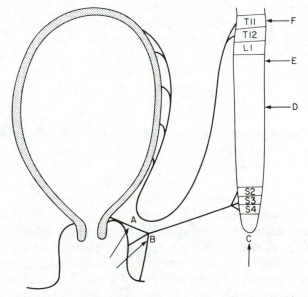

Figure 11. Sites at which regional block may be performed for the relief of pain in labour and/or delivery. A, paracervical block. B, pudendal nerve block. C, caudal epidural block. D, lumbar epidural and subarachnoid block. E, sympathetic block at L2. F, paravertebral block of T11 and T12.

SOME PHYSIOLOGICAL CONSIDERATIONS

Cardiovascular effects of epidural and subarachnoid analgesia

The haemodynamic changes associated with epidural or subarachnoid analgesia represent the greatest hazard of these techniques for mother and child. These changes may be further compounded by the effects of caval occlusion in the supine position and by hypovolaemia resulting from the loss of blood or other fluids. The cardiovascular complications of epidural and subarachnoid block are often preventable, are always amenable to the correct treatment and should no longer cause maternal or fetal death. The attainment of this level of safety demands the highest standards of anaesthetic, obstetric and nursing care and the rigorous application of the now well-documented observations concerning the haemodynamic consequences of extensive preganglionic sympathetic block in the pregnant woman.

Caval occlusion in the supine position is the rule rather than the exception in the final weeks of pregnancy (Kerr et al, 1964) although venous return is usually maintained by the alternative vertebral venous route and the azygos vein. Even if venous return is reduced in the supine position a normal arterial pressure is usually maintained by an increase in peripheral resistance. Quite large reductions in cardiac output can occur without a fall in mean arterial pressure because of this compensatory vasoconstriction. Normotension is therefore far from indicative of a normal cardiac output. Supine hypotension (revealed caval occlusion) occurs in only 2 or 3% of pregnant women and is then usually associated with bradycardia (Holmes, 1960).

Epidural and subarachnoid blocks reduce peripheral resistance by 30% or more and there is little alteration in cardiac output during high epidural block in non-pregnant subjects when plain lignocaine is used (Ward et al, 1965), but Greene (1981) argues that the cardiovascular responses to epidural blockade are not identical to those accompanying spinal anaesthesia, even if the block extends to the same dermatome. The two-segment zone seen with spinal anaesthesia (the segmental sympathetic spread following spinal anaesthesia is at least two segments higher than the sensory block), is not seen with epidural analgesia, the sympathetic block being less extensive. Greene also believes that extensive epidural blockade with local anaesthetic solutions results in substantial blood levels which are pharmacologically active, unlike those following spinal anaesthesia.

In pregnant women, in contrast to the non-pregnant subject, the addition of adrenaline often fails to increase cardiac output (Akamatsu and Bonica, 1975). The situation in the pregnant woman who has caval occlusion may be very different if she has received an epidural or subarachnoid block. Cardiac output may fall by up to 30% as the result of caval occlusion, and the abolition of the normal vasoconstrictor response by conduction analgesia may result in a severe fall in blood pressure.

In an earlier series of continuous epidural blocks in labour the patients were managed in the supine position and the incidence of hypotension (systolic blood pressure 90 mmHg (12.0 kPa or lower) was almost 20% (Moir and Willocks, 1968). It has been our policy to employ the lateral position during epidural analgesia in labour since 1970 and the current incidence of hypotension is under 5%. In the presumed absence of caval occlusion the present incidence of hypotension is probably attributable mainly to the sympathetic blockade. All of these patients receive intravenous fluids and it is thought that absolute hypovolaemia is unlikely. Hypotension was usually of brief duration and no mother and no infant suffered clinically recognizable permanent harm as the result. The sympathetic block is probably more extensive than the sensory block which usually reaches to between the tenth and eighth thoracic dermatome. Heavner and De Jong (1974) have demonstrated that the small, myelinated preganglionic sympathetic β-fibres are the most readily blocked.

It was recognized by Assali and Prystowsky in 1950 that hypotension was commoner in pregnant patients than in other women during subarachnoid and epidural blocks. The incidence varies very widely from 1 to 25% in recorded series of epidural blocks (Chaplin and Renwick, 1958; Hehre and Sayig, 1960; Cowles, 1965; Hellman, 1965; Crawford, 1972a; Moore et al, 1974). Comparisons are difficult because of the various definitions of hypotension, the assiduousness of patient monitoring, the probable influence of caval occlusion in the early series and the various intravenous fluid regimens employed. Moore et al (1974) observed hypotension in 6% of their patients, who were all in the lateral position, a figure which agrees with the writers' experiences in similar circumstances. Crawford (1978) states that only 3 or 4% of his patients developed hypotension which was not due to caval occlusion. Hypotension may occur more suddenly and perhaps more frequently during subarachnoid analgesia in comparison with epidural analgesia (Forthman and Adriani, 1957; Bonica, 1967). Blood pressure and cardiac output reductions are greatest under epidural block with adrenaline in the solution, less severe under subarachnoid block and least extensive under epidural block with plain solutions (Ueland et al, 1972; Akamatsu and Bonica, 1975). The severity and frequency of the hypotension following epidural block is proportional to the extent of the block and the circulating blood volume. The extensive block required for caesarean section is associated with a 25–44% incidence of hypotension (Antoine and Young, 1982; Dutton et al, 1984), which is presumably not related to caval occlusion, as the patients were placed in the modified supine position. Although maternal hypotension does not apparently affect the fetus adversely if the episode is brief, if fetal lactic acidosis does develop then it will persist, despite rapid correction of the hypotension (Antoine and Young, 1982).

Transient fetal bradycardia may follow maternal hypotension (Maltau, 1975; Raabe and Belfrage, 1976; Collins et al, 1978) and uterine contractions may diminish in strength or cease entirely for a brief period of time (Raabe and Belfrage, 1976; Schellenberg, 1977). The placental vasculature is thought to lack sympathetic vasoconstrictor nerves (Greiss, 1967) and placental blood flow probably falls along with cardiac output. Maternal and fetal 'unexplained' deaths during spinal and epidural analgesia are almost certainly due to severe reductions in cardiac output and blood pressure resulting from caval occlusion and sympathetic blockade, and in some instances are associated with hypovolaemia. Wollman and Marx (1968) and Marx et al

(1969) have stressed that blood pressure and cardiac output can be maintained by the liberal administration of crystalloid solutions before and during conduction analgesia. An adequate circulating blood volume can be maintained in the presence of a temporary increase in the volume of the vascular compartment resulting from the sympathetic blockade. In hypotensive ewes under subarachnoid analgesia an impaired uteroplacental circulation could be improved by the administration of intravenous fluids. In the absence of maternal hypotension placental blood flow is not reduced during lumbar epidural analgesia in labour or during caesarean section (Jouppila et al, 1978a,b; Husemeyer and Crawley, 1979).

Hypovolaemia. An important study by Bonica et al (1972) in healthy non-pregnant volunteers has demonstrated the sometimes disastrous effects of high epidural block in the presence of hypovolaemia. Blood loss of the order of 13% of the blood volume transformed individuals who were little affected by high epidural block into 'poor risk' subjects who were highly vulnerable to the cardiovascular depressant effects of extensive vasomotor blockade and also to the depressant effect of lignocaine upon the myocardium. The adverse response to epidural block was greater with plain solutions of lignocaine. The addition of adrenaline 1 : 200 000 partly opposed the myocardial depressant action of lignocaine. The authors were strongly of the opinion that high epidural block should normally be avoided in patients with existing hypovolaemia. The dangers of epidural block in the presence of hypovolaemia have been confirmed by Morikawa et al (1974). In the absence of a coagulation defect resulting from a complication of pregnancy such as abruptio placentae (an absolute contraindication), the benefits of conduction analgesia must be carefully assessed in any patient with a history of antepartum haemorrhage. If bleeding occurs during established epidural or subarachnoid analgesia, then vigorous and early replacement with blood substitute or blood is mandatory. Reliance on the arterial pressure as a guide is totally inadequate, and replacement should commence before the blood loss is reflected in a change in arterial pressure. These observations reinforce the recommendation usually made that epidural and subarachnoid analgesia should be avoided in patients who have bled, unless blood volume has been restored and further bleeding is not anticipated. It should be recalled that blood loss at caesarean section and at forceps delivery under epidural analgesia is approximately halved in comparison with the losses measured when general anaesthesia is used (Moir and Wallace, 1967; Moir, 1970).

Prevention and treatment of hypotension. In clinical practice the anaesthetist will normally rely upon blood pressure readings for assessment of the cardiovascular effects of epidural or subarachnoid block. It will be appreciated that a reduction in cardiac output in the presence of a reduced peripheral resistance is the real cause for concern. The relationship between blood pressure, cardiac output and peripheral resistance is expressed as:

Mean arterial pressure = cardiac output × peripheral resistance

The avoidance of caval occlusion and the maintenance or restoration of an adequate circulating blood volume are the primary measures for the prevention and treatment of hypotension and the maintenance of cardiac output.

It is recommended that the lateral position be used during labour for all patients who have received epidural analgesia. The tone of the vascular compartment will be reduced as the result of the sympathetic blockade, with a reduced vascular resistance and an increase in the venous capacitance. These effects are reduced by compensatory sympathetically mediated vasoconstriction of the unblocked segments. Maternal stability can be maintained by the avoidance of caval occlusion and the infusion of adequate volumes of balanced salt solutions. The addition of glucose to these solutions should be strictly limited. It has been suggested that not more than 6 g glucose should be infused per hour (Kenepp et al, 1982) with a maximum of 25 g of glucose during labour (Rutter et al, 1980). The ketosis associated with labour may be normal (Dumoulin and Foulkes, 1984) and energetic efforts to treat this with glucose solutions may induce neonatal hypoglycaemia (Mendiola et al, 1982). The use of solutions containing 5% dextrose only is unsatisfactory. The antidiuretic effects of the administration of oxytocin and the concomitant infusion of more than 3.5 litres of 5% dextrose has been associated with hyponatraemic convulsions (Feeny, 1982).

It is our practice at the Queen Mother's Hospital, when intravenous therapy commences, to prescribe alternate 500 ml units of Ringer lactate solution and 5% dextrose. In the first 12 hours 2.5 litres are infused; this is then reduced to a rate of 2.5 litres in the succeeding 24 hours. In the Queen Mother's Hospital it is our policy to withhold food and drink from mothers in labour; the intravenous fluid regimen is designed to correct any mild dehydrating effects resulting from a limited oral intake. These precautions will limit the severity and frequency of maternal hypotension during epidural analgesia for pain relief. If, however, hypotension does occur, it is important to examine the patient and exclude inadvertent subarachnoid injection of local anaesthetic by confirming that the block is not more extensive than might have been anticipated. Mild hypotension responds rapidly to turning the patient on to her side (if not already in this position). Rapid infusion of intravenous fluids, 200–300 ml, and an injection of intravenous ephedrine 5–10 mg may be required if the block is extensive. Vasopressor drugs will rarely be required if caval occlusion is avoided and the plasma volume is adequately maintained. The anaesthetist initiating the block must assess and be satisfied with the effects of the initial injection, and the first injection through the catheter, before leaving the patient.

Hypotension and caesarean section

The increasing popularity of epidural analgesia for caesarean section and the extensive block required for satisfactory and painfree surgery, have increased the frequency and severity of maternal hypotension and the incidence of adverse effects on the fetus. Hypotension occurs in 25–45% of patients, despite preloading with intravenous fluids, and the avoidance of caval occlusion (Dutton et al, 1984; Antoine and Young, 1982). Preloading with an infusion of 1 litre of crystalloid solution half an hour before surgery was popularized by Marx et al (1969). Increasing the volume of the 'preload' to 2 litres, infused during institution of epidural block, reduces the frequency of hypotension to 6.6% (as defined by a decrease in arterial systolic pressure of >21%, Lewis et al, 1983). This was also associated with an increase in central venous pressure of 5 cm of water following delivery. While the majority of healthy patients will tolerate this, a lingering doubt of its safety must remain if some unsuspected cardiovascular abnormality exists. The preload fluid should not contain more than 6 g glucose, as discussed previously (Kenepp et al, 1982), and Peng et al (1981) noted that the infusion of Ringer's lactate solution containing 1% glucose prior to caesarean section was associated with improved maternal and neonatal stability. The use of colloid solutions prior to caesarean section is attractive as the extravascular loss is less rapid than that associated with the use of crystalloid solutions (gelatin solutions should not be used, as serious sensitivity reactions may occur if administered to normovolaemic patients). However, albumin-containing solutions are very expensive, and their efficacy controversial (Gibbs et al, 1981; Mathru et al, 1980). The benefits are not sufficiently clear to justify routine use. The use of prophylactic intravascular injections of ephedrine before initiating epidural analgesia for caesarean section has been investigated by Rolbin et al (1982). They noted that the incidence of hypotension was 12% when defined as a fall in arterial systolic pressure to 70% of control values, and an unpredictably high and unacceptable incidence of hypertension was associated with the use of 50 mg of ephedrine i.m. 30 minutes before inserting the epidural block. Gutsche (1976) advocates ephedrine prophylaxis for hypotension during spinal anaesthesia. Craft et al (1982) observed that 64% of patients who received epidural analgesia for caesarean section became hypotensive when ephedrine prophylaxis was omitted. It is interesting to note the relationship of the maximum reduction in arterial blood pressure to time, and in the author's experience, the maximum change in arterial pressure occurs during or just after transfer of the patient to theatre. Movement of the extensively sympathetically blocked patient, no matter how carefully carried out, is undesirable and should be avoided if possible. Needless to say, the technique demands scrupulous attention to detail, the avoidance of caval occlusion and rapid action if hypotension occurs including the liberal use of intravenous ephedrine. Hypotension is a significant risk, current therapy is not entirely satisfactory and the claim by Gibbs et al (1983), that wrapping the legs in elastic bandages of patients undergoing caesarean section with epidural analgesia significantly reduced the frequency of hypotension is attractive as a simple and safe technique.

Uterine action

Uterine action in the first stage of labour is usually assessed either by the continuous recording of intra-amniotic pressures or by graphic analysis of the rate of cervical dilatation by the construction of a partogram. It is now agreed that in the absence of hypotension and aortocaval occlusion, lumbar and caudal epidural analgesia and subarachnoid analgesia do not alter the overall rate of progress in the first stage of normal labour (Friedman, 1955; Vasicka and Kretchmer, 1961; Cibils and Spackman, 1962). Schellenberg (1977) has confirmed these observations and suggests that the temporary reduction in uterine activity which some observers have recorded was due to aortocaval occlusion. Phillips et al (1977) observed only progressive cervical dilatation in patients already in active labour.

There are two occasions during epidural analgesia when uterine contractions may be temporarily inhibited. A hypotensive episode may be associated with cessation of contractions due, presumably, to inadequacy of the uterine circulation. Restoration of a normal blood pressure and cardiac output quickly leads to the return of uterine contractions. A vasoconstrictor drug (α-adrenergic) should not be used to restore blood pressure because tetanic uterine contractions may be produced (Senties et al, 1970). These comments are probably also applicable to hypotension caused by subarachnoid analgesia, caval occlusion or hypovolaemia.

Although high concentrations of adrenaline given by intravenous infusion can inhibit uterine action (Pose et al, 1962; Zuspan et al, 1964) the addition of adrenaline 1 : 200 000 to local anaesthetic solutions does not affect the progress of labour or the intensity of contractions (Moore, 1964; Bonica, 1967; Craft et al, 1972). The inhibitory effect apparently observed during caudal analgesia by Gunther and Bauman (1969) may have been due to the relatively large volumes injected or more probably to the hypotension which occurred in 20% of these patients. Jouppila et al (1977) thought that 1 : 200 000 adrenaline might have contributed to a reduction in uterine activity lasting for 60 minutes after injection into the epidural space with 0.5% bupivacaine and thought that adrenaline should not be used. Caval occlusion in the supine position can inhibit uterine contractions even in the absence of overt hypotension (Caldeyro-Barcia, 1960).

The effect of epidural analgesia on labour is not clear, but the earlier fear of it abolishing spontaneous labour is no longer thought to be correct. The changes in obstetric practice, the more liberal use of oxytocin, and the current trend to reduce the frequency of artificial induction of labour has put an end to the unnecessarily arbitrary and rigid criteria governing the earlier use of epidural analgesia. The indication for epidural analgesia is pain, whatever the extent of cervical dilatation.

The concept of incoordinate uterine action is less prevalent as a result of the changing patterns in the obstetric management of labour. The benefits of epidural analgesia for the relief of pain in the management of accelerated labour by oxytocin stimulation are substantial. The definitive study of the effects of epidural analgesia will probably never be published, as most obstetricians and anaesthetists would consider the required randomization and withholding epidural analgesia from patients in labour as unethical. To this extent, present studies are a compromise, but they do suggest that epidural analgesia has little effect on the progress of normal labour, and may be of considerable benefit if labour is abnormal (Moir and Willocks, 1966; Raabe and Belfrage, 1976; Studd et al, 1980).

With the current liberal use of oxytocin and the tendency to limit the duration of labour the benefits of epidural analgesia on abnormal uterine action are less obvious, although the relief of pain in these unusually painful labours remains of great benefit. The explanation for the onset of a more normal type of uterine action after epidural block is uncertain. It has been suggested that in these patients fear and anxiety and associated high sympathetic tone are the cause of the abnormality and that epidural analgesia, by interrupting the preganglionic sympathetic fibres, allows the uterus to act more normally without higher control. Uterine blood flow is much reduced where uterine action is incoordinate and, in 1955, Johnson and Clayton demonstrated a restoration of placental blood flow following continuous caudal analgesia.

In the third stage of labour the uterus retracts powerfully under subarachnoid or epidural analgesia and blood loss is usually reduced by about 50% at forceps delivery and caesarean section (Moir and Wallace, 1967; Moir, 1970).

Respiration and acid–base balance

High epidural analgesia has almost no effect on maximal ventilatory capacity, blood pH, P_{CO_2}, P_{O_2} and the base excess in non-pregnant subjects who are not undergoing surgery (Moir, 1963; Moir and Mone, 1964; Ward et al, 1965). The implication of these findings is that the power of the respiratory muscles is not seriously impaired by epidural block with 1.5% lignocaine. The retention of normal maximal expiratory power confirms the clinical impression that voluntary expulsive efforts can be fully effective and that spontaneous delivery is possible under epidural analgesia when obstetric factors permit (Doughty, 1969; Matouskova et al, 1975). High subarachnoid block reduces maximal expiratory capacity by almost 50%, although resting ventilation remains adequate (Egbert et al, 1961; Freund et al, 1967) and blood–gas values are normal in non-pregnant patients not undergoing surgery (Ward et al, 1965).

Hyperventilation is usual in painful labour (Cole and Nainby-Luxmore, 1962; Crawford and Tunstall, 1968; Pearson and Davies, 1973) and the maternal P_aCO_2 is likely to average about 25 mmHg (3.3 kPa), with further reductions during the hyperventilation associated with painful contractions. Epidural analgesia reduces or abolishes this hyperventilation and hypocapnia is prevented or reduced (Fisher and Prys-Roberts, 1968; Pearson and Davies, 1973). When labour is managed under continuous epidural analgesia maternal metabolic acidosis is less severe in comparison with the acidosis which occurs when pethidine is used (Pearson and Davies, 1973). In the second stage voluntary expulsive efforts usually produce a considerable maternal metabolic acidosis. If pushing is not permitted during epidural analgesia the acidosis does not develop. Involuntary expulsive efforts are abolished if perineal anaesthesia is present. Not surprisingly the maternal blood–gas and metabolic changes are usually reflected in the fetus. Epidural analgesia does not cause fetal bradycardia in the absence of hypotension and loss of beat-to-beat variability of the heart rate is uncommon (Maltau, 1975; Raabe and Belfrage, 1976; Crawford, 1979a). These observations are consistent with the finding that placental blood flow is unaltered by normotensive epidural analgesia (Jouppila et al, 1978a). The incidence of hypotension and fetal heart rate abnormalities may be substantially reduced by intravenous fluid loading in labour (Collins et al, 1978).

Seven per cent of healthy pregnant women exhibit ketosis (Dumoulin and Foulkes, 1984); ketonuria may occur in normal labour and its onset and severity is related to the duration of labour. Efforts to abolish it completely are unwise as the infusion of large quantities of dextrose can readily saturate the maternal metabolic pathways inducing hyperglycaemia, resulting in a fetal infusion of glucose and consequently neonatal hypoglycaemia (Kenepp et al, 1982; Mendiola et al, 1982). During labour it is essential to maintain adequate hydration with a balanced salt solution, but the amount of dextrose should be limited to <6 g/h as discussed previously.

Fetal welfare

The mechanisms whereby regional analgesia might affect the condition of the fetus at birth include:

Alterations in placental blood flow.
Alterations in uterine contractions and tone.
Direct action of local anaesthetics on the fetus.
Alterations in maternal respiratory and acid–base status.
Relaxation of the pelvic floor muscles.
Provision of optimal conditions for controlled delivery.

Not all of these mechanisms are necessarily harmful to the fetus. Some are undoubtedly beneficial.

Reductions in uteroplacental blood flow may be anticipated if maternal hypotension develops and may also result from caval occlusion in the absence of hypotension (concealed caval occlusion). Epidural and subarachnoid analgesia are especially likely to cause hypotension if the cardiac output is reduced by caval occlusion or hypovolaemia. It is not possible to nominate a critical maternal blood pressure below which placental circulation becomes inadequate for fetal wellbeing. The critical pressure must vary from patient to patient and must be affected by the pre-existing blood pressure and factors such as pre-eclampsia and placental insufficiency. Hypotension accompanied by alteration in the fetal heart rate calls for urgent treatment by posture, fluids and, if these are ineffective, then an intravenous injection of ephedrine 5 mg or 10 mg.

It is thought that placental blood flow may be improved by the careful use of epidural analgesia in pre-eclampsia. If cardiac output is maintained (by avoiding caval occlusion) then the sympathetic blockade may result in an improvement in blood flow in the uterine arteries. Certainly the condition of the infant of the severely toxaemic mother is often clinically satisfactory in these circumstances (Moir et al, 1972).

The use of α-adrenergic vasoconstrictors such as methoxamine to treat hypotension is totally condemned because they further reduce uterine artery blood flow (Ralston et al, 1974).

The progressive fetal acidosis which occurs in painful labour when pain is inadequately relieved by pethidine does not occur with epidural analgesia (Pearson and Davies, 1974).

Alterations in uterine tone and in the intensity and frequency of contractions are not usually associated with uncomplicated epidural analgesia in normal established labour. Hypertonicity and tetanic contractions may follow the injection of an α-adrenergic drug and there will be an associated severe reduction in uteroplacental blood flow (Cibils et al, 1962) in addition to that already resulting from constriction of the uterine arteries. The restoration of a more normal pattern of uterine contractions and reduction of resting uterine tone following the institution of an epidural block during incoordinate labour is accompanied by an improvement in placental blood flow (Johnson and Clayton, 1955). This together with earlier delivery is beneficial to the fetus.

The mechanism by which paracervical block is followed by fetal bradycardia in a high percentage of cases is uncertain but may involve hypertonicity of the uterus with a consequent reduction in placental blood flow (Liston et al, 1973).

The placental transfer of local anaesthetic drugs has been discussed in chapter 3. In summary the concentrations of lignocaine and prilocaine in the blood of the umbilical vein are usually about 70% of the concentration in the maternal venous blood during epidural analgesia. The fetal concentration of mepivacaine may be close to 100% of the maternal concentration. In striking contrast the concentration of bupivacaine in the umbilical vein is only 20–35% of the maternal venous concentration. The reduced placental transfer of bupivacaine is attributable largely to binding of the drug to maternal plasma proteins (Tucker et al, 1970). It is this feature of bupivacaine, together with its longer duration of action, which makes it the agent of choice for continuous epidural analgesia in labour. The placental transfer of etidocaine appears to be comparable to that of bupivacaine (Bromage et al, 1974).

Neurobehavioural assessment has become part of the armamentarium in assessing the neonatal effects of drugs given to the mother and subsequently transferred to the fetus. While detectable effects can be noted for many drugs given during labour, including analgesics and general anaesthetics, the significance of these effects on the baby is not clear and may sometimes have been exaggerated. Nevertheless it provides a mechanism whereby an evaluation can be made of some of the more subtle effects of maternally administered drugs on the neonate.

An early study by Scanlon et al (1974) noted that neonates whose mothers received epidural lignocaine during labour had reduced muscle tone, but Apgar scores were high, and metabolic acidosis was absent. However, Abboud and her colleagues (1982, 1983, 1984), Kileff et al (1984) and Kuhnert et al (1984) have failed to attribute adverse fetal effects to the epidural administration of lignocaine for either caesarean section or pain relief in labour. Fetal transfer of 2-chloroprocaine is negligible, and the neonatal effects attributable to 2-chloroprocaine will be minimal. In an elegant study, Kuhnert et al (1984) compared the neonatal effects of 2-chloroprocaine and lignocaine when used for caesarean section. The neurobehavioural scores of the neonates whose mothers received 2-chloroprocaine were slightly higher than the lignocaine group, but the conclusion was that the effects were subtle and other influences were more important. The use of epidural bupivacaine, with its reduced placental transfer, has not been associated with reduced neonatal muscle tone, and neurobehavioural scores were normal (Scanlon et al, 1976; Kileff et al, 1984). It should also be noted that similar neurological testing of infants whose mothers had received pethidine revealed a high incidence of reflex depression (Brackbill et al, 1974). These tests are refined, and biochemically and clinically the infants were in satisfactory condition. One is forced to conclude that no methods of analgesia (except perhaps psychological methods) are free of side-effects, although carefully conducted epidural analgesia comes close to this ideal.

It has been widely believed that the explanation for the fetal bradycardia which occurs during upwards of 20% of paracervical blocks, and usually within 20 minutes of injection, lies in rapid and extensive placental transfer of the local anaesthetic drug. The fetal bradycardia is almost invariably associated with fetal acidosis (Asling et al, 1970; Teramo and Rajamaki, 1971) and must therefore be presumed to indicate fetal hypoxia. It was postulated that the local anaesthetic agent depressed the fetal myocardium. Beat-to-beat variability increases after paracervical block and is thought to indicate fetal hypoxia (Miller et al, 1978).

In a critical review of the theories put forward in explanation of fetal bradycardia during paracervical block, Liston et al (1973) emphasize that the concentrations of local anaesthetic drug in the fetal scalp blood during labour are well below those usually regarded as toxic in adults (Beazley et al, 1972; Thiery and Vroman, 1972). Rather higher levels were recorded by Asling et al (1970) who suggest that absorption of the drug may take place directly into the uterine artery. Such a mechanism seems contrary to all orthodox theories concerning the absorption of drugs from tissues and the hypothesis that paracervical block impairs placental circulation is more attractive. A direct vasoconstrictor action of lignocaine upon the uterine artery is possible (Gibbs and Noel, 1977), and bupivacaine has a powerful constrictor action on the uterine artery (Greiss et al, 1976). However, Van Dorsten et al (1981) noted that if the sites of the paracervical injections were carefully spaced and the patient suitably laterally tilted to avoid caval occlusion, no significant fetal bradycardia was seen. Fetal bradycardia was attributed to the effect of peak fetal and maternal concentrations of the local anaesthetic agent used.

The harmful effects of paracervical block are probably dose-related, and the use of small volumes and low concentrations of local anaesthetic agents and a superficial injection site away from the uterine artery reduce the incidence of fetal heart rate changes (Cibils and Santonja-Lucas, 1978).

Direct injection of the local anaesthetic into the fetus is a possibility during caudal, paracervical and pudendal blocks and during infiltration of the perineum. Finster et al (1965) have recorded massive injection of the fetus during caudal analgesia with mepivacaine concentrations of up to 75 μg/ml at birth. The writers know of two instances of injection of the fetus during perineal infiltration by an inexperienced midwife. The occurrence of such a catastrophe indicates prompt delivery of the child. Efforts must then be made to rid the infant of a potentially lethal concentration of local anaesthetic by exchange transfusion and perhaps by gastric lavage along with general resuscitative measures.

The occurrence of methaemoglobinaemia in mother and child after the use of prilocaine for continuous epidural analgesia or for repeated paracervical blocks contributes to fetal hypoxia. Prilocaine should not be used for repeated injections in labour, although it is a very suitable agent for pudendal nerve block and perineal infiltration.

It has for many years been believed that the incidence of fetal malposition and the need for instrumental delivery is increased during epidural analgesia since relaxation of the pelvic floor muscles results in failure of the descending fetal head to rotate. The maternal expulsive powers are also likely to be impaired as a consequence of the motor and sensory block, however slight, on the maternal voluntary expulsive effort. Utilizing a segmental block, in which analgesia is restricted to T11 and T12, a spontaneous delivery rate of 80% has been claimed. Doughty (1969) and Jouppila et al (1979) did not observe an increase in the frequency of fetal malposition. The use of larger volumes and more concentrated solutions such as 0.5% bupivacaine substantially increased the frequency of both rotational and non-rotational forceps deliveries (Hoult et al, 1977; Husemeyer, 1983). The excellent analgesia associated with the use of epidural analgesia makes it the technique of choice for the more prolonged, difficult and painful labours—labours which intuitively one would believe to be more likely to require instrumental delivery. It is impossible to distinguish clearly which has the most significant effect, the expulsive forces of labour, the relationship between the presenting part and the birth canal or the effects of epidural analgesia. A further important factor is the permitted duration of the second stage of labour and there is a welcomed trend to allow adequate time for descent of the fetal head with a consequent lessening of the need for difficult and rotational forceps delivery. Lumbar epidural analgesia with bupivacaine 0.5% provides excellent pain relief, more than 70% of patients experiencing complete relief of pain. The use of 0.25% bupivacaine for epidural analgesia does not produce quite such excellent relief, but the majority find the pain relief satisfactory, with the additional benefit of a significant reduction in the frequency and severity of motor block and a substantial increase in the frequency of spontaneous delivery (Thorburn and Moir, 1981). This important observation is probably due to the fact that a weaker solution of bupivacaine has less effect on motor function and that the duration of the second stage of labour is not arbitrarily limited in the absence of fetal distress.

Despite the numerous potential hazards which may be associated with epidural analgesia in labour the detailed studies of Pearson and Davies (1973, 1974) clearly illustrate the real benefits of the technique, not only in terms of pain relief but also in providing a more normal biochemical environment for mother and child. The impressive catalogue of complications of regional analgesia is presented with the hope that an understanding of their causes will lead to their prevention, and that if a complication does occur then treatment will be prompt, rational and effective.

The techniques of regional analgesia are best learned in the labour room and operating theatre from an expert. It is hoped that the following descriptions will nevertheless be helpful to the anaesthetist who may be denied this privilege and may augment the practical tuition received by the more fortunate learner.

LUMBAR EPIDURAL ANALGESIA

There are many methods of identifying the epidural space, and success depends more upon the skill of the anaesthetist than upon any special virtues of a particular method. Because there is a positive pressure of 4.6–10 cmH$_2$O (0.8–1.8 kPa) in the lumbar epidural space in active labour (Galbert and Marx, 1974) a technique which depends upon the existence of a negative pressure for success is unsuitable. The loss of resistance technique (Dogliotti technique) is deservedly popular and the detailed and vivid descriptions by Bromage (1954, 1978) are commended to anyone learning the technique of epidural puncture. Other recommended descriptions, differing only in points of detail, have been given by Moore (1964), Bonica (1967) and Doughty (1978).

The patient should be on a firm, tilting obstetric bed. A brief history should be taken and the absence of any contraindications to epidural analgesia should be confirmed. The patient should of course consent to the procedure and verbal permission will normally be acceptable. The three United Kingdom Medical Defence Societies have agreed that verbal consent after a simple explanation of the purpose of epidural analgesia is acceptable and they recommend that the fact of verbal agreement should be recorded in the case sheet. Access to an open vein is essential. An intravenous infusion must be in place before undertaking the block, and the anaesthetist should confirm that it is running satisfactorily. A full surgical scrub should be carried out and a mask, cap and gown should be worn. Although transatlantic and some British opinion (Crawford, 1978) considers that a sterile gown need not be worn, the trainee frequently, in the writers' experience, finds difficulty in passing the epidural catheter without risking contamination if a gown is not worn and efforts to keep the bare arms out of contact with the sterile area may create an awkward posture.

Most anaesthetists work with the patient in the lateral lumbar puncture position and this is usually perfectly satisfactory. Injection in the lateral position gives earlier onset, more extensive spread and much more prolonged analgesia on the dependent side (Grundy et al, 1978), but this influence is thought to be of insufficient magnitude to be important (Merry et al, 1983). The authors prefer that the patient be in the sitting position. The patient sits on the edge of the bed and rests her arms on the shoulders of an assistant who stands face to face with the patient. It is thought that greater spinal flexion can sometimes be achieved in this position. A useful sterile working surface is acquired on the bed and extreme flexion of the thighs on the abdomen with possible obstruction of the femoral veins is avoided.

The anaesthetist now applies an antiseptic solution to an area of the back extending vertically from the lower border of the scapulae to the natal cleft and laterally well out over the iliac crests. A solution of 0.5% chlorhexidine in alcohol is used. A suitable alternative is iodine, but there is then a slight risk of a sensitivity reaction. A detergent is not used in case it should come into contact with nerve tissue. The antiseptic solution is not allowed to come into contact with the gloved hand or with any of the equipment. A large towel is now draped from the iliac crests, downwards over the buttocks, across the bed and allowed to hang over the edge of the bed, thus providing a sterile working surface. If the lateral position is preferred then a fenestrated towel is used.

The anaesthetist next palpates the iliac crests through the sterile towel. A line joining the iliac crests transects the fourth lumbar interspace (L4–L5) or the fourth lumbar spinous process. The L2–L3 or L3–L4 interspace is usually most suitable for epidural puncture but if these spaces seem narrow or difficult to identify then another lumbar interspace may be chosen. A small intradermal weal is raised with a 25 gauge needle at the proposed site of entry. The subcutaneous tissues are next infiltrated with about 1 ml of local anaesthetic solution, taking care not to obscure the landmarks by injecting too large a volume. Infiltration of the spinal ligaments is difficult and unnecessary. The skin is now pierced with a Sise introducer, a wide bore needle or a small scalpel blade. This facilitates insertion of the epidural needle and avoids carrying a plug of skin and antiseptic into the epidural space with the possibility of later development of an implantation dermoid tumour and chemical irritation of nerve tissue.

A 16 or 18 gauge Tuohy needle with stilette is now inserted until its tip passes through the tough and sometimes sensitive supraspinous ligament. The patient should be warned that supraspinous puncture may be painful. A common cause of failure is the advancement of the needle on to one or other side of the midline. A few experienced anaesthetists advocate a paramedian approach as being less painful. The supraspinous ligament is felt as a rounded ridge running between the spinous processes and it is essential to use controlled, steady pressure to pierce this ligament and not allow the needle to be deflected to one side. The stilette is now withdrawn and a well lubricated glass syringe with free-moving plunger is firmly attached to the needle. A 5 ml or a 10 ml syringe may be used. Opinions differ over the contents of this syringe. If air is used then certainly any liquid which later emerges must be cerebrospinal fluid and the novice may feel secure in this knowledge. A possible additional advantage of air may be that the injection of fragments of glass from the ampoule is avoided. Others use sterile saline so that if an intradural injection is made then subarachnoid analgesia will not result. One author has used local anaesthetic solution for over 25 years and has never been in serious doubt as to whether any emergent liquid was cerebrospinal fluid or local anaesthetic. It is believed that the jet of liquid which emerges from the needle point on entering the epidural space briefly pushes the dura away and may avoid a dural puncture on an incalculable number of occasions and therefore the use of air is not advocated (see Figure 12).

The hub of the epidural needle is gripped firmly between the thumb and index finger of the left hand. The ulnar border of the left hand rests against the patient's back and maintains stability. The thumb of the right hand maintains a constant moderate pressure on the plunger of the syringe. This is the sole function of the right hand; it is not used to advance the needle. Using only the left hand, the needle is slowly and steadily advanced through the interspinous ligament. The bevel of the needle should point towards the patient's head. Progress should be smooth and resistance is not great at this stage. If a gritty sensation is experienced the needle is grating against a spinous process, success is unlikely in this plane and the needle should be reinserted, taking care to locate it in a position equidistant from each adjacent spinous process and in the midline. A false positive loss of resistance is occasionally met with in the interspinous ligament and is due to the presence of small cavities within the ligament (Sharrock, 1979).

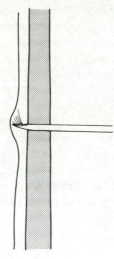

Figure 12. The dura being briefly 'tented' by the epidural needle as it enters the epidural space while using the loss of resistance method. The risk of dural puncture is probably thereby diminished.

As the steady, smooth advance continues, an increased resistance to progress will be appreciated. The needle point now lies within the ligamentum flavum and success is imminent. The ligamentum flavum is usually about 1 cm thick but may vary considerably, and it lies at an average depth of about 7 cm from the skin but this too varies widely. If bone is encountered at this depth the needle should be partly withdrawn and then redirected in a more cephalad direction until it enters the ligamentum flavum. Occasionally a more caudad inclination is successful.

Maintaining a firm grip with the left hand the needle is cautiously but steadily advanced and pressure is maintained on the plunger. Injection is almost impossible while the needle remains within the ligamentum flavum. Entry into the epidural space is heralded by a sudden 'give' which is appreciated by the left hand and the sudden loss of resistance to injection. The volume of liquid injected at this time should be limited to perhaps 1.0 ml. The needle in the epidural space is illustrated in Figure 13 and Figure 14.

Stability and firmness are essential at the moment of epidural puncture. Occasionally a degree of force is necessary if the ligamentum flavum is abnormally tough and the use of force calls for even greater steadiness. Throughout the entire process the anaesthetist should concentrate his thoughts on his left hand which is advancing the needle and he should try to picture in his mind the structures through which the tip of the needle is passing.

When an apparently successful epidural puncture has been performed the syringe should be detached from the needle. If more than a few drops of liquid emerge from the hub of the needle a dural puncture must be suspected.

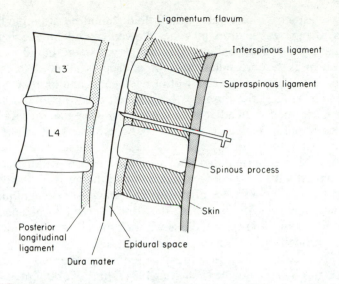

Figure 13. Longitudinal section of spine at L3–L4 showing needle in the epidural space. The needle is roughly parallel with the upper border of the spinous process of L4.

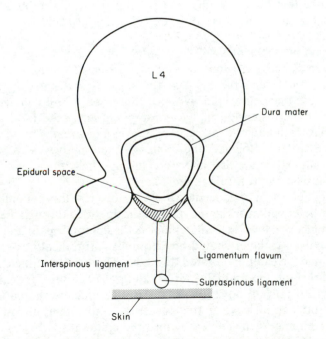

Figure 14. Transverse section through upper part of body of L4 vertebra showing structures traversed by the epidural needle.

In that case aspiration of cerebrospinal fluid should be attempted. If liquid continues to emerge, a drop may be allowed to fall on the back of the anaesthetist's hand, after pulling back his glove. If the liquid is warm and flows freely it is cerebrospinal fluid. If a drop is allowed to fall onto a Dextrostix, the presence of sugar will provide confirmation that the liquid is cerebrospinal fluid. If the dura has been penetrated, an epidural puncture should be performed at an adjacent interspace and the patient should receive continuous epidural analgesia. The further measures to be taken for the prevention or treatment of spinal headache are discussed later.

Having satisfied himself that the needle point lies within the epidural space the anaesthetist's next moves depend upon the needs of the patient and the circumstances in which he practises. If a single-shot technique is to be used because delivery is imminent, then the dose of local anaesthetic is injected quite slowly and the needle is withdrawn. The routine injection of a test dose through the needle is considered unnecessary, but unusually extensive blockade has been reported following the injection of local anaesthetic through the needle (Pearson, 1984). In case of doubt, an injection of 3 ml of local anaesthetic solution may be given, and the epidural catheter inserted carefully. It has been suggested that intravascular injections will go unrecognized unless the solution contains adrenaline (Moore and Batra, 1981). After a 5-minute interval the patient is asked to move her toes. Paralysis indicates subarachnoid injection. The absence of a motor block does not guarantee that the needle has not pierced the dura, because experience has shown that 3 ml of 0.25% or even 0.5% bupivacaine solution will not always cause paralysis of the leg muscles.

A continuous technique will be used in the great majority of epidural blocks. Even in these circumstances the injection of the initial full dose of local anaesthetic through the needle at this stage has much to commend it, if it is not proposed to allow midwives to administer top-up injections. It is believed that the distension of the epidural space by the local anaesthetic solution may facilitate the passage of the epidural catheter. The Central Midwives Board for England and Wales permits midwives to give top-up injections only where the first injection through the catheter has been given by a doctor. The Scottish rule is similar.

With the bevel of the needle directed towards the patient's head an epidural catheter with markings at intervals is threaded through the needle. A slight resistance is felt as the catheter enters the epidural space and a further 3 or 4 cm length of catheter should be introduced. If difficulty is encountered the needle may be carefully rotated through 180° when the cather may pass in a caudad direction. Occasionally a fresh and presumably stiffer catheter may pass. Crawford (1972b) advises that in case of difficulty the patient should slowly extend her hips while the anaesthetist maintains pressure on the catheter which may then slide easily into the epidural space.

The needle is now withdrawn over the catheter by maintaining pressure on the catheter during withdrawal. When the needle has emerged from the skin, the catheter is gripped between finger and thumb at its point of entry into the skin while the needle is slid along the catheter. On no account should the catheter ever be pulled back through the needle if the catheter has entered the epidural space. The risk of shearing off the end of the catheter is considerable in these circumstances.

There is little doubt that the incidence of paravertebral placement of the catheter and unilateral analgesia increases as the length of catheter within the epidural space increases (Sanchez et al, 1967; Bridenbaugh et al, 1968; Usubiaga et al, 1970; Doughty, 1975). A technique has been described by Doughty (1974) which permits the insertion of a measured length of catheter. Doughty recommends the insertion of only 2 cm of catheter but agrees that some anaesthetists might consider the risk of displacement of the catheter rather high in these circumstances and might prefer to insert 3 or 4 cm of catheter. A modified Portex catheter with markings at 1 cm intervals is used along with a needle with graduations at the same intervals.

It is now necessary to arrange for the administration of sterile top-up doses of local anaesthetic solution. A growing body of opinion supports the use of a bacterial filter as the sole precaution against infection. Protagonists of this regimen attach the filter (the Millex filter is suitable) to the catheter while wearing sterile gloves. Thereafter no other aseptic or antiseptic precautions are taken. The local anaesthetic solution used for top-ups is drawn into a syringe held in unsterile hands and the solution is drawn from ampoules, the exterior of which is unsterile. The syringe may be left attached to the filter between injections or the open end of the filter may be closed by a rubber cap. The Millex filter is disposable and is claimed to prevent the passage of all particles greater than 0.22 μm.

Conscious of the potentially disastrous consequences of an epidural abscess, the author continues to use the well-tried syringe in bag method for the administration of sterile top-up injections (Cole, 1964). While scrubbed-up (and usually before embarking on epidural puncture) the anaesthetist fills a 50 ml sterile syringe from autoclaved ampoules of local anaesthetic. The syringe is attached to the catheter and then enclosed within a sterile transparent bag which has been made from a length of plastic sleeving, heat-sealed at one end. The neck of the bag is sealed around the catheter. Top-up injections can then be given without handling the syringe directly, and the anaesthetist is entirely responsible for correct identification of the contents of the syringe.

It is now recognized that the opening of ampoules results in the contamination of the contents with glass and other matter in most instances (Furgang, 1974) and it is possible that these particles might act as irritants to nerve tissue when injected. It is therefore recommended that a Millex filter be inserted between syringe and catheter to trap these particles of glass, whether or not the sterile syringe in bag method is used.

Dural puncture by the epidural catheter is a rare but recognized occurrence (Moir and Hesson, 1965; Moore, 1969; Dawkins, 1972) and it is therefore a wise precaution to inject a 3 ml test dose of local anaesthetic through the catheter after placement. After a 5-minute interval a full dose may be given, if this has not already been administered through the needle. As already indicated, a 3 ml test dose is not infallible, and there are now several reports of an unexpectedly extensive block following the initial or subsequent standard top-up injection during labour, despite normal responses to the initial injections (Park, 1984; Brindle Smith et al, 1984; Soni and Holland, 1981; Collier, 1982). Possible explanations for this dangerous phenomenon are dural perforation by the epidural catheter during labour, or the use of a three eye catheter, when the distal eye is in the subarachnoid space. The authors have personal experience of three such episodes, and now advocate the use of a preliminary injection of 3 ml bupivacaine, waiting for at least 5 minutes, and then assessing motor function by asking the patient to move her legs, before injecting the remainder of the prescribed dose. Rees and Rosen (1979) believe that every top-up should be given by the anaesthetist, because absolute certainty about the position of the catheter is not possible. In the Queen Mother's Hospital and in many other centres with a resident obstetric anaesthetist about 50% of top-ups are given by the anaesthetists, but in less well-staffed hospitals the obstetric epidural service relies heavily upon the midwives. Some types of epidural catheter have two side-openings, and the distal opening may be in the subarachnoid space while the proximal opening is in the epidural space (Ward et al, 1978). Rapid, forceful injections may then produce accidental subarachnoid block and a slower injection may result in a purely epidural block (Finucane, 1979). There were two deaths due to subarachnoid injection through a catheter in England in 1975.

The catheter is now securely fixed to the skin at the point of emergence by a gauze swab and waterproof tape. The catheter is then led upwards and over the shoulder and may be pinned to the gown. If the syringe-in-bag method is in use the catheter may be led onto the abdominal wall where the syringe is secured. The catheter should not be kinked. If the patient was in the sitting position she should now lie on her side.

Disposable epidural sets are now available from several manufacturers in the UK. In principle their arrival is welcomed. In practice some of the individual items in these sets are not always of the most appropriate design, at least in the writers' opinion. Some sets make no provision for sterile topping-up and, probably inevitably, none of the sets includes a local anaesthetic drug.

Choice of local anaesthetic drug. The placental transfer of the local anaesthetic drugs has been discussed elsewhere. Bromage (1962) found that the dose requirements for lumbar epidural analgesia were reduced by about one-third in pregnancy and the suggested explanation is that the engorged epidural veins occupy more of the epidural space and so a given volume spreads further. Recently it has been shown that the dose requirements are unaltered in pregnancy if caval occlusion is prevented (Grundy et al, 1978). Of the generally available drugs bupivacaine is without doubt the local anaesthetic of choice for continuous epidural analgesia in labour. Bupivacaine is preferred because it is fairly long-acting, has a high protein-binding capacity and a low fetal/maternal concentration ratio. Motor weakness is minimal or absent with concentrations of up to 0.375%, although the 0.5 and 0.75% solutions cause severe lower limb paralysis in 11 and 20% of mothers respectively (Littlewood et al, 1977). These workers found that analgesia lasted no longer with 0.375 than with 0.25% bupivacaine (mean 65 and 73 minutes). The use of 0.75% bupivacaine is no longer recommended for obstetric patients. The circumstances surrounding this decision are not clear, but deaths relating to the use of 0.75% bupivacaine were cited from Transcripts of the Fifth Meeting of Anesthetic and Life Support Drug Advisory Committee (Albright, 1984).

Weakness of the legs is disliked by most mothers, and pain relief in labour following the use of 0.25% bupivacaine is almost as effective as that of 0.5% bupivacaine. The reduced leg weakness and the increase in spontaneous delivery rate makes it the solution of choice for normal labour (Thorburn and Moir, 1981). The use of dilute solutions reduces the total dose of bupivacaine and the plasma concentration (Tucker et al, 1972), a benefit which may be important if the epidural block is to be extended to allow delivery by caesarean section (Thorburn and Moir, 1984). Top-up injections of bupivacaine 0.25% may have to be given slightly more frequently than is the case with the more concentrated solution, and motor block increases pari passu with the number of injections. According to Littlewood et al (1977), increasing the concentration of the local anaesthetic increases the duration of analgesia, reduces the onset time, increases motor block but does not increase segmental spread. A dose of 5–6 ml of 0.25% bupivacaine is adequate for analgesia in the first stage of labour. This volume may be increased if necessary and the concentration increased if a more extensive block is required, particularly if the sacral roots are to be blocked.

Bupivacaine 0.125% with 1 : 400 000 adrenaline has been successfully used by Vanderick et al (1974) but has not gained wide acceptance, although maternal and fetal plasma concentrations are low (Geerinckx et al, 1974). The addition of adrenaline has almost no effect on the duration of analgesia, the placental transfer of bupivacaine or the toxicity of bupivacaine (Reynolds et al, 1973) and is therefore not necessary.

Etidocaine, although long-acting, is associated with a high degree of motor block in the concentration (0.5%) necessary for good relief of pain (Bromage et al, 1974) and as far as can be assessed at present, this agent is unlikely to rival bupivacaine for obstetric epidural analgesia. Edelist and Perera (1976) did not achieve adequate analgesia with 0.5% etidocaine in a small series of obstetric patients, and 1% etidocaine was abandoned because of its high incidence of severe motor block. Littlewood et al (1977) noted a

38% incidence of severe motor block with 1% etidocaine, and analgesia lasted for 86 minutes.

Lignocaine hydrochloride may be used in 1.5% or 2% concentration. Analgesia lasts for about 70 minutes with plain solutions and about 120 minutes with added adrenaline. The addition of adrenaline increases the incidence of motor block. Tachyphylaxis develops after the first four or five top-ups and makes lignocaine unsuitable for prolonged analgesia (Moir and Willocks, 1966, 1967). Prilocaine is not advocated for continuous blocks because methaemoglobinaemia will develop and mepivacaine is relatively toxic for the infant (Morishima et al, 1966). Mepivacaine has high fetal/maternal concentration ratios, is not extensively bound to serum protein and causes neonatal hypotonia (Scanlon et al, 1974). Bupivacaine does not affect muscle tone or reflex activity in the neonate (Scanlon et al, 1976). Although the placental transfer of procaine and 2-chloroprocaine is minimal or non-existent owing to breakdown by cholinesterase, the short action of these drugs makes them inconvenient for prolonged use. Recently, reports have been published in which relatively large volumes of 2 or 3% 2-chloroprocaine intended for epidural injection were inadvertently injected intrathecally, with resulting total spinal anaesthesia and severe motor and sensory deficits which lasted several weeks (Covino et al, 1980; Covino, 1983). The relatively low pH of 2-chloroprocaine is no longer implicated as a contributing factor (Ravindran et al, 1982). Animal work suggests that neurological damage following the subarachnoid injection of large volumes of local anaesthetic solutions is related to the volume and concentration of the solution used (Lundy et al, 1933, Ravindran et al, 1982, Rosen et al, 1983). Barotrauma from the force of injection and the preservative used in 2-chloroprocaine have also been implicated (Ready et al, 1983; Rosen et al, 1983). Consensus opinion is that, despite the impressive list of reports of neurological damage, the incidence of damage is so low that a frequency proportion cannot be stated with any confidence. 2-Chloroprocaine is unavailable in the UK. Carbonated lignocaine has been claimed to be an excellent agent for obstetric epidural analgesia and to almost eliminate unblocked segments (Bromage, 1972) but this was not confirmed in a large series by an author and his colleagues (Moir et al, 1976).

Continuous infusion epidural analgesia

Continuous infusion of local anaesthetic solution into the epidural space was first described by Scott and Walker (1963) and would appear to offer many advantages. A lower concentration of local anaesthetic solution may be used, with the provision of a more stable level of analgesia and the avoidance of painful episodes while waiting for a top-up injection. The major disadvantage, which is theoretical at present, is the possibility of failure to identify an inadvertent subarachnoid injection. Despite its undoubted advantages, the technique has not yet proved universally popular, and in the UK, continuous epidural analgesia is usually maintained by intermittent top-up injections of local anaesthetic agents.

The objective of continuous epidural infusion is to achieve effective pain relief with minimal segmental spread and to avoid motor block and hypotension without the need for supplementary bolus injections. To achieve this, various concentrations of bupivacaine solution infused at differing rates have been investigated. Davis and Fettes (1981) and Taylor (1983) utilized a simple Intraflow device delivering 6 ml/h, and Taylor noted the optimal concentration of bupivacaine to be 0.30% plain solution. However, although simple and safe to operate, the Intraflow device cannot be adjusted and is thus inflexible. In the interests of safety the red tail, which when pulled allows a rapid flow, was removed. Until recently the majority of reports advocated the use of an accurate volumetric infusion pump, with an infusion rate of 10 ml/h of 0.25% bupivacaine. Tunstall and Ramamoorthy (1984) found that 44% of mothers receiving 20–25 ml of 0.08% bupivacaine per hour did not require any top-up injections. Analgesia was initiated with an injection of 9 ml (in divided doses of 3 and 6 ml) of 0.5% bupivacaine. A reduction in blood pressure was noted in 13% of mothers following the initial injection. It is essential to initiate the block with an effective dose of local anaesthetic, and follow on with the infusion, since Matouskova et al (1979) noted that an infusion of a radio-opaque dye into the epidural space at a rate of 10 ml/h required 30 minutes to achieve a three-segment spread.

Kenepp et al (1983) investigated the efficacy of an infusion of 20 mg/h of bupivacaine in concentrations of 0.125%, 0.25% and 0.5%. Bupivacaine 0.125% was found to be the most effective; the motor block was related to the number of dermatomes blocked rather than the concentration of the drug used. Li et al (1985) also investigated various concentrations and infusion rates of bupivacaine, and recommend an infusion of 10 ml/h of 0.125%. This appeared to offer the best compromise as 69% of mothers required only one top-up injection, effectively relieving pain but retaining some sensation, which patients like. Rosenblatt et al (1983) infused 25 mg/h of bupivacaine 0.25%, and occasionally observed transient hypotension. Slow spread of the block to T4 has been observed during infusion of 0.25% bupivacaine at 5 ml/h (Matouskova et al, 1979).

Clearly there is no single infusion volume and concentration which will be ideal for all patients, reflecting the range of doses required to produce effective analgesia when intermittent top-up injections are given. Flexibility is essential either by the provision of top-up injections, if required, or changing the infusion rates as necessary. The optimum infusion rate would appear to lie between 12.5 and 20 mg/h of 0.125% bupivacaine. The use of large volumes of more dilute bupivacaine requires further investigation.

Meticulous observation of the mother is essential. The extent of the block should be noted at least every 2 hours by testing and plotting the upper limit of sensory loss (Li et al, 1985). North American practice is to identify and mark dermatome level T8 and plot the upper limit of sensory loss with either a pin prick or a cold swab every half hour. If the block reaches T8, the rate of infusion is reduced. The degree of motor impairment should also be assessed and noted at regular intervals. Taylor (1983) argues that the intermittent top-up injection technique is extremely labour-intensive and time-consuming, as it requires aspiration of the catheter before and after each injection, test dose injection and its assessment followed by frequent blood pressure measurements, and the fact that top-up injections may be delayed if staff are busy. In her opinion, supervision of epidural infusions is much more simple and less time-consuming. However, differences in obstetric practice and the regulations governing the administration of analgesia in obstetrics are emphasized by the increasing popularity of epidural infusions in North America. A lingering doubt remains regarding the safety of the technique. Adequate and accurate supervision of an epidural infusion that will permit early detection of excessive dermatome spread, and motor block that may follow inadvertent subarachnoid infusion, is mandatory.

Complications of epidural analgesia

Hypotension. Hypotension is probably the commonest complication of obstetric epidural analgesia. The systolic pressure is likely to fall briefly to 90 mmHg (12.0 kPa) or lower in approximately 4 or 5% of patients, even when managed in the lateral position. The hypotension following the extensive block required for caesarean section is much more profound and common. Vigilance and early detection, followed by vigorous treatment, are the most important elements in its management. The aetiology, prevention and management of hypotension have been considered earlier in this chapter.

Dural puncture. The incidence of dural puncture varies largely with the experience of the anaesthetist. In the hands of the beginner the rate may be as high as 20% (Crawford, 1972a) while the very experienced individual may attain a personal figure of about 0.2%. In the authors' hospital, where many blocks are performed by registrars in training, the overall rate is between 2 and 3%.

Hodgkinson (1981) reviewed 2603 epidural caesarean sections, and noted a dural puncture incidence of 2.3%; in 31 of the 58 cases, the epidural was resited in an adjacent interspace. Three patients developed a total spinal, despite the use of a test dose, and 5-minute interval before injecting the main dose. If caesarean section is being undertaken and inadvertent dural puncture has occurred, Hodgkinson advises abandoning the epidural anaesthesia and inducing general or spinal anaesthesia. If the epidural block is for the relief of the pain of labour, the dose should be reduced and the patient carefully assessed. Collier (1982) cites similar experiences, but ascribes them to subdural placement of the catheter, although he was unable to demonstrate this. These experiences are substantially at variance with that of Crawford (1983), who did not observe total spinal in 302 patients following epidural injections in an adjacent interspace after dural puncture, and this is similar to the authors' experiences. Nevertheless, the evidence suggests that careful assessment should follow insertion of an epidural block in an interspace adjacent to one in which an inadvertent dural puncture has occurred.

The incidence of lumbar puncture headache after dural puncture with a 16 or 18 gauge Tuohy needle was 76% in one series (Craft et al, 1973). Headache usually develops within 48 hours, and most frequently on the second day after delivery. Because of the frequency and severity of the headache, it is strongly recommended that active measures be taken to prevent its development. Merely confining the patient to bed in a recumbent position is not very effective (Jones, 1974) although there is reason to believe that the prone position may be more effective than the supine position in prophylaxis (*British Medical Journal*, 1975). The following regimen is recommended if the dura is punctured:

(1) Perform epidural puncture at an adjacent lumbar interspace and proceed with a continuous epidural block in the usual manner. Delivery by forceps is recommended because straining is inadvisable.

(2) After delivery, leave the catheter in place and inject 40–60 ml of sterile Ringer lactate solution or normal saline solution through the catheter.

(3) Allow 1 litre of sterile Ringer lactate solution to drip slowly into the epidural space over the next 24 hours or so under the influence of gravity. Very occasionally severe interscapular pain of unknown origin has caused the anaesthetist to stop the epidural drip.

(4) Keep the patient in bed for 24 hours and encourage her to lie in the prone position whenever possible.

(5) If headache has not developed after 36 hours the catheter may be removed.

It is usually believed that the above regimen works by raising the pressure in the epidural space, thus stopping the leakage of cerebrospinal fluid and encouraging closure of the dural puncture. This simple explanation was questioned by Usubiaga et al (1970) who pointed out that the epidural pressure falls quite swiftly after a single injection of saline. The epidural drip may maintain a higher pressure. According to Craft et al (1973) a rather similar regimen was successful in about 90% of patients in the prevention of lumbar puncture headache. A single injection of 30 ml of sterile saline solution into the epidural space was ineffective in the treatment of headaches following dural puncture with 17 gauge needles and is not recommended in this circumstance (Bart and Wheeler, 1978).

If the preceding regimen is unsuccessful, or if severe headache develops at a later time, then an epidural injection of autologous blood may be given. Although it has been argued that epidural blood patch should not be introduced at the time of dural puncture because the failure rate is then as high as 70% (Loeser et al, 1978), Bali (1984) has suggested that the immediate injection of 2 ml of autologous blood will reduce the frequency of subsequent headaches. However, the use of epidural blood patch is not without some morbidity, although reports are rare (Ostheimer et al, 1974; Abouleish, 1978), and radicular back pain (Cornwall and Dolan, 1975) has been described. The changes in cerebrospinal fluid dynamics following dural puncture may result in slight descent of the pons and medulla, which then stretches the sixth cranial nerve over the sharp apex of the petrous temporal bone with resultant temporary sixth nerve palsy (Bonica, 1967; Greene, 1961; Heyman et al, 1982). The immediate injection of autologous blood would entail its administration to significantly more patients than would eventually require a blood patch. Only a small proportion of patients develop a headache of such severity that blood patch is required. A testimony to the safety of blood patches lies in the fact that it is now used in outpatients in some centres (Ravindran, 1984). Restriction of spread of epidural solutions has been reported following epidural blood patch (Rainbird and Pfitzner, 1983). Bacteraemia may occur during labour or shortly after delivery. Abouleish (1978) has successfully treated post lumbar puncture headache of up to 180 days duration by epidural blood patch. The anaesthetist performs an epidural puncture while a colleague withdraws a sample of the patient's venous blood under sterile conditions. This blood is now injected slowly into the epidural space until 20 ml have been given. If the patient complains of pain or paraesthesiae the injection is stopped immediately. A success rate of between 91 and 100% is claimed (Gormley, 1960; Di Giovanni and Dunbar, 1970; Di Giovanni et al, 1972). The collaborative evaluation carried out by the Society of Obstetric Anaesthesiologists and Perinatologists in the USA indicated a success rate of 91% (Ostheimer et al, 1974). Relief may be instantaneous or may be delayed for up to 24 hours. A blood patch may be repeated if unsuccessful or if headache returns. It is claimed that the 'blood patch' merely acts as a 'gelatinous tamponade' and that arachnoiditis does not occur. Clot fibrosis does not occur until long after the headache has been cured (Di Giovanni et al, 1972).

Epidural analgesia has been successfully performed from 7 to 380 days after a blood patch (Abouleish et al, 1975; Naulty and Herold, 1978) and the spread of solutions was apparently normal, suggesting that adhesions had not formed. In experimental goats the blood patch had been absorbed two weeks after injection and no adhesions formed (Di Giovanni et al, 1972). Nevertheless the clinician will fear the introduction of infection and possible neurological sequelae from nerve root involvement. Cornwall and Dolan (1975) report the following sequelae in 185 patients:

Persistent backache   2%
Transient pyrexia   5%
Facial paralysis   0.5%
Tinnitus, vertigo and ataxia   0.5%

Although a blood patch is usually safe and dramatically successful, it is a lingering doubt about its total safety which causes the writer to reserve it as a second line of treatment for use if an epidural drip has failed. Other methods of treatment include intravenous fluid therapy, injections of pitressin, applications of a tight abdominal binder and inhalations of carbon dioxide (Sikh and Agerwal, 1974) but are relatively ineffective.

It is perhaps worth stating that epidural analgesia does not, if uncomplicated by dural puncture, cause headache and that headache occurred in 14% of recently delivered women who had not received epidural analgesia (Moir and Davidson, 1972), although Ravindran et al (1980) have identified typical low pressure spinal headaches in 1% of patients following successful continuous epidural analgesia.

Accidental (total) spinal injection. Three potentially dangerous phenomena may occur during epidural analgesia:

The subarachnoid injection of an epidural dose of local anaesthetic may produce a disastrously extensive block, which must be recognized early and treated promptly if necessary. This follows unrecognized subarachnoid placement of the catheter, or the migration of an epidurally placed catheter during an effective epidural block (Park, 1984). A further possible mechanism may be related to the use of a three-hole catheter, where the catheter tip containing the distal hole pierces the dura and lies within the subarachnoid space. If the local anaesthetic agent is injected forcefully, a major proportion of the dose will emerge from the distal hole, producing a subarachnoid block, the extent of the block being related to the volume of local anaesthetic leaving the distal hole. If less force is used, less fluid will exit from the distal hole and more will exit from the two proximal holes, thus producing a block which is indistinguishable from an epidural block. This may be the mechanism by which total spinal may follow a top-up injection during an effective epidural block.

A second type of reaction follows subdural placement of the catheter. Here, the catheter is inserted and lies between the dura and arachnoid membranes. Extra-arachnoid or subdural placement of the catheter occurs in 5% of patients undergoing myelography (Jones and Newton, 1963). The events following subdural injection are characteristic, with the slow onset of an extensive block (Boys and Norman, 1975; Brindle Smith et al, 1984).

Subdural injection may be identified by the mode of onset of the block, and Collier (1982) has drawn attention to the following points:

(1) Hypotension is moderate.
(2) The onset of symptoms is slow (15–20 minutes).
(3) The onset of respiratory symptoms is progressive and slow.
(4) Complete recovery occurs within 2 hours.

The X-ray appearance of the subdural injection of contrast medium is characteristic, and if subdural injection is suspected, the epidural catheter can be retained until after delivery and contrast medium injected to confirm its position. Respiratory and cardiovascular support are not usually necessary.

The third rare, but potentially serious, consequence is 'massive epidural injection'. This concept was first described by Dawkins (1969), and in many respects may be similar to subdural injection or subarachnoid injection. The concept is rather nebulous, and defies accurate assessment of the mechanism. There are, however, a sufficient number of bizarre events following epidural injection of local anaesthetic (Maycock, 1978; Kritz and Jouppila, 1980; Carter, 1984) which may be explained by partial subarachnoid blockade. These reports describe the anomalous onset of sensory blockade, involving the upper limbs and head, sometimes associated with reduced respiratory function and moderate hypotension. The mechanism is obscure, and the anaesthetist should be concerned with assessing respiratory and cardiovascular function, and the provision of ventilatory and circulatory support if necessary.

Treatment of total spinal blockade

Fortuna (1981) in a review of 13 872 epidural blocks claims that total spinal blockade occurs in approximately 1 : 2000. As discussed above, total spinal blockade may occur after the second or other top-up injection. The injection is followed by a fall in maternal arterial pressure and ascending paralysis of the legs and trunk, eventually leading to respiratory difficulties and possibly apnoea. The speed of onset is probably related to the dose of local anaesthetic injected into the subarachnoid space. If the appropriate steps are taken to provide respiratory and cardiovascular support, sequelae should be minimal. Hypotension should be treated as already outlined. If necessary the trachea should be intubated, preferably following the induction of general anaesthesia, taking the same precautions as for an emergency caesarean section, and ventilatory support undertaken. Fetal monitoring should confirm fetal welfare, and precipitate delivery is unnecessary.

Early recognition is essential, as it will allow sufficient time to summon the anaesthetist who then has sufficient time to assess the patient properly and to take the appropriate steps, without undue emphasis on speed (or panic). The patient is usually terrified at the slow and apparently relentless ascent of muscle weakness, particularly when breathing becomes difficult, and general anaesthesia should be induced if necessary.

Deaths from this cause continue to be reported, and they emphasize the need both for some form of simple assessment following each top-up injection, and the relative proximity of personnel, usually the anaesthetist, capable of adequate resuscitation. This must include the ability to pass an endotracheal tube and to ventilate the lungs. It is our practice at the Queen Mother's Hospital to teach the midwives to make a simple assessment of the patient's motor function following each top-up injection. Merely asking the patient to move her legs 5 minutes after the injection of 3 ml bupivacaine should be sufficient. Weakness, if associated with a fall in arterial pressure, should alert staff to the unusual response to the injection. Early detection of a subarachnoid block is mandatory.

Bloody tap. Puncture of a blood vessel in the epidural space occurs in 2.8% of epidural blocks according to Dawkins (1969). In the obstetric patient the incidence of bloody taps is considerably higher and in our experience is almost 10%. Damage to the engorged epidural veins is probably caused more often by the catheter than by the needle. The incidence of vessel puncture by the insertion of the epidural catheter is reduced if, following the insertion of the epidural needle into the epidural space, 10 ml of fluid is injected. This has been shown to reduce the incidence of vessel puncture from 9% to 3% (Verniquet, 1980). Frequently there is merely a slight red tinge to the solution in the catheter, indicating that a vessel has been scratched. In this case the anaesthetist should pause for 2 or 3 minutes to allow bleeding to cease and after careful further aspiration for blood, he may proceed with the block. If frank blood emerges from the catheter, it must be repositioned. It is sometimes possible to push the catheter onwards until it no longer lies within the vessel, as confirmed by repeated negative aspiration for blood. If this cannot be done, then the catheter and needle should be withdrawn together and a second epidural injection performed at an adjacent interspace.

Epidural haematoma. The occurrence of spontaneous epidural haemorrhage and the creation of an intraspinal space-occupying lesion is well documented in patients receiving anticoagulant drugs (Alexander, 1955; Winer et al, 1959; Jacobson et al, 1966; Sreerama et al, 1973) and, not surprisingly, damage to epidural veins during epidural analgesia in patients on anticoagulant therapy has occurred (Gingrich, 1968; Butler and Green, 1971; Helperin and Cohen, 1971; De Angelis, 1972; Varkey and Brindle, 1974), although uneventful epidural analgesia and the administration of anticoagulants has been described in an extensive non-obstetric series (Odoom and Sih, 1983). Clearly therefore epidural analgesia is contraindicated if a patient has received or is about to receive anticoagulant drugs or if she suffers from a coagulopathy. Low-dose subcutaneous heparin injections (mini-heparin) contraindicate epidural analgesia. Severe pre-eclampsia may be associated with a platelet-consumption coagulopathy. An early sign of epidural haematoma formation is severe back pain, and this should call for a careful neurological assessment (Helperin and Cohen, 1971; Varkey and Brindle, 1974).

Toxic reactions. The incidence of toxic reactions to the local anaesthetic drug has been stated to be 0.2% (Dawkins, 1969). Minor sequelae such as dizziness, tinnitus, drowsiness and mild disorientation are occasionally observed and may be attributable to the local anaesthetic drug or to other drugs administered during labour. Serious toxic reactions should not occur if intravascular injection is avoided and the correct dosage is adhered to. Doses as large as 30 ml of 0.75% bupivacaine (225 mg) did not result in blood concentration higher than 4 μg/ml, which is thought to be the threshold for convulsions (Moore et al, 1977), and almost 50% of the patients receiving 0.75% bupivacaine for caesarean section were given a dose in excess of that recommended by the manufacturer (McGuiness et al, 1978; Dutton et al, 1984). In the UK, the manufacturer's recommended maximum dose of bupivacaine is 2 mg/kg every 4 hours, but many have thought this to be too restrictive (Moore et al, 1978; Crawford, 1985). Convulsions have been reported following the epidural administration of bupivacaine substantially in excess of the manufacturer's recommendation (Thorburn and Moir, 1984). The risk of toxic reactions is increased with the larger doses required for caesarean section. If, in an attempt to provide effective analgesia for caesarean section, the recommended maximum dose is approached, consideration should be given to changing the local anaesthetic solution used, from bupivacaine to lignocaine (with adrenaline 1:200 000), for example. The toxicity of two amide local anaesthetic agents may be additive, but lignocaine is recommended in the treatment of bupivacaine-induced toxicity (Batra et al, 1984; Conklin and Ziadlou-Rad, 1983). Carrie (1985) recommends the insertion of a thoracic epidural catheter or spinal anaesthesia if difficulty is experienced in extending the block. While it is true that the manufacturer's recommendation has been frequently exceeded, and blood levels have not been in the convulsive range (Dutton et al, 1984), this should not be taken to mean that the manufacturer's limit may be exceeded with impunity.

A major toxic reaction to the local anaesthetic drug usually takes the form of generalized convulsions, which may be preceded by premonitory twitchings. Treatment consists of maintenance of the airway and the administration of oxygen. Diazepam may be used to control the convulsions, but they are usually of brief duration and may have ceased before an anticonvulsant can be given. In the unlikely event of the convulsions persisting, they may be controlled by the intravenous injection of thiopentone and a muscle relaxant by a person skilled in the management of the apnoeic patient.

The withdrawal of the recommendation for the use of 0.75% bupivacaine in obstetrics has highlighted the dangers of toxic reactions, particularly the identification of inadvertent intravenous injection through the catheter. The function of an epidural 'test dose' is to allow identification of the position of the epidural catheter with safety and certainty by the injection of a small dose of local anaesthetic. If the catheter tip lies either in the subarachnoid space or in a vein, a 'test dose' would produce signs and symptoms which could be interpretable with accuracy and certainty. At present, there is no agreement regarding the choice of solution which would effectively achieve these objectives. Further, the toxic response would appear to be related to the dose injected. Physiological systems have different thresholds. Central nervous system toxicity (convulsions) is usually the first manifestation of toxicity, followed by cardiovascular toxicity, if the injected dose is excessive. Bupivacaine-induced cardiovascular toxicity is refractory and difficult to treat. This has followed the sudden deflation of tourniquet, when bupivacaine is used for Bier's block (Reynolds, 1984), but it has also been reported following epidural analgesia (Albright, 1984), with fatal results. UK experience and that of Fortuna (1981) would suggest that subarachnoid migration or insertion of the catheter is more likely than inadvertent intravascular injection, unlike Moore's observations (Moore et al, 1978).

Moore has argued (Moore and Batra, 1981) that lignocaine 2% with the addition of adrenaline 1 : 200 000 is the test solution of choice, as injection of a local anaesthetic solution containing 0.015 mg of adrenaline causes a significant tachycardia and a slight rise in blood pressure, within 25 seconds. These signs last for up to 3 minutes. This is a brief effect and would perhaps be difficult to detect. Marx (1984) does not advise the use of adrenaline in the test dose as there is evidence to suggest that adrenaline may reduce placental blood flow, and she advocates lignocaine as a test dose because its use has not been associated with refractory cardiovascular effects (Morishima et al, 1983; Kotelko et al, 1984). There is no doubt about the increasing concern regarding inadvertent intravenous injection, and great care should be taken on insertion of the catheter to ensure that it has not entered a vein; it should not be possible to aspirate blood through the catheter. (Millipore filters will allow aspiration without damage to the filter.) Abouleish and Bourke (1984) recommend the injection of 5 ml of bupivacaine as a test dose. This may satisfactorily detect an intravenous injection, but if subdural or subarachnoid, this would produce an undesirably extensive block.

The detection of subarachnoid and subdural injections has been discussed previously and only a brief outline will be given here. The use of bupivacaine 0.5% plain solution for spinal anaesthesia in obstetrics has been investigated by Russell (1983), and 3 ml was found to produce a block which was sufficiently extensive for caesarean sections (perhaps occasionally too extensive) (Russell, 1983, 1985; Stonham and Moss, 1983). The onset time of the block varies slightly, and could be more than 10 minutes. Therefore, waiting 5 minutes to assess a test dose would not necessarily confirm a subarachnoid injection, but in the majority of cases, leg weakness would be evident. It is important to attempt to elicit leg weakness following the test dose and to detect hypotension, although hypotension is not always present.

It is the authors' opinion that all top-up injections should be made in divided doses. The effect of the preliminary injection of 3 ml (if bupivacaine plain solution is used) should be simply assessed by asking the patient to move her legs before injecting the subsequent dose, in the absence of hypotension. Successful treatment of major toxic reactions with cardiovascular involvement has included adrenaline, 0.1–0.2 mg, 500 mg calcium chloride, manual systole, cardioversion and lignocaine and cardioversion (Conklin and Ziadlou-Rad, 1983; Batra et al, 1984; Mallampti et al, 1984).

Methaemoglobinaemia of mother and fetus due to prilocaine may be reversed by the intravenous injection of methylene blue, a substance which crosses the placenta.

Allergy to local anaesthetics. True allergy to local anaesthetics is very rare, and it is believed that only one case in which an immunological mechanism has been invoked has been described (Brown et al, 1981). The majority of episodes described, often associated with the intra-oral injection of local anaesthetic drugs, are thought to be related to the rapid absorption of the drug and the vasoconstrictor used. However, a suggestive history should not be ignored. Skin testing is of controversial value. The topic has been well reviewed by Incaudo et al (1978) who consider that the advantages of local or regional analgesia may often justify investigation. Skin testing was usually unhelpful; only 5 out of 50 patients gave positive intradermal tests. Much more helpful was a subcutaneous challenge by injecting increasing doses of a chemically dissimilar local anaesthetic drug at 15-minute intervals. These provocative tests were safe and correctly determined which agent could safely be used. IgE-mediated reactions were considered to be rare.

Breakage of catheter or needle. It has been estimated that breakage of the epidural catheter occurs in 0.1% of continuous epidural blocks (Dawkins, 1972). A catheter has broken twice in 12 000 epidural blocks in the Queen Mother's Hospital (0.017%) and it may be that the quality of catheters has improved in recent years, making breakage less common. The vulnerable point is at the lateral openings. It is, of course, mandatory that the catheter which has entered the epidural space should never be pulled back through the needle, lest the terminal portion of catheter be sheared off by the bevel of the needle.

Most authorities are of the opinion that attempts to remove a portion of catheter from the epidural space should not be made (Moore, 1964; Bonica, 1967; Dawkins, 1969). Epidural catheters are usually not radio-opaque, become soft at body temperature and may migrate within the epidural space, so attempts at removal might well result in failure. Plastic catheters are made of non-irritant materials and the authorities referred to above have all had knowledge of several patients in whom retention of a segment of catheter for several years has caused no apparent harm. The author knows of two such instances. It is therefore suggested that if a breakage occurs then the fact should be recorded in the case notes, the remainder of the catheter should be kept and the patient and her general practitioner should be informed. If it is considered that the patient would be seriously disturbed by this information then her husband and her general practitioner should be notified.

Knotting of an epidural catheter has been reported (Brown and Politi, 1979). The catheter was removed by steady traction by a pair of artery forceps and it was thought that the knot was thereby tightened and made small enough to be pulled out. If only 2 or 3 cm of catheter are inserted, then knotting is very unlikely.

Breakage of a metal needle calls for surgical removal and retention of the broken parts.

Horner's syndrome. A surprisingly high incidence of this harmless complication has been reported by Carrie and Mohan (1976), who observed Horner's syndrome in 75% of obstetric lumbar epidural blocks when the cutaneous analgesia was of normal extent, and it is thought to be common following thoracic epidural or extensive blocks (Evans, 1975; Carrie and Mohan, 1976; Sakredof and Datta, 1981). The explanation for this unexpected phenomenon is uncertain, and Bromage (1978) questions whether the cause may lie not with the epidural block, but with some other factor such as the oxytocin infusion.

Inadequacy of analgesia

Analgesia is complete throughout over 80% of obstetric epidural blocks in which bupivacaine is used (Crawford, 1972a; Moore et al, 1974; Moir et al, 1976). When analgesia is deficient in a localized area or over the whole of one side there will often be a technical explanation, and simple remedial measures will often be successful. Two of the major forms of inadequate analgesia are the unblocked segment and unilateral analgesia.

Unblocked segments. One or more spinal segments are unanaesthetized during between 6% and 8% of epidural blocks (Ducrow, 1971; Moir et al, 1976). Most frequently, pain is experienced during contractions in one groin (usually the right groin) during an otherwise satisfactory block. Other areas may be affected. Usually, although not always, the skin in the painful area remains sensitive to pinprick while the adjacent areas are analgesic. It is usually presumed that one or more nerve roots have not been blocked although, as Crawford (1972a) points out, the ileohypogastric nerve which supplies the skin of the groin forms outwith the epidural space, so this explanation is not entirely satisfactory. Pain in the affected area is often severe and in the patient's view analgesia has failed. Fortunately in about two-thirds of these patients the pain can be relieved by the injection of a further 3 or 4 ml of local anaesthetic solution while the patient lies on the painful side. Bromage (1972) found that the choice of local anaesthetic drug strongly influenced the incidence of unblocked segments. He confirmed that incidence of this complication with bupivacaine is about 8% and recorded that the incidence of unblocked segments could be reduced to 1% by using a carbonated solution of lignocaine with 1 : 200 000 adrenaline. Unfortunately a controlled trial failed to confirm this observation (Moir et al, 1976) and in our experience the incidence of unblocked segments is about 8% with bupivacaine hydrochloride and carbonated lignocaine. If a further epidural injection in the appropriate position is ineffective and the pain is severe, then infiltration of the subcutaneous tissues in the painful area may be tried. The unblocked segment continues to be an enigma (Crawford, 1980b).

Unilateral analgesia. Although Ducrow (1971) noted this complication in only 1.5% of blocks the incidence in our experience may be as high as 12% (Moir et al, 1976), and Caseby (1974) observed unilateral analgesia in 21% of blocks. This complication usually responds well to simple remedial measures. Unilateral analgesia is probably associated in most instances with the insertion of an excessive length of catheter into the epidural space. It is believed that in some patients an anterior septum exists within the epidural space and that if the tip of the catheter lies in the anterior compartment then passage of solution to the opposite side involves a longer and circuitous course where this barrier is present (Usubiaga et al, 1970). It is therefore recommended that unilateral analgesia be treated by first withdrawing the catheter until it is estimated that only 1 or 2 cm remain within the epidural space and then injecting a further 4 ml of solution while the patient lies on the painful side. Prevention consists in the insertion of no more than 2 cm catheter into the epidural space (Doughty, 1975).

Paravertebral passage of the catheter. Although up to 6% of catheters may pass through an intervertebral foramen (Sanchez et al, 1967; Bridenbaugh et al, 1968), the incidence of this complication is very much lower if the length of catheter inserted is restricted to 2 cm or so. When the tip of the catheter lies in a paravertebral space, analgesia will be limited to a very localized area and will probably be unilateral. Treatment consists in partial withdrawal of the catheter and the injection of a further dose of local anaesthetic solution.

Total failure. Failure to identify the epidural space occurs in less than 1% of patients in the hands of an experienced anaesthetist.

Other causes of incomplete analgesia. Backache is sometimes a prominent feature of the more protracted and painful labours and is therefore commonly associated with occipitoposterior positions of the vertex and incoordinate uterine action. On occasions this backache persists when the abdominal pains of the first stage have been relieved and in these patients the injection of a further 3 or 4 ml of local anaesthetic while the patient sits up is often effective. According to Bonica (1979), this type of backache originates in intrapelvic structures other than the uterus. If pain persists then the local infiltration of the painful area by a subcutaneous injection of 0.5% lignocaine may be tried.

Suprapubic pain may be associated with retention of urine and may be relieved by catheterization of the bladder. Rectal pain is occasionally severe during an otherwise effective epidural block, and is often associated with descent of the presenting fetal part, heralding full dilatation of the cervix. It can be regarded as an unblocked segment (S1), and further injections of local anaesthetic may provide satisfactory relief.

It should be realized that analgesia is complete in about 80% of epidural blocks in labour (Crawford, 1972a; Moore et al, 1974; Moir et al, 1976). A further 15% of patients classify epidural analgesia as helpful and in these patients there has often been a temporary inadequacy of analgesia due to an unblocked segment, or unilateral analgesia which has responded to a further injection and to suitable positioning of the patient. In approximately 5% analgesia continues to be inadequate. Doughty (1975) has proposed a useful practical classification of pain relief as (1) completely satisfactory, (2) satisfactory after adjustment (by top-up and positioning or other manoeuvre) and (3) unsatisfactory. There can be no doubt that, although epidural analgesia may on occasion fail to give complete relief of pain, the reasons for this inadequacy are often of a simple technical nature and can be overcome by the experienced anaesthetist or midwife, and that epidural analgesia is vastly superior to narcotic or inhalational analgesia (Beazley et al, 1967; Cole et al, 1970; Holdcroft and Morgan, 1974). If pain persists, repuncture at another space may succeed.

Postpartum sequelae

Among the many symptoms of which the puerperal patient may complain are headache, backache, difficulties of micturition and neurological complications. When these symptoms occur in a patient who has received epidural analgesia in labour there is a natural, although not necessarily logical, tendency to look for the cause of the symptoms in the method of analgesia. The evidence which will now be reviewed supports the view that the sequelae

Table 10. The incidence (%) of headache, backache and disturbances of micturition after forceps delivery, with and without analgesia

Analgesic	Headache	Backache	Disturbance of micturition
Epidural			
Crawford, 1972a	not stated	45	26
Moir and Davidson, 1972	18	22	34
Moir et al, 1976	8	14	38
No epidural			
Moir and Davidson, 1972	10	32	20
Grove, 1973	25	25	37

are the result of pregnancy, labour and delivery and are in most cases not causally related to the use of epidural analgesia, being an example of the dictum of '*post hoc, sed non ergo propter hoc*'. The results of four studies (summarized in Table 10) showing the incidence of headache, backache and disturbances of micturition were recorded following forceps delivery under epidural analgesia and other forms of analgesia (excluding subarachnoid analgesia).

Backache. Lumbosacral pain has been noted in 14–45% of recently delivered women and the incidence is not obviously related to the method of pain relief employed. This common symptom is probably related to the laxity of ligaments which develops in pregnancy and to the use of the lithotomy position for forceps delivery. Local tenderness at the site of skin puncture is a common minor complaint after epidural blockade. Although Tunstall (1972) believes that bachache may be commoner if a true midline approach to the epidural space is used, there is little evidence to substantiate this opinion.

Headache. There is of course no reason why an uncomplicated epidural block should cause headache and this symptom is present in 8–25% of women in the early puerperium. Headache due to dural puncture is discussed earlier in this chapter.

Perineal pain. It is quite widely believed that postpartum pain at the site of episiotomy is more severe if epidural analgesia was used for labour, although in Moir and Davidson's (1972) series pain was equally severe after epidural analgesia and pudendal nerve block. If epidural analgesia is indeed followed by more pain in the perineum, the explanation may be that a painless labour makes the woman less tolerant of subsequent pain. Crawford (1978) suggests that sutures may be tied more tightly if the wound is not swollen by local anaesthetic solution.

Disturbances of micturition. Upsets of micturition usually take the form of painless retention of urine and hesitancy and are not associated with infection. Upsets of micturition occur approximately twice as frequently after forceps delivery as after spontaneous delivery and this statement is true whether or not epidural analgesia is used. After forceps delivery between 26% and 38% of patients may have a disturbance of micturition (see Table 10) while from 14 to 21% of women who have spontaneous deliveries may be expected to have difficulty with micturition (Grove, 1973; Moir et al, 1976).

Although in one series (Moir and Davidson, 1972) upsets of micturition were more common after forceps delivery under epidural analgesia than after forceps delivery under pudendal nerve block, it was considered that this difference was explicable by the much greater duration of labour and the more frequent use of Kielland's forceps and manual rotation of the fetal head in the epidural group. It is considered that trauma to bladder and urethra during delivery and perhaps during labour constitutes the principal cause of postpartum upsets of micturition. Loss of bladder sensation for one or two days is very common after epidural analgesia and does not in itself call for bladder catheterization.

Delayed recovery. An interval of 3 or 4 hours between delivery and the return of full sensation and power is quite common and is regarded as normal. Very occasionally full recovery may take from 24 to 72 hours. There may be a local area of hypoaesthesia and reflexes may be reduced (Pathy and Rosen, 1975; Cuerden et al, 1977; Ramanathan et al, 1978). Recovery is complete and the cause is uncertain. Adrenaline may so reduce the vascularity of neural tissue as to prolong the block unduly, and it has been suggested that the catheter tip may have lain close to or within an intervertebral foramen, so that the local anaesthetic was deposited alongside the dural cuffs where penetration is easy.

Neurological sequelae. According to Dawkins (1972) neurological damage follows approximately 0.02% of epidural blocks. The cause may sometimes be unrelated to the use of epidural analgesia. The causes of neurological sequelae to epidural analgesia have been well reviewed by Edmonds (1972) and Kane (1981) and classified as epidural, spinal and obstetric cases. The majority of the complications described occurred during or immediately following the epidural block, and were related to local spinal root trauma or involvement. Very rarely, intracranial complications have been described following inadvertent dural puncture in the course of an epidural analgesia and blood patch. Although an impressive list of complications following vertebral blocks has been described (Hargrove, 1981), the rarity of significant neurological complications following careful administration of the epidural and the injection of the correct solution has meant that the majority of reports are anecdotal. The true incidence is unknown (Ballin, 1981).

Epidural causes of neurological damage

Damage to a nerve root by needle or catheter may explain phenomena such as an area of hypoaesthesia on the lateral surface of thigh with spontaneous recovery after a few weeks, and was reported by Birkhahn and Heifetz (1961), Moir and Willocks (1968) and Crawford (1972a). Pressure upon a nerve root has resulted from the foreign body reaction to a piece of foam rubber carried into the epidural space by the needle whose tip had been inserted into the rubber (Crawford et al, 1975).

Two cases of arachnoiditis have been reported after epidural analgesia (Braham and Saia, 1958) and may possibly have been due to chemical *contamination*. Severe flaccid paraplegia with extensive sensory loss and recovery after 16 months has followed the injection of 1.5% benzyl alcohol as a preservative in a saline solution injected into the epidural space for the prevention of a dural puncture headache in a obstetric patient (Craig and Habib, 1977). There is now one documented case of paraplegia due to epidural abscess following epidural analgesia in a surgical patient and the infection was thought to have been carried in the blood to an epidural haematoma (Saady, 1976). Crawford (1975a) has postulated a similar haematogenous spread of infection to an epidural haematoma in an obstetric patient in whom the development of an abscess was prevented by antibiotic therapy. The possibility of contamination of solution by minute fragments of glass is now well recognized and the possibility exists that these particles might act as irritants to nerve tissue (Furgang, 1974). The use of a Millex filter is advised in order to prevent this complication.

Epidural haematoma has been discussed earlier in this chapter and the inadvisability of performing epidural puncture in patients receiving anticoagulants is reiterated.

It is probable that *ischaemia of the cord* has resulted from impairment of blood flow in the spinal arteries in two elderly patients who suffered from arteriosclerosis and who developed profound hypotension during epidural analgesia. Adrenaline was used in these cases (Davies et al, 1958; Urquhart-Hey, 1969). Dawkins (1972) agrees that adrenaline may be dangerous in these circumstances. He advises that plain solutions of bupivacaine should be used and points out that adrenaline is unnecessary with bupivacaine.

Intracranial lesions have been reviewed by Jack (1979), who associates such lesions following dural puncture with altered cerebrospinal fluid dynamics, and suggests the early use of epidural blood patch to reduce the cerebrospinal leak.

Durocutaneous leaks of cerebrospinal fluid have followed dural puncture and have responded to epidural blood patch (Longmire and Joyce, 1984).

Obstetric causes of neurological damage

Obstetric palsy is well-recognized after delivery in which neither epidural nor subarachnoid analgesia has been used and is generally thought to be due to pressure of the fetal head or the forceps blade upon a nerve of the lumbosacral plexus. Foot-drop is commonly the result and recovery often takes place in six or eight weeks (Moir and Myerscough, 1971) although permanent damage has occurred. According to Hill (1962) obstetric palsy occurs once in every 2500 deliveries. Edmonds (1972) states that the incidence may be as high as 1 in 600 or 1 in 900 deliveries without epidural analgesia, and suggests that many of these cases may be due to the development of an acute disc lesion during labour or delivery.

Pressure on the lateral popliteal nerve by a lithotomy pole is recognized and will cause no pain during epidural analgesia. Labour and delivery have been thought to cause subarachnoid haemorrhage and exacerbation of spinal tumours. Very rarely, general anaesthesia has been followed by neurological damage (Sinclair, 1954; Ditzler and McIver, 1956). A spontaneous exacerbation of existing disease of the nervous system may be wrongly attributed to epidural analgesia.

Indication for epidural analgesia

There are at present two schools of thought concerning the indications for continuous epidural analgesia in labour. The more traditional approach to the use of epidural analgesia in labour is that one of a number of specific obstetric indications should exist. Increasingly this view has been replaced by the concept that epidural analgesia is outstandingly the most effective method of pain relief in labour and should therefore be available to all women in painful labour. Epidural analgesia should not be forced upon a woman against her wishes and it should be noted that only 2% of women who received epidural analgesia in labour subsequently experienced a sense of deprivation of the experience of natural, and therefore often painful, labour (Billewicz-Driemel and Milne, 1976).

In practice, the policy implemented in a particular hospital will be influenced by many considerations including the views of obstetricians and anaesthetists, the availability of anaesthetists and the frequency with which labour is electively induced and accelerated. Epidural analgesia is never entirely free of risk, and undoubtedly the risk is lowest where the method is extensively used and anaesthetists, obstetricians and midwives are entirely familiar with the safe management of labour and delivery under epidural analgesia.

While it is desirable to have epidural analgesia available to all labouring women, in terms of economic efficiency it is difficult to reconcile the provision of expensive and underutilized anaesthetic services in the smaller maternity units. Amalgamation of small units is not always possible, as the distances women may then have to travel are too great. For some women, epidural analgesia is a therapeutic measure as well as a method of pain relief. In practice, because of the shortage of anaesthetists and the consequent absence of a 24-hour obstetric epidural service, epidural analgesia is sometimes available only on an elective basis to women who may desire this service, and may not be available to those whose need is greatest.

The following are the generally accepted indications for epidural analgesia in obstetrics: pain; pre-eclampsia; prolonged labour; premature labour; cardiovascular and respiratory disease; diabetes mellitus; recent abdominal operation; breech presentation; multiple pregnancy; forceps delivery; caesarean section. To this list one might add manual removal of the placenta and postpartum tubal ligation.

Pain. The primary reason for administering epidural analgesia is, of course, pain, and epidural analgesia is by far the most effective method of pain relief in labour. In consequence there will be a tendency to use epidural analgesia for the more painful and prolonged labours. Labours of this type are often associated with obstetric abnormalities such as occipitoposterior positions and incoordinate uterine action.

It will often be possible to predict that labour is likely to be more than usually prolonged or painful and to these patients an epidural block may be given as soon as contractions become painful. If a narcotic analgesic has been given, an epidural block should be substituted for a second injection of analgesic drug if this should be required. It should be recalled that Holdcroft and Morgan (1974) observed that only 22% of patients obtained satisfactory pain relief from pethidine.

There is absolutely no need to withhold epidural analgesia until the cervix has reached some predetermined dilatation. American authorities were formerly of the opinion that the cervix should be 6 or 7 cm dilated before epidural analgesia could be given to a primigravida and that earlier administration would inhibit uterine contractions. The current management of labour with oxytocin makes such restrictions groundless. Epidural analgesia should be given whenever pain makes it necessary. The indication for any form of analgesia is pain rather than cervical dilatation.

In centres it is the practice to insert an epidural catheter before amniotomy. Some anaesthetists administer a dose of local anaesthetic solution before amniotomy (Caseby, 1974) while others await the onset of painful labour before injecting the first dose of local anaesthetic (Green, 1972). Amniotomy is sometimes a worrying and occasionally an embarrassing experience but it is not always painful. In Caseby's series only 22% of patients who did not have an epidural block found amniotomy painful. As Green (1972) pointed out, the patient who is allowed to feel a few strong contractions has a greater appreciation of the pain relief then provided. There can be little objection to the placement of the epidural catheter as an elective procedure when it is accepted that approximately 98% of patients experience pain in labour. In hospitals where shortage of staff precludes the organization of a 24-hour epidural service, the policy of offering induction of labour at a time when epidural analgesia is available may be the only way of ensuring that such services are provided to some of those who desire it.

Pre-eclampsia. Continuous lumbar epidural analgesia is indicated in the management of labour in patients with pre-eclampsia (Moir et al, 1972). Blood pressure can usually be maintained at a safe level by the sympathetic blockade and epidural analgesia effectively suppresses that contribution which pain and distress may make to a rise in blood pressure. If cardiac output is maintained and caval occlusion is avoided than placental and renal blood flow should be maintained and may even be improved as the result of vasodilatation. Delivery by forceps or vacuum extractor is often indicated in pre-eclampsia, and epidural analgesia is the preferred method of analgesia for these procedures. In severe, fulminating pre-eclampsia a coagulopathy may contraindicate epidural analgesia. The management of pre-eclampsia and eclampsia is discussed further in chapter 9.

Prolonged labour. Maternal distress was formerly a prominent feature of prolonged labour, and tachycardia, pyrexia, dehydration, electrolyte depletion, ketosis, vomiting and gastrointestinal dilatation were frequently present. If due to incoordinate uterine action, the normal pattern of synchronous contraction of the upper uterine segment and relaxation of the lower segment is lost. It was observed that when epidural analgesia was administered in the course of incoordinate and painful labour, the rate of cervical dilatation increased substantially in 70% of women (Moir and

Willocks, 1966, 1967). Concomitant administration of oxytocics and the prevention of dehydration by intravenous fluids have almost banished incoordinate uterine action as a cause of prolonged labour. Cephalopelvic disproportion was often a complicating factor.

The abnormal uterine contractions are thought to arise from ectopic foci in the myometrium instead of originating from the normal pacemakers near the mouths of the Fallopian tubes. The normal pattern of synchronous contraction of the upper uterine segment and relaxation of the lower segment is lost. This loss of uterine polarity causes the cervix to dilate very slowly and descent of the presenting part of the fetus is delayed.

It was observed that when epidural analgesia was administered in the course of incoordinate and painful labour the rate of cervical dilatation increased substantially in 70% of patients (Moir and Willocks, 1966, 1967). Failure of the cervix to dilate was usually associated with cephalopelvic disproportion. The onset of a more normal type of uterine action after epidural blockade in incoordinate labour has been demonstrated by intra-amniotic manometry (Caldeyro-Barcia and Alvarez, 1952). The relief of pain and the isolation of the uterus from higher control seem to allow the uterus to act more normally.

Happily such labours are now almost unknown in advanced countries. Labour is rarely allowed to last for longer than 12 hours. Incoordinate uterine action is treated by intravenous oxytocin, and dehydration and ketosis are prevented by intravenous fluid therapy. If these measures fail then caesarean section is performed. Epidural analgesia remains a valuable adjunct in the management of these painful labours although it is now only one of the therapeutic measures employed.

Premature labour. Epidural analgesia is valuable in premature labour because it is likely that the stress of labour and delivery upon the infant is lessened. The liberal use of episiotomy and forceps delivery is indicated in the fetal interest and order to reduce the incidence of intracranial haemorrhage, and under epidural analgesia these procedures can be readily undertaken in order to shorten the second stage of labour. The Ontario Perinatal Mortality Study Committee demonstrated that when conduction analgesia is used the perinatal mortality rate is dramatically reduced in premature infants. David and Rosen (1976) also noted a lower perinatal mortality rate among immature infants delivered under epidural analgesia and considered that the probable explanation was the increased use of forceps delivery. Epidural analgesia is usually available in the better staffed and equipped hospitals, and obstetric, paediatric and anaesthetic care of high quality all contribute to these findings.

For similar reasons epidural analgesia is indicated where the infant is dysmature (small-for-dates) due to poor placental function.

Cardiovascular and respiratory disease. The effective relief of pain afforded by continuous epidural analgesia can be of value in patients with congenital or acquired heart disease where the tachycardia which results from pain and anxiety may prevent adequate diastolic filling of the heart. In patients with mitral valve disease episodes of acute left ventricular failure apparently precipitated by distress and tachycardia have responded rapidly to the institution of epidural analgesia (Moir and Willocks, 1968). Muscular effort is reduced in the first and second stages of labour and elective delivery by forceps or vacuum extractor can be undertaken. The dangers of intravenous ergometrine in patients with heart disease are discussed in chapter 3. In patients with cerebrovascular disease the avoidance of stress and expulsive efforts by epidural analgesia should also be beneficial (Amias, 1970).

It would appear that the maintenance of cardiac output by the avoidance of caval occlusion in the supine position may be of the greatest importance in patients with heart disease who receive an epidural block. A sudden reduction in venous return in a patient with mitral or aortic valvular disease might be disastrous for mother and child. If cardiac output is maintained then, in certain circumstances, the vasodilatation of epidural blockade might be expected to improve placental circulation.

The management of heart disease in labour is further discussed in chapter 9. Severe respiratory disease is uncommon in women in labour but the absence of respiratory depression and the reduction in muscular effort make epidural analgesia the method of choice.

Diabetes mellitus. The management of diabetes mellitus has changed radically in the past 20 years. Strict control of the maternal diabetic state by the introduction of diabetic clinics for pregnant women, the introduction of home blood glucose testing, and abandoning urinary glucose estimations as satisfactory monitoring, have transformed the outlook for the baby. The object is to attempt to maintain normal maternal blood glucose levels throughout the pregnancy, yet avoiding hypoglycaemia. The majority of diabetic mothers can now anticipate a normal pregnancy and delivery, as opposed to the planned delivery of macrosomic infants of yesteryear. To achieve this, strict control and combined care by obstetricians and diabetic physicians are essential. During labour, the blood glucose is maintained at a normal level, and glucose and insulin is administered as a continuous infusion to ensure this. Epidural analgesia reduces the frequency of maternal and neonatal acidosis during labour (Pearson and Davies, 1973) and is the analgesic method of choice. Despite the improved care and prognosis, there is still an increase in maternal morbidity and fetal abnormality. Fetal macrosomia still occurs, but the improvements in fetal monitoring should allow early detection and delivery, often by caesarean section, at 36–38 weeks under epidural analgesia. Spinal anaesthesia for caesarean section in diabetic mothers has been associated with a high incidence of acidosis (Datta et al, 1982), but this may be avoided by scrupulous control of blood pressure.

Recent abdominal operation. Emergency abdominal surgery and occasionally the removal of an ovarian cyst in late pregnancy may result in the presence of a painful, recent abdominal wound in a woman in labour. Epidural analgesia is useful in these circumstances because it relieves pain and permits elective forceps delivery.

Breech delivery. It had for long been feared that the perineal anaesthesia associated with a complete epidural or subarachnoid block would inhibit the maternal expulsive efforts and so increase the need for breech extraction instead of assisted breech delivery. Breech extraction carries a high fetal mortality. Bonica (1965) rejected this line of reasoing and advocated the use of conduction analgesia for vaginal breech delivery. Crawford (1974) has analysed a series of 162 vaginal breech deliveries, 56 of which were conducted under lumbar epidural analgesia. The higher Apgar scores and the improved general condition of the infants delivered under epidural analgesia strongly suggested that epidural analgesia was associated with a reduction in the incidence of severe neonatal depression in mature and premature infants. Although the second stage was somewhat prolonged by epidural analgesia, the incidence of breech extraction was not increased by the existence of perineal anaesthesia. Others have confirmed that fetal acid–base status and Apgar scores are improved and perinatal mortality is lowered by the use of epidural analgesia for breech delivery (Bowen-Simpkins and Fergusson, 1974; Donnai and Nicholas, 1975; Darby et al, 1976; Breeson et al, 1978). The risks of breech delivery are greatest in infants of low birth weight and it is for these infants that controlled delivery in a patient who is relaxed and free of pain may be of greatest value. It is essential that a skilled obstetrician should conduct every assisted breech delivery and it is equally important that the adequacy of the maternal pelvis be carefully vetted before allowing labour to proceed in any breech presentation. During the course of labour there should be no hesitancy in resorting to delivery by caesarean section for failure of progress or fetal distress. It is now advocated that epidural analgesia should be used in every woman in whom vaginal breech delivery is planned. It is now common practice in many hospitals to use caesarean section for all breech deliveries. It is believed that the fetal risks are slightly increased by vaginal breech delivery, as are the maternal risks by caesarean section. Many obstetricians will only allow parous women in normal spontaneous labour to undertake vaginal breech delivery.

Other techniques of analgesia and anaesthesia are discussed in chapter 8.

Multiple births. It is universally agreed that the mortality is greater among second twins, but current methods of fetal monitoring and its interpretation are providing safer conditions which perhaps challenge earlier work. Current obstetric opinion emphasizes the need to deliver the second twin without delay in a controlled manner, and effective epidural analgesia makes a significant contribution to this objective. Complications of pregnancy are common in multiple pregnancies and those factors which predispose to fetal asphyxia include pre-eclampsia, placental insufficiency, hydramnios and premature labour. Many of these complications are an indication for epidural analgesia and reports have confirmed its benefit. Labour is not prolonged and the metabolic state of the first twin is as good as that of a singleton fetus, although inevitably the second twin is more acidotic (Crawford, 1975*b*; James et al, 1977; Jashcevatzky et al, 1977; Weekes et al, 1977).

Forceps delivery. Epidural analgesia is one of the preferred techniques for forceps delivery. The use of 0.5% bupivacaine plain solution makes a positive contribution to increasing the need for forceps delivery, but provides optimum analgesia (Thorburn and Moir, 1981). The use of 0.25% bupivacaine solution, conversely, increases the frequency of spontaneous delivery, but analgesia is not quite as effective. If the perineum remains sensitive to pain it will often be effective to infiltrate the perineum with a local anaesthetic solution. The relaxation of the pelvic floor muscles facilitates rotation of the fetal head by Kielland's forceps or by hand.

To provide effective muscle relaxation and analgesia if more difficult and painful forceps delivery is being undertaken, increasing the volume and the concentration of bupivacaine will usually prove satisfactory. If speed is necessary, 2% lignocaine with adrenaline 1:200000 will have a more rapid onset. The belief that allowing epidural analgesia to wear off will allow a spontaneous delivery is to be condemned since current evidence does not support this (Phillips and Thomas, 1983). The abrupt onset of the pain of labour following regression of effective epidural analgesia is very distressing. If vaginal delivery is not achieved, instrumental delivery is undertaken, often with urgency, as maternal or fetal distress has supervened. It is then impossible in the time available to provide effective epidural analgesia if the block has been allowed to regress completely. The distressed mother is then subjected to a painful instrumental delivery. This practice must be vigorously discouraged. Arbitrary limitation of the second stage is unnecessary if fetal monitoring confirms fetal well-being. Time may convert a difficult forceps delivery to a simple outlet forceps delivery, or even a vaginal delivery. An increase in spontaneous delivery rate and no increase in neonatal acidosis has been observed when the time of onset of maternal pushing was delayed (Maresh, 1983).

It has been demonstrated that pudendal nerve blocks are successful in only 50% of patients (Scudamore and Yates, 1966). In the view of these writers, outlet forceps delivery can be satisfactorily performed after local infiltration of the vulva and perineum with local anaesthetic, and mid-cavity forceps deliveries are best performed under lumbar or caudal epidural block, subarachnoid analgesia or general anaesthesia.

A most important benefit which arises out of the extensive use of epidural analgesia is that general anaesthesia need hardly ever be given for operative vaginal delivery. In the Queen Mother's Hospital, Glasgow, in 1964, almost 300 general anaesthetics were given for forceps delivery and assisted breech delivery. In 1978 only 10 general anaesthetics were given for these reasons.

Naturally the diminished use of general anaesthesia must decrease the likelihood of a mother dying from the pulmonary aspiration of stomach contents. A subarachnoid block is recommended for forceps delivery if the patient has not already received epidural analgesia. The technique is discussed later in this chapter.

Caesarean section. There is a growing interest in the use of epidural analgesia for caesarean section, arising out of a keen awareness of the risks of general anaesthesia in obstetrics. In the authors' hospital epidural analgesia is used for over 70% of elective caesarean sections and it is hoped that this figure will increase.

The advantages of epidural analgesia for caesarean section include:

1. The avoidance of the hazards of inhalation of stomach contents and failed intubation.
2. The absence of neonatal depression of respiration and reflex responses (Hollmen et al, 1978; McGuiness et al, 1978).
3. Participation by the mother and perhaps the father in the birth.
4. The early establishment of breast feeding if this is desired.
5. A reduction in blood loss (Moir, 1970).
6. Elimination of the problem of awareness associated with general anaesthesia.
7. A possible reduction in the incidence of deep venous thrombosis (Cousins and Wright, 1971).

The major problems associated with caesarean section under epidural analgesia are hypotension and the provision of an adequate block for intrapelvic surgery. The frequency of hypotension varies from 7 to 45%, depending on its definition. The satisfactory management of hypotension constitutes one of the important challenges during epidural analgesia for caesarean section. The management has been considered in detail earlier in this chapter and consists of:

1. meticulous attention to the technique, maintaining the laterally tilted or wedged position
2. intravenous preload of at least 1.5 litres of crystalloid solution immediately preceding the block
3. careful and frequent monitoring of the arterial pressure
4. avoiding movement of the patient when the block is extensive
5. liberal use of ephedrine if hypotension does occur.

Placental blood flow is unaltered during caesarean section under epidural analgesia in the absence of hypotension, but failure to maintain blood pressure results in a reduction in placental blood flow and a depression of neurobehavioural responses in the neonate (Hollmen et al, 1978; Jouppila et al, 1978*b*). Analgesia was inadequate and required general anaesthesia or intravenous analgesia in 12% (Milne and Murray Lawson, 1973) to 13% of cases (Baheti et al, 1975) using 8–18 ml of 2% lignocaine solution, and Bridenbaugh et al (1976) noted that 20% of women experience pain if traction is applied to the uterus under epidural block. The intravenous injection of ergometrine causes vomiting or retching in over 40% of patients, whereas intravenous oxytocin has no emetic action and is equally effective in preventing bleeding (Milne and Murray Lawson, 1973; Moodie and Moir, 1976). If ergometrine is not used, then pain and vomiting are usually associated with intrapelvic manipulations after the delivery of the child and can be avoided by the provision of adequate sacral blockade.

The incidence of inadequate pain relief is under 2% when blockade of all nerves from S5 to T6 is ensured (Moir and Thorburn, 1980). Higher figures for awareness are associated with some techniques of general anaesthesia! A recommended technique is as follows.

Technique of epidural analgesia for caesarean section. Before and during the initiation of the block at least 1.5 litres of Ringer lactate solution are infused and a further 1 litre of this solution is infused during surgery to maintain circulating blood volume and placental blood flow (Wollman and Marx, 1968). If hypotension occurs despite these measures, a further rapid infusion of fluid is given and an intravenous injection of ephedrine 10 mg may be required. If bradycardia accompanies hypotension, then atropine should be given.

With the patient in the sitting position the epidural space is entered at L2–L3 or L3–L4 interspace and 10–12 ml of 0.5% plain bupivacaine solution is injected. An epidural catheter is inserted. The upper level of analgesia is now ascertained and a further dose of 0.5% bupivacaine is injected on a basis of 1.5 ml of solution for every unblocked segment below T6 dermatome. The mean volume of 0.5% bupivacaine required in total is 23 ml (115 mg). A top-up injection of 6–8 ml is given after delivery of the infant to ensure maintenance of the block from S5 to T6. The circulation is more stable if adrenaline is avoided (Ueland et al, 1972).

At delivery 5 units of oxytocin are injected intravenously and an infusion of 20 units in 500 ml of fluid is initiated. The mother breathes a mixture of 70–80% of oxygen with nitrous oxide through a nasal mask and thereby obtains the benefit of a high F_IO_2 and relative analgesia.

The importance of a sacral block is paramount. A disadvantage of the above technique is the time required, which usually exceeds 30 minutes for an elective caesarean section if bupivacaine is used. The use of lignocaine 2.0% with 1:200000 adrenaline can substantially reduce the onset time. If the mother has already received epidural analgesia in labour, then much less time is required and the anaesthetist must ensure that the block is sufficiently extensive by a further injection and the use of posture.

A larger mean dose (168 mg) of bupivacaine had no toxic effect upon mother or infant (McGuiness et al, 1978) and Apgar scores, times to sustained respiration and the acid–base state of the infants are at least as good as those of infants delivered under general anaesthesia (Downing et al, 1979; Moir and Thorburn, 1980).

Blood loss at caesarean section under epidural analgesia is approximately halved in comparison with general anaesthesia (Moir, 1970). Even so, it is essential that compatible blood be available for transfusion.

The successful conduct of caesarean section under epidural analgesia is a rewarding experience for the mother, the anaesthetist and the obstetrician and the condition of the infant at birth is usually excellent. The problems are recognized and the solution of them calls for the highest standards of care and meticulous attention to every detail. Not all patients (and perhaps not all anaesthetists and obstetricians) will accept abdominal surgery while conscious and no undue pressure should be brought to bear upon the patient. In a hospital where the technique is practised, the initial resistance by patients and by staff disappears as experience enlarges.

Contraindications to epidural analgesia

There are perhaps surprisingly few contraindications to epidural analgesia in obstetrics and some of these are relative rather than absolute. As experience has enlarged, conditions such as breech delivery and probably also the delivery of twins are now seen as positive indications for epidural analgesia rather than as contraindications. Epidural analgesia may be contraindicated for anaesthetic or obstetric reasons or simply because the patient does not wish to receive this form of pain relief.

Other contraindications to epidural analgesia may be as follows:

Anticoagulant therapy.
Obstetric defibrination.
Haemorrhage and hypovolaemia.
Local sepsis.
Disease of the nervous system.
Gross deformity of the spine.
Objection by the patient.

Many of these contraindications are self-explanatory and need not be further discussed. The possibility of producing extensive bleeding within the epidural space when the patient is receiving anticoagulants has been discussed earlier in this chapter; epidural analgesia is contraindicated in these circumstances. Defibrination would also constitute a bar to epidural analgesia for the same reason.

The possibility of a disastrous reduction in cardiac output and blood pressure if epidural or subarachnoid analgesia is used in the patient who is hypovolaemic is well-recognized and has been recently confirmed by Bonica et al (1972) and Morikawa et al (1974). It may be prudent to avoid epidural analgesia in patients with a history of antepartum haemorrhage because of the possibility of sudden severe bleeding, and in the case of abruptio placentae, there is the further possibility of defibrination. The pain of abruptio placenta may be detectable during epidural analgesia. Crawford (1976) suggested that an 'epidural sieve' might allow the perception of pathological pain. This is no more than a hypothesis, and the perception of pain may be related to the quality of the block.

The customary warning to avoid epidural and subarachnoid analgesia in patients with existing disease of the nervous system is of course issued on medico-legal grounds. There is in fact no reason to believe that conduction analgesia can exacerbate disease of the nervous system but a relapse in a disease such as multiple sclerosis which followed an epidural block could be, by faulty logic, attributed to the block. Nevertheless, the use of lumbar epidural analgesia in women with disseminated sclerosis has been reported (Warren et al, 1982; Crawford et al, 1981). Bamford et al (1978) have suggested that spinal anaesthesia in patients with multiple sclerosis may be followed by temporary deterioration. There is, however, no need to withhold epidural analgesia in patients with a past history of poliomyelitis or meningitis and in those with an intervertebral disc lesion or epilepsy.

The advisability of using epidural analgesia during labour in patients with a uterus scarred from a previous caesarean section, hysterotomy or myomectomy depends largely on the presence or absence of cephalopelvic disproportion. Where the previous caesarean section was performed for a reason such as antepartum haemorrhage or fetal distress and no mechanical problem exists, the dangers of missing a 'silent' uterine rupture under epidural analgesia are probably not great (Cooper, 1972; Meehan et al, 1972). Careful obstetric management with monitoring of the strength and frequency of uterine contractions and the control of oxytocin dosage should enhance the safety of epidural analgesia in these circumstances. Exploration of the uterus for evidence of dehiscence of the old scar may be advisable at delivery. The dangers of overstimulation of the uterus have been emphasized by Brudenell and Chakravarti (1975), and Carlsson et al (1980) have reviewed the use of epidural analgesia in women who have previously undergone caesarean section. Carlsson noted uterine rupture in 2 out of 98 women. In the Queen Mother's Hospital epidural analgesia was used for 46 labours after previous lower-segment caesarean section. No mothers died but there were six uterine ruptures and four fetal deaths. Rupture was not always a dramatic event and on three occasions was first diagnosed on exploring the uterus after forceps delivery. Five of the ruptures were incomplete dehiscences. The risks of labour after caesarean section are real but there need be no further increase in that risk if epidural analgesia is used with care and labour is not prolonged.

Manual removal of placenta

If the patient has already received epidural analgesia, then manual removal of the placenta can be performed painlessly if the block extends from S4 to T10. In order to avoid the administration of general anaesthesia a single-shot epidural block may be given, although a subarachnoid block has many advantages in this situation in the absence of haemorrhage.

Postpartum sterilization

Epidural analgesia is an excellent choice for this procedure, which carries a risk of Mendelson's syndrome if performed under general anaesthesia. If sterilization has been decided upon, the epidural catheter inserted during labour may be left in position and used to provide epidural analgesia for sterilization some 12–36 hours after delivery. Breast feeding is not interrupted.

The organization and management of labour under epidural analgesia

Much of the detailed management of the patient in labour under epidural analgesia has been discussed earlier in this chapter and the following is a summary presented for the convenience of the reader.

Staffing requirements. A 24-hour resident anaesthetic service is essential if a full epidural service is to be provided. The Obstetric Anaesthetists Association recommends that a maternity hospital or department should have the services of two or three consultant anaesthetists who should have a specific allocation of sessions for obstetric anaesthesia and analgesia. An anaesthetist should be present in the hospital at all times and he should have no commitment to any other branch of anaesthesia while on duty for obstetrics. It is also recommended that no anaesthetist should administer obstetric anaesthesia or analgesia without direct supervision until he has had at least one year's experience as an anaesthetist.

An obstetric anaesthesia service which does not provide epidural analgesia on a 24-hour basis is an incomplete service, yet it is logistically unreasonable to attempt to provide an epidural service where there are fewer than perhaps 2500 deliveries per annum. This is one of several reasons for the closure or amalgamation of small maternity units in all but the most isolated communities (Hunter and Moir, 1979). An anaesthetic staff such as described above should cope with up to 4000 deliveries each year and maintain a balance between the boredom of under-employment for a resident anaesthetist and excessive fatigue, which also leads to loss of interest and perhaps even to dangerous situations.

An anaesthetist who practises obstetric anaesthesia should be technically competent in general and regional techniques and should be familiar with the modern management of labour. An important duty of the consultant anaesthetist is the teaching of epidural analgesia to trainees and for this purpose he should be physically present with the trainee. With the complete novice it is often helpful if the teacher inserts the needle into the interspinous ligament. In this way the beginner will often be successful with his first epidural puncture to his own benefit and to the benefit of the patient.

Midwifery and nursing staff must be adequate for the constant supervision of patients under epidural analgesia, and all midwives and nurses must be familiar with epidural analgesia and be fully aware of the dangers of hypotension and of caval occlusion. The obstetric staff too must be of high calibre and the organization of the labour suite must be first-class. Without all these things an epidural service can only be a potential hazard. The converse is true, for there is no place for the occasional obstetric epiduralist in the modern labour ward.

Equipment. Sterile equipment is of course essential and this can be obtained by the use of one of the several disposable epidural sets now available or by the preparation of sterile epidural packs in the hospital Central Sterile Supply Department. Whichever method is used it will be advisable to autoclave ampoules of local anaesthetic solution.

Equipment must be available for the immediate treatment of complications, and among the necessary items are ephedrine, oxygen, a bag and mask, suction apparatus and equipment for tracheal intubation. The presence of staff skilled in the use of these facilities is, of course, essential and epidural analgesia should only be performed by, or in the presence of, someone skilled in resuscitation. The patient should be on a tilting bed.

Care of the patient. Every patient should have an intravenous infusion running and a suitable fluid regime prescribed. No patient should ever be in the supine or dorsal position without a lateral tilt or the elevation of the right buttock by a wedge. The lateral position should be used during all labours and the assumption of the supine position avoided as far as possible.

Frequent blood pressure readings are essential and a suitable schedule is the taking of readings at intervals of 5 minutes for 20 minutes after each epidural injection and thereafter readings may be taken at intervals of 10 minutes. The use of automatic blood pressure monitors is valuable, but care should be taken since the cuff can damage the skin of the arm if its position is not altered from time to time, and the pressure recorded with unnecessary frequency. Continuous monitoring of the fetal heart rate and uterine contractions throughout labour is recommended in every case.

Ice may be given to suck. Painless retention of urine should be looked for and the bladder should be catheterized if necessary. Attempts should be made to encourage the patient to pass urine before a top-up injection.

Progress in labour should be monitored by careful observation for signs of descent of the fetal head, and evidence of full dilatation. Vaginal examination should be performed as required.

Top-up injections. Top-up injections are given as soon as pain returns. The National Board for Nursing, Midwifery and Health Visiting has authorized the administration of top-up injections by experienced midwives and has issued the following statement of policy. 'The Board would raise no objection to an experienced midwife undertaking the topping-up procedure (not the primary dose through the catheter) in the maintenance of an epidural block provided that the following safeguards are observed:

1. That the ultimate responsibility for such a technique should be clearly stated to rest with the doctor.
2. That written instructions as to the dose should be given by the doctor concerned.
3. That in all cases the dose given by the midwife should be checked by one other person.
4. That instructions should be given by the doctor as to the posture of the patient at the time of injection, observation of blood pressure etc., and measures to be taken in the event of any side-effect.
5. That the midwife should have been thoroughly instructed in the technique so that the doctor concerned is satisfied as to her ability.'

It should be noted that the anaesthetist must inject the first dose which is administered through the catheter in order to confirm that the catheter has not punctured the dura. It will often be convenient for the anaesthetist to make this injection when he performs the epidural block. The enlightened attitude of the National Boards for Nursing, Midwifery and Health Visiting has already allowed epidural analgesia to be used in smaller hospitals where a full-time obstetric anaesthesia service is not available. The involvement of the midwife in the administration of the pain-relieving injection is of considerable psychological value to the midwife and to her patient. It is, of course, an important aspect of the training of the junior anaesthetist that he should observe the course of labour in the patient to whom he has administered epidural analgesia, and in the teaching hospital it will be advisable that the anaesthetic registrars administer many of the top-up injections. As has been discussed previously, there are considerable advantages in terms of safety in giving top-up injections in divided doses and assessing the effects of the initial dose before injecting the remainder. This will allow early detection of the rare, but worrying, complication of subdural or subarachnoid injection of local anaesthetic during what is apparently successful epidural analgesia.

In 1978 the Central Midwives Board for Scotland gave restricted approval to the giving of top-up injections by midwives. This is now permitted in the small number of hospitals where a 24-hour resident obstetric anaesthesia service exists. The rules are otherwise similar to those stated above.

Delivery. The anaesthetist should be present at every operative delivery conducted under epidural analgesia. The anaesthetist and his obstetric colleagues must decide whether a policy of elective forceps delivery is to be pursued or whether spontaneous delivery is to be the aim whenever possible. The requirements of a training school for midwives for spontaneous deliveries may have to be taken into account along with the wishes of the mother.

As has been stressed elsewhere (Moir and Willocks, 1968; Moir, 1971), if epidural analgesia is used selectively for patients with obstetric abnormalities such as incoordinate uterine action, pre-eclampsia and occipitoposterior position, then the operative delivery rate will be high. Conversely, if epidural analgesia is used extensively for pain relief in normal labour and if the block is confined to the region of the eleventh and twelfth thoracic nerves, then spontaneous delivery may be achieved in 80% of patients (Doughty, 1969) or over 50% if epidural analgesia is conducted with 0.25% bupivacaine plain solution or 30% with 0.5% bupivacaine (Thorburn and Moir, 1981). Where perineal anaesthesia exists because the block extends to the sacral nerve roots, the operative delivery rate will also be high because the reflex urge to push will be abolished through interruption of Ferguson's reflex. Extensive lumbar epidural blockade with 0.5% bupivacaine substantially increases the percentage of rotational forceps deliveries (Hoult et al, 1977) and should be avoided. Although caudal analgesia, by relaxing the pelvic floor muscles, may cause failure of rotation of the fetal head from occipitoposterior or transverse positions (Hingson et al, 1961), this is less likely to occur under lumbar epidural block which will often exclude the sacral nerves. Traditional obstetric teaching may be modified. If continuous monitoring of the fetal heart rate indicates that the fetus is in good condition, there is no need to set an arbitrary time limit on the second stage of labour. Safe prolongation of the second stage might allow descent and rotation of the fetal head. Such a policy, together with avoidance of motor block of the sacral nerve roots, might reduce the incidence of potentially hazardous rotational forceps deliveries, although O'Driscoll et al (1981) have argued eloquently that all forceps deliveries are potentially hazardous, even in the hands of experts.

The arguments on the benefits to the fetus of outlet forceps delivery versus spontaneous delivery are of long standing. Recent work seems to suggest that a more important consideration may be the avoidance of caval occlusion in the first and second stages of labour. Where the spontaneous delivery takes place in the unmodified dorsal position, there is a progressive and quite severe fetal acidosis which develops during the second stage to the extent of 0.25 of a pH unit in 30 minutes (Humphrey et al, 1974); thus a short second stage is desirable (Wood et al, 1973). The introduction of a left lateral tilt in the dorsal position prevents fetal acidosis in the second stage (Humphrey et al, 1974). If acceptable to obstetricians and midwives then delivery may safely be conducted in the lateral or Sims' position. Outlet forceps delivery carries no more risk for the fetus than spontaneous delivery when allowance is made for the duration of the second stage of labour, according to Livnat et al (1978).

If intravenous ergometrine is given at forceps delivery under epidural analgesia then almost 50% of patients will experience nausea, retching or vomiting. The use of a single intravenous injection of oxytocin (Syntocinon) 5 units followed by an injection of 500 ml of a fluid containing 20 units of oxytocin will usually avoid this unpleasant complication and will be an equally effective uterine stimulant (Moodie and Moir, 1976).

Caesarean section will sometimes be necessary during labour. In the Queen Mother's Hospital, Glasgow, 14% of patients receiving epidural analgesia are delivered by caesarean section. The performance of caesarean section under epidural analgesia has been discussed earlier in this chapter and where this procedure is acceptable to the patient and is skilfully managed then the well-recognized risks of general anaesthesia for emergency obstetrics can be circumvented. For successful caesarean section the block must extend from T6 to S5 segments. The sensory blockade for the relief of pain in labour is not so extensive, and it may take some time to allow the block to be extended. It is only if the need for delivery is urgent that time may not be available to permit extension of the block. In the Queen Mother's Hospital, 27% of women undergoing caesarean section required delivery within 30 minutes of the decision being made. Thus, for the majority, sufficient time is available to permit insertion of an epidural block or the extension of an existing one. Occasionally, the need for delivery may be so urgent that general anaesthesia is appropriate. It is the authors' experience that the use of 2% lignocaine with 1:200000 adrenaline allows surgery to be undertaken within 30 minutes. If general anaesthesia is to be used it is strongly recommended that the standard anaesthetic technique described in detail in chapter 6 be used without modification. Although there might appear to be a likelihood of severe hypotension arising out of the combination of sympathetic blockade, general anaesthesia and intermittent positive pressure ventilation, considerable clinical experience suggests that the risk is not great if blood volume is maintained and caval occlusion is avoided. It is quite often possible to time the operation to take place when the epidural blockade has just worn off. The temptation to supplement the epidural block either with a light general anaesthetic without tracheal intubation or with heavy sedation should be resisted in the interests of maternal and fetal safety.

Epidural and intrathecal administration of opiates

Since the discovery of opioid receptors in nerve tissue by Pert and Snyder (1973), considerable excitement has been generated by the vision of producing selective analgesia without the sympathetic and motor block which accompanies the non-selective blocks associated with epidural and spinal injection of local anaesthetic agents. β-Endorphin is thought to be one of the neuromodulatory substances involved in pain perception and has been shown to produce analgesia to noxious stimuli (Bradbury et al, 1976). Plasma β-endorphin-like activity has also been shown to increase during labour reaching a maximum at the second stage of labour, correlating with the duration of labour, and activity is significantly reduced in those patients receiving pethidine (Thomas et al, 1982). Intrathecal and epidurally administered opiates are thought to act on the substantia gelatinosa of the spinal cord, selectively blocking pain pathways (Kitahata and Collins, 1981). Bowsher (1978) has suggested that uterine pain is largely conducted by A gamma fibres, some of which bypass the substantia gelatinosa containing the opioid receptors. This may in part explain the conflicting reports of the benefits of exogenously administered opiates in labour.

The qualities required of an opiate for effective intrathecal and epidural action are also conflicting. Intrathecal analgesia requires a drug with a high affinity for the receptors with a slow dissociation. Thus morphine is very effective intrathecally. However, morphine has low lipid solubility, a property which is required for rapid uptake following epidural administration. Because of its hydrophilicity it may remain in the cerebrospinal fluid for many hours, with the risk of delayed effects. In contrast, fentanyl is much more lypophilic, produces reliable analgesia, but has a short duration of action because of its rapid dissociation from receptors and subsequent redistribution.

Although a large series with a low incidence of side-effects has been reported following administration of extradural and intrathecal opiates (Gustaffsson et al, 1982), cases of severe respiratory depression following both intrathecal and epidural morphine have been recorded. The majority of reports relate to intrathecal morphine and the respiratory depression occurring 2–12 hours after administration (Christensen, 1980; Reiz and Westberg, 1980; Chambers et al, 1981; Torda and Pybus, 1981).

The pharmacokinetics of epidurally administered morphine are similar to those of intramuscular morphine (Nordberg et al, 1983), the plasma half-life is similar (Brunke and Delle, 1974; Kafer et al, 1983), but the cerebrospinal fluid morphine levels are considerably higher following epidural administration (Weddell and Ritter, 1981).

Clearly, intrathecally placed opiates will have a faster and more direct action with a different mode of onset than epidurally sited opiates, but intrathecal injection carries with it the risk of headache and many obstetric patients have an epidural catheter inserted for pain relief in labour. Thus ready access to the epidural space is often available. Kafer et al (1983) proposed three different mechanisms for the actions of epidurally injected morphine:

1. Early pain relief and respiratory depression are the results of rapid absorption of morphine into the epidural veins and recirculatory distribution to the brain.
2. The continuing and prolonged pain relief is the result of morphine diffusing through the dura and subarachnoid membrane into cerebrospinal fluid and so to the dorsal horn where its high receptor affinity prolongs the action.
3. The late respiratory depression is the result of cephalad movement of cerebrospinal fluid containing morphine, where, 2–12 hours after injection, the morphine concentration is sufficient to depress the respiratory centres. Jorgensen et al (1981) have demonstrated relatively high concentrations of morphine within the cerebrospinal fluid.

Many investigations of the effects of intrathecal and epidurally administered opiates have been reported, particularly for post-surgical pain relief. The subject has been reviewed in detail recently by Cousins and Mather (1984). The following is a brief account of opiate use in obstetrics.

Disadvantages reported following the intrathecal and epidural use of morphine are pruritus, the incidence varying from slight (Bromage et al, 1980), to almost 100% (Bromage et al, 1982), nausea and vomiting have also proved troublesome (Cohen and Woods, 1983), with doses varying from 2 to 10 mg of preservative-free morphine. Booker et al (1980) investigated the effects of 2.5 and 4 mg of epidural morphine, and noted effective pain relief, but pruritus proved annoying, while Husemeyer et al (1980) found 2 mg of morphine to be ineffective in relieving the pain of labour, and Justins et al (1982) observed a more rapid onset and complete analgesia when fentanyl was added to the first dose of epidural bupivacaine. Husemeyer et al (1981) attributed the superior analgesia of pethidine 100 mg injected into the epidural space to the higher blood pethidine concentration rather than to that observed following the intramuscular injection of 100 mg, although the duration of effective analgesia was relatively brief.

Currently, however, no drug provides effective analgesia of adequate duration without the risk of side-effects. Fentanyl would appear to have the lowest frequency of undesirable side-effects, but its high lipid solubility results in a short duration of action. Morphine is not suitable. Despite the obvious attractions of this method of administration, the high frequency of adverse reactions severely limits its value in obstetrics at present. Future developments are awaited with interest.

CAUDAL ANALGESIA

Historically caudal analgesia preceded lumbar epidural analgesia, having been performed by Sicard and Cathélin in Paris in 1901 and first used in obstetrics by Stoeckel of Marburg in 1909. Continuous caudal analgesia was introduced by Hingson and Edwards in the USA in 1942 and made painless labour a practical possibility. Although still used in a few centres in the USA, caudal analgesia has to a large extent been replaced by lumbar epidural analgesia. Caudal analgesia has never been extensively favoured in the UK, although it was used in Oxford until about 1970.

Technique of continuous caudal analgesia

The lateral or semi-prone position is used and the thighs are flexed on the abdomen. The knee–chest position gives good access to the sacral hiatus but is disliked by many women.

The anaesthetist scrubs up, puts on sterile gown and gloves and applies an antiseptic solution such as 0.5% chlorhexidine in alcohol to a wide area of skin over the buttocks, sacrum and coccyx. A suitably placed swab keeps irritant solutions such as alcohol away from the sensitive perianal skin. A fenestrated sterile towel is positioned to allow access to the sacral hiatus.

The sacral cornua should now be palpated. These are two slight bony prominences which lie one on either side of the hiatus and are therefore the key to success. If the cornua cannot be identified then the sacral hiatus may be presumed to be some 5 cm from the tip of the coccyx and in the midline. If the patient is in the lateral position the median skin crease may sag and the true midline should be identified by palpation. The hiatus commonly lies beneath the upper end of the natal cleft, but this is an unreliable guide. Unfortunately obesity and oedema frequently make precise location of the sacral hiatus a matter of difficulty during pregnancy.

An intradermal weal of local anaesthetic solution is now raised over the sacral hiatus and a small volume of this solution is infiltrated beneath the skin. A straight 16 or 18 gauge thin-walled caudal needle is now inserted at an angle of 70° to the skin while the thumb of the other hand rests over the hiatus. A Tuohy needle may be used. A plastic intravenous cannula is suitable for continuous caudal analgesia. The needle is introduced with its bevel facing anteriorly. The sacrococcygeal membrane which covers the sacral hiatus is now identified by the tip of the needle and the membrane is pierced so that the point of the needle now lies against the bony anterior wall of the sacral canal. The needle is now withdrawn very slightly and the hub of the needle is depressed until the shaft of the needle makes an angle of some 20° with the skin and is directed in line with the sacral canal. After rotating the needle through 180° so that its bevel now faces posteriorly, the needle is now advanced for 2 cm upwards within the canal. It is important that the needle point does not rub against the anterior wall of the sacral canal where there are frequently bony ridges and where venous plexuses lie. Painful subperiosteal injections must also be avoided. Upward advance must be restricted to 2 cm in order to avoid puncture of the dural sac which descends to the level of the second sacral foraminae. These manoeuvres are illustrated in Figures 15 and 16.

A true loss of resistance technique is not used to identify the sacral canal but advance of the needle should be unrestricted and any injection should meet with no resistance. When it is considered that the needle is correctly placed then aspiration for blood and cerebrospinal fluid should be carried out. In the knee–chest position the cerebrospinal fluid pressure in the sacral part of the dural sac may be very low and dural puncture may go undetected at this stage. A common difficulty is superficial placement of the needle in the subcutaneous tissues and this is detected by an air-injection test. The fingertips of one hand rest over the lower part of the sacrum while a rapid injection of a few millilitres of air is made. Crepitus will be felt if the needle is superficially placed. A sharp tap on the plunger of a 2 ml syringe containing air will be followed by rebound of the plunger if the needle lies outwith the sacral canal.

An epidural catheter is now passed through the needle. A stiff catheter made of Teflon or even one containing a wire stilette (Rubin, 1972) will encourage the advance of the catheter unit until its tip lies in the cephalad

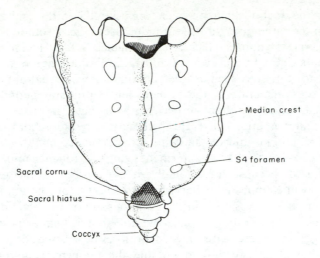

Figure 15. Posterior surface of sacrum showing sacral cornua and sacral hiatus (covered in life by the sacrococcygeal membrane) (from *Obstetric Therapeutics* (1974) by D.D. Moir, edited by D.F. Hawkins and published by Baillière Tindall, London).

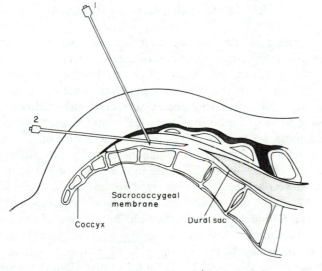

Figure 16. Caudal analgesia. Longitudinal section of sacrum showing (1) the needle piercing the sacrococcygeal membrane and (2) the needle having been depressed and advanced within the sacral canal. The needle has been rotated through 180° to facilitate advancement. The dural sac reaches the lower border of S2 (from *Obstetric Therapeutics* (1974) by D.D. Moir, edited by D.F. Hawkins and published by Baillière Tindall, London).

portion of the sacral canal or even opposite the fifth lumbar vertebra. Insertion of the catheter to this extent reduces leakage of solution through the anterior sacral foraminae which are not sealed off by ligament and also facilitates blockade of the eleventh and twelfth thoracic nerve roots. The use of an ultrastiff catheter, such as one containing a wire stilette, may increase the risk of dural puncture by the catheter and is probably better avoided.

The needle is now withdrawn leaving the catheter in place and a Millex (Millipore) filter is attached to the catheter. A test dose of 3 ml of local anaesthetic solution is injected and after an interval of 5 minutes the ability of the patient to move her feet is confirmed. Complete reliance upon a test dose is not advised because occasionally it will produce no evidence of subarachnoid injection. A further 17 ml of solution are now injected, to a total of 20 ml. It is necessary to inject 20 ml of solution to obtain pain relief in the first stage of labour and to make the injection as high as possible within the sacral canal. Some care must therefore be exercised to avoid the administration of an excessive dose, and the preferred solution is 0.25% bupivacaine plain. Alternatively 1% lignocaine with 1:200000 adrenaline may be used. The onset of analgesia may take up to 30 minutes and is usually rather slower than is the case after a lumbar epidural injection where the injection is made closer to the lower pairs of thoracic nerve roots.

A COMPARISON OF CAUDAL AND LUMBAR EPIDURAL ANALGESIA

Almost everything which has been written elsewhere in this chapter concerning lumbar epidural analgesia is applicable to caudal analgesia. In particular the incidence of hypotension is broadly similar with both techniques and although the incidence of dural puncture is probably lower with caudal analgesia, the incidence of accidental subarachnoid injection is not, according to some authorities, very different (Bush, 1959; Nellermoe et al, 1960; De Jong, 1961; Ellis and DeVita, 1962; Evans et al, 1962) and one would agree with Dawkins (1972) when he questions the frequently made assumption that caudal analgesia is safe in the hands of the obstetrician who may not be fully competent to resuscitate an apnoeic, hypotensive mother. Moore (1964) records dural puncture by the caudal catheter and subsequent total subarachnoid block and the writer has knowledge of three such cases.

The caudal technique requires the injection of considerably larger doses of local anaesthetic solution and so the risk of a maternal toxic reaction is greater (Russell and Coakley, 1964; Gunther and Bauman, 1969). For the same reason the placental transfer of local anaesthetic is increased, particularly if an agent with a free placental transfer such as lignocaine is used (Shnider and Way, 1968). Bupivacaine is preferred because its placental transfer is restricted by its binding to plasma proteins.

273

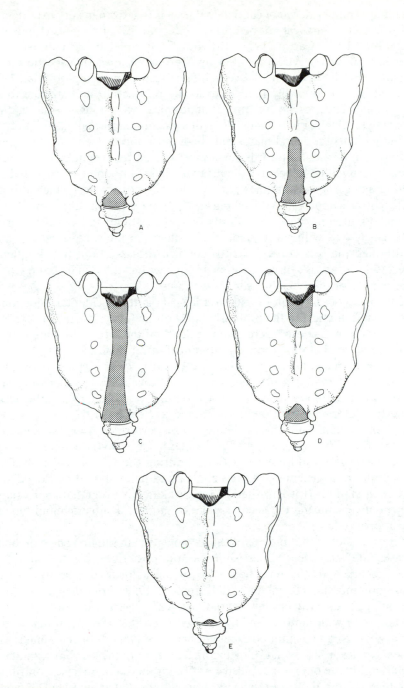

Figure 17. Some abnormalities of the sacrum. A = normal sacrum; B = upward extension of the hiatus; C = complete failure of fusion of laminae with an open sacral canal; D = failure of fusion of SI laminae; E = abnormally small hiatus due to complete fusion of all laminae.

An important criticism of caudal analgesia is that even in very experienced hands the sacral canal cannot be entered in about 5% of patients (Lindstrom and Moore, 1957; Carrie, 1972; Rubin, 1972) while in the context of an obstetric analgesia service provided by a group of anaesthetists the failure rate is likely to lie between 10% and 20% (Bush, 1959; Hingson et al, 1961; Carrie, 1972). Many of the failures to locate the sacral canal are due to the frequent and occasionally extensive anatomical variations of the sacrum. According to Black (1949) almost 30% of sacra are abnormal (see Figure 17). In some patients the sacral hiatus may be almost non-existent while in others the hiatus may extend upwards for almost the entire length of the sacrum. Having successfully injected a local anaesthetic into the sacral canal the resulting analgesia is sometimes patchy and may not reach the eleventh and twelfth thoracic nerves. As Nicholas (1972) pointed out there may be a tendency to attempt caudal block only on those patients in whom the cornua can be easily felt, with consequent improvement in the success rate.

Although there is no evidence to confirm the assertion, it is frequently suggested that the risk of infection is greater with caudal analgesia owing to the proximity of the puncture site to the anus.

A bizarre complication of caudal analgesia is the accidental injection of the local anaesthetic into the presenting part of the fetus. The injection of this relatively enormous dose has resulted in death of the fetus, although survival has been recorded after vigorous treatment (Finster et al, 1965; Sinclair et al, 1965). Treatment consists of immediate delivery of the child followed by general resuscitative measures and exchange transfusion in order to remove the drug from the blood. This disastrous complication occurs when the needle is inserted lateral to the sacrum or coccyx (Rubin, 1972). It has been recommended that caudal block should not be performed when the fetal head is low in the pelvis (Bonica, 1970*a*), and Moore (1964) recommends that caudal analgesia should not be instituted during the second stage of labour and that anterior placement of the needle or catheter should be excluded by rectal examination. If it is wished to provide effective regional analgesia for forceps delivery during the second stage of labour, a subarachnoid block is more appropriate.

It is often stated that the use of caudal analgesia in the first stage of labour increases the incidence of persistent occipitoposterior positions and deep transverse arrest of the fetal head due to the associated relaxation of the pelvic floor muscles (Ritmiller and Rippman, 1957; Friedman et al, 1960; Hingson et al, 1961). Certainly caudal analgesia reverses the order of nerve blockade seen with lumbar epidural analgesia so that the sacral nerve roots are blocked first and cannot be excluded from the block. For the same reason perineal anaesthesia is an inevitable feature of caudal block and, by eliminating the involuntary expulsive efforts of the second stage, contributes to the high forceps delivery rate associated with caudal analgesia. The type of selective blockade used by Doughty (1969) to relieve only the uterine pain and which can achieve a spontaneous delivery rate of 80% in normal patients is unobtainable with caudal analgesia. It is probable that caudal analgesia, like lumbar epidural analgesia, does not alter the rate of progress of normal labour in the absence of hypotension (Friedman and Sachtleben, 1959) and there is no need to adhere to the older view that caudal analgesia should not be induced until the cervix was 7–8 cm dilated in the primigravida and 6–7 cm dilated in the parous woman (Moore, 1964).

In most circumstances the evidence is quite strongly in favour of lumbar epidural analgesia. It is the writers' practice to use the lumbar technique almost exclusively, despite (or perhaps because of) quite extensive experience with caudal analgesia in the USA. Caudal analgesia is used in the occasional patient who has deformity of the lumbar spine, a localized septic lesion in the lumbar area or who objects to an injection in the lumbar spine but who will accept a caudal injection.

SPINAL (SUBARACHNOID) ANALGESIA

The introduction of bupivacaine 0.5% plain, and 8% dextrose spinal solutions, has rekindled interest in spinal anaesthesia in the UK. Despite the obvious enthusiasm in many centres, it is too early to be certain of the place of

Table 11. A comparison of the advantages and disadvantages of spinal and epidural anaesthesia

Advantages	Disadvantages
Spinal	
Rapid onset	Single shot
Small dose	Hypotension
Arguably faster to perform	No control of spread
Local trauma negligible	Headaches—up to 20%
No risk of toxicity	
No risk of catheter breakage	
Epidural	
Continuous technique	Large dose
Good control of spread	Relatively traumatic
Slow onset of hypotension	Slow onset
	Headaches—severe in 1–2%
	Risk of drug toxicity

spinal anaesthesia in the anaesthetic armamentarium of the obstetric anaesthetist. Experiences in North America, where spinal anaesthesia has long been popular, suggests that the use of spinal anaesthesia is declining although it still has a significant place. Epidural analgesia both for pain relief in labour and for caesarean section is becoming more popular, apparently at the expense of spinal anaesthesia for delivery. This is not to deny that subarachnoid anaesthesia offers certain advantages over epidural blocks, but it also carries certain penalties (Table 11). What is required is a spinal anaesthetic drug with an entirely controllable onset and spread, the upper limit of the block being directly and predictably dose-related. Over the next few years one can prophesy with confidence that the effects of bupivacaine spinal solutions in pregnancy will be known and consequently the place of spinal anaesthesia in obstetrics, particularly for caesarean section, will be made clear.

At the time of writing, only two drugs are available for use, and approved by the Committee on Safety of Medicines: cinchocaine (dibucaine), and bupivacaine plain and in 8% glucose solution. Cinchocaine is too long-acting to be suitable for use in obstetrics, where the operations tend to be of relatively short duration.

Dibucaine withdrawn

The rapid onset of hypotension and the uncertainty of the block height are the two main anxieties concerning the use of spinal anaesthesia. Headache is frequent, though usually mild, even when fine spinal needles are used. Many experienced anaesthetists can recall subarachnoid blocks which were either inadequate or too extensive for comfort, despite attempts to control some of the variables. Adjusting the dose to the height of the patient has not proved reliable. The position of the patient, the time taken to complete the injection and the position adopted by the patient following injection may all influence the extent of the block. The effects of an intrathecal injection of local anaesthetic agent would appear to be quite different in the pregnant patient from those in the non-pregnant patient. In the non-pregnant, it is unusual to experience very high blocks, despite the injection of relatively large volumes of local anaesthetic agent. Intrathecal injection of 3 ml of bupivacaine plain solution proved inadequate for gynaecological surgery (Chambers et al, 1981). In the pregnant, relatively small doses can be associated with alarmingly extensive blocks, and 2 ml of bupivacaine has produced a total spinal block (Russell, 1985). It is clear that the cerebrospinal fluid dynamics are different, but they are also unpredictable. The effect of pregnancy on the contents of the epidural space and the increased flow of venous blood etc. may also play a part in altering cerebrospinal fluid dynamics. In this respect, spinal analgesia is similar to epidural analgesia in that the relationship between dose and effect is not clear. Epidural analgesia has the advantage that it is administered incrementally, unlike spinal anaesthesia. The spread of analgesia is of particular interest for caesarean section, where, for satisfactory operating conditions, the upper limit of the block should be at T4–T6. It would appear that to block to precisely this segmental level with certainty in all women is difficult, although the majority of blocks may be satisfactory (Russell, 1983; Santos et al, 1984).

The rapid onset of subarachnoid block is commonly associated with hypotension, though this may be modified by the use of adequate preloading, as for epidural block, and by the use of adequate doses of intravenous ephedrine, as the block develops (Kang et al, 1982). The incidence of headaches following spinal anaesthesia in obstetrics is relatively high. Dripps and Vandam (1954) noted an overall incidence of headache of 6% following the use of small bore spinal needles. Crawford (1979b) observed that the incidence of post spinal headaches ranged from 16 to 20%, and was not influenced by needle diameters of 22 or 25 gauge. However, there is a distinct clinical impression that the severity of headaches following the use of 25 gauge needles is significantly less severe. The practice of keeping the patient in bed for 24 hours following spinal anaesthesia does not appear to reduce the frequency of post-spinal headaches (Carbaat and Van Crevel, 1981). Preliminary reports suggest that if a 26 gauge spinal needle is used, the incidence and severity of headaches is reduced, but this is a very fine needle and can be difficult to use. An introducer is required, and it can be difficult to identify the end-point, as cerebrospinal fluid may be reluctant to flow through the needle. When comparing the incidence of headaches between epidural and spinal blocks, it should not be forgotten that, although dural puncture is rare during epidural block (1–2%), it is not negligible, and the subsequent headache following dural puncture with a 16 gauge Tuohy needle can be very severe. As has already been discussed, hypotension is a significant problem in patients undergoing caesarean section with epidural analgesia, and Caritis et al (1980) have demonstrated that if the volume of preload is increased to 1.5 litres of crystalloid solution before inducing spinal anaesthesia, the fetal acidosis is then similar to that following epidural analgesia, and the hypotension is easier to treat.

The use of continuous catheter techniques is of historical interest only (Elam, 1970).

Three techniques of subarachnoid analgesia have been described in obstetrics, but the divisions into (1) saddle block, (2) low spinal analgesia and (3) mid-spinal analgesia are rather artificial and cannot be achieved with precision.

Saddle block

Spinal analgesia is used for operative delivery or to allow examinations and manipulations, e.g. manual removal of placenta, which would otherwise be too painful to be performed. It is therefore essential to provide adequate analgesia. The use of saddle block analgesia may provide satisfactory analgesia for outlet forceps delivery, but will be inadequate for any more extensive manipulations. It is therefore of limited value, and offers little to current obstetric practice. It consists of the subarachnoid injection of <1 ml of a hyperbaric spinal solution with the patient in the sitting position. The patient remains in this position for at least 3 minutes until the solution has become fixed to the sacral nerves. The injection is made without barbotage. As the block is confined to the sacral roots, anaesthesia is confined to the perineal skin (the saddle area) and the vagina. Hypotension is not a feature of this block, but the patient remains aware of her uterine contractions and the block is not suitable for anything other than an outlet forceps delivery. Saddle block provides inadequate conditions for manual removal of placenta, and because of its limited value, a so-called 'low-spinal' block offers a great deal more in terms of pain relief and enables more extensive operative procedures.

Low-spinal anaesthesia

This block extends from the sacral roots to T10, and so provides adequate analgesia for mid-cavity and rotation forceps delivery and also manual removal of placenta and breech delivery. As has been stated earlier, it is difficult to define precisely the upper limit of block height; the physiological effects of the block will relate to the extent of the sympathetic block, and hypotension may occur. The reduction in the arterial pressure will be in proportion to the extent of the sympathetic block and the state of the patient's hydration. While a deliberately extensive block is not sought, the spread may be greater than anticipated and it is good practice to precede this block with an intravenous fluid load of at least 1.5 litres in the 15 minutes prior to injection of the local anaesthetic.

Mid-spinal anaesthesia

Subarachnoid anaesthesia from the sacral roots to the level of the sixth thoracic dermatome will permit the performance of caesarean section.

Solutions and doses

Currently cinchocaine (dibucaine) 0.5% in 5% dextrose, bupivacaine 0.5% plain and bupivacaine 0.5% plain in 8% dextrose are available in the UK and are the only solutions approved by the Committee on Safety of Medicines. Lignocaine and amethocaine are not commercially available, but spinal solutions may be produced by the hospital pharmacist. Prilocaine and mepivacaine are no longer available. The recent introduction of the bupivacaine spinal solutions has provided agents with a rapid onset, adequate duration of action and a reassuring record of safety. The onset of analgesia is rapid with all solutions, but the duration of action varies quite widely being longest with cinchocaine. Crawford (1979b) used hyperbaric solutions of cinchocaine and states that evidence of blockade could be found after 8.8 hours. Durations of action of this length, especially if associated with motor block, are disliked by women. Amethocaine (tetracaine, Pontocaine), which is very popular in the United States, and has been safely given to a vast number of patients, is supplied as a 1% solution which is mixed with equal volumes of 10% dextrose solution before injection to create a 0.5% solution of amethocaine in 5% dextrose. Lignocaine 'spinal' is supplied as a 5% solution in 7.5% dextrose. It would appear that lignocaine, amethocaine and cinchocaine (dibucaine) are equipotent when used in equal volumes. Differences in onset times and extent of the block may be primarily related to the position of the patient during and following the injection of the local anaesthetic solution and the rate of injection. Preliminary studies with bupivacaine in pregnant women (Russell, 1983) suggest that a greater volume is required to produce a block of similar extent to that produced by the other local anaesthetic agents. In contrast, the results of comparison of bupivacaine and tetracaine (both in glucose) revealed no differences in spread (Ekblom and Widman, 1966), although Moore (1980) in a similar study noted a significantly longer motor block with amethocaine.

Santos et al (1984) found that 7.5–10 mg subarachnoid bupivacaine in dextrose produced anaesthesia to T3 within 10–15 minutes for caesarean section. Russell (1983) recommends the use of 10–15 mg of bupivacaine plain solution for caesarean section, but has recorded total spinal blockade using 10 mg (1985), and Stonham and Moss (1983) observed a total spinal block following the subarachnoid injection of 15 mg of the plain solution. Yet 15 mg of bupivacaine plain solution provied inadequate for gynaecological surgery (Chambers et al, 1981). It is evident that the spread of bupivacaine within the subarachnoid space is not always predictable.

Table 12. Dose requirements for cinchocaine and amethocaine in subarachnoid analgesia

	Saddle block	Low spinal	Mid-spinal
Heavy cinchocaine, 0.5% (dibucaine, Nupercaine)	0.6 ml	0.8–1 ml	1.2–1.6 ml
Heavy amethocaine 0.5% (tetracaine, Pontocaine)	0.6 ml	0.8–1 ml	1.2–1.6 ml

Technique of lumbar puncture

Absolute asepsis and antisepsis are essential and all equipment, including the solutions for injection, must have been autoclaved or obtained from a sterilized disposable set. Although North American practice permits the anaesthetist to perform lumbar puncture after simply pulling on sterile gloves, orthodox British practice insists upon a full surgical scrub and the wearing of gown and gloves.

Undoubtedly lumbar puncture is easier when the needle is of 22 or 23 gauge. Crawford (1979b) did not find a relationship between the frequency of headaches and the diameter of the needle in an obstetric population, but significant differences have been recorded in non-obstetric populations (Dripps and Vandam, 1954). It seems probable that the use of fine bore spinal needles will reduce, if not the frequency, then the severity of any subsequent post-spinal headache, and their use should be encouraged. The flexible nature of the fine needles of 25 and 26 gauge makes the use of an introducer advisable. A suitable introducer is a 19 gauge Butterfly needle, with the plastic extension tube cut short at the hub, thus simplifying entrance of the needle to the introducer. The Butterfly needle is an ideal length. It can enter the interspinous ligament but cannot puncture the dura. Local anaesthesia

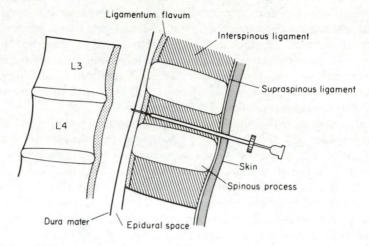

Figure 18. Longitudinal section showing 25 gauge spinal needle in subarachnoid space, having been passed through a Sise introducer.

need not be used to infiltrate the skin since insertion of the 19 gauge needle is no more uncomfortable than the injection of the local anaesthetic.

The introducer is inserted into the supraspinous ligament, and the spinal needle inserted through the introducer (Figure 18). Careful but steady and reasonably rapid advance will enable the operator to identify ligamentum flavum. The rate of advance is then reduced, as the dura is approximately 0.5 cm from the needle point as it enters ligamentum flavum. Subarachnoid entry should be slow lest the advancing needle damages nerve roots. Advancing the needle through the interspinous ligament at a reasonable speed permits ready distinction between bone and ligamentum flavum. If bone is detected, both the spinal needle and the introducer require to be resited. Cerebrospinal fluid does not flow freely through small diameter needles. Aspiration may be required, but even this may fail to demonstrate cerebrospinal fluid. In the authors' opinion, no injection of local anaesthetic should be made if cerebrospinal fluid is not identified, and, ideally, cerebrospinal fluid should again be identified following injection of local anaesthetic. Before injecting local anaesthetic, the anaesthetist should ensure that the cerebrospinal fluid is clear. If frank blood is obtained, the needle should be withdrawn and puncture repeated at another interspace. If a slight reddish tinge of blood is obtained, this should be allowed to clear before the injection is made. As the initial pressure is put on the plunger of the syringe, the patient should be asked if any pain is felt. If any suggestion of nerve root discomfort is elicited, administration should cease immediately because root damage may occur. Nerve root trauma is unlikely to occur if free flow of cerebrospinal fluid is obtained prior to injection. If pain is elicited, the needle should be repositioned by advancing it or withdrawing it slightly. The procedure should be abandoned if pain persists.

The patient may be in the lateral or sitting position for spinal anaesthesia, the preferred position being that which is most comfortable for the patient and most familiar to the anaesthetist. While the position of the patient may affect the speed of onset and the final segmental extent of the block, particularly if glucose-containing solutions are used, insufficient evidence is available to identify predictive elements with certainty.

Hypotension has been discussed at length previously, but following subarachnoid block, hypotension may develop very rapidly despite adequate preloading. Prophylactic infusions of ephedrine (Kang et al, 1982) have been effectively used to prevent hypotension, as has intramuscular ephedrine, although the latter has been shown to produce an unacceptably high incidence of hypertensive episodes.

Contraindications to subarachnoid block are similar to those for epidural anaesthesia, as discussed previously. The risk of vascular damage is very small when a fine needle is inserted into the subarachnoid space in the mid-line, and spinal analgesia may be acceptable when specially indicated in the presence of a coagulation defect.

Precautions for spinal anaesthesia for delivery, other than saddle block

1. Ensure i.v. infusion running, and preload at least 1.5 litre fluid for caesarean section and vaginal procedures.
2. Position of patient for injection is that of choice, but the right buttock must be on a wedge or the operating table laterally tilted when placed in the supine position.
3. Hypotension develops rapidly; consider prophylactic ephedrine, detect early and treat vigorously.
4. Plot ascent of block and be prepared to induce general anaesthesia and intubate the trachea if too extensive or inadequate.
5. The cardiovascular system must be monitored continuously.

Marx et al (1984) have reviewed the use of epidural and spinal anaesthesia for emergency caesarean section. They concluded that spinal anaesthesia offered significant advantages to the fetus and the mother, and was considered to be the most suitable in experienced hands.

Postoperative care

Traditionally, women have been kept in bed for 24 hours following spinal anaesthesia, but Carbaat and van Crevel (1981) did not observe any difference in the frequency headaches following lumbar puncture in ambulant patients and in those kept in bed. Following delivery, enforced bed rest is undesirable. Postural manoeuvres have not prevented the onset of headaches

(Smith, 1980; Hilton-Jones et al, 1982). Neurologists do not recommend the use of blood patches (Pearce, 1982), and recommend laying flat until recovery after diagnostic lumbar puncture. The very rare sequelae to lumbar puncture have been reviewed by Meeke (1983) and Rudehill et al (1983); Jack (1979) recommends the early administration of epidural blood patch to stop the leak of cerebrospinal fluid and so prevent any complications which could be attributed to the altered cerebrospinal fluid dynamics. Severe headaches usually have an early onset, and if the headache occurs after three or four days, it is unlikely to be severe. The headache should be assessed and the patient examined. If the headache is severe enough to necessitate bed rest for more than two days, blood patch should be considered. The application of external pressure to the abdominal wall can give dramatic transient relief, and longer duration of relief can be obtained by the inflation of a blood pressure cuff within an abdominal binder.

Permanent neurological sequelae. Permanent damage to the spinal cord, nerve roots or meninges has been reported from time to time and has been reviewed by Greensite and Katz (1980), Kane (1981) and Hargrove (1981). The neurological toxicity of local anaesthetic agents has been reviewed by Covino (1983) and Rosen et al (1983). The subject has been discussed earlier in the chapter. Reports of damage before 1950 (Ericson, 1947; Thorsen, 1947; Kennedy et al, 1950) were thought to have been possibly due to the injection of chemically contaminated solutions. After 1950 several very large series of subarachnoid blocks were reported with careful long-term follow-up, and no serious neurological sequelae were recorded (Arner, 1952; Dripps and Vandam, 1954; Sadove and Levin, 1954; Moore and Bridenbaugh, 1968; Philips et al, 1969; Noble and Murray, 1971). It is tempting to conclude that the use of autoclaved equipment and drugs, and more recently the use of disposable equipment, has eliminated this type of 'unexplained' damage to the cord and its coverings.

There remain several other factors which might act as rare and often preventable causes of nerve damage. The injection of vasoconstrictor agents into the subarachnoid space may cause avascular necrosis, and efforts to prolong analgesia by this means are condemned (Moore, 1955). The possibility of creating an epidermoid tumour of the meninges by the introduction of a plug of skin in the needle is prevented by the use of an introducer or a scalpel blade to puncture the skin. Antiseptic solution should not come into direct contact with the needle because it too could conceivably damage nerve tissue. Subdural haematoma with permanent paralysis has followed lumbar puncture in patients with coagulation defects, and subarachnoid analgesia is contraindicated in such patients (de Angelis, 1972). Bacterial meningitis is avoided by scrupulous technique, and local sepsis at the puncture site contraindicates subarachnoid analgesia. There remains the recently recognized possibility of injecting minute fragments of glass from the ampoule of anaesthetic solution with resulting damage to nerve tissue

(Furgang, 1974). This possibility could be eliminated by injecting through a Millipore filter or by passing the solution through a filter before making the injection.

It should be pointed out that neurological sequelae can follow both epidural and subarachnoid analgesia and the opposition to subarachnoid analgesia by some protagonists of epidural analgesia may not be fully justified. It is also worth recalling that obstetric palsy occurs in about 1 out of 2500 deliveries in which conduction analgesia has not been used (Hill, 1962) and that a neurological defect which follows subarachnoid analgesia may have an obstetric cause. Permanent neurological damage has even followed general anaesthesia (Ditzler and McIver, 1956) and Sinclair (1954) reported a patient who developed ascending spinal paralysis after hysterectomy under general anaesthesia.

The place of subarachnoid analgesia in obstetrics

It is often asked 'if a spinal, why not an epidural?' and certainly where continuous epidural analgesia has been instituted earlier in labour there will be no need for subarachnoid analgesia. The question is then only relevant when a patient who is not under epidural analgesia requires an operative vaginal delivery, or perhaps a caesarean section. The question often implies that epidural analgesia is safer for the patient. Although this implication will sometimes be justified, it is possible with skill and care to reduce the risks of subarachnoid analgesia to a very low level. Given the requisite knowledge, equipment and skill it seems to the writers that the widespread fear of subarachnoid analgesia among British anaesthetists can no longer be justified and that, after an absence of nearly 30 years, subarachnoid analgesia merits a restored place in British obstetric anaesthesia.

The analgesia of subarachnoid blockade is very intense. Motor block is also more intense and paralysis of the lower limbs and abdominal muscles is commonly seen. While the profound relaxation may be helpful during caesarean section, it causes distress to some patients. A very important advantage of subarachnoid blockade is the rapidity with which analgesia develops. Surgery is usually possible within a short time of injection, and perhaps the greatest benefit is that it is a swift and effective alternative to a hazardous general anaesthetic in the second or third stage of labour.

Pudendal nerve block is at present extensively used for forceps delivery in the UK. As Scudamore and Yates (1966) demonstrated, the block fails completely in approximately 50% of patients, and delivery is conducted under the limited analgesia provided by infiltration of the perineum. Undoubtedly many women suffer a good deal of pain, although perhaps briefly, during forceps delivery and the apparent popularity of pudendal nerve block may merely result from the unavailability of an effective alternative. A spinal block creates a tranquil patient, free of all pain, and operating conditions are excellent. Occasionally the descent of the fetal head through the vagina causes a feeling of distension which may be relieved by nitrous oxide analgesia. Uterine retraction is excellent and bleeding is usually reduced. The very small quantity of local anaesthetic used for subarachnoid analgesia eliminates the possibility of a direct toxic action of the drug upon mother and child.

Subarachnoid analgesia has been successfully used for assisted breech delivery (Sears, 1959; Moore, 1964; Salvatore et al, 1965). The arguments in favour of subarachnoid analgesia for breech delivery are essentially the same as those previously presented in favour of epidural analgesia, and it will usually be preferable to perform a continuous epidural block early in labour.

For caesarean section the advantages and disadvantages are essentially those presented for epidural analgesia, and the avoidance of caval occlusion and the maintenance of blood volume are of prime importance (Marx et al, 1969; Clark et al, 1976). The quality of analgesia may be rather greater with subarachnoid block, and the muscular relaxation is superb. Bleeding is significantly reduced (Williams, 1969). Postoperative analgesia cannot be maintained and this is a disadvantage.

Subarachnoid block is recommended for urgent caesarean section if the patient does not already have an epidural block and it is desired to avoid a hazardous general anaesthetic.

Williams (1969) has been a rare enthusiast for subarachnoid analgesia among British obstetricians for many years and he pleads for a reappraisal of the technique and for the rejection of prejudice against the method. In the words of Lake (1958) concerning subarachnoid analgesia, 'like all other anaesthetic techniques it has its risks, but it also has great merits which are plain to see unless one is unduly biased'.

PARACERVICAL BLOCK

This method of providing pain relief in the first stage of labour has several advantages including simplicity, suitability for use by obstetricians and the avoidance of hypotension. Until recently paracervical block was extensively used in North America, continental Europe and Scandinavia. The method was less widely used in Great Britain. Unfortunately this otherwise useful technique has now been shown to be associated with a very high incidence of fetal bradycardia and fetal acidosis and very occasionally with fetal death in labour. Consequently the continued use of paracervical block is difficult to justify in most circumstances.

Paracervical block satisfactorily relieves the pain of uterine contractions in 55–90% of patients (Spanos and Steel, 1959; Baken et al, 1962; Seeds et al, 1962; Gudgeon, 1968). Unilateral analgesia may occur and a failure rate of about 25% would be representative. Failure may be due to misplacement of the needle or to the existence in some patients of sensory nerve fibres alongside the ovarian vessels.

A successful bilateral paracervical block affects only the uterus. The vagina, perineum and vulva remain sensitive to pain. Some obstetricians perform pudendal nerve blocks for delivery. A disadvantage of paracervical block was the need for repeated injections during labour. With the availability of bupivacaine and the tendency to accelerate labour with oxytocin, this disadvantage has become less important. Bupivacaine 0.25% gives pain relief of 90–210 minutes duration (Cooper et al, 1968; Gudgeon, 1968) but has the important disadvantage of causing substantial reductions in uteroplacental blood flow. Catheter techniques were introduced by Baggish and by Burchell and Sadove in 1964. Catheters with hooked ends were used in the hope of preventing displacement but these techniques were frequently unsuccessful and are not recommended. Paracervical block can of course be used safely in patients who are not in labour and has been used for minor gynaecological surgery and for evacuation of the uterus in the course of spontaneous or therapeutic abortion (Littlepage et al, 1969; Chatfield et al, 1970; McKenzie and Shaffer, 1978) and may be indicated for outpatient surgery or in the absence of a skilled anaesthetist.

Technique of paracervical block

The sensory nerves emerging from the uterus pass laterally in the parametrial tissues on each side of the cervix near the base of the broad ligaments; it is at this site that they may be blocked. The patient is placed in the dorsal position and aseptic and antiseptic routines are followed. It is essential that a paracervical block needle with a blunt outer guard is used in order to limit penetration by the needle. The Kobak, Freeman, Brittain, Oxford or Iowa trumpet needles may be used and in their absence the use of a sterile drinking straw has been suggested. The Oxford needle which restricts penetration to about 1 cm is perhaps the safest needle.

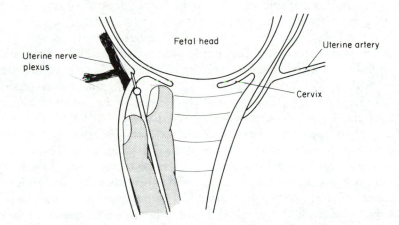

Figure 19. The paracervical block needle is correctly placed and further advance is prevented by the blunt guard. Note the proximity of the uterine artery.

The guard is pressed into the lateral fornix, the needle is advanced for 0.5–1 cm and, after careful aspiration for blood, an injection of 5–10 ml of 0.25% bupivacaine is made. The injection is repeated on the other side. Injections are usually made at 3 o'clock and 9 o'clock in relation to the cervical os. Injections may be made at the 4 o'clock and 8 o'clock positions to reduce the risk of injection into the uterine artery. This modification is sometimes referred to as uterosacral block because of the proximity of the uterosacral ligament to the injection site. Both sites are probably equally successful because solutions spread freely in the loose parametrial tissues to reach the nerves of the paracervical plexus (see Figure 19). According to Jagerhorn (1975) the incidence of adverse effects upon the fetus can be reduced by making the injections at a depth of only 3 mm, by using two injection sites in each lateral fornix and by reducing the total dose of 0.25% bupivacaine to 10 ml. These modifications seem well advised.

Paracervical block should be performed when labour is established and painful. If labour is far advanced or the presenting part is very low then the injection may be technically difficult or even impossible.

Complications

Fetal bradycardia. Fetal bradycardia is the outstanding hazard of an otherwise safe technique. The reported incidence of fetal bradycardia has varied from 1% to about 50% (Cooper and Moir, 1963; Nyirjesy et al, 1963; Teramo, 1969; Asling et al, 1970; Teramo and Rajamaki, 1971; Vasicka et al, 1971). Explanations for the wide variations in the incidence of fetal bradycardia may include varying definitions of bradycardia, the use of different local anaesthetic drugs, the use of adrenaline and, perhaps most important of all, the intensity with which the fetal heart-rate has been monitored. It is noticeable that the higher incidences of bradycardia have usually been reported in the more recent series where continuous monitoring has been used. Fetal tachycardia has less often been noted.

Earlier workers tended to discount fetal bradycardia. This attitude cannot now be upheld because fetal bradycardia (and probably tachycardia) during paracervical block is almost invariably associated with fetal acidosis (Asling et al, 1970; Rogers, 1970; Teramo and Rajamaki, 1971; Liston et al, 1973). Death of the fetus has been reported (Nyirjesy et al, 1963). There is an increase in beat-to-beat variability of the fetal heart-rate and this is interpreted as evidence of intrauterine hypoxia (Miller et al, 1978).

Fetal bradycardia usually occurs from 2 to 10 minutes after injection and the heart rate usually returns to normal after a further 20–30 minutes. The alterations in heart-rate are often uninfluenced by uterine contractions. The causation of the fetal bradycardia is disputed but its invariable innocence can no longer be accepted. In favour of a direct depressant action of the local anaesthetic drug upon the fetal myocardium with resulting tissue hypoxia are the abnormally high concentrations of local anaesthetic measured in the fetal blood by Asling et al (1970). Other workers have failed to detect unusually high concentrations of anaesthetic drug in the fetus (Beazley et al, 1972; Thiery and Vroman, 1972; Liston et al, 1973) and the last-named authors favour the hypothesis that the uterine hypotonus which may follow paracervical block interferes with placental circulation. A more acceptable explanation for a reduction in uteroplacental blood flow lies in the vasoconstrictor action of local anaesthetic agents on the uterine arteries (Greiss et al, 1976; Gibbs and Noel, 1977). The concentration of local anaesthetic agent will be high alongside the uterine artery.

It is with regret that it is concluded that this otherwise safe and quite effective technique cannot be recommended unless no other method of pain relief is available or appropriate. If the method is used, despite these comments, continuous monitoring of the fetal heart-rate and uterine contractions should be employed and estimations of the pH of the fetal scalp blood undertaken if variations in the fetal heart-rate are observed. The modified technique described above should be used so that a relatively small dose of local anaesthetic agent is placed superficially, and therefore as far away as possible, from the uterine arteries. Adrenaline should not be used because it is a vasoconstrictor, and according to Cibils and Santonja-Lucas (1978), bupivacaine should be avoided because it is especially likely to cause spasm of the uterine arteries. Paracervical block should not be used in the presence of placental insufficiency or if the fetus is premature.

Other complications. The other complications of paracervical block are relatively infrequent and should be avoidable with reasonable care. They include injection into a uterine artery, injection into the fetus, overdosage, infection and laceration of the vagina.

Uterine contractibility is unaltered or sometimes increased after paracervical block (Miller et al, 1978).

PUDENDAL NERVE BLOCK

The pudendal nerve is derived from the anterior roots of the second, third and fourth sacral nerves and is a mixed motor and sensory nerve. It is the principal sensory nerve to the perineum, vulva and all but the upper portion of the vagina and is the motor nerve to the perineal muscles and to the external anal sphincter. The levator ani muscles are not supplied by the pudendal nerve but receive their motor innervation from the fourth sacral nerve. Pudendal nerve block does not relieve pain of uterine origin. Successful block of both pudendal nerves will usually permit delivery by forceps although the patient will continue to appreciate the pain of her uterine contractions.

Technique of pudendal nerve block

Pudendal nerve block is almost always performed by the obstetrician. The nerve is blocked where it lies in or close to the pudendal canal on the lateral wall of the ischiorectal fossa and is closely associated with the pudendal artery and vein. There are two principal methods of performing bilateral pudendal nerve block:

(1) *The transvaginal method* which is the simpler and more successful method and is the recommended technique unless the presenting part is already too low to permit its use. The patient is placed in the lithotomy position and antiseptic and aseptic procedures are observed. A pudendal block needle of gauge 20 or 22 and some 12.5 cm length is attached to a 20 ml syringe containing local anaesthetic solution. Some obstetricians prefer to use a guarded needle of the type used for paracervical block in order to limit penetration and to avoid the risk of lacerating the vagina. The needle is placed along the second and third fingers of one hand and is introduced carefully into the vagina. The ischial spine is palpated with the tips of the fingers and the needle is advanced through the vaginal wall immediately behind the ischial spine to a depth of about 1.25 cm. The needle should have been felt to enter the tough sacrospinous ligament. The needle is now advanced continuously until its tip is felt to emerge from this ligament. A loss of resistance will be appreciated and the needle is held in this position while aspiration for blood is performed. Puncture of the adjacent pudendal vessels is common and injection into a vessel may cause a serious toxic reaction. An injection of 10 ml of local anaesthetic solution is now made. The procedure is repeated on the other side. Most obstetricians routinely follow pudendal nerve block by infiltration of the line of proposed episiotomy. A subcutaneous injection of 2 ml of solution may also be made along the skin folds at the outer attachments of the labia.

(2) *The transperineal approach* which is the older and less successful method should only be used when the presenting part of the fetus is too low to permit the use of the transvaginal approach. An unguarded needle is inserted through the perineal skin at a point halfway between the fourchette and the ischial tuberosity. Two fingers of the other hand are placed within the vagina and the ischial spine is identified. The needle is advanced until its point lies just behind the ischial spine. After careful aspiration for blood, 10 ml of local anaesthetic solution are injected. The procedure is repeated on the other side. The line of episiotomy is usually then infiltrated.

Choice of local anaesthetic solution

In order to avoid maternal toxicity it is necessary to exercise some care over the solution to be used for pudendal nerve block. Some obstetricians inject up to 40 ml of solution when performing bilateral pudendal nerve blocks accompanied by perineal and labial infiltration, although such a volume is normally unnecessary. Lignocaine, prilocaine and mepivacaine are the agents commonly used and 1% solutions are suitable. If the solution used is 1% plain lignocaine then there is a risk of causing a toxic reaction if the volume injected greatly exceeds 20 ml (200 mg), and the addition of adrenaline 1 : 200000 to this solution is recommended in order to reduce its toxicity. The addition of adrenaline to 1% prilocaine and mepivacaine solutions is not necessary. In the Queen Mother's Hospital, Glasgow, during a six-month period in 1964 a 1% plain lignocaine solution was (wrongly) used in quantities of up to 40 ml for pudendal nerve blocks and five major, convulsive reactions occurred. Since then a 1% plain prilocaine solution has been used and there have been no reactions.

Surprisingly little information is available about the placental transfer of local anaesthetics when used for pudendal nerve block. It is probable that fetomaternal concentration ratios for lignocaine, prilocaine and mepivacaine will lie between 0.5 and 1.0 (Burt, 1971). Belfrage et al (1973) have assessed the placental transfer of bupivacaine 0.25% with 1 : 200000 adrenaline following pudendal nerve block and found a mean fetomaternal ratio of 0.25 (range 0.11–0.55). These workers suggest that bupivacaine 0.25% may be the preferred solution because of its relatively inextensive placental transfer. It may be noted, as far as can be judged from the limited evidence available, that the placental transfer of local anaesthetic after pudendal nerve block seems comparable to that which is known to occur after epidural injection.

Adequacy of analgesia

In 1966 Scudamore and Yates recorded a disturbingly low success rate for pudendal nerve blocks in a series of non-pregnant women. With the transvaginal approach, 50% of the blocks were successful on both sides. With the transperineal approach the bilateral success rate was only 25%. These women were not in labour and the stimulus was the prick of a pin or the grasp of tissue forceps on the perineal skin and not the birth of a baby. Although many experienced obstetricians would claim better results, there can be no doubt that a substantial number of women experience a considerable degree of pain at forceps delivery with this technique and that the sometimes vigorous movements of the mother must add to the dangers of the delivery. The conclusions of Scudamore and Yates demand attention. They suggested that most low forceps deliveries can be performed after infiltration of the perineum and labia, without pudendal nerve block, and that mid-cavity forceps should be performed under an entirely different technique such as epidural, caudal, subarachnoid or (rarely) general anaesthesia. Pudendal nerve block may often be a misnomer and could become obsolete. Does this rather inefficient technique survive because anaesthetists are failing to provide a satisfactory and safe alternative? It may be possible to mask inadequate analgesia by the intravenous injection of a mixture of pethidine and a phenothiazine, as was advocated by Crawford (1965). This sort of supplementation of an unsatisfactory regional block cannot usually create perfect conditions and must inevitably negate one of the principal advantages of regional analgesia by causing some degree of neonatal depression. It is obviously preferable to use an effective method of regional analgesia. A comprehensive obstetric anaesthesia service should include the provision of subarachnoid analgesia as an effective alternative to pudendal nerve block for mid-cavity forceps deliveries.

PARAVERTEBRAL BLOCK

There are two types of paravertebral blocks capable of relieving the pains associated with uterine contractions but not the pain of delivery. Paravertebral block of the second lumbar sympathetic ganglion on each side will block the passage of impulses in the sympathetic chain. Bilateral blockade of the eleventh and twelfth thoracic somatic nerves will also relieve the pains of the first stage of labour (Cleland, 1933). These techniques involve repeated, multiple injections and there is a considerable risk of drug overdose and accidental subarachnoid injection.

Meguiar and Wheeler (1978) have performed bilateral paravertebral lumbar sympathetic blocks by injecting 10 ml of 0.5% bupivacaine with 1 : 200 000 adrenaline. A 10 cm 22 gauge needle was inserted 4.5 cm lateral to the spinous process of L2 vertebra and advanced in a 20° cephalad direction until the transverse process of that vertebra was identified. The needle was then pulled back and redirected to pass beneath, and 4.5 cm beyond, the transverse process with a 10° medial inclination and the local anaesthetic solution was injected at that point, close to the body of the vertebra. First stage analgesia was complete in 31 out of 40 mothers and lasted for an average of 283 ± 103 minutes. Another form of analgesia was provided for the delivery. It was concluded that the technique gives good and prolonged analgesia but is technically difficult, sometimes painful to perform and requires supplementary analgesia in the second stage. Hypotension was absent and Apgar scores were good.

INFILTRATION OF THE GROINS AND LUMBOSACRAL REGION

The pains of uterine contractions are referred to the lower abdomen, groins and lumbosacral region, mainly in the area of skin supplied by the eleventh and twelfth thoracic nerves and first lumbar nerves and occasionally in areas supplied by adjacent nerves. The extensive infiltration of up to 100 ml of a 0.5% solution of prilocaine or lignocaine may relieve the pains of labour. The technique was used by Abrams (1950) but success is uncertain and there is a rather high incidence of toxic reactions. Injections may have to be repeated during labour. The method is not recommended for general use. The local infiltration of the area of referred pain, associated with a persistent unblocked segment occurring during continuous epidural analgesia, has occasionally been successful in relieving pain.

REFERENCES

Abboud, T.K., Khoo, S.S., Miller, F., Doan, T. and Henrikson, E. (1982) Maternal, fetal and neonatal responses after epidural anesthesia with bupivacaine, 2-chloroprocaine or lidocaine. *Anesth. Analg.*, **61**, 638.

Abboud, T.K., Kim, K.C., Noueihed, R. et al (1983a) Epidural bupivacaine, chloroprocaine or lidocaine for Cesarean section, maternal and neonatal effects. *Anesth. Analg.*, **62**, 914.

Abboud, T.K., Sarkis, F., Ablikian, A. et al (1983b) Lack of adverse neonatal neurobehavioral effects of lidocaine. *Anesth. Analg.*, **62**, 473.

Abboud, T.K., Afrasiabi, A., Sarkis, F. et al (1984) Continuous infusion of epidural analgesia in parturients receiving bupivacaine, chloroprocaine or lidocaine—maternal, fetal and neonatal effects. *Anesth. Analg.*, **63**, 421.

Abouleish, E. (1978) Epidural blood patch for the treatment of chronic post-lumbar-puncture cephalgia. *Anesthesiology*, **49**, 291.

Abouleish, E. and Bourke, D. (1984) Concerning the use and abuse of test doses for epidural anesthesia. *Anesthesiology*, **61**, 344.

Abouleish, E., Wadhwa, R.K., DeLa Vega, S., Tan, R.N. and Uy, N.T.L. (1975) Regional analgesia following epidural blood patch. *Anesth. Analg. curr. Res.*, **54**, 634.

Abrams, A.A. (1950) Obliteration of pain at the site of reference by infiltration anesthesia in the first stage of labor. *New Engl. J. Med.*, **243**, 636.

Akamatsu, T.J. and Bonica, J.J. (1975) Extradural analgesia for labor and vaginal delivery. In *Clinics in Obstetrics and Gynaecology: Obstetric Anaesthesia and Analgesia*, **2**, 605. London: W.B. Saunders.

Albright, G.A. (1984) Epinephrine should be used with the therapeutic dose of bupivacaine in obstetrics. *Anesthesiology*, **61**, 217.

Alexander, B. (1955) Coagulation—hemorrhage and thrombosis. *New Engl. J. Med.*, **252**, 432.

Amias, A.G. (1970) Cerebral vascular disease in pregnancy. 1. Haemorrhage. *J. Obstet. Gynaec. Br. Commonw.*, **77**, 110.

Antoine, C. and Young, B.K. (1982) Fetal lactic acidosis with epidural anesthesia. *Am. J. Obstet. Gynec.*, **142**, 55.

Arner, O. (1952) Complications following spinal anesthesia. *Acta chir. scand.*, Suppl. **167**.

Asling, J.H., Shnider, S.M., Margolis, A.J., Wilkinson, G.L. and Way, E.L. (1970) Paracervical block anesthesia in obstetrics. *Am. J. Obstet. Gynec.*, **107**, 626.

Assali, N.S. and Prystowsky, H. (1950) Studies on autonomic blockade. I. Comparison between the effects of tetraethylammonium chloride and high selective spinal anesthesia on the blood pressure of normal and toxemic pregnancy. *J. clin. Invest.*, **29**, 1354.

Baggish, M. (1964) Continuous paracervical block. *Am. J. Obstet. Gynec.*, **88**, 968.

Baheti, D.K., Pandit, S.K., Devi, P.K. and Mirakhur, R.K. (1975) Epidural analgesia with left lateral tilt for Caesarean section. *Anaesthesia*, **30**, 396.

Baken, M. jr., Freeman, D. and Barno, A. (1962) Transvaginal regional blocks. *Surg. Gynec. Obstet.*, **114**, 375.

Bali, I.M. (1984) Epidural blood patch. *Anaesthesia*, **39**, 718.

Ballin, N.C. (1981) Paraplegia following epidural analgesia. *Anaesthesia*, **36**, 952.

Bamford, D., Sibley, W. and Laguna, J. (1978) Anaesthesia in multiple sclerosis. *Can. J. Neurol. Sci.*, **5**, 41.

Bart, A.J. and Wheeler, A.S. (1978) Comparison of saline placement and epidural blood placement in the treatment of post-lumbar-puncture headache. *Anesthesiology*, **48**, 221.

Batra, M.S., Bridenbough, L.D., Caldwell, R.B. et al (1984) Bupivacaine cardiotoxicity in a patient with mitral valve prolapse: an example of improperly administered epidural block. *Anesthesiology*, **60**, 170.

Beazley, J.M., Leaver, E.P., Morewood, J.H.M. and Bircumshaw, J. (1967) Relief of pain in labour. *Lancet*, **i**, 1033.

Beazley, J.M., Taylor, G. and Reynolds, F. (1972) Placental transfer of bupivacaine after paracervical block. *Obstet. Gynec.*, **39**, 2.

Belfrage, P., Berlin, A., Lindstedt, M. and Raabe, N. (1973) Plasma levels of bupivacaine following pudendal block in labour. *Br. J. Anaesth.*, **45**, 1067.

Billewicz-Driemel, A.M. and Milne, M.D. (1976) Long-term assessment of extradural analgesia for the relief of pain in labour. II. Sense of 'deprivation' after extradural analgesia in labour: relevant or not? *Br. J. Anaesth.*, **48**, 139.

Birkhahn, H.J. and Heifetz, M. (1961) A complication following epidural anesthesia. *Anesth. Analg. curr. Res.*, **40**, 650.

Black, M.G. (1949) Anatomic reasons for caudal anesthesia failure. *Anesth. Analg. curr. Res.*, **28**, 33.

Blogg, C.E. and Simpson, B.R. (1974) Obstetric analgesia and the newborn baby. *Lancet*, **i**, 1283.

Bonica, J.J. (1965) *Clinical Anesthesia: Obstetric Complications.* Oxford: Blackwell.

Bonica, J.J. (1967) *Principles and Practice of Obstetric Analgesia and Anesthesia*, vol. I. Oxford: Blackwell.

Bonica, J.J. (1970a,b) In *Obstetrical Anaesthesia: Current Concepts and Practice*, ed. Shnider, S.M., p. 75 and p. 174. Baltimore: Williams and Wilkins.

Bonica, J.J. (1979) Peripheral mechanisms and pathways of parturition pain. *Br. J. Anaesth.*, **51**, 38.

Bonica, J.J., Kennedy, W.F. jr., Akamatsu, T.J. and Gerbershagen, H.U. (1972) Circulatory effects of peridural block. III. Effects of acute blood loss. *Anesthesiology*, **36**, 219.

Booker, P.D., Wilkes, R.G. and Bryson, T.L.H. (1980) Obstetric pain relief using epidural morphine. *Anaesthesia*, **35**, 377.

Bowen-Simpkins, P. and Fergusson, I.L.C. (1974) Lumbar epidural block and the breech presentation. *Br. J. Anaesth.*, **46**, 420.

Bowsher, D. (1978) Pain pathways and mechanism. *Anaesthesia*, **33**, 935.

Boys, J.E. and Norman, P.F. (1975) Accidental subdural. *Br. J. Anaesth.*, **49**, 1111.

Brackbill, Y., Kane, J., Manniello, R.L. and Abramson, D. (1974) Obstetric meperidine usage and assessment of neonatal status. *Anesthesiology*, **40**, 116.

Bradbury, A.F., Smyth, D.G., Snell, C.R., Birdsall, N.J.M. and Hulme, E.C. (1976) C fragment lipoprotein has a high affinity for brain opiate receptors. *Nature (Lond)*, **260**, 793.

Braham, J. and Saia, A. (1958) Neurological complications of epidural analgesia. *Br. med. J.*, **ii**, 657.

Breeson, A., Kovacs, G.T., Pickles, B.G. and Hill, J.G. (1978) Epidural analgesia—the preferred method of analgesia for vaginal breech delivery. *Br. J. Anaesth.*, **50**, 1227.

Bridenbaugh, L.D., Moore, D.C., Bagdi, P. and Bridenbaugh, P.O. (1968) The position of plastic tubing in continuous block techniques: an x-ray study of 522 patients. *Anesthesiology*, **29**, 1047.

Bridenbaugh, P.O., Balfour, R.I., Bridenbaugh, L.D. and Lysons, D.F. (1976) Bupivacaine and etidocaine for intra-abdominal pelvic surgery, a double-blind study. *Anesthesiology*, **45**, 560.

Brindle Smith, G. Barton, F.L. and Watt, J.M. (1984) Extensive spread of local anaesthetic solution following subdural injection of an epidural catheter in labour. *Anaesthesia*, **39**, 355.

British Medical Journal (1975) Leading article. Lumbar Puncture. *Br. med. J.*, **i**, 3.

Bromage, P.R. (1954) *Spinal Epidural Analgesia.* Edinburgh: Livingstone.

Bromage, P.R. (1962) Spread of analgesic solutions in the epidural space and their site of action. *Br. J. Anaesth.*, **34**, 61.

Bromage, P.R. (1969) An evaluation of bupivacaine in epidural analgesia for obstetrics. *Can. Anaesth. Soc. J.*, **16**, 46.

Bromage, P.R. (1972) Unblocked segments in epidural analgesia for relief of pain in labour. *Br. J. Anaesth.*, **44**, 676.

Bromage, P.R. (1978) *Epidural Analgesia.* Philadelphia: W.B. Saunders.

Bromage, P.R., Datta, S. and Dunford, L.A. (1974) Etidocaine: an evaluation in epidural analgesia for obstetrics. *Can. Anaesth. Soc. J.*, **21**, 535.

Bromage, P.R., Camporesi, E. and Chestnut, D. (1980) Epidural narcotics for postoperative pain. *Anesth. Analg.*, **59**, 473.

Bromage, P.R., Camporesi, E., Durrant, P.A.C. and Neilson, C.H. (1982) Non-respiratory side effects of epidural morphine. *Anesth. Analg.*, **61**, 491.

Brown, R.A. and Politi, V.L. (1979) Knotting of an epidural catheter: a case report. *Can. Anaesth. Soc. J.*, **26**, 142.

Brown, D.T. Beamish, D. and Wildsmith, J.A.W. (1981) Allergic reaction to an amide local anaesthetic. *Br. J. Anaesth.*, **53**, 435.

Brudenell, M. and Chakravarti, S. (1975) Uterine rupture in labour. *Br. med. J.*, **ii**, 122.

Brunke, S.F. and Delle, M. (1974) Morphine metabolism in man. *Clin. Pharmac. Ther.*, **16**, 51.

Burchell, R. and Sadove M. (1964) Continuous paracervical block in obstetrics. *Obstet. Gynec.*, **23**, 112.

Burt, R.A.P. (1971) The foetal and maternal pharmacology of some drugs used for the relief of pain in labour. *Br. J. Anaesth.*, **43**, 824.

Bush, R.C. (1959) Caudal analgesia for vaginal delivery. *Anesthesiology*, **20**, 31.

Butler, A.B. and Green, C.D. (1971) Haematoma following epidural anaesthesia. *Can. Anaesth. Soc. J.*, **17**, 635.

Caldeyro-Barcia, R. (1960) Effect of position changes on the intensity and frequency of uterine contractions during labor. *Am. J. Obstet. Gynec.*, **80**, 284.

Caldeyro-Barcia, R. and Alvarez, H. (1952) Abnormal uterine action in labour. *J. Obstet. Gynaec. Br. Emp*, **59**, 646.

Carbaat, P.A.T. and van Crevel, H. (1981) Lumbar puncture headache: a controlled trial on the preventive effects of 24 h bed rest. *Lancet*, **ii**, 1133.

Caritis, S.N., Abouleish, E., Edelstone, D.I. and Mueller-Heubach, E. (1980) Fetal acid base status following spinal or epidural anesthesia for Cesarean section. *Obstet. Gynec.*, **58**, 3.

Carlsson, C., Nybell-Lindahl, G. and Ingemarsson, I. (1980) Extradural block in patients who have previously undergone Caesarean section. *Br. J. Anaesth.*, **52**, 827.

Carrie, L.E.S. (1972) In *Proceedings of the Symposium on Epidural Analgesia in Obstetrics*, ed. Doughty, A., p. 99. London: Lewis.

Carrie, L.E.S. (1985) 0.75% bupivacaine. *Br. J. Anaesth.*, **57**, 241.

Carrie, L.E.S. and Mohan, J. (1976) Horner's syndrome following obstetric extradural block. *Br. J. Anaesth.*, **48**, 611.

Carter, A. (1984) A rare complication of extradural analgesia. *Anaesthesia*, **39**, 1033.

Caseby, N.G. (1974) Epidural analgesia for the surgical induction of labour. *Br. J. Anaesth.*, **46**, 747.

Chambers, W.A., Edstrom, H.H. and Scott, D.B. (1981) Effect of baricity on spinal anaesthesia with bupivacaine. *Br. J. Anaesth.*, **52**, 827.

Chambers, W.A., Sinclair, C.J. and Scott, D.B. (1981) Extradural morphine for pain after surgery. *Br. J. Anaesth.*, **53**, 921.

Chaplin, R.A. and Renwick, W.A. (1958) Lumbar epidural analgesia for vaginal delivery. *Can. Anaesth. Soc. J.*, **5**, 414.

Chatfield, W.R., Suter, P.E.N. and Kotonya, A.O. (1970) Paracervical block anaesthesia for the evacuation of incomplete abortion: a controlled trial. *J. Obstet. Gynaec. Br. Commonw.*, **77**, 462.

Christensen, V. (1980) Respiratory depression after extradural morphine. *Br. J. Anaesth.*, **52**, 841.

Cibils, L.A. and Santonja-Lucas, J.J. (1978) Clinical significance of fetal heart rate patterns during labor. III. Effect of paracervical block anesthesia. *Am. J. Obstet. Gynec.*, **130**, 95.

Cibils, L.A. and Spackman, T.J. (1962) Caudal analgesia in first stage labor. *Am. J. Obstet. Gynec.*, **84**, 1042.

Cibils, L.A., Pose, S.V. and Zuspan, F.P. (1962) Effect of L-norepinephrine infusion on uterine contractility and cardiovascular system. *Am. J. Obstet. Gynec.*, **84**, 307.

Clark, R.B., Thompson, D.S. and Thompson, C.H. (1976) Prevention of spinal hypotension association with Cesarean section. *Anesthesiology*, **45**, 670.

Cleland, J.G.P. (1933) Paravertebral anesthesia in obstetrics. *Surgery Gynec. Obstet.*, **57**, 51.

Cohen, S.E. and Woods, W.A. (1983) The role of epidural morphine in the post caesarean section patient: efficacy and the effects of bonding. *Anesthesiology*, **58**, 500.

Cole, P.V. (1964) Continuous epidural lignocaine: a safe method. *Anaesthesia*, **19**, 562.

Cole, P.V. and Nainby-Luxmoore, R.C. (1962) Respiratory volumes in labour. *Br. med. J.*, **i**, 118.

Cole, P.V., Crawford, J.S., Doughty, A.G. et al (1970) Specifications and recommendations for nitrous oxide/oxygen apparatus to be used in obstetric analgesia. *Anaesthesia*, **25**, 317.

Collier, C.B. (1982) Total spinal or massive subdural block? *Anaesthesia and Intensive Care*, **10**, 92.

Collins, K.M., Bevan, D.R. and Beard, R.W. (1978) Fluid loading to reduce abnormalities of fetal heart rate and maternal hypotension during epidural analgesia in labour. *Br. med. J.*, **ii**, 1460.

Conklin, K.A. and Ziadlou-Rad, F. (1983) Bupivacaine cardiotoxicity in a pregnant patient with mitral valve prolapse. *Anesthesiology*, **58**, 596.

Cooper, K. (1972) In *Proceedings of the Symposium on Epidural Analgesia in Obstetrics*, ed. Doughty, A., p. 82. London: Lewis.

Cooper, K. and Moir, J.C. (1963) Paracervical nerve block: a simple method of pain relief in labour. *Br. med. J.*, **i**, 1372.

Cooper, K., Gilroy, K.J. and Hurry, D.J. (1968) Paracervical block in labour using bupivacaine. *J. Obstet. Gynaec. Br. Commonw.*, **75**, 863.

Cornwall, R.D. and Dolan, W.M. (1975) Radicular back pain following lumbar epidural blood patch. *Anesth. Analg. curr. Res.*, **54**, 459.

Cousins, M.J. and Mather, L.E. (1984) Intrathecal and epidural administration of opioids. *Anesthesiology*, **61**, 276.

Cousins, M.J. and Wright, C.J. (1971) Graft, muscle and skin blood flow after epidural block in vascular surgical procedures. *Surgery Gynec. Obstet.*, **133**, 59.

Covino, B.J. (1983) Potential neurotoxicity of local anaesthetic agents. *Can. Anaesth. Soc. J.*, **30**, 111.

Covino, B.J., Marx, G.F., Finster, M. and Zsigmond, E.K. (1980) Prolonged sensory/motor deficits following inadvertent spinal anaesthesia. *Anesth. Analg.*, **59**, 399.

Cowles, G.T. (1965) Experiences with lumbar epidural blocks. *Obstet. Gynec.*, **26**, 734.

Craft, J.B., Epstein, B.S. and Coakley, C.S. (1972) Effect of lidocaine with epinephrine versus lidocaine (plain) on induced labor. *Anesth. Analg. curr. Res.*, **51**, 243.

Craft, J.B., Epstein, B.S. and Coakley, C.S. (1973) Prophylaxis of dural puncture headache with epidural saline. *Anesth. Analg. curr. Res.*, **52**, 228.

Craft, J.B., Roizen, M.F. Dao, S.D., Edward, M. and Gilman, R. (1982) A comparison of T4 and T7 dermatomal levels of analgesia for Caesarean section using the lumbar technique. *Can. Anaesth. Soc. J.*, **29**, 264.

Craig, D.B. and Habib, G.G. (1977) Flaccid paraparesis following obstetrical epidural anesthesia: possible role of benzyl alcohol. *Anesth. Analg. curr. Res.*, **56**, 219.

Crawford, J.S. (1965) *Principles and Practice of Obstetric Anaesthesia*, 2nd ed., p. 204. Oxford: Blackwell.

Crawford, J.S. (1972a) Lumbar epidural block in labour: a clinical analysis. *Br. J. Anaesth.*, **44**, 66.

Crawford, J.S. (1972b) *Principles and Practice of Obstetric Anaesthesia*, 3rd ed. Oxford: Blackwell.

Crawford, J.S. (1974) An appraisal of lumbar epidural blockade in patients with a singleton fetus presenting by the breech. *J. Obstet. Gynaec. Br. Commonw.*, **81**, 867.

Crawford, J.S. (1975a) Pathology in the extradural space. *Br. J. Anaesth.*, **47**, 412.

Crawford, J.S. (1975b) An appraisal of lumbar epidural blockade in labour in patients with multiple pregnancy. *Br. J. Obstet. Gynaec.*, **82**, 929.

Crawford, J.S. (1976) The epidural sieve and MBC (minimum blocking concentration): an hypothesis. *Anaesthesia*, **31**, 1277.

Crawford, J.S. (1978) *Principles and Practice of Obstetric Anaesthesia*, 4th ed. Oxford: Blackwell.

Crawford, J.S. (1979a) Continuous lumbar epidural analgesia for labour and delivery. *Br. med. J.*, **i**, 72.

Crawford, J.S. (1979b) Experience with spinal analgesia in a British obstetric unit. *Br. J. Anaesth.*, **51**, 531.

Crawford, J.S. (1980a) Experiences with epidural blood patches. *Anaesthesia*, **35**, 513.

Crawford, J.S. (1980b) The enigma of the missed segment. *Can. Anaesth. Soc. J.*, **27**, 594.

Crawford, J.S. (1983) Collapse after epidural injection following inadvertent dural perforation. *Anesthesiology*, **59**, 78.

Crawford, J.S. (1985) Bupivacaine toxicity. *Br. J. Anaesth.*, **57**, 240.

Crawford, J.S. and Tunstall, M.E. (1968) Notes on respiratory performance during labour. *Br. J. Anaesth.*, **40**, 612.

Crawford, J.S., Williams, M.E. and Veales, S. (1975) Particulate matter in the extradural space. *Br. J. Anaesth.*, **47**, 807.

Crawford, J.S., James, F.M., Nolte, H., van Steenberge, A. and Shah, J.L. (1981) Regional anaesthesia for patients with chronic neurological disease and similar conditions. *Anaesthesia*, **36**, 821.

Cuerden, C., Buley, R. and Downing, J.W. (1977) Delayed recovery after epidural block in labour. *Anaesthesia*, **32**, 773.

Darby, S., Thornton, C.A. and Hunter, D.J. (1976) Extradural analgesia in labour when the breech presents. *Br. J. Obstet. Gynaec.*, **83**, 35.

Datta, S., Kitzmiller, J.L., Naulty, J.S., Ostheimer, G.W. and Wiess, J.B. (1982) Acid base status of diabetic mothers and their infants following spinal anesthesia for Cesarean section. *Anesth. Analg.*, **61**, 662.

David, H. and Rosen, M. (1976) Perinatal mortality after epidural analgesia. *Anaesthesia*, **31**, 1054.

Davies, A., Solomon, B. and Levene, A. (1958) Paraplegia following epidural anaesthesia. *Br. med. J.*, **ii**, 654.

Davis, F.O. and Fettes, I.W. (1981) A simple safe method for continuous infusion epidural analgesia. *Can. Anaesth. Soc. J.*, **28**, 484.

Dawkins, C.J.M. (1969) An analysis of the complications of extradural block. *Anaesthesia*, **24**, 554.

Dawkins, C.J.M. (1972) In *Proceedings of the Symposium on Epidural Analgesia in Obstetrics*, ed. Doughty, A., p. 67. London: Lewis.

De Angelis, J. (1972) Hazards of subdural and epidural anesthesia during anticoagulant therapy. *Anesth. Analg. curr. Res.*, **51**, 676.

De Jong, R.H. (1961) Anesthetic complications during continuous caudal analgesia for obstetrics. *Anesth. Analg. curr. Res.*, **40**, 384.

Department of Health and Social Security (1979) *Report on Confidential Enquiries into Maternal Deaths in England and Wales*. London: H.M.S.O.

Di Giovanni, A.J. and Dunbar, B.S. (1970) Epidural injection of autologous blood for postlumbar-puncture headache. *Anesth. Analg. curr. Res.*, **49**, 268.

Di Giovanni, A.J., Galbert, M.W. and Wahle, W.M. (1972) Epidural injection of autologous blood for postlumbar-puncture headache. *Anesth. Analg. curr. Res.*, **51**, 226.

Ditzler, J.W. and McIver, G. (1956) Paraplegia following general anaesthesia. *Anesth. Analg. curr. Res.*, **35**, 501.

Donnai, P. and Nicholas, A.D.G. (1975) Epidural analgesia, foetal monitoring and the condition of the baby at birth with breech presentation. *Br. J. Obstet. Gynaec.*, **82**, 360.

Doughty, A. (1969) Selective epidural analgesia and the forceps rate. *Br. J. Anaesth.*, **41**, 1058.

Doughty, A. (1972) In *Proceedings of the Symposium on Epidural Analgesia in Obstetrics*, ed. Doughty, A., p. 10. London: Lewis.

Doughty, A. (1974) A precise method of cannulating the lumbar epidural space. *Anaesthesia*, **29**, 63.

Doughty, A. (1975) Lumbar epidural analgesia—the pursuit of perfection. *Anaesthesia*, **30**, 741.

Doughty, A. (1978) Epidural analgesia in labour: the past, the present and the future. *J. R. Soc. Med.*, **71**, 879.

Doughty, A. (1978) The relief of pain in labour. In *A Practice of Anaesthesia*, ed. Churchill-Davidson, H.C., 4th ed. London: Lloyd-Luke.

Downing, J.W., Houlton, P.C. and Barclay, A. (1979) Extradural analgesia for Caesarean section: a comparison with general anaesthesia. *Br. J. Anaesth.*, **51**, 367.

Dripps, R.D. and Vandam, L.D. (1954) Long term follow-up of patients who received 10098 spinal anesthetics: failure to discover major neurological sequelae. *J. Am. med. Ass.*, **156**, 1486.

Ducrow, M. (1971) The occurrence of unblocked segments during continuous lumbar epidural analgesia for pain relief in labour. *Br. J. Anaesth.*, **43**, 1172.

Dumoulin, J.G. and Foulkes, J.E.B. (1984) Ketonuria during labour. *Br. J. Obstet. Gynaec.*, **91**, 97.

Dutton, D.A., Moir, D.D., Howie, H.B., Thorburn, J. and Watson, R. (1984) Choice of local anaesthetic drug for extradural caesarean section. *Br. J. Anaesth.*, **56**, 1361.

Edelist, G. and Perera, E. (1976) Comparison of etidocaine and lidocaine for obstetrical analgesia. *Can. Anaesth. Soc. J.*, **23**, 459.

Edmonds, J. (1972) In *Proceedings of the Symposium on Epidural Analgesia in Obstetrics*, ed. Doughty, A., p. 57. London: Lewis.

Egbert, L.D., Tamersoy, K. and Deas, T.C. (1961) Pulmonary function during spinal anesthesia. *Anesthesiology*, **22**, 882.

Ekblom, L. and Widman, B. (1966) LAC-43 and tetracaine in spinal anaesthesia. *Acta anaesth. scand.*, Suppl. XXIII, 419.

Elam, J.O. (1970) Catheter subarachnoid block for labor and delivery: a differential segmental technic employing hyperbaric lignocaine. *Anesth. Analg. curr. Res.*, **49**, 1007.

Ellis, G.J. and De Vita, M.R. (1962) Continuous caudal anesthesia in obstetrics by means of lidocaine 1 per cent. *Am. J. Obstet. Gynec.*, **84**, 1057.

Ericson, N.O. (1947) On frequency of complications, especially those of long duration after spinal anesthesia. *Acta chir. scand.*, **95**, 167.

Evans, J.M. (1975) Horner's syndrome as a complication of epidural block. *Anaesthesia*, **30**, 774.

Evans, T.N., Morley, G.W. and Helder, L. (1962) Caudal anesthesia in obstetrics. *Obstet. Gynec.*, **20**, 726.

Feeny, J.G. (1982) Water intoxication and oxytocin. *Br. med. J.*, **285**, 243.

Finster, M., Poppers, P.J., Sinclair, J.C., Morishima, H.O. and Daniels, S.S. (1965) Accidental intoxication of the fetus with local anesthetic drug during caudal anesthesia. *Am. J. Obstet. Gynec.*, **92**, 922.

Finucane, B.T. (1979) Safety of double-orifice epidural catheters. *Can. Anaesth. Soc. J.*, **26**, 146.

Fisher, A. and Prys-Roberts, C. (1968) Maternal pulmonary gas exchange. *Anaesthesia*, **23**, 350.

Forthman, H.J. and Adriani, J. (1957) Blood pressure changes during cesarean section. *Anesth. Analg. curr. Res.*, **36**, 63.

Fortuna, G. (1981) Test doses. *Anesth. Analg.*, **60**, 616.

Fox, G.S. and Houle, G.L. (1971) Acid–base studies in elective caesarean sections during epidural and general anaesthesia. *Can. Anaesth. Soc. J.*, **18**, 60.

Freund, F.G., Bonica, J.J., Ward, R.J., Akamatsu, T.J. and Kennedy, W.F. (1967) Ventilatory reserve and level of motor block during high spinal and epidural anesthesia. *Anesthesiology*, **28**, 834.

Friedman, E.A. (1955) Primigravid labor: a graphico-statistical analysis. *Obstet. Gynec.*, **6**, 567.

Friedman, E.A. and Sachtleben, M.R. (1959) Caudal anesthesia. *Obstet. Gynec.*, **13**, 442.

Friedman, E.A., Schantz, S. and Pace, H.R. (1960) Continuous caudal analgesia and anesthesia in obstetrics. A critical evaluation of 510 cases. *Am. J. Obstet. Gynec.*, **80**, 1181.

Furgang, F.A. (1974) Glass particles in ampules. *Anesthesiology*, **41**, 525.

Galbert, M.W. and Marx, G.F. (1974) Extradural pressures in the parturient patient. *Anesthesiology*, **40**, 499.

Geerinckx, K., Vanderick, G., Van Steenberge, A.L., Bouche, R. and De Muylder, E. (1974) Bupivacaine 0.125% in epidural block analgesia during childbirth: maternal and foetal plasma concentrations. *Br. J. Anaesth.*, **46**, 939.

Gibbs, C.P. and Noel, S.C. (1977) Response of arterial segments from gravid human uterus to multiple concentrations of lignocaine. *Br. J. Anaesth.*, **49**, 409.

Gibbs, C.P., Spohr, L., Petrakis, J., Paulus, D. and Schultetus, R. (1981) Prevention of hypotension with hydration. *Anesthesiology*, **55**, A308.

Gibbs, C.P., Werba, J.V., Banner, R.C., James, C.F. and Hill, C.R. (1983) Leg wrapping prevents hypotension. *Anesthesiology*, **59**, A405.

Gingrich, T.F. (1968) Spinal epidural hematoma following epidural anesthesia. *Anesthesiology*, **29**, 162.

Gormley, J.B. (1960) Treatment of post spinal headache. *Anesthesiology*, **21**, 565.

Greene, N.M. (1961) Preganglionic sympathetic blockade in man: a study of spinal anaesthesia. *Acta anaesth. scand.*, **25**, 463.

Greensite, F.S. and Katz, J. (1980) Spinal subdural haematoma associated with epidural analgesia. *Anesth. Analg.*, **59**, 72.

Green, R. (1972) In *Proceedings of the Symposium on Epidural Analgesia in Obstetrics*, ed. Doughty, A., p. 47. London: Lewis.

Greiss, F.C. (1967) A clinical concept of uterine blood flow during pregnancy. *Obstet. Gynec.*, **30**, 595.

Greiss, F.C., Still, J.C. and Anderson, S.G. (1976) Effects of local anesthetic agent on the uterine vasculatures and myometrium. *Am. J. Obstet. Gynec.*, **124**, 889.

Grove, L.H. (1973) Backache, headache and bladder dysfunction after delivery. *Br. J. Anaesth.*, **45**, 1147.

Grundy, E.M., Rao, L. and Winnie, A.P. (1978) Epidural anesthesia and the lateral position. *Anesth. Analg. curr. Res.*, **57**, 95.

Grundy, E.M., Zamora, A.M. and Winnie, A.P. (1978) Comparison of spread of epidural anesthesia in pregnant and nonpregnant women. *Anesth. Analg. curr. Res.*, **57**, 544.

Gudgeon, D.H. (1968) Paracervical block with bupivacaine 0.25 per cent. *Br. med. J.*, **ii**, 403.

Gunther, R.E. and Bauman, J. (1969) Obstetrical caudal anesthesia. *Anesthesiology*, **31**, 5.

Gustaffsson, L.L., Schildt, B. and Jacobsen, K. (1982) Adverse effects of extradural and intrathecal opiates: report on a nationwide survey in Sweden. *Br. J. Anaesth.*, **54**, 479.

Gutsche, B.B. (1976) Prophylactic ephedrine preceding spinal anesthesia for Cesarean section. *Anesthesiology*, **45**, 462.

Hargrove, R.L. (1981) The neurological complications of spinal and epidural analgesia. *Anaesthesia*, **36**, 454.

Heavner, J.E. and De Jong, R.H. (1974) Lidocaine blocking concentrations for B- and C-nerve fibres. *Anesthesiology*, **40**, 228.

Hehre, F.W. and Sayig, J.M. (1960) Continuous lumbar peridural anesthesia in obstetrics. *Am. J. Obstet. Gynec.*, **80**, 1173.

Hellman, K. (1965) Epidural anaesthesia in obstetrics: a second look at 26 127 cases. *Can. Anaesth. Soc. J.*, **12**, 398.

Helperin, S.W. and Cohen, D.D. (1971) Hematoma following epidural anesthesia: report of a case. *Anesthesiology*, **35**, 641.

Heyman, H.J., Salem, M.R. and Klimov, I. (1982) Persistent sixth cranial nerve paresis following blood patch for post dural puncture headache. *Anesth. Analg.*, **61**, 948.

Hill, E.C. (1962) Maternal obstetric paralysis. *Am. J. Obstet. Gynec.*, **38**, 1452.

Hilton-Jones, D., Harrad, R.A., Gill, M.W. and Warlow, C.P. (1982) Failure of postural manoevres to prevent lumbar puncture headache. *J. Neurol. Neurosurg. Psychiat.*, **45**, 743.

Hingson, R.A. and Edwards, W.B. (1942) Continuous caudal anesthesia during labour and delivery. *Anesth. Analg. curr. Res.*, **21**, 301.

Hingson, R.A. and Hellman, L.M. (1956) *Anesthesia for Obstetrics*, p. 251. Philadelphia: Lippincott.

Hingson, R.A., Cull, W.A. and Benzinger, M. (1961) Continuous caudal analgesia in obstetrics. *Anesth. Analg. curr. Res.*, **40**, 119.

Hodgkinson, R.J. (1981) Total spinal block after epidural injection into an interspace adjacent to an inadvertent dural perforation. *Anesthesiology*, **55**, 593.

Holdcroft, A. and Morgan, M. (1974) An assessment of the analgesic effect in labour of pethidine and 50 per cent nitrous oxide in oxygen (Entonox). *J. Obstet. Gynaec. Br. Commonw.*, **81**, 603.

Hollmen, A.I., Jouppila, R., Koivisto, M. et al (1978) Neurologic activity of infants following anesthesia for Cesarean section. *Anesthesiology*, **48**, 350.

Holmes, F. (1960) Incidence of the supine hypotensive syndrome in late pregnancy. *J. Obstet. Gynaec. Br. Emp.*, **67**, 254.

Hoult, I.J., MacLennan, A.H. and Carrie, L.E.S. (1977) Lumbar epidural analgesia in labour: relation to fetal malposition and instrumental delivery. *Br. med. J.*, **i**, 14.

Humphrey, M.D., Chang, A., Wood, E.C., Morgan, S. and Hounslow, D. (1974) A decrease in fetal pH during the second stage of labour when conducted in the dorsal position. *J. Obstet. Gynaec. Br. Commonw.*, **81**, 600.

Hunter, A.R. and Moir, D.D. (1979) Maternity services and the anaesthetist. *Br. J. Anaesth.*, **51**, 169.

Husemeyer, R.P. (1983) Epidural analgesia and assisted delivery. *Br. J. Obstet. Gynaec.*, **90**, 594.

Husemeyer, R.P. and Crawley, J.C.W. (1979) Placental intervillous blood flow measured by inhaled ^{133}Xe clearance in relation to induction of epidural analgesia. *Br. J. Obstet. Gynaec.*, **86**, 426.

Husemeyer, R.P., O'Conner, M.C. and Davenport, H.T. (1980) Failure of epidural morphine to relieve pain in labour. *Anaesthesia*, **35**, 161.

Husemeyer, R.P., Davenport, H.T., Cummings, A.J. and Rosankiewicz, J.R. (1981) Comparison of epidural and intramuscular pethidine for analgesia in labour. *Br. J. Obstet. Gynaec.*, **88**, 711.

Incaudo, G., Schatz, M., Patterson, R. et al (1978) Administration of local anesthetics to patients with a history of prior adverse reaction. *J. Allergy clin. Immunol.*, **61**, 339.

Jack, T.M. (1979) Post-partum intracranial subdural haematoma: a possible complication of epidural analgesia. *Anaesthesia*, **34**, 176.

Jacobson, J., MacCabe, J.J. and Harris, P. (1966) Spontaneous spinal epidural haemorrhage during anticoagulation therapy. *Br. med. J.*, **i**, 522.

Jagerhorn, M. (1975) Paracervical block in obstetrics: an improved injection method. *Acta obstet. gynec. scand.*, **54**, 9.

James, F.M., Crawford, J.S., Davies, P. and Naiem, H. (1977) Lumbar epidural analgesia for labor and delivery of twins. *Am. J. Obstet. Gynec.*, **127**, 176.

Jaschevatzky, O.E., Shalit, A., Levy, Y. and Grunstein, S. (1977) Epidural analgesia during labour in twin pregnancy. *Br. J. Obstet. Gynaec.*, **84**, 327.

Johnson, G.T. and Clayton, S.G. (1955) Studies in placental action during prolonged dysfunctional labours using radioactive sodium. *J. Obstet. Gynaec. Br. Emp.*, **62**, 513.

Jones, M.D. and Newton, T.H. (1963) Inadvertent extra-arachnoid injection in myelography. *Radiology*, **80**, 818.

Jones, R.J. (1974) The role of recumbency in the prevention and treatment of postspinal headache. *Anesth. Analg. curr. Res.*, **53**, 788.

Jorgenson, B.C., Anderson, H.B. and Engquist, A. (1981) CSF and plasma morphine after epidural and intrathecal application. *Anesthesiology*, **55**, 714.

Jouppila, P., Jouppila, R., Kaar, K. and Merila, M. (1977) Fetal heart rate patterns and uterine activity after segmental epidural analgesia. *Br. J. Obstet. Gynaec.*, **84**, 481.

Jouppila, R., Jouppila, P., Hollmen, A. and Kuikka, J. (1978a) Effect of segmental extradural analgesia on placental blood flow during normal labour. *Br. J. Anaesth.*, **50**, 563.

Jouppila, R., Jouppila, P., Kuikka, J. and Hollmen, A. (1978b) Placental blood flow during Caesarean section under lumbar extradural analgesia. *Br. J. Anaesth.*, **50**, 275.

Jouppila, R., Jouppila, P., Karinen, J.-M. and Hollmen, A. (1979) Segmental epidural analgesia in labour: related to the progress of labour, fetal malposition and instrumental delivery. *Acta obstet. gynec. scand.*, **59**, 135.

Justins, D.M., Francis, D., Houlton, P.G. and Reynolds, F. (1982) A controlled trial of epidural fentanyl. *Br. J. Anaesth.*, **54**, 409.

Kafer, E.R., Brown, J.T., Scott, D. et al (1983) Biphasic ventilatory response to CO_2 followig epidural morphine. *Anesthesiology*, **58**, 418.

Kane, R.E. (1981) Neurological deficits after spinal and epidural anaesthesia. *Anesth. Analg.*, **60**, 150.

Kang, Y.G., Abouleish, E. and Caritis, S. (1982) Prophylactic intravenous ephedrine infusion during spinal Cesarean section. *Anesth. Analg.*, **61**, 839.

Kenepp, N., Kumar, K., Shelley, W.C. et al (1982) Fetal and neonatal hazards of maternal hydration with 5% dextrose before Caesarean section. *Lancet*, **i**, 1150.

Kenepp, N.B., Cheek, T.G. and Gutsche, B.B. (1983) Bupivacaine continuous infusion epidural analgesia for labour. *Anesthesiology*, **59**, A407.

Kennedy, F., Effron, A.S. and Perry, G. (1950) Grave spinal cord paralyses caused by spinal anesthesia. *Surgery Gynec. Obstet.*, **91**, 385.

Kerr, M.G., Scott, D.B. and Samuel, E. (1964) Studies of the inferior vena cava in pregnancy. *Br. med. J.*, **i**, 532.

Kileff, M., James, F.M., Denan, D.M. and Floyd, H. (1984) Neonatal neurobehavioral responses after epidural anesthesia for Cesarean section using lidocaine or bupivacaine. *Anesth. Analg.*, **63**, 413.

Kitahata, L.M. and Collins, J.G. (1981) Spinal actions of narcotic analgesics. *Anesthesiology*, **54**, 153.

Kotelko, D.M., Shnider, S.M., Dailey, P.A. et al (1984) Bupivacaine induced cardiac arrythmia in sheep. *Anesthesiology*, **60**, 10.

Kritz, M. and Jouppila, R. (1980) Subarachnoid block after a 'top-up' dose during continuous segmental epidural analgesia in labour. *Acta anaesth. scand.*, **24**, 495.

Kuhnert, B.J., Harrison, M.J., Linn, P.L. and Kuhnert, P.M. (1984) Effects of maternal epidural anesthesia on neonatal behavior. *Anesth. Analg.*, **63**, 301.

Lake, N.C. (1958) Spinal anaesthesia: the present position. *Lancet*, **i**, 387.

Lancet (1975) Leading article. Diabetes and the fetus. *Lancet*, **i**, 669.

Lewis, M., Thomas, P. and Wilkes, R.G. (1983) Hypotension during epidural analgesia for Caesarean section. *Anaesthesia*, **38**, 250.

Li, D.F., Rees, G.A.D. and Rosen, M. (1985) Continuous extradural infusion of 0.0625% or 0.125% bupivacaine for pain relief in primigravid labour. *Br. J. Anaesth.*, **57**, 264.

Lindstrom, C. and Moore, D.C. (1957) Trends in obstetrical anesthesia following the acceptance of a twenty-four hour physician anesthesia service. *West. J. Surg. Obstet. Gyn.*, **65**, 63.

Liston, W.A., Adjepon-Yamoah, K.K. and Scott, D.B. (1973) Foetal and materal lignocaine levels after paracervical block. *Br. J. Anaesth.*, **45**, 750.

Littlepage, B.N.C., Daniel, D.G., Ahmad, S. and Turnbull, A.C. (1969) Paracervical block anaesthesia for minor gynaecological operations. *J. Obstet. Gynaec. Br. Commonw.*, **76**, 163.

Littlewood, D.G., Scott, D.B., Wilson, J. and Covino, B. (1977) Comparative anaesthetic properties of various local anaesthetic agents in extradural block for labour. *Br. J. Anaesth.*, **49**, 75.

Livnat, E.J., Fejgin, M., Scommegna, A., Bieniarz, J. and Burd, L. (1978) Neonatal acid–base balance in spontaneous and instrumental vaginal deliveries. *Obstet. Gynec.*, **52**, 549.

Loeser, E.A., Hill, G.A., Bennett, G.M. and Sederberg, J.H. (1978) Time vs success rate for epidural blood patch. *Anesthesiology*, **49**, 147.

Longmire, S. and Joyce, T.H. (1984) Durocutaneous fistula. *Anesthesiology*, **60**, 63.

Lundy, J.S., Essex, H.E. and Kernohan, J.W. (1933) Experiments with anesthetics, lesions produced in the spinal cord of dogs by a dose of procaine hydrochloride sufficient to cause permanent and fatal paralysis. *J. Am. med. Ass.*, **101**, 1546.

Mallampti, S.E., Liu, P.L. and Knapp, R.M. (1984) Convulsions and ventricular tachycardia from bupivacaine with epinephrine. *Anesth. Analg.*, **63**, 856.

Maltau, J.M. (1975) The frequency of fetal bradycardia during selective epidural anaesthesia. *Acta obstet. gynec. scand.*, **54**, 357.

Maresh, M., Choong, K.-H. and Beard, R.W. (1983) Delayed pushing with lumbar epidural in labour. *Br. J. Obstet. Gynaec.*, **80**, 623.

Marx, G.F. (1984) The plot thickens. *Anesthesiology*, **60**, 3.

Marx, G.F., Cosmi, E.V. and Wollman, S.B. (1969) Biochemical status and clinical condition of mother and infant at cesarean section. *Anesth. Analg. curr. Res.*, **48**, 986.

Marx, G.F., Luykx, W.M. and Cohen, S. (1984) Fetal–neonatal status following Caesarean section for fetal distress. *Br. J. Anaesth.*, **56**, 1004.

Mathru, M., Rao, T.L.K. and Kartha, R.K. (1980) Intravenous albumin administration for prevention of spinal hypotension during Caesarean section. *Anesth. Analg.*, **59**, 655.

Matouskova, A., Dottori, O., Forssman, L. and Victorin, L. (1975) An improved method of epidural analgesia with reduced instrumental delivery rate. *Acta obstet. gynec. scand.*, **54**, 231.

Matouskova, A., Hanson, B. and Elman, H. (1979) Continuous mini-infusion of bupivacaine into the epidural space during labour. III. A clinical study of 225 parturients. *Acta obstet. gynec. scand.*, **83**, 43.

Maycock, E. (1978) An epidural anaesthetic with unusual complications. *Anaesthesia and Intensive Care*, **6**, 263.

McGuiness, G.A., Merkow, A.J., Kennedy, R.L. and Erenberg, A. (1978) Epidural anesthesia with bupivacaine for Cesarean section. *Anesthesiology*, **49**, 270.

McKenzie, R. and Shaffer, W.L. (1978) A safer method for paracervical block in therapeutic abortions. *Am. J. Obstet. Gynec.*, **130**, 317.

Meehan, F.P., Moolgaoker, A.S. and Stallworthy, J. (1972) Vaginal delivery under caudal analgesia after caesarean section and other major uterine surgery. *Br. med. J.*, **ii**, 740.

Meeke, R. (1983) Hazards of lumbar puncture. *Br. med. J.*, **286**, 143.

Meguiar, R.V. and Wheeler, A.S. (1978) Lumbar sympathetic block with bupivacaine: analgesia for labor. *Anesth. Analg. curr. Res.*, **57**, 486.

Mendiola, J., Grylack, L.J. and Scanlon, J.W. (1982) Effects of intrapartum maternal glucose infusion on the normal fetus and newborn. *Anesth. Analg.*, **61**, 32.

Merry, A.F., Cross, J.A., Mayadeo, S.V. and Wild, C.J. (1983) Posture and spread of extradural analgesia in labour. *Br. J. Anaesth.*, **55**, 303.

Miller, F.C., Quesnel, G., Petrie, R.H., Paul, R.H. and Hon, E.H. (1978) The effects of paracervical block on uterine activity and beat-to-beat variability of the fetal heart rate. *Am. J. Obstet. Gynec.*, **130**, 284.

Milne, M.K. and Murray Lawson, J.I. (1973) Epidural analgesia for caesarean section. *Br. J. Anaesth.*, **45**, 1206.

Moir, D.D. (1963) Ventilatory function during epidural analgesia. *Br. J. Anaesth.*, **35**, 3.

Moir, D.D. (1970) Anaesthesia for caesarean section: an evaluation of a method using low concentrations of halothane and 50 percent oxygen. *Br. J. Anaesth.*, **42**, 136.

Moir, D.D. (1971) Recent advances in pain relief in childbirth. II. Regional anaesthesia. *Br. J. Anaesth.*, **43**, 849.

Moir, D.D. and Davidson, S. (1972) Postpartum complications of forceps delivery performed under epidural and pudendal nerve block. *Br. J. Anaesth.*, **44**, 1197.

Moir, D.D. and Hesson, W.R. (1965) Dural puncture by epidural catheter. *Anaesthesia*, **20**, 373.

Moir, D.D., McLaren, R. and Slater, P. (1974) Experience with carbonated lignocaine in obstetric epidural analgesia. *Anaesthesia*, **29**, 305.

Moir. D.D. and Mone, J.G. (1964) Acid–base balance during epidural analgesia. *Br. J. Anaesth.*, **36**, 480.

Moir, D.D., Slater, P.J., Thorburn, J., McLaren, R. and Moodie, J. (1976) Epidural analgesia in obstetrics: a controlled trial of carbonated lignocaine and bupivacaine HCl solutions, with and without adrenaline. *Br. J. Anaesth.*, **48**, 129.

Moir, D.D. and Thorburn, J. (1980) Epidural analgesia for Caesarean section: evaluation of an improved technique. In *Proceedings of the Second Symposium on Epidural Analgesia in Obstetrics, Coventry*, ed. Doughty, A. London: H.K. Lewis.

Moir, D.D., Victor-Rodrigues, L. and Willocks, J. (1972) Epidural analgesia during labour in patients with pre-eclampsia. *J. Obstet. Gynaec. Br. Commonw.*, **79**, 465.

Moir, D.D. and Wallace, G. (1967) Blood loss at forceps delivery. *J. Obstet. Gynaec. Br. Commonw.*, **74**, 424.

Moir, D.D. and Willocks, J. (1966) Continuous epidural analgesia in inco-ordinate uterine action. *Acta anaesth. scand.*, Suppl., **23**, 144.

Moir, D.D. and Willocks, J. (1967) Management of inco-ordinate uterine action under continuous epidural analgesia. *Br. med. J.*, **iii**, 396.

Moir, D.D. and Willocks, J. (1968) Epidural analgesia in British obstetrics. *Br. J. Anaesth.*, **40**, 129.

Moir, J.C. and Myerscough, P.R. (1971) *Munro Kerr's Operative Obstetrics*, 8th ed., p. 923. London: Baillière Tindall.

Moodie, J.E. and Moir, D.D. (1976) Ergometrine, oxytocin and epidural analgesia. *Br. J. Anaesth.*, **48**, 571.

Moore, D.C. (1955) *Complications of Regional Block*. Springfield, Ill.: Charles C. Thomas.

Moore, D.C. (1964) *Anesthetic Techniques for Obstetrical Anesthesia and Analgesia*. Springfield, Ill.: Charles C. Thomas.

Moore, D.C. (1969) *Regional Block*, 4th ed., p. 467. Springfield, Ill.: Charles C. Thomas.

Moore, D.C. (1980) Spinal anesthesia: bupivacaine compared with tetracaine. *Anesth. Analg.*, **59**, 743.

Moore, D.C. and Batra, M.S. (1981) Components of a test dose prior to epidural block. *Anesthesiology*, **55**, 693.

Moore, D.C. and Bridenbough, L.D. (1968) Present status of spinal (subarachnoid) and epidural (peridural) block. *Anesth. Analg. curr. Res.*, **47**, 40.

Moore, D.C., Mather, L.E., Bridenbough, L.D. et al. (1977) Bupivacaine (Marcaine): an evaluation of its tissue and systemic toxicity in humans. *Acta anaesth. scand.*, **21**, 109.

Moore, D.C., Bridenbough, L.D., Thompson, G.E., Balfour, R.I. and Horton, W.G. (1978) Bupivacaine: a review of 11,080 cases. *Anesth. Analg.*, **57**, 42.

Moore, J., Murnaghan, G.A. and Lewis, M.A. (1974) A clinical evaluation of the maternal effects of extradural analgesia for labour. *Anaesthesia*, **29**, 537.

Morgan, B., Bulpitt, C.J., Clifton, P. and Lewis, P.J. (1982) Effectiveness of pain relief in labour: a survey of 1000 mothers. *Br. med. J.*, **285**, 689.

Morikawa, K.I., Bonica, J.J., Tucker, G.T. and Murphy, T.M. (1974) Effect of acute hypovolaemia on lignocaine absorption and cardiovascular response following epidural block in dogs. *Br. J. Anaesth.*, **46**, 631.

Morishima, H.O., Daniel, S.S., Finster, M., Poppers, P.J. and James, L.S. (1966) Transmission of mepivacaine hydrochloride (Carbocaine) across the human placenta. *Anesthesiology*, **27**, 147.

Morishima, H.O., Pedersen, H., Finster, M. et al (1983) Is bupivacaine more toxic than lidocaine? *Anesthesiology*, **59**, A409.

Naulty, J.S. and Herold, R. (1978) Successful epidural anesthesia following epidural blood patch. *Anesth. Analg. curr. Res.*, **57**, 272.

Nellermoe, C.W., Moore, D.C., Bridenbaugh, L.D., Casady, G.N. and Braly, B. (1960) A clinical appraisal of 2-chloroprocaine in continuous caudal obstetrical anesthesia. *Anesthesiology*, **21**, 269.

Nicholas, A.D.G. (1972) In *Proceedings of the Symposium on Epidural Analgesia in Obstetrics*, ed. Doughty, A., p. 98. London: Lewis.

Noble, A.B. and Murray, J.J. (1971) A review of the complications of spinal anaesthesia with experience in Canadian teaching hospitals from 1959–1969. *Can. Anaesth. Soc. J.*, **18**, 5.

Nordberg, G., Hedner, T., Mellstrand, T. and Dahlstrom, B. (1983) Pharmacokinetic aspects of epidural morphine. *Anesthesiology*, **58**, 545.

Nyirjesy, I., Hawks, B.L., Herbert, J.E., Hopwood, H.G. and Falls, H.C. (1963) Hazards of the use of paracervical block anesthesia in obstetrics. *J. Am. Obstet. Gynec.*, **87**, 231.

Odoom, J.A. and Sih, I.L. (1983) Epidural analgesia and anticoagulant therapy. Experience with 1000 cases of continuous epidural. *Anaesthesia*, **38**, 254.

O'Driscoll, K., Meagher, D., MacDonald, D. and Geoghegan, F. (1981) Traumatic intracranial haemorrhage in first born infants and delivery with forceps. *Br. J. Obstet. Gynaec.*, **88**, 577.

Ostheimer, G.W., Palahniuk, R.J. and Shnider, S.M. (1974) Epidural blood patch for post-lumbar-puncture headache. *Anesthesiology*, **41**, 307.

Park, R. (1984) Migrating epidural cannula. *Anaesthesia*, **39**, 289.

Pathy, G.V. and Rosen, M. (1975) Prolonged block with recovery after extradural analgesia for labour. *Br. J. Anaesth.*, **47**, 520.

Pearce, J.M.S. (1982) Hazards of lumbar puncture. *Br. med. J.*, **285**, 1521.

Pearson, J.F. and Davies, P. (1973) The effect of continuous epidural analgesia on the acid–base status of maternal arterial blood during the first stage of labour. *J. Obstet. Gynaec. Br. Commonw.*, **80**, 218.

Pearson, J.F. and Davies, P. (1974). The effect of continuous lumbar epidural analgesia upon fetal acid–base status during the first stage of labour. *J. Obstet. Gynaec. Br. Commonw.*, **81**, 971.

Pearson, R.M.G. (1984) A rare complication of epidural analgesia. *Anaesthesia*, **39**, 460.

Peng, A.T.C., Shamsi, H.H., Blancato, L.S., Chervenak, F.A. and Castro, J.L. (1981) Euglycaemic hydration prior to epidural block for Caesarean section. *Anesthesiology*, **55**, A307.

Pert, C.B. and Snyder, S.H. (1973) Opiate receptors: demonstration in nerve tissue. *Science*, **179**, 1011.

Phillips, K.C. and Thomas, T.A. (1983) Second stage labour with or without extradural analgesia. *Anaesthesia*, **38**, 972.

Philips, O.C., Ebner, J., Nelson, A.T. and Black, M.H. (1969) Neurological complications following spinal anesthesia with lidocaine. *Anesthesiology*, **30**, 284.

Phillips, J.C., Hochberg, C.J., Petrakis, J.K. and Van Winkle, J.D. (1977) Epidural analgesia and its effects on the 'normal' progress of labor. *Am. J. Obstet. Gynec.*, **129**, 316.

Pose, S.V., Cibils, L.A. and Zuspan, F.P. (1962) Effect of L-epinephrine infusion on uterine contractility and the cardio-vascular system. *Am. J. Obstet. Gynec.*, **84**, 297.

Raabe, N. and Belfrage, P. (1976) Epidural analgesia in labour. IV. Influence on uterine activity and fetal heart rate. *Acta obstet. gynec. scand.*, **55**, 305.

Rainbird, A. and Pfitzner, J. (1983) Limitation of spread of analgesia after blood patch. *Anaesthesia*, **38**, 481.

Ralston, D.H., Shnider, S.M. and Lorimer, A.A. (1974) Effects of equipotent ephedrine, metaraminol, mephentermine and methoxamine on uterine blood flow in the pregnant ewe. *Anesthesiology*, **40**, 354.

Ramanathan, S., Chalon, J., Richards, M., Patel, K. and Turndorf, H. (1978) Prolonged spinal nerve involvement after epidural anesthesia with etidocaine. *Anesth. Analg. curr. Res.*, **57**, 361.

Ravindran, R.S. (1984) Epidural autologous blood patch on an out-patient basis. *Anesth. Analg.*, **63**, 692.

Ravindran, R.S., Albrecht, W.H. and Tasch, M. (1980) Low pressure headache after successful continuous epidural analgesia. *Anesth. Analg.*, **59**, 799.

Ravindran, R.S., Turner, M. and Muller, J. (1982) Neurological effects of subarachnoid administration of 2-chloroprocaine-CE, Bupivacaine and low pH normal saline in dogs. *Anesth. Analg.*, **61**, 279.

Ready, B., Plummer, M.H., Fink, B.R. and Sumi, S.M. (1983) Intrathecal local anesthetic toxicity in rabbits. *Anesthesiology*, **59**, A187.

Rees, G.A.D. and Rosen, M. (1979) Test dose in extradural analgesia. *Br. J. Anaesth.*, **51**, 71.

Reiz, S. and Westberg, M. (1980) Side effects of epidural morphine. *Lancet*, **i**, 203.

Reynolds, F. (1984) Bupivacaine and intravenous regional anaesthesia. *Anaesthesia*, **39**, 105.

Reynolds, F., Hargrove, R.L. and Wyman, J.B. (1973) Maternal and foetal plasma concentrations of bupivacaine after epidural block. *Br. J. Anaesth.*, **45**, 1049.

Ritmiller, L.F. and Rippman, E.T. (1957) Caudal analgesia in obstetrics: report of thirteen years experience. *Obstet. Gynec.*, **9**, 25.

Robinson, J.O., Rosen, M., Evans, J.M. et al (1980) Maternal opinion about analgesia for labour. *Anaesthesia*, **35**, 510.

Rogers, R.E. (1970) Fetal bradycardia associated with paracervical block anesthesia in labor. *Am. J. Obstet. Gynec.*, **106**, 913.

Rolbin, S.H., Cole, A.F.D., Hew, E.M., Pollard, A. and Virgint, S. (1982) Prophylactic IM ephedrine before epidural anaesthesia for Caesarean section: efficacy and actions on fetus and newborn. *Can. Anaesth. Soc. J.*, **29**, 148.

Rosen, M.A., Curtis, C.L., Shnider, S.M. et al (1983) Valuation of neurotoxicity after subarachnoid injection of large volumes of local anesthetic solutions. *Anesth. Analg.*, **62**, 802.

Rosenblatt, R., Wright, R., Denson, D.A. and Raj, P. (1983) Continuous epidural infusion for obstetric analgesia. *Req. Anaesthesia*, **8**, 10.

Rubin, A.P. (1972) In *Proceedings of the Symposium on Epidural Analgesia in Obstetrics*, ed. Doughty, A., p. 91. London: Lewis.

Rudehill, A., Gordon, E. and Rahn, T. (1983) Subdural haematoma. A rare but life-threatening complication after spinal anaesthesia. *Acta anaesth. scan.*, **27**, 376.

Russell, I.F. (1983) Spinal anaesthesia for Caesarean section; the use of 0.5% bupivacaine. *Br. J. Anaesth.*, **55**, 309.

Russell, I.F. (1985) High spread after 2 ml of bupivacaine plain solution. *Anaesthesia*, **40**, 199.

Russell, P.H. and Coakley, C.S. (1964) Re-evaluation of continuous caudal anesthesia for obstetrics. *Surgery Gynec. Obstet.*, **119**, 531.

Rutter, N., Spence, A., Mann, N. and Smith, M. (1980) Glucose during labour. *Lancet*, **ii**, 155.

Saady, A. (1976) Epidural abscess complicating thoracic epidural analgesia. *Anesthesiology*, **44**, 244.

Sadove, M.S. and Levin, M.J. (1954) Neurological complications of spinal anesthesia. *Illinois med. J.*, **105**, 169.

Salvatore, C.A., Cigivizzo, E. and Turatti, S. (1965) Breech delivery with saddle-block anesthesia. *Obstet. Gynec.*, **26**, 261.

Sanchez, R., Acuna, L. and Rocha, F. (1967) An analysis of the radiological visualization of the catheters placed in the epidural space. *Br. J. Anaesth.*, **39**, 485.

Santos, A., Pedersen, H., Finster, N. and Edstrom, H.H. (1984) Hyperbaric bupivacaine for spinal anesthesia in Caesarean section. *Anesth. Analg.*, **63**, 1009.

Scanlon, J.W., Brown, W.U., Weiss, J.B. and Alper, M.H. (1974) Neurobehavioral responses of newborn infants after maternal epidural anesthesia. *Anesthesiology*, **40**, 121.

Scanlon, J.W., Ostheimer, G.W., Lurie, A.O. et al (1976) Neurobehavioral responses and drug concentrations in newborns after maternal epidural anesthesia with bupivacaine. *Anesthesiology*, **45**, 400.

Schellenberg, J.C. (1977) Uterine activity during lumbar epidural analgesia with bupivacaine. *Am. J. Obstet. Gynec.*, **127**, 26.

Scott, D.B. and Walker, L.R. (1963) Administration of continuous epidural analgesia. *Anaesthesia*, **18**, 82.

Scudamore, J.H. and Yates, M.J. (1966) Pudendal block—a misnomer? *Lancet*, **i**, 23.

Sears, R.T. (1959) Use of spinal analgesia in forceps and breech deliveries. *Br. med. J.*, **i**, 755.

Seeds, A.E., Stein-Messinger, P. and Dorsey, M.J. (1962) Paracervical blocks: results of a double-blind evaluation. *Obstet. Gynec.*, **20**, 462.

Senties, G.L., Arellano, G., Casellas, F.A., Ontiveros, E. and Santos, J. (1970) Effects of some vasopressor drugs upon uterine contractility in pregnant women. *Am. J. Obstet. Gynec.*, **107**, 892.

Sharrock, N.E. (1979) Recordings of and an anatomical explanation for false positive loss of resistance during lumbar extradural analgesia. *Br. J. Anaesth.*, **51**, 253.

Shnider, S.M. and Way, E.L. (1968) Plasma levels of lidocaine (Xylocaine) in mothers and newborn following obstetrical conduction anesthesia. *Anesthesiology*, **29**, 951.

Sikh, S.S. and Agarwal, G. (1974) Post-spinal headache. A preliminary report on the effect of inhaled carbon dioxide. *Anaesthesia*, **29**, 297.

Sinclair, R.N. (1954) Ascending spinal paralysis following hysterectomy under general anaesthesia. *Anaesthesia*, **9**, 286.

Sinclair, J.C., Fox, H.A., Lentz, J.F., Fuld, C.L. and Murphy, J. (1965) Intoxication of the fetus by a local anesthetic. *New Engl. J. Med.*, **273**, 1173.

Skaredof, M.N. and Datta, S. (1981) Horner's syndrome during epidural anaesthesia for elective Caesarean section. *Can. Anaesth. Soc. J.*, **28**, 82.

Smith, F.R. (1980) Posture and headache after lumbar puncture. *Lancet*, **ii**, 1133.

Soni, N. and Holland, R. (1981) An extensive lumbar epidural block. *Anaesthesia and Intensive Care*, **9**, 150.

Spanos, W. and Steel, J.C. (1959) Uterosacral block. *Obstet. Gynec.*, **13**, 129.

Sreerama, V., Ivan, L.P., Dennery, J.M. and Richard, M.T. (1973) Neurosurgical complications of anticoagulant therapy. *Can. med. Ass. J.*, **108**, 305.

Stonham, J. and Moss, P. (1983) The optimal test dose. *Anesthesiology*, **58**, 389.

Studd, J.W., Crawford, J.S., Duignan, N.M., Rowbotham, C.J. and Hughes, A.O. (1980) The effect of lumbar epidural analgesia in the rate of cervical dilatation and the outcome of labour of spontaneous onset. *Br. J. Obstet. Gynaec.*, **87**, 1015.

Taylor, H.J.C. (1983) Clinical experiences with continuous infusion of bupivacaine at 6 ml/hr in obstetrics. *Can. Anaesth. Soc. J.*, **30**, 277.

Teramo, K. (1969) Foetal acid–base balance and heart rate during labour with bupivacaine paracervical block anaesthesia. *J. Obstet. Br. Commonw.*, **76**, 881.

Teramo, K. and Rajamaki, R. (1971) Foetal and maternal plasma levels of mepivacaine and foetal acid–base balance and foetal heart rate after paracervical block during labour. *Br. J. Anaesth.*, **43**, 300.

Thiery, M. and Vroman, S. (1972) Paracervical block analgesia during labor. *Am. J. Obstet. Gynec.*, **113**, 988.

Thomas, T.A., Fletcher, J.E. and Hill, R.G. (1982) Influence of medication, pain and progress in labour on plasma β endorphin-like immunoreactivity. *Br. J. Anaesth.*, **54**, 401.

Thompson, E.M., Wilson, C.M., Moore, J. and McClean, E. (1985) Plasma bupivacaine levels associated with extradural anaesthesia for Caesarean section. *Anaesthesia*, **40**, 427.

Thorburn, J. and Moir, D.D. (1981) Extradural analgesia: the influence of volume and concentration of bupivacaine on the mode of delivery, analgesic efficacy and motor block. *Br. J. Anaesth.*, **53**, 933.

Thorburn, J. and Moir, D.D. (1984) Bupivacaine toxicity in association with extradural analgesia for Caesarean section. *Br. J. Anaesth.*, **56**, 551.

Thorsen, G. (1947) Neurological complications after spinal anaesthesia. *Acta chir. scand.*, **46**, Suppl. 121.

Torda, T.A. and Pybus, D.A. (1981) Clinical experience with epidural morphine. *Anaesthesia and Intensive Care*, **9**, 129.

Tucker, G.T. Boyes, R.N., Bridenbaugh, P.O. and Moore, D.C. (1970) Binding of anilide-type local anesthetics in human plasma: relationships between binding, physicochemical properties and anesthetic activity. *Anesthesiology*, **33**, 287.

Tucker, G.T., Moore, D.C., Bridenbough, P.O., Bridenbough, L.D. and Thompson, G.E. (1972) Systemic absorption of mepivacaine in commonly used regional block procedures. *Anesthesiology*, **37**, 277.

Tunstall, M.E. (1972) In *Proceedings of the Symposium on Epidural Analgesia in Obstetrics*, ed. Doughty, A., p. 64. London: Lewis.

Tunstall, M.E. and Ramamoorthy, C. (1984) Continuous epidural infusion with 0.08% bupivacaine. *Anaesthesia*, **39**, 939.

Ueland, K., Akamatsu, T.J., Bonica, J.J. and Hansen, J.M. (1972) Cesarean section under epidural anesthesia without epinephrine. *Am. J. Obstet. Gynec.*, **114**, 775.

Urquhart-Hay, D. (1969) Paraplegia following epidural anaesthesia. *Anaesthesia*, **24**, 461.

Usubiaga, J.E., dos Reis and Usubiaga, L.E. (1970) Epidural misplacement of catheters and mechanisms of unilateral blockade. *Anesthesiology*, **32**, 158.

Vanderick, G., Geerinckx, K., Van Steenberge, A.L. and De Muylder, E. (1974) Bupivacaine 0.125% in epidural block analgesia during childbirth: clinical evaluation. *Br. J. Anaesth.*, **46**, 838.

Van Dorsten, J.P., Miller, F.C. and Yeh, S. (1981) Spacing the injection interval with paracervical block: a randomised study. *Obstet. Gynec.*, **58**, 696.

Varkey, G.P. and Brindle, G.F. (1974) Peridural anaesthesia and anticoagulant therapy. *Can. Anaesth. Soc. J.*, **21**, 106.

Vasicka, A. and Kretchmer, H.E. (1961) Effect of conduction and inhalational anesthesia on uterine contractions. *Am. J. Obstet. Gynec.*, **82**, 600.

Vasicka, A., Robertazzi, R., Raji, M. et al (1971) Fetal bradycardia and paracervical block. *Obstet. Gynec.*, **38**, 500.

Verniquet, A.J.W. (1980) Vessel puncture with epidural catheter. *Anaesthesia*, **35**, 660.

Wall, P.D. (1967) The laminar organization of dorsal horn and effects of descending impulses. *J. Physiol., Lond.*, **188**, 403.

Ward, C.F., Osborne, R., Beaumof, J.L. and Saidman, L.J. (1978) A hazard of double-orifice epidural catheters. *Anesthesiology*, **48**, 362.

Ward, R.J., Bonica, J.J., Freund, F.G. et al (1965) Epidural and subarachnoid anesthesia: cardiovascular and respiratory effects. *J. Am. med. Ass.*, **191**, 275.

Warren, T.M., Datta, S. and Ostheimer, G.W. (1982) Lumbar epidural anesthesia in patients with multiple sclerosis. *Anesth. Analg.*, **61**, 1022.

Weddel, S.J. and Ritter, R.R. (1981) Serum levels following epidural administration of morphine and correlation with relief of post surgical pain. *Anesthesiology*, **54**, 210.

Weekes, A.R.L., Cheridjian, V.E. and Mwanje, D.K. (1977) Lumbar epidural analgesia in labour in twin pregnancy. *Br. med. J.*, **ii**, 730.

Williams, B. (1969) The present place of spinal subarachnoid analgesia in obstetrics. *Br. J. Anaesth.*, **41**, 628.

Winer, B.M., Horenstein, S. and Starr, A.N. (1959) Spinal epidural haematoma during anticoagulation therapy. *Circulation*, **19**, 735.

Wollman, S.B. and Marx, G.F. (1968) Acute hydration for prevention of hypotension of spinal anesthesia in parturients. *Anesthesiology*, **29**, 374.

Wood, C., Ng, K.H., Hounslow, D. and Benning, H. (1973) Time—an important variable in normal delivery. *J. Obstet. Gynaec. Br. Commonw.*, **80**, 295.

Zuspan, F.P., Nelson, G.H. and Ahlquist, R.P. (1964) Epinephrine infusion in normal and toxemic pregnancy. *Am. J. Obstet. Gynec.*, **90**, 88.

8

The Selection of Anaesthesia

In this, as in other chapters, it is assumed that the reader has a basic knowledge of anaesthetics and obstetrics and therefore only selected aspects will be considered.

There are a number of obstetric procedures for which the anaesthetist is required to provide anaesthesia or analgesia and the selection of the most appropriate technique can sometimes influence the outcome for mother or child, perhaps even to the extent of determining survival. The obstetric anaesthetist should be competent in the techniques of general anaesthesia, inhalational analgesia, lumbar epidural and caudal analgesia and in subarachnoid analgesia. The obstetrician usually performs pudendal nerve blocks, paracervical blocks and local infiltration of the perineum. Midwives are permitted to infiltrate the perineum with local anaesthetic solution and to perform episiotomy. A few obstetricians have learned to perform epidural, caudal or subarachnoid blocks and they have usually done this where anaesthetists have not provided an epidural analgesia service (Cooper, 1972; Brown and Vass, 1977; Taylor et al, 1977). Any doctor who accepts responsibility for the safety of women in labour under epidural analgesia must be proficient in cardiopulmonary resuscitation. Accidental total subarachnoid block calls for intubation of the trachea, artificial ventilation and circulatory support as a matter of urgency.

Spontaneous delivery

In the UK spontaneous vertex deliveries are usually conducted by midwives and are generally managed with great expertise. Frequently neither the obstetrician nor the anaesthetist is directly involved in a normal delivery, so most British women at present receive a narcotic analgesic followed by inhalational analgesia in the second stage of labour. Some form of psychological preparation for labour is widely practised. When allowance is made for the duration of the second stage of labour and the occiput is anterior, then the neonatal acid–base status is similar after spontaneous delivery, low forceps delivery and vacuum extraction (Livnat et al, 1978). The woman's desire to have a spontaneous delivery should be taken into account when selecting the method of analgesia and delivery. Doughty (1969) has demonstrated that it is possible to achieve spontaneous delivery in about 80% of obstetrically normal patients by using a selective epidural block restricted to the eleventh and twelfth thoracic dermatomes and immediately adjacent

305

areas, and excluding the sacral nerve roots. With this selective block, analgesia of the lower birth canal is absent and reflex, involuntary, expulsive efforts are not abolished. Using 0.25% plain bupivacaine and placing the catheter tip close to the eleventh and twelfth thoracic nerve roots, instrumental delivery was required in only 15% of mothers (Matouskova et al, 1975). In sharp contrast the Oxford workers Hoult et al (1977) found that instrumental delivery was required in 70% of primigravidae and 40% of multigravidae who received epidural analgesia with 0.5% plain bupivacaine. There was a 20% incidence of rotational forceps delivery due, it was thought, to relaxation of the pelvic floor muscles. The concentration of the local anaesthetic solution, and therefore the incidence of motor blockade, clearly influences the method of delivery and a significant increase in rotational forceps deliveries is an important criticism of any technique of analgesia. An important variable is the duration of the second stage. In the absence of fetal distress, time will allow descent and possible rotation of the presenting part. The use of 0.25% bupivacaine is associated with an increased frequency of spontaneous delivery, a reduction in the frequency and severity of motor blockade and the provision of acceptable pain relief, although not as complete as that provided by the use of 0.5% bupivacaine (Thorburn and Moir, 1981). Maresh et al (1983) did not observe any increase in fetal acidosis if the onset of pushing was deliberately delayed to allow further descent of the presenting part in the second stage of labour. Recent work has emphasized the importance of avoiding caval occlusion during spontaneous delivery in the dorsal position. Quite severe falls in fetal pH were demonstrated during the second stage when the unmodified dorsal position was used. Elevation of the right buttock prevented fetal acidosis (Humphrey et al, 1974). Presumably the use of Sims' position would also prevent the adverse effects of caval occlusion on the fetus. Motor weakness, which is unwelcome to most mothers, can be minimized by the use of 0.25% or 0.375% bupivacaine plain (Crawford, 1975; Littlewood et al, 1977).

Forceps delivery

Pain during forceps delivery arises from the uterine contractions, from the descent of the fetal head and from the episiotomy. Regional analgesia can therefore only be completely effective when the eleventh and twelfth thoracic and first lumbar nerve roots and the second, third and fourth sacral nerve roots are blocked. Ideal conditions for forceps delivery require relaxation of the muscles of the pelvic floor and perineum. Hypotension, hypoxia and drug-induced respiratory depression must be avoided.

The following techniques are used for forceps delivery although not all of them are capable of fulfilling all the foregoing requirements:

Lumbar epidural analgesia.
Caudal analgesia.

Subarachnoid analgesia.
Pudendal nerve block.
Local infiltration.
General anaesthesia.

Lumbar epidural analgesia. If the patient has received continuous lumbar epidural analgesia with bupivacaine 0.5% earlier in labour then forceps delivery will be completely painless in 75% of patients and analgesia will be satisfactory in a further 18% (Moir et al, 1976). If 0.25% bupivacaine is used, 38% of mothers experience complete relief of pain and 41% find the analgesia provided helpful. This is significantly different from the effect produced by 0.5% bupivacaine, but linear analogue scores indicate a smaller difference than suggested by the proportion of patients experiencing complete relief of pain (Thorburn and Moir, 1981). A feeling of dragging or distension is quite common during an otherwise effective epidural block and can be eased by the administration of an analgesic concentration of nitrous oxide in oxygen. If perineal anaesthesia is absent when forceps delivery is to be undertaken then a further epidural injection of 4 or 5 ml of local anaesthetic solution should be made with the patient in a semi-sitting position. If immediate delivery is indicated, then the obstetrician should infiltrate the perineum with 1% lignocaine or prilocaine solution. Caval occlusion must be avoided by elevation of the right buttock in the lithotomy position.

One of the consequences of providing an epidural analgesia service is that a high proportion of the patients who require forceps delivery will already have received epidural analgesia in labour. This is because prolonged and painful labour, occipitoposterior position, incoordinate uterine action, pre-eclampsia and many medical diseases in which forceps delivery is often indicated are also conditions in which epidural analgesia is administered during labour. In the 1960s when only about 10% of the patients in the Queen Mother's Hospital, Glasgow, received continuous epidural analgesia in labour, single-shot lumbar epidural analgesia was quite frequently given in the second stage of labour for forceps delivery (see Figure 20). This practice has now been abandoned because almost all patients who require mid-cavity forceps delivery and forceps delivery with rotation of the fetal head have already received continuous epidural analgesia. Subarachnoid analgesia is preferred if a single-injection technique is indicated. The use of general anaesthesia for forceps delivery has been almost abandoned in the absence of a contraindication to local anaesthetic blocks in the Queen Mother's Hospital, Glasgow.

An intravenous infusion should be running during forceps delivery under conduction analgesia. The intravenous injection of ergometrine following forceps delivery under epidural analgesia is followed by retching, nausea or vomiting in about half of the patients who receive this drug. The substitution of an intravenous injection of 5 units of oxytocin (Syntocinon) followed by an infusion of 20 units of oxytocin in 500 ml of fluid is recommended as an

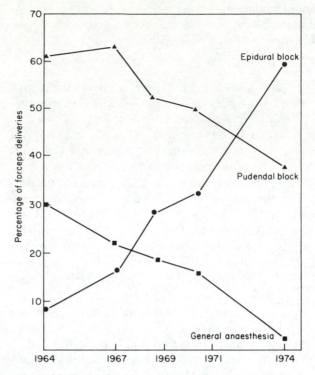

Figure 20. Percentage of forceps deliveries performed under epidural analgesia, pudendal nerve block and general anaesthesia in the Queen Mother's Hospital between 1964 and 1974.

effective and non-emetic uterine stimulant (Moodie and Moir, 1976). An intramuscular injection of Syntometrine 1 ml may also be used. Manual removal of the placenta can be performed under epidural block. Uterine retraction is usually excellent and blood loss is reduced (Moir and Wallace, 1967).

Caudal analgesia. Most of the preceding comments concerning lumbar epidural analgesia are applicable to the performance of forceps delivery under caudal analgesia. Perineal anaesthesia will always be present during a successful caudal block because the injection is made among the nerves of the cauda equina. It may sometimes be difficult to obtain upward spread to the lower thoracic nerve roots.

A single-injection caudal block is favoured by a few anaesthetists and obstetricians for forceps delivery. Failure is likely in 10% or more of patients, except in very experienced hands, and perhaps only then after prior exclusion of the obese or 'difficult' patients. When the fetal head is low in the pelvis there is a risk of direct injection of the fetus (Finster et al, 1965) and a rectal examination should be made in order to avoid this hazard. Where a single-injection technique is required to give rapid and effective analgesia and muscular relaxation, a subarachnoid block is a preferable alternative. A delay of 20 minutes before caudal analgesia develops is quite common.

Subarachnoid analgesia. It is arguable that subarachnoid analgesia is the technique of choice for forceps delivery when the patient has not already received continuous epidural analgesia. The analgesia of subarachnoid block is usually profound and is of rapid onset. Skeletal muscular relaxation is excellent and uterine retraction is powerful. Hypotension is unlikely to be a problem with the relatively limited blocks required for vaginal delivery, but is frequently associated with the extensive blocks required for Caesarean section.

Although outlet forceps delivery can be satisfactorily performed under saddle block (subarachnoid analgesia confined to the sacral nerve roots) the conditions for low- and mid-cavity forceps delivery and for rotation of the fetal head will be much improved if analgesia extends to the level of the tenth thoracic dermatome. As with epidural analgesia, so do some patients experience a sensation of distension or dragging during forceps delivery under subarachnoid analgesia and these patients may receive inhalational analgesia if required.

Where a full-time resident service exists for obstetric anaesthesia, then subarachnoid analgesia could be introduced with benefit to mothers, infants and obstetricians as a superior alternative to pudendal nerve block for use in the second stage of labour. Crawford (1979) argues for the reintroduction of subarachnoid analgesia into British obstetrics. If the patient does not have an epidural block, then subarachnoid analgesia is excellent for use in the second stage of labour. In the Queen Mother's Hospital subarachnoid analgesia is now used for 9% of forceps deliveries, although the majority of these deliveries are conducted under epidural analgesia. The persistent British resistance to spinal analgesia in obstetrics is difficult to justify in the light of greater understanding of the physiology of subarachnoid block, the inefficiency of pudendal nerve block and the hazards of general anaesthesia.

Pudendal nerve block and local infiltration. The regrettable frequency with which pudendal nerve block fails to reduce the pain for forceps delivery is being increasingly recognized. Scudamore and Yates (1966) demonstrated that half of all bilateral pudendal blocks were ineffective on one or both sides and suggested that the term pudendal nerve block was a misnomer. It is still only too often that one sees patients in obvious pain during forceps delivery under 'pudendal block'. Many of these deliveries appear to be conducted solely under the modicum of analgesia provided by the perineal infiltration which commonly accompanies pudendal nerve block. It is also, in the authors' experience, rather uncommon for obstetricians to allow time for pudendal nerve block to develop before proceeding with the delivery.

Ideally, therefore, pudendal nerve block should be replaced by a rapidly effective technique such as subarachnoid analgesia for mid- and low-cavity forceps deliveries. Outlet forceps delivery can be satisfactorily accomplished after local infiltration of the perineum and labia. Nevertheless, obstetricians will of choice or necessity continue to use pudendal nerve blocks, and where pain relief is absent or incomplete, the patient should receive supplementary inhalational analgesia. The pain of the uterine contractions is uninfluenced by pudendal nerve block. This pain may be relieved by paracervical block if this has been performed during the first stage of labour.

General anaesthesia. If general anaesthesia is used for forceps delivery then the technique should not differ in any way from the technique advocated for emergency caesarean section, because the risks of anaesthesia for mother and child are essentially the same whenever any emergency obstetric anaesthetic is administered. The patient should be in the laterally tilted supine position at induction of anaesthesia. Anaesthesia should not be induced in the lithotomy position because the intragastric pressure is further elevated in this position (Spence et al, 1967).

In many centres there has been a welcome reduction in the number of general anaesthetics administered for forceps delivery in recent years. This reduction is probably due mainly to an awareness of the risk of general anaesthesia among obstetricians and anaesthetists. A further reduction can be achieved by the provision of a satisfactory alternative to general anaesthesia. As Noble (1972) pointed out, the introduction of an epidural service can reduce the proportion of patients receiving general anaesthesia for forceps delivery to a fraction of 1% and this has also been our experience in the Queen Mother's Hospital (see Figure 20). Paradoxically therefore the provision of a high quality obstetric anaesthesia service reduces the demand for dangerous general anaesthetics and this is one of the benefits of an epidural service which is not always fully recognized.

It is important to respect the mother's wishes regarding the choice of anaesthetic technique. It is in her interest and those of the anaesthetist that the risks associated with general anaesthesia are explained in some detail. In the absence of an absolute contraindication to local blocks, the use of general anaesthesia should be discouraged. If anaesthesia is required for a 'trial' of forceps delivery, with the provision of suitable operating conditions for immediate caesarean section, epidural analgesia with lignocaine 2% with 1 : 200000 adrenaline will allow surgery within 30 minutes in over 50% of mothers. Fetal distress may call for immediate delivery, and Marx et al (1984) advocate the use of spinal anaesthesia as it offers speed, safety and better conditions for the baby. It is hoped that with the growing recognition of the need for training all junior anaesthetists in obstetric anaesthesia, anaesthetists will be experienced in the techniques of both epidural and subarachnoid blocks for labour and delivery. Anticipation of the need for perhaps urgent operative delivery should indicate the institution of epidural analgesia in labour.

Vacuum extraction

The vacuum extractor or ventouse is used to supplement the natural forces of parturition and, unlike the forceps, the vacuum extractor may be applied when the cervix is less than fully dilated. Many obstetricians require the patient to make expulsive efforts in time with her uterine contractions and the pull of the vacuum extractor. The patient should therefore be conscious, free of pain and cooperative. Delivery by the ventouse frequently takes longer than delivery by forceps. These factors, together with the well-recognized risks of vomiting and regurgitation, contraindicate the use of general anaesthesia. Epidural analgesia with dilute solutions will provide good conditions although it may be difficult to eliminate pain without some impairment of voluntary effort. If spinal anaesthesia eliminates pain, muscle tone will also be lost and patient cooperation will be less effective. Pudendal nerve blocks, when successful, will relieve the pain of delivery but not the pain of the contractions. Inhalational analgesia may be administered during painful contractions.

Assisted breech delivery

Breech delivery presents many problems to obstetricians and anaesthetists and most of these problems are related to the hazards of breech delivery for the infant. Some experienced obstetricians now consider that the dangers of vaginal breech delivery are sufficiently great to justify delivery by elective caesarean section in the fetal interest in every case where the infant is normal and presents by the breech. About 3% of infants would come into this category. Breech deliveries account for 0.6% of all vaginal deliveries in the Queen Mother's Hospital, the majority being delivered by caesarean section. Almost every obstetrician now advocates elective caesarean section if there is any suspicion of cephalopelvic disproportion. Caesarean section is often preferred if the infant is premature or weighs under 2.5 kg and presents by the breech (Lyons and Papsin, 1978). Preterm infants who underwent vaginal breech delivery had a neonatal mortality rate of 14.6% and a 24% incidence of neurological or developmental abnormality at one year of age. Comparable infants delivered electively by caesarean section had a 4.8% neonatal mortality and a 2.5% incidence of abnormality at one year (Ingemarrson et al, 1978). Caesarean section should therefore be freely used (Lyons and Papsin, 1978).

Although the uncorrected perinatal mortality for breech delivery is high, many of the infants die as the result of prematurity or fetal abnormality, conditions which are commonly associated with breech presentation. It is postulated that assisted breech delivery may carry an acceptable perinatal mortality and morbidity when skilfully performed, when the infant is normal and mature, when the pelvis is adequate, when the mother is cooperative and free of pain and when the obstetrician is willing to perform caesarean section at any stage in the labour.

The following are among the requirements for assisted breech delivery:

A skilled obstetrician.
A skilled anaesthetist.
A pain-free, conscious, calm and cooperative mother who is capable of voluntary expulsive efforts.
Absence of cephalopelvic disproportion.
Good uterine action, augmented if necessary by oxytocin.

Whatever method of pain relief is selected there should be a competent anaesthetist and obstetrician present at every breech delivery. Assisted breech delivery is no longer a procedure for the house surgeon or midwife. The anaesthetist should be in the delivery room and be fully prepared to administer anaesthesia immediately. The fact that his services may not always be utilized should be a cause for relief rather than resentment to the anaesthetist.

The choice of anaesthesia for assisted breech delivery has for long been heavily influenced by the fear of abolishing the mother's expulsive efforts lest this should necessitate delivery by breech extraction, a procedure carrying a high perinatal mortality. Many anaesthetists and obstetricians have avoided epidural, caudal and subarachnoid analgesia because it was believed that the associated perineal anaesthesia would abolish the involuntary, reflex expulsive effects of the second stage. Although this effect does occur in some women, the ability to perform voluntary expulsive efforts is not lost. Moreover there will usually be a need for perineal analgesia for the performance of episiotomy at delivery of the buttocks. The importance of maternal effort may have sometimes been exaggerated because it is principally uterine action which produces descent of the presenting part. Failure of descent is likely to be attributable to poor uterine action or to mechanical difficulty associated with disproportion. Uterine action may be improved by oxytocin, and the obstetrician must be prepared to perform caesarean section even in the second stage in case of hitherto unsuspected disproportion.

Crawford (1974) has used continuous lumbar epidural analgesia for 56 vaginal breech deliveries and has found that the incidence of severe and prolonged neonatal depression was reduced among normal and low birthweight infants. The satisfactory condition of most of these infants was attributed mainly to the ability to perform a careful, controlled assisted breech delivery without trauma to the infant because the mother was calm, relaxed and free of pain. Although perineal anaesthesia was usually present, the second stage of labour was prolonged only slightly and the number of breech extractions was not increased. Bowen-Simpkins and Fergusson (1974) used epidural analgesia for 72 breech deliveries and agree that epidural analgesia is the technique of choice, even though the second stage may be prolonged. Donnai and Nicholas (1975) have used epidural analgesia for 138 singleton breech labours with benefit for the fetus. Conditions for delivery were excellent and breech extraction was required in only 6% of patients. Continuous fetal heart monitoring was helpful and some doubt was cast on the validity of fetal blood sampling from the breech. Continuous lumbar epidural analgesia was used by Breeson et al (1978) for 51 breech presentations. Labour was not prolonged, the frequency of breech extraction was decreased and the condition of the infants was improved as assessed by fetal blood sampling during labour and the Apgar score at delivery. Caesarean section was performed in 15 cases (29%) during labour. These writers also strongly recommend epidural analgesia.

Others have advocated the use of conduction analgesia for breech delivery (Daily and Rogers, 1957; Boyson and Simpson, 1960; Bonica, 1965; Salvatore et al, 1965) and it is now the author's opinion that continuous epidural analgesia is positively indicated and should be initiated early in labour. Where this has not been done, then subarachnoid or epidural block may be performed when the cervix is fully dilated. Occasionally a woman whose infant presents by the breech will make repeated expulsive efforts at a relatively early stage in labour. These efforts are exhausting to the mother and may cause oedema of the cervix and even harm the infant. These premature expulsive efforts are prevented or abolished by epidural analgesia. The use of epidural analgesia eliminates the hazardous induction of general anaesthesia for the delivery of the aftercoming head, which is sometimes requested by the obstetrician when less effective methods of analgesia are employed.

Alternative techniques include the use of pudendal nerve block and local infiltration for episiotomy and delivery of the body. Supplementary inhalational analgesia will usually be helpful. Nevertheless the conditions for atraumatic delivery of the head may be far from ideal. Controlled delivery of the head is the key to successful breech delivery and for this reason it may be necessary to administer general anaesthesia. The dangers of inducing 'instant' anaesthesia in the lithotomy position while the mother struggles in pain and her infant is half-delivered are very real. The procedure calls for expert anaesthesia and the technique used should be that advocated for forceps delivery and caesarean sections.

Many obstetricians are turning to caesarean section as the preferred method of breech delivery for all patients. This inevitably impairs the teaching and experience of junior obstetricians in the management of vaginal breech delivery. Some obstetricians may never acquire the skill to perform vaginal breech deliveries with confidence. Caesarean section is widely regarded as a safe and relatively simple operation. It is, however, not as safe for the mother as vaginal delivery, as the morbidity and mortality associated with caesarean section is considerably in excess of that relating to vaginal delivery. Understandably, no satisfactorily conclusive study has been performed, and the obstetrician faces the uncomfortable dilemma that whatever method of delivery is chosen in the interests of the one patient, the baby or the mother, it may not be in the best interests of the other.

Breech extraction

When internal version and breech extraction are to be performed, it is usually advisable to perform these procedures under general anaesthesia. Uterine relaxation may be required and can be obtained by the addition of 2% of halothane to the nitrous oxide and oxygen mixture. The use of halothane in this concentration carries a risk of promoting atonic postpartum haemorrhage and maternal hypotension, and these risks must be weighed against the value of uterine relaxation. Certainly halothane should be administered in a 2% concentration for the shortest possible time during the intrauterine manipulations. It is usually stated that the performance of intrauterine manipulations under subarachnoid and epidural analgesia carries a risk of uterine rupture. Breech extraction, without version, can often be performed under conduction analgesia.

Delivery of twins

The anaesthetic requirements for the delivery of twins are influenced by the presentation of each infant and by the recognition of the need to avoid delay in delivering the second twin. Skilful antenatal care utilizing ultrasound monitoring and cardiotocography will enable the obstetrician to assess with accuracy the condition and presentation of both babies. This information permits the obstetrician to select the optimal time and method for delivery. The value of epidural analgesia for twins delivery is now established. It offers excellent pain relief and allows the mother to cooperate in the delivery. Placental blood flow is maintained in the absence of hypotension, and caval occlusion and fetal acidosis is avoided. It is now our practice to conduct every twins delivery under epidural analgesia. The critical stage in the delivery of twins is the delivery of the second child. Ideally the second twin should be delivered more than 10 minutes (avoiding precipitate delivery) and less than 20 minutes after the first infant, minimizing the risks associated with possible separation of the placenta. Current management of labour with oxytocin augmentation allows control of the second stage. Recourse to caesarean section is preferable to hazardous intrauterine manipulations. An anaesthetist should always be present at twins delivery. Personnel and facilities for the resuscitation of two infants will be required.

James and his colleagues (1977) found that the acid–base status of the first twin was the same as that of singleton fetuses also delivered under epidural analgesia. The acidosis of the second twin, although greater than that of the first twin, was not severe in vertex presentations. Weekes et al (1977) noted no prolongation of the first and second stages of labour by epidural analgesia, and the incidence of instrumental deliveries and breech extractions was unaltered. A note of caution was sounded by Jaschevatzky et al (1977), who found that oxytocin was more often required for hypotonic uterine dysfunction, that instrumental delivery was more often needed and that perinatal mortality was increased in preterm infants when epidural analgesia was used. The hazards of caval occlusion are even greater when the uterus contains two fetuses.

Triplets and quadruplets

Triplets occur approximately once in 8000 pregnancies and quadruplets occur approximately once in 700000 pregnancies. The incidence increases with maternal age, and triplets are common in negroes. The use of clomiphene increases the possibility of a multiple pregnancy.

The many anaesthetic and obstetric hazards include the increased risk of aortocaval occlusion by the very large uterus, a high incidence of pre-eclampsia, hydramnios and premature labour. Epidural and subarachnoid analgesia may be difficult because lumbar lordosis is often marked and the risk of hypotension is increased. Intragastric pressure may be very high, increasing the risk of regurgitation under general anaesthesia, and there may be respiratory difficulty due to upward displacement of the diaphragm and airway closure.

Abouleish (1976) chose continuous caudal analgesia for the vaginal delivery of quadruplets because it avoided a difficult lumbar injection, gave good analgesia and allowed intrauterine manipulations. Craft et al (1978) used lumbar epidural analgesia for elective caesarean section for the delivery of quadruplets and accepted the higher risk of supine hypotension. The writers have used this technique on five occasions for the delivery of triplets by caesarean section.

Uterine atony is common, and oxytocin should be available and adequate supplies of blood should be at hand because there is a high risk of postpartum haemorrhage.

As each fetus is delivered, the infants remaining in the uterus are at increased risk of hypoxia due to further placental separation, uterine contraction and obstruction to blood flow in the umbilical cord. There must be adequate numbers of personnel to resuscitate all the infants.

Few obstetricians recommend vaginal delivery of triplets today, caesarean section being the method of choice.

Caesarean section

The techniques which may be used to provide anaesthesia or analgesia for caesarean section include:

General anaesthesia.
Lumbar epidural analgesia.
Caudal analgesia.
Subarachnoid analgesia.
Local infiltration of the abdominal wall.

In the past obstetricians have been compelled to perform caesarean section with local infiltration due to the unavailability of other forms of anaesthesia. One author's brief and long-past experience of the technique was far from satisfactory. Infiltration is performed in stages and time is allowed for analgesia to develop before incising the underlying structures. First skin and subcutaneous tissues, then muscle, then the posterior rectus sheath and parietal peritoneum are infiltrated. The peritoneal cavity is opened and the tissues under the peritoneum overlying the lower uterine segment are infiltrated. A 0.5% solution of lignocaine or prilocaine is used and up to 100 ml are infiltrated. There is therefore some risk of a toxic reaction. Intraperitoneal manipulations are liable to provoke pain, hypotension, nausea and sweating. A detailed description of this type of technique has been given by Ranney and Stanage (1975) and the interested reader is referred to this. Suture of the uterine incision and closure of the parietal peritoneum may be painful, and Ranney and Stanage routinely induce general anaesthesia with 'intravenous pentothal supplemented by gas' after the delivery. The potential hazards of this type of general anaesthesia will be obvious. There should no longer be any necessity for this type of 'anaesthesia'.

It is sometimes possible to perform caesarean section under caudal analgesia, especially if a Pfannenstiel incision is used. Lumbar epidural block is usually preferred because a more extensive block can be obtained.

There are therefore three techniques which merit serious consideration for use under good, modern conditions: (1) general anaesthesia, (2) lumbar epidural analgesia and (3) subarachnoid analgesia.

The correct choice in any given circumstance must take account of the emergency or elective nature of the oepration, the skill of the anaesthetist with the various techniques, the physical condition of the patient and the wishes of the patient and the obstetrician.

General anaesthesia. In favour of general anaesthesia are the presumed familiarity of the anaesthetist with the basic technique, the preference of some patients, obstetricians and anaesthetists for general anaesthesia for abdominal surgery and the rapidity with which anaesthesia can be induced in an emergency. Unlike conduction analgesia, general anaesthesia is capable of being fully effective in every patient if measures are taken to avoid awareness. General anaesthesia is relatively safe for the patient who is hypovolaemic, severely anaemic and for whom epidural and subarachnoid analgesia are contraindicated.

The dangers of vomiting and regurgitation are a very substantial argument against the use of general anaesthesia, and general anaesthesia has now become an important cause of maternal death. The increase in maternal mortality from anaesthetic causes is due almost entirely to a rise in the number of deaths from Mendelson's syndrome. Technical difficulties with tracheal intubation cannot always be foreseen and, in an obstetric population, failed intubation occurs in approximately 1 in 300 general anaesthetics. For the infant there is the possibility of drug-induced respiratory depression at birth. Where hypotension develops under spinal analgesia the condition of the infant is likely to be worse than that of the infant delivered under general anaesthesia. The use of a relatively high inspired oxygen concentration necessitates the addition of a low concentration of a volatile agent to eliminate the risk of awareness. In the post-operative period there is probably a greater incidence of nausea and vomiting after general anaesthesia and certainly postoperative pain is less well relieved by narcotic analgesics than by continuous epidural analgesia.

The satisfaction afforded the mother and the subsequent development of the mother–child relationship is arguably reduced by caesarean section under general anaesthesia, as immediate contact is lost. Loss of this 'bonding' is seen as a disadvantage, but the long-term effects of this and the effects of general anaesthesia on the development of the child are not known. Closely related to the establishment and development of this bond is the neurological and behavioural status of the neonate. It is now evident that infants born under general anaesthesia take longer to establish spontaneous respiration than those born under regional anaesthesia (James et al, 1977; Downing et al, 1979; Moir and Thorburn, 1980). The acid–base status of infants delivered under general anaesthesia is not significantly different from that of those born under epidural or subarachnoid analgesia if caval occlusion and hypotension are avoided (James et al, 1977; Palahniuk et al, 1977; Hollmen et al, 1978; Downing et al, 1979; Moir and Thorburn, 1980). If the incision of the uterus–delivery (U-D) interval is >3.5 minutes, fetal acidosis occurs (Datta et al, 1981), although Crawford et al (1972) suggest that fetal acidosis increases after 90 seconds under general anaesthesia, but not so rapidly if epidural analgesia is employed. Hypotension however, as discussed previously, occurs in up to 40% of patients undergoing caesarean section with epidural analgesia (Antoine and Young, 1982; Dutton et al, 1984). Hypotension occurs with greater rapidity following subarachnoid block for caesarean section, but Marx et al (1984) advocate this technique for fetal distress when delivery is urgent. Detailed neurobehavioural testing has demonstrated that babies delivered under epidural or subarachnoid analgesia are more active and better able to establish feeding in the first 24–48 hours of life (Palahniuk et al, 1977; Hodgkinson et al, 1978; Hollmen et al, 1978).

Following upon the lead given by Milne and Murray Lawson (1973), other British anaesthetists are giving up general anaesthesia for epidural analgesia in caesarean section. Epidural analgesia is at present used for over 70% of elective caesarean sections in the Queen Mother's Hospital, Glasgow. General anaesthesia was used for 43% of caesarean sections in American teaching hospitals in 1975 (Hicks et al, 1976).

Epidural analgesia. The most compelling argument for performing caesarean section under epidural analgesia is the virtual elimination of the risk of pulmonary aspiration of stomach contents. The superior condition of the infant delivered under properly managed conduction analgesia has been referred to above and is presumed to be due to the avoidance of drug-induced respiratory depression. The alert and pain-free condition of the mother who has epidural analgesia maintained in the postoperative period is in striking contrast to the picture presented by some of the patients who received general anaesthesia and then narcotic analgesics.

Some mothers welcome the opportunity to be awake at the birth of their infant, even when delivery is by caesarean section. This emotional experience is of great importance to some women and encourages 'bonding' between mother and child. A woman may feel deprived by being delivered under general anaesthesia and others may believe themselves to have failed when delivered by caesarean section. These emotions may sometimes be lessened in intensity by being awake at the birth of the child. The authors have quite frequently given epidural analgesia to women who had previously been delivered by caesarean section under general anaesthesia and who very much wanted to be awake at the delivery of a subsequent infant by elective caesarean section. Many patients are unaware that caesarean sections can be performed without general anaesthesia. As this knowledge spreads in a community, the number of patients requesting epidural analgesia increases. In a number of centres the father is present in the operating theatre and shares the experience. He should sit at the mother's head and should not come into the theatre until analgesia and normotension are established.

There are a number of arguments against the use of epidural analgesia. Some are valid, some are more in the nature of prejudices and many can be overcome with skill, experience, teamwork and good patient care. The possibility of a serious reduction in cardiac output with hypotension and impairment of placental blood flow is an ever-present threat when caesarean section is performed under epidural block. The avoidance of caval occlusion, the maintenance of blood volume and the occasional injection of ephedrine will usually prevent this complication. There will then be no reduction in placental blood flow (Jouppila et al, 1978). There has been a failure to eliminate all pain in at least 4% of patients (Shnider, 1970; Milne and Murray Lawson, 1973) and it is this element of uncertainty which has marred an otherwise useful technique. The incidence of inadequate analgesia can be reduced to 2% (Moir and Thorburn, 1980). Surgery should not commence until the sensory block extends from T6 to S5 spinal segments. Compartments have been described within the epidural space (Husemeyer and White, 1980) and this may explain failure of epidural blockade to extend, despite the injection of adequate doses of local anaesthetic. The administration of excessive doses should be avoided by resiting the epidural catheter or by abandoning the technique and utilizing a subarachnoid block (Carrie, 1985). The performance of abdominal surgery in a conscious and unpremedicated patient is a most severe test of an epidural block, and success demands kindness and gentleness as well as the highest standard of technique by anaesthetist and obstetrician. The intravenous injection of ergometrine should be avoided in the absence of haemorrhage, as it induces vomiting in almost 50% of patients (Moodie and Moir, 1976). If ergometrine is avoided, then retching after the delivery is usually due to stimuli arising within the pelvis. Prevention lies in the provision of a complete block from S5 to T6 spinal segments. The technique of analgesia is described in chapter 7. If the patient is not already under continuous epidural analgesia, then the time needed to produce analgesia may preclude the use of epidural block when urgent delivery is indicated. 2-Chloroprocaine will give a rapid onset of analgesia which can be continued with bupivacaine. Unfortunately chloroprocaine is not marketed in the UK. Epidural analgesia is usually contraindicated if there is haemorrhage, hypovolaemia, severe anaemia or a coagulation defect. Undue pressure should never be put upon a patient to accept epidural analgesia for caesarean section, but equally the method should be available to patients who request it. Many patients undergo epidural caesarean section because they believe it to be the technique of choice. Despite the absence of pain and the benefits of being awake, a proportion of patients experience distress. It is the authors' practice to ask the patient if she would like some sedation following delivery, even in the absence of evidence of pain or distress. Few accept this offer. Sosis and Ahmad (1984) advocate the epidural injection of a single bolus of 0.5% bupivacaine claiming this allows surgery to commence within 15 minutes. However, Thompson et al (1985) have shown that the highest peak blood levels of local anaesthetic are obtained following bolus injections of local anaesthetic agents into the epidural space, and advocate an incremental injection technique to achieve a satisfactory block; this is the authors' preference. Epidural analgesia with 2% lignocaine with adrenaline 1:200000 provides satisfactory operating conditions within 30 minutes in 50% of patients, a considerably greater proportion than that receiving bupivacaine 0.5% using an identical technique. Safe and effective epidural analgesia demands a meticulous and painstaking technique.

Subarachnoid analgesia. Almost everything which has just been written about the use of epidural analgesia for caesarean section is equally applicable to subarachnoid analgesia. The quality of the analgesia associated with subarachnoid block is probably marginally superior and the motor block is certainly more intense. Abdominal relaxation is profound but the inability to move the legs is distressing to some patients and calls for reassurance. Analgesia develops more rapidly after subarachnoid injection and this may sometimes be advantageous. Although hypotension occurs under subarachnoid and epidural block, the blood pressure may fall more swiftly and perhaps more profoundly under subarachnoid analgesia. The incidence of, and measures to control spinal headache have been discussed in chapter 7. Its incidence is approximately 20% and it is not significantly altered by the use of 22 or 25 gauge spinal needles. However, the incidence of debilitating headache is low. Inadvertent dural puncture complicates 1–2% of epidural blocks and the resulting headache is severe and prostrating in over half of the patients, despite the use of an infusion of epidural fluids. The incidence of debilitating headache requiring bed rest for 24 hours is more common after spinal anaesthesia than that following epidural analgesia, but headache requiring bed rest for more than 24 hours is very rare. The authors have a conservative approach to epidural blood patch in the management of post-spinal headache and approximately the same number of patients are treated with epidural blood patch after spinal anaesthesia as after epidural analgesia in the Queen Mother's Hospital. Anecdotal accounts of neurological damage following spinal and epidural anaesthesia have exaggerated the fear of permanent damage (Kane, 1981). Large prospective and retrospective studies have confirmed their safety (Dripps and Vandam, 1954; Phillips et al, 1969; Noble and Murray, 1971). The technique requires meticulous and aseptic preparations, and the injection must not be given if clear cerebrospinal fluid is not obtained or if pain is experienced by the patient at the commencement of the injection of the local anaesthetic. If caval occlusion, hypotension and hypovolaemia are prevented, then the acid–base status of the neonate is at least as good as that of infants delivered under general anaesthesia (Marx et al, 1969) and neurobehavioural scores are better after subarachnoid analgesia (Hodgkinson et al, 1978).

Subarachnoid analgesia is specially indicated as an alternative to general anaesthesia for urgent section where the patient has not already received continuous epidural analgesia. Because subarachnoid block is unsuitable for continuous analgesia by catheter, the inability to obtain prolonged postoperative analgesia is a disadvantage in comparison with epidural block. A single-injection technique does not offer the facility to manipulate volumes, concentrations and types of local anaesthetic agent and to make full use of positional changes to ensure perfect analgesia. The introduction of bupivacaine spinal solutions has rekindled interest in subarachnoid techniques in the UK, but their precise role for caesarean section is yet to be established. The rapid onset and occasional report of undesirably extensive blocks resulting from the subarachnoid injection of 2–3 ml of bupivacaine (Stonham and Moss, 1983; Russell, 1985) indicate the need for caution, and careful evaluation of the technique is awaited.

Manual removal of the placenta and postpartum haemorrhage

The modern management of the third stage of labour almost always includes the administration of an oxytocic drug and frequently the placenta is delivered by controlled cord traction (modified Brandt–Andrews method). Undoubtedly the routine use of oxytocic drugs has reduced blood loss at delivery. For example, Martin and Dumoulin (1953) reduced the incidence of postpartum haemorrhage from 13.3 to 1.2% by this practice.

The time taken to produce contraction of the puerperal uterus depends upon the drug and the route of injection. Embrey (1961) gives the following onset times:

ergometrine (i.v.)   41 seconds
ergometrine (i.m.)   7 minutes
oxytocin (i.m.)   2 minutes 32 seconds
Syntometrine (i.m.)   2 minutes 37 seconds

Syntometrine is a combination of oxytocin and ergometrine and combines the more rapid onset of oxytocin with the longer action of ergometrine when given by intramuscular injection. Leeton (1974) in his review of the subject concluded that controlled cord traction and intramuscular Syntometrine give results as good as those found with intravenous ergometrine.

It was formerly believed that the routine use of oxytocic drugs, while greatly reducing the incidence of postpartum haemorrhage, increased the need for manual removal of the placenta. Later studies failed to confirm this belief (Francis et al, 1965; Gate and Noel, 1967; Mathie and Snodgrass, 1967). The emetic and pressor actions of intravenous ergometrine cause unpleasant and occasionally dangerous side-effects (Baillie, 1963; Johnstone, 1972; Williams et al, 1974; Moodie and Moir, 1976) and intravenous oxytocin or intramuscular Syntometrine are acceptable substitutes.

There are three principal types of postpartum haemorrhage: (1) bleeding from the placental site, often because placental separation is incomplete, fragments of placenta or membranes are retained in utero or because the uterus is atonic, (2) bleeding as the result of trauma to the perineum, vagina, cervix or lower uterine segment and (3) bleeding due to relatively rare blood dyscrasias such as hypoprothrombinaemia or thrombocytopoenia. According to Dewhurst and Dutton (1957) the risk of postpartum haemorrhage is 1 in 5 after one previous haemorrhage and 1 in 3 after two previous haemorrhages. Clearly such a history demands hospital confinement with cross-matched blood available, an intravenous infusion running through a suitable cannula at delivery and preparedness for general anaesthesia.

The Report on Confidential Enquiries into Maternal Deaths in England and Wales 1976–78 (Department of Health and Social Security, 1982) emphasizes the need for a simple protocol as a guide to junior obstetricians and anaesthetists. The treatment of postpartum haemorrhage is based upon the intravenous administration of 0.5 mg of ergometrine or 5 units of oxytocin, perhaps followed by the infusion of 20 units of oxytocin in 500 ml of fluid and the administration of blood or blood substitutes. Central venous pressure monitoring may be helpful in severe or problem cases, but the insertion of a CVP line should not be attempted during the acute phase when management of the haemorrhage has overriding priority, and attention must not be distracted from this priority. A sharp rise in central venous pressure after the rapid infusion of 200 ml of fluid suggests that blood volume is adequate. The obstetrician may wish to perform manual removal of the placenta or to inspect and suture lacerations of the birth canal, and general anaesthesia or suitable regional analgesia will frequently be required. In case of severe trauma to the uterus, laparotomy and sometimes hysterectomy may be necessary. Packing of the uterus is sometimes an effective if apparently old-fashioned treatment. Uncontrollable bleeding may indicate ligation of the uterine or internal iliac arteries in the moribund patient. Compression of the abdominal aorta through the abdominal wall has temporarily reduced potentially fatal uterine bleeding.

The anaesthetist is frequently required to provide anaesthesia for manual removal of the placenta. With the routine administration of oxytocic drugs at delivery, serious bleeding is now relatively uncommon, but the risk of haemorrhage is always present. Where bleeding has occurred, resuscitative measures will have been undertaken before anaesthesia and every patient should have an intravenous infusion running. Rarely, adequate control of bleeding may prove difficult or impossible. In such circumstances it is preferable to compromise, induce anaesthesia and explore the uterus before the results of failure to replace the blood volume adequately are reflected by significant deterioration in the maternal condition. Blood should be available. In the Queen Mother's Hospital, Glasgow, it has been the practice to arrange for the cross-matching of blood by the 'emergency' method when the placenta is undelivered 20 minutes after delivery of the child. This blood is usually available after a further 20 or 30 minutes. Manual removal of the placenta is then performed and this relatively 'unsafe' blood is transfused only in the event of severe haemorrhage. Screened O-negative blood is also available for use in any life-threatening emergency and is probably the safer product. Plasma volume expanders will often suffice, but blood should be available if at all possible.

The placenta may be firmly adherent (to the uterus), partially separated or separated but 'trapped' in the lower segment. Manual removal of a trapped placenta is usually straightforward and can sometimes be performed under pudendal nerve block, inhalational analgesia or intravenous hypoaesthesia with a mixture of pethidine and promazine. Dickins and Michael (1966) claimed that 86% of patients who had the placenta removed manually under pudendal nerve block accompanied by an intravenous injection of 50 mg of pethidine experienced no pain. Combined pudendal and paracervical blocks will render the lower birth canal and the uterus insensitive. These techniques are useful in the absence of a skilled anaesthetist or sometimes in domiciliary practice, particularly where the placenta is merely trapped. Subarachnoid block is indicated in the absence of haemorrhage if the delivery has not been conducted with epidural analgesia. If difficulty is anticipated, or blood loss is occurring, general anaesthesia is preferable. Uterine relaxation should be avoided by restricting the use of inhalational agents, or by avoiding them altogether and using intravenous anaesthesia and analgesia. Subarachnoid block to spinal segment T10 is necessary to provide adequate analgesia for manual removal of placenta. Manual removal of the placenta can turn out to be unexpectedly difficult and time-consuming. An adherent placenta may require to be removed piecemeal. The location and suture of cervical lacerations can be very difficult without good anaesthesia. The cervix may have closed down, making the insertion of the obstetrician's hand difficult. For this emergency procedure, a technique of anaesthesia based upon an intravenous induction agent, suxamethonium, and tracheal intubation should be used. Uterine relaxation should usually be avoided. The gentle and experienced *main d'accoucheur* can usually be gradually introduced through the cervix without recourse to halothane.

If the patient has already received an epidural, caudal or subarachnoid block then manual removal can be easily and painlessly performed without additional anaesthesia. Subarachnoid analgesia to the level of T10 is very suitable for manual removal of the placenta (Crawford, 1979) and it is the writers' practice to use subarachnoid analgesia rather than general anaesthesia for this procedure if the patient has not already received epidural analgesia in her labour. Although the intragastric pressure may be assumed to have fallen after the delivery of the child, it cannot be assumed that gastric emptying times are now normal and that the pH of the gastric juice is above 2.5. Blouw et al (1976) found that the volume of gastric contents was normal 8 hours after delivery, but did not investigate very recently delivered patients. Rennie et al (1979) found that 54% of patients for postpartum sterilization had a gastric pH below 2.5. It is clear that if general anaesthesia is used for manual removal of the placenta, then all the precautions which are taken before any other obstetric anaesthetic must be taken and a risk of Mendelson's syndrome must be presumed to exist.

Acute inversion of the uterus

Acute inversion of the uterus is a rare and dramatic complication of the third stage of labour which occurs once in approximately 20 000 deliveries. Cord traction or fundal pressure when the uterus is relaxed and the placental site is at the fundus are said to cause acute inversion, and the condition may occur if the uterus is relaxed by general anaesthesia. The death rate varies from 23 to 80% (Lee et al, 1978). Urgent treatment is required in this dire emergency. Unless the uterus is repositioned and shock is swiftly treated, then the mortality rate is high. Shock develops rapidly and may be out of all proportion to the haemorrhage. Pain is often severe. It is thought that the inverted uterus exerts traction on the sympathetic nerves and creates 'neurogenic shock'. If bleeding occurs from the placental site it may be exaggerated due to restriction of the venous outflow from the inverted uterus. Treatment comprises early reduction of the inversion and the infusion of blood or blood substitutes. General anaesthesia will be required for the replacement of the uterus and light, endotracheal anaesthesia, including the use of a muscle relaxant, is suitable. If an intravenous induction agent is used the dose should be much reduced. It may be necessary to relax the uterus briefly to permit replacement and 2% halothane may be administered for about 1 minute if replacement is impossible without uterine relaxation. If the uterus can be replaced within a few minutes, then a successful outcome is likely. Delay leads to profound shock and death. Delay increases uterine engorgement; laparotomy may then be required so that traction can be applied to the round ligaments to assist replacement (Lee et al, 1978).

Examination under anaesthesia

A frequent indication for the administration of a general anaesthetic in late pregnancy is the need to confirm or exclude placenta praevia in patients with a history of antepartum haemorrhage or unstable lie of the fetus. This is usually an elective procedure in a prepared patient although occasionally the examination may be necessary in emergency circumstances. The examination may occasionally provoke severe or even torrential haemorrhage and there should therefore be at least two units of cross-matched blood available in theatre and an intravenous infusion should be running. Severe haemorrhage or the presence of a major degree of placenta praevia will indicate immediate delivery by caesarean section. Everything should be ready for immediate section. This is the North American 'double set-up' for section or amniotomy.

Placental localization by ultrasonography has now reached a high degree of accuracy. Where this technique together with the history and clinical examination all suggest that the placenta is normally situated, it is permissible to examine the patient in theatre, without general anaesthesia. The anaesthetist should be standing by, the patient prepared for anaesthesia, an intravenous infusion running and blood immediately available. Where placentography has not been performed or where placenta praevia is considered a probable diagnosis on clinical grounds or by placentography, then general anaesthesia should be administered for the examination.

The standard obstetric anaesthetic should be used. Relaxation may be maintained with suxamethonium until the examination has been completed. If caesarean section is to be performed then a non-depolarizing relaxant may be given. Because of the risk of sudden severe haemorrhage, epidural and subarachnoid analgesia are unsuitable.

External cephalic version

External version under general anaesthesia carries a risk of fetal death from partial separation of the placenta and of course there is a maternal risk from any general anaesthetic. These risks must be measured against the risks of breech delivery or of delivery by elective caesarean section. Proper selection of patients for assisted breech delivery, higher standard of obstetrics and anaesthesia for breech delivery and delivery by elective caesarean section, where there is any possibility of cephalopelvic disproportion, have reduced the hazards of breech presentation for the fetus. If external version is performed under general anaesthesia there is a possibility that breech presentation will recur before term. The arguments for and against version under anaesthesia have been considered in depth by Bonnar et al (1968).

General anaesthesia has not been given for external cephalic version in the Queen Mother's Hospital since 1967. If external version cannot be performed easily under sedation then the attempt is abandoned. External version is usually attempted between weeks 32 and 34 of pregnancy.

If the obstetrician considers external version under general anaesthesia to be justified, then an intravenous induction agent and suxamethonium should be used. The trachea is intubated and anaesthesia is maintained with nitrous oxide, oxygen and further increments of suxamethonium or a suxamethonium drip. Obstetric opinion differs on the desirability of providing uterine relaxation. It is the view of most obstetricians that relaxation should be confined to the skeletal musculature. Others consider that 2% halothane should be administered for about 1 minute before attempting version. It is likely that the use of halothane in this concentration will increase the risk of placental separation and, as has been pointed out, breech presentation is quite likely to recur if version has required uterine relaxation. The fetal heart-rate should be monitored. Evidence of fetal distress or vaginal bleeding may indicate immediate caesarean section. It is therefore appropriate to carry out external cephalic version under general anaesthesia in the operating theatre, and blood should have been cross-matched.

Postpartum tubal ligation

In many obstetric units tubal ligation soon after delivery has been replaced by laparoscopic sterilization six weeks postpartum. A delay of six weeks allows the mother to recover from the very common postpartum psychological depression and perhaps to make a more reasoned decision about sterilization. Sterilization by the laparoscope requires only a brief stay in hospital, and the postponement of the procedure for six weeks permits the reversal of the hypercoagulability of the blood which exists in pregnancy and in the early puerperium and predisposes to thrombosis.

The alternative approach is to perform tubal ligation within 48 hours of delivery. McKenzie (1977) states that 24–36 hours postpartum is optimal because the mother is then rested, the risk of bleeding is reduced and bacteria are not usually found in the uterus for the first 48 hours after delivery. Tubal ligation may be done as a semi-urgent procedure during daylight hours and within 48 hours of delivery. The risks of general anaesthesia remain high for at least 48 hours after delivery (James et al, 1984). It is important that the infant should be healthy before sterilization is performed. Laparoscopic sterilization in the early puerperium carries the same risk as tubal ligation (Clark et al, 1974) and allows earlier mobility and discharge from hospital. Laparoscopic sterilization is usually avoided before the fifth postpartum day because it is technically difficult.

General anaesthesia may be given for early postpartum tubal ligation. A cuffed endotracheal tube should be passed, because the risk of Mendelson's syndrome exists (Blouw et al, 1976; Rennie et al, 1979). General anaesthetic agents may appear in the milk of the lactating mother, and the establishment of lactation may be interrupted by a general anaesthetic. For these reasons subarachnoid or epidural analgesia may be preferred. McKenzie (1977) recommends subarachnoid block to T10 or slightly above this level with 60–90 mg (mean 75 mg) of 5% lignocaine in dextrose or 6–9 mg of amethocaine in 10% dextrose or 10–15 mg of bupivacaine. Epidural analgesia is a satisfactory alternative. If epidural analgesia has been used in labour, then the epidural catheter may be left in place and the block can be reinstated after a test dose. It is sometimes claimed that the operation can be performed through a small incision after infiltration of the abdominal wall. Access may be difficult and traction on the Fallopian tubes is likely to cause unpleasant symptoms. The possibility of ligating a structure other than the Fallopian tube may be increased.

Spontaneous abortion and termination of pregnancy

Spontaneous abortion is of course common in early pregnancy and termination of pregnancy within the terms of the Abortion Act is frequently performed in many British hospitals. The anaesthetist has the right to refuse to administer anaesthesia for the legal termination of pregnancy.

Spontaneous abortion is often incomplete and evacuation of the uterus is then necessary. General anaesthesia is usually given and halothane and other powerful uterine relaxants such as methoxyflurane, ether and chloroform should be avoided. Cullen et al (1970) noted that the use of halothane caused increased bleeding at therapeutic abortion. An intravenous induction with thiopentone and maintenance of anaesthesia with nitrous oxide, oxygen and trichloroethylene will usually prove satisfactory. Fentanyl 0.1 mg intravenously, followed by thiopentone, nitrous oxide and oxygen is usually adequate. Cross-matched blood should be available and ergometrine 0.25 mg or oxytocin 5 units is usually given intravenously during the procedure.

Therapeutic abortion is usually performed by dilatation of the cervix and removal of the uterine contents by curette or by suction when the pregnancy is of not more than 14 weeks' duration. Termination at a more advanced stage of pregnancy is more hazardous and has until recently usually entailed abdominal hysterectomy. Recently prostaglandins have proved to be safe and effective in inducing labour to terminate a pregnancy in the second trimester. It is now extremely rare to have to resort to abdominal hysterotomy. However, labour induced by this method may make slow progress, despite augmentation with oxytocin. Analgesia is usually required. The unfortunate patient's natural anxiety and distress can be treated with freely administered intramuscular sedation, but epidural analgesia is frequently necessary. Oxytocics should be administered as a concentrated solution by a volumetric pump to reduce the problems associated with the anti-diuretic effects of oxytocin, and the intravenous infusion of large volumes of dextrose solutions must be avoided.

Many techniques of anaesthesia have been used for the termination of pregnancy in the first trimester. The technique chosen is sometimes influenced by the facilities available and by the practice, undesirable in the writers' view, of discharging the patient from the hospital or clinic a few hours after surgery. It is not rarely that such patients are readmitted to another hospital with potentially dangerous bleeding. Filshie and colleagues (1977) used a slow intravenous injection of pethidine 50 mg and diazepam 10 mg for the evacuation of retained products of conception and only 3% found the procedure painful. Filshie and Sanders (1977) used injections of local anaesthetic into the cervix for surgical termination of early pregnancy. Twelve per cent found dilatation of the cervix painful, and tinnitus or convulsion occurred in 3.6% due to the injection of local anaesthetic into the vascular, pregnant cervix. Vomiting or vasovagal attacks occurred in 5%. Vaginal termination can be satisfactorily performed under general anaesthesia in which the use of halothane is minimized. Bilateral paracervical block will make dilatation of the cervix painless in most patients (Chatfield et al, 1970) and has been used for abortion and minor gynaecological surgery. McKenzie and Shaffer (1978) have used a jet injector for paracervical block before termination of pregnancy and have reduced blood lignocaine concentrations to one-third of those recorded after needle injections. It is sometimes helpful to have an infusion of 20 units of oxytocin in 500 ml of fluid running during the procedure and ergometrine 0.5 mg is usually given intravenously. If given to the conscious patient ergometrine may have an emetic action. Abdominal hysterotomy requires essentially the same technique of anaesthesia as is used for caesarean section. Placental transfer is no longer a cause for concern and general anaesthesia is usually preferred. If epidural or subarachnoid block is chosen then heavy premedication should be given.

Anaesthesia for the obstetric flying squad

At the time of writing 2% of confinements in the UK take place in the home and therefore true domiciliary obstetric anaesthesia has almost ceased to exist. For many years in several large cities, including Glasgow, obstetricians have transferred patients to hospital in preference to administering anaesthesia in the home. The Queen Mother's Hospital flying squad has neither a senior nor a junior anaesthetist as a member. Anaesthetic equipment is not provided and the objective is to transfer the patient to hospital as rapidly as possible. An experienced obstetrician is present who can assess and deal with the majority of emergencies. Over 20 years experience has shown that disastrous emergencies are so rare that the provision of adequate mobile resources is not necessary, and would not be cost-effective, as no patient's life has been lost by the absence of these facilities. It might reasonably be argued that if these facilities are available, hasty and ill-considered assessment may lead to their inappropriate use. Many deliveries now take place in general practitioner units. Most of these units are equipped with anaesthetic apparatus but it may occasionally be necessary for an anaesthetist to use the apparatus belonging to the flying squad in a general practitioner unit or nursing home. Davies (1969) recorded that between 1962 and 1968 general anaesthesia was used on 47 occasions by his obstetric flying squad and that the indication for anaesthesia was almost always a retained placenta or other complication of the third stage. One-third of these anaesthetics were given in the home and the remainder were administered in general practitioner units.

Stabler (1957) laid down two sound principles for obstetric flying squads. First, the full facilities of the hospital should be brought to the patient and, second, flying squad duties should not be delegated solely to junior staff. One might question whether the full facilities of the hospital can ever be brought to the patient. It was noted by Fraser and Tatford (1961) that a senior anaesthetist was rarely available to the flying squad and they considered that patients should therefore be transferred to hospital. There is, of course, no place for the very junior or occasional anaesthetist or obstetrician on the flying squad. If an anaesthetist is to be available for the limited volume of flying squad work still performed then a separate call list of experienced anaesthetists should be drawn up. The person on call should not be on call for other purposes and he should be able to rendezvous with the flying squad and its equipment at the patient's house.

Anaesthetic and resuscitation equipment for obstetric flying squads has been considered in detail by Davies (1969) and Whitford et al (1973). Essential items include a portable anaesthetic apparatus allowing the administration of nitrous oxide, oxygen and a volatile agent, and intermittent positive pressure ventilation, intubation equipment, drugs, infusion fluids (including screened O negative blood), a foot-operated suction apparatus and equipment for neonatal resuscitation, including an incubator and a source of oxygen. Portability is essential because, although the equipment will normally be transported by ambulance, it may have to be carried up several flights of stairs in the home. A simple and suitable apparatus can be constructed using a cylinder of Entonox, an Oxford Miniature Vaporizer, an inflating bellows and a non-return valve. Whitford et al (1973) used this apparatus to maintain endotracheal anaesthesia with nitrous oxide, oxygen, 0.25% trichloro-ethylene and intermittent injections of suxamethonium. Davies (1969) used a Portanaest apparatus which had been modified to include an extra oxygen input to allow the use of the oxygen cylinder carried by the ambulance (these cylinders did not have the pin-index system). A technique was described by Dallas (1967) which did not require an anaesthetic machine and cylinders. Intermittent injections of thiopentone and suxamethonium were given, the trachea was intubated and an Ambu bag was used to inflate the lungs with air.

Older techniques such as open chloroform (Adamson et al, 1960) and intermittent injections of thiopentone with spontaneous ventilation (Laing, 1963) would not be considered acceptable today and would not be consistent with the principle that the full facilities of the hospital should be brought to the patient. Such techniques are unfamiliar to many anaesthetists who should use methods based on sound hospital practice. Finally it should be remembered that it will often be possible to perform uncomplicated manual removal of the placenta under hypoaesthesia with pethidine, and a phenothiazine or diazepam given intravenously, and perhaps accompanied by inhalational analgesia. These techniques may be accompanied by pudendal nerve block (Dickins and Michael, 1966) for analgesia of the lower birth canal and by paracervical block to render the uterus insensitive to pain. Manual removal of the placenta has been performed after a single intravenous injection of 100 mg ketamine given by the obstetrician (Roopnarinesingh and Kalipersadsingh, 1974).

The use of ketamine in obstetrics

The exceptional properties of ketamine merit an attempt to evaluate the place of this phencyclidine derivative in obstetric anaesthesia. The use of ketamine in obstetrics was proposed by Chodoff and Stella in 1966 and the drug has since then been used in North America and in continental Europe, mainly for the provision of brief anaesthesia for outlet forceps delivery (Stolp et al, 1968; Galbert and Gardner, 1973; Akamatsu et al, 1974). Although Moore et al (1971) reported the use of ketamine in British obstetric practice, it appears that most British anaesthetists have, with justification, preferred to rely on now well-tried methods based upon tracheal intubation and intermittent positive pressure ventilation with nitrous oxide, oxygen and the administration of a muscle relaxant. A further explanation may be found in the frequent use of elective low-forceps delivery by many North American obstetricians and the desire for brief, light anaesthesia for this procedure.

Ketamine increases blood pressure, heart rate, central venous pressure and cardiac output (Savege et al, 1973). Respiration is only slightly depressed and it is often claimed that the protective laryngeal reflexes are maintained and that upper respiratory obstruction does not occur. While this is often the case it is not invariable (Morgan et al, 1971) and Penrose (1972) has reported aspiration pneumonitis after ketamine.

The incidence of unpleasant and alarming dreams on awakening from ketamine anaesthesia has influenced many anaesthetists against the drug. Among the many factors which appear to affect the incidence of unpleasant dreams are the type of premedicant drugs given, the age and sex of the patient, the circumstances surrounding recovery and the extent of pre- and postoperative anxiety. Nevertheless Galbert and Gardner (1973) and Moore et al (1971) noted unpleasant dreams in only 4% and 8% respectively of their patients and the first-named authors stressed the need for verbal reassurance before and after anaesthesia. In contrast Knox et al (1970) recorded unpleasant dreams in 33% of gynaecological patients receiving ketamine.

The clinical condition of the infant at birth has been good in most series of vaginal deliveries and at caesarean section (Peltz and Sinclair, 1973), although Moore et al (1971) recorded hypertonicity in some infants. The experiences of Downing et al (1976) were less favourable. These workers noted neonatal depression which appeared to be dose-related. Ketamine crosses the placental barrier and large or repeated doses would be expected to cause neonatal depression. More recent studies indicate that ketamine does cause dose-dependent neonatal depression (Eng et al, 1975; Downing et al, 1976; Akamatsu and Bonica, 1977). Blood loss has been reported as normal or reduced at delivery after ketamine and contractility of the murine uterus is increased by ketamine (Jawalekar et al, 1972). It is conceivable that uterine hypertonicity could impair placental blood flow to the detriment of the fetus. The analgesic properties of ketamine should prove useful in obstetrics.

Ketamine has been compared favourably with thiopentone as an induction agent for caesarean section when followed by conventional nitrous oxide, oxygen and relaxant anaesthesia (Peltz and Sinclair, 1973). Although the incidence of neonatal depression, excessive bleeding, dreaming and postpartum psychosis was the same with each agent, the authors considered that awareness was less likely and that postoperative analgesia was better after ketamine.

There is widespread agreement that ketamine should be avoided in patients with pre-eclampsia because it is likely to aggravate hypertension. Where there is a requirement to provide narcosis of short duration for outlet forceps delivery, then ketamine may be useful. An intravenous injection of a solution containing 5 mg ketamine/ml is injected until the eyes assume a fixed and staring look (Galbert and Gardner, 1973). This takes about 60 seconds to develop. Attention to the airway is essential, and vomiting and regurgitation can occur, albeit rarely. The patient should breathe oxygen or a nitrous oxide and oxygen mixture with a high oxygen content. Most British anaesthetists would prefer to administer endotracheal anaesthesia with a muscle relaxant and intermittent positive pressure ventilation, or better still, to use epidural or subarachnoid analgesia for forceps delivery. Ketamine may be successfully substituted for thiopentone for the induction of conventional anaesthesia for caesarean section or operative vaginal delivery in the normotensive patient, and its analgesic properties may contribute to the patient's wellbeing. Ketamine is reported to be suitable for the asthmatic patient because of its bronchodilator action (Corssen et al, 1972) and in the shocked patient its cardiovascular stimulant properties may be valuable and the patient may be given 100% oxygen to breathe. Despite the possibility of aggravating existing hypertension, ketamine has been successful in the treatment of eclampsia when given as a single intravenous injection of 50 mg followed by an infusion of 250 mg in 500 ml of 5% glucose solution (Rucci and Caroli, 1974). This observation is rather surprising in view of the fast activity produced in the electroencephalographic tracing by ketamine (Schwartz et al, 1974) although ketamine was found to suppress seizure-like EEG discharges in epileptic patients (Corssen et al, 1974). Ketamine is valuable when short procedures such as manual removal of the placenta or evacuation of the uterus must be undertaken in difficult circumstances and without an anaesthetic apparatus; it may then be used as the sole agent. An intravenous injection of 100 mg (or 2 mg/kg) will provide anaesthesia lasting for 5–10 minutes and increments may be given if necessary. This valuable property of ketamine in maintaining the airway is utilized in situations where other forms of anaesthesia are difficult or impractical. Small children for focal linear accelerator radiotherapy may receive ketamine as the sole anaesthetic agent. The authors have used ketamine to anaesthetize patients with severe ankylosing spondylitis where conventional endotracheal intubation is impossible. Endotracheal intubation with the fibreoptic laryngoscope is not always possible, and is certainly not the method of choice for emergency surgery.

REFERENCES

Abouleish, E. (1976) Caudal analgesia for quadruplet delivery. *Anesth. Analg. curr. Res.*, **55**, 61.
Adamson, T.L., Brown, R., Myerscough, P.R. and Loudon, J.D.O. (1960) The Edinburgh flying squad: a review 1948–1957. *J. Obstet. Gynaec. Br. Emp.*, **67**, 243.
Akamatsu, R.J. and Bonica, J.J. (1977) Ketamine for obstetric delivery. *Anesthesiology*, **46**, 78.
Akamatsu, T.J., Bonica, J.J., Rehmet, R., Eng, M. and Ueland, K. (1974) Experiences with the use of ketamine for parturition. *Anesth. Analg. curr. Res.*, **53**, 284.
Antoine, C. and Young, B.K. (1982) Fetal lactic acidosis with epidural anesthesia. *Am. J. Obstet. Gynec.*, **142**, 55.
Baillie, T.W. (1963) Vasopressor activity of ergometrine maleate in anaesthetised parturient women. *Br. med. J.*, **i**, 585.
Blouw, R., Scatliff, J., Craig, D.B. and Palahniuk, R.J. (1976) Gastric volume and pH in postpartum patients. *Anesthesiology*, **45**, 456.
Bonica, J.J. (1965) *Obstetric Complications*, p. 171. Oxford: Blackwell.
Bonnar, J., Howie, P.W. and MacLennan, H. (1968) External cephalic version with anesthesia. *J. Am. med. Ass.*, **205**, 97.
Bowen-Simpkins, P. and Fergusson, I.L.C. (1974) Lumbar epidural block and the breech presentation. *Br. J. Anaesth.*, **46**, 420.
Boyson, W.D. and Simpson, J.W. (1960) Breech management with caudal anesthesia. *Am. J. Obstet. Gynec.*, **79**, 1121.
Breeson, A.J., Kovacs, G.T., Pickles, B.G. and Hill, J.G. (1978) Extradural analgesia: the preferred method of analgesia for vaginal breech delivery. *Br. J. Anaesth.*, **50**, 1227.
Brown, S.E. and Vass, A.C.R. (1977) An extradural service in a district general hospital. *Br. J. Anaesth.*, **49**, 243.
Carrie, L.E.S. (1985) 0.75% bupivacaine. *Br. J. Anaesth.*, **57**, 241.
Chatfield, W.R., Suter, P.E.N. and Kotonya, A.O. (1970) Paracervical anaesthesia for the evacuation of incomplete abortion: a controlled trial. *J. Obstet. Gynaec. Br. Commonw.*, **77**, 462.
Chodoff, P. and Stella, J.G. (1966) Use of CI-581, a phencyclidine derivative for obstetric anesthesia. *Anesth. Analg. curr. Res.*, **45**, 527.
Clark, D.H., Schneider, J.T. and McManus, S. (1974) Tubal sterilization: comparison of outpatient laparoscopy and postpartum ligation. *J. reprod. Med.*, **13**, 69.
Cooper, K. (1972) In *Proceedings of the Symposium on Epidural Analgesia in Obstetrics*, ed. Doughty, A., p. 108. London, Lewis.
Corssen, G., Gutierrez, J. and Reves, J.G. (1972) Ketamine in the anesthetic management of asthmatic patients. *Anesth. Analg. curr. Res.*, **51**, 588.
Corssen, G., Little, S.C. and Tavakoli, M. (1974) Ketamine and epilepsy. *Anesth. Analg. curr. Res.*, **53**, 319.
Craft, J.B., Levinson, G. and Shnider, S.M. (1978) Anaesthetic considerations in Caesarean section for quadruplets. *Can. Anaesth. Soc. J.*, **25**, 236.
Crawford, J.S. (1972) Principles and Practice of Obstetric Anaesthesia, 3rd edn. Oxford: Blackwell.

Crawford, J.S. (1974) An appraisal of lumbar epidural blockade in patients with a singleton fetus presenting by the breech. *J. Obstet. Gynaec. Br. Commonw.*, **81**, 867.

Crawford, J.S. (1975) Patient management during extradural anaesthesia for obstetrics. *Br. J. Anaesth.*, **47**, 273.

Crawford, J.S. (1979) Experience with spinal analgesia in a British obstetric unit. *Br. J. Anaesth.*, **51**, 531.

Cullen, B.F., Margolis, A.J. and Eger, E.I. (1970) The effects of anesthesia and pulmonary ventilation on blood loss during elective therapeutic abortion. *Anesthesiology*, **32**, 108.

Daily, H.I. and Rogers, S.F. (1957) Saddle-block anesthesia in breech delivery. *Surgery Gynec. Obstet.*, **105**, 620.

Dallas, S.H. (1967) A method of domiciliary anaesthesia. *Br. J. Anaesth.*, **39**, 969.

Datta, S., Ostheimer, G.W., Weiss, J.B., Brown, W.U. and Alper, M.H. (1981) Neonatal effects of prolonged anesthetic induction for Cesarean section. *Obstet. Gynec.*, **58**, 331.

Davies, C.K. (1969) Anaesthesia for an obstetric flying squad. *Br. J. Anaesth.*, **41**, 545.

Department of Health and Social Security (1982) *Report on Confidential Enquiries into Maternal Deaths in England and Wales, 1976–78*. London: HMSO.

Dewhurst, C.J. and Dutton, W.A. (1957) Recurrent abnormalities of the third stage of labour. *Lancet*, **ii**, 764.

Dickins, A.M. and Michael, C.A. (1966) Manual removal of the placenta without general anaesthesia. *J. Obstet. Gynaec. Br. Commonw.*, **73**, 460.

Donnai, P. and Nicholas, A.D.G. (1975) Epidural analgesia, fetal monitoring and the condition of the baby at birth with breech presentation. *Br. J. Obstet. Gynaec.*, **82**, 360.

Doughty, A. (1969) Selective epidural analgesia and the forceps rate. *Br. J. Anaesth.*, **41**, 1058.

Downing, J.W., Mahomedy, M.C., Jeal, D.E. and Allen, P.J. (1976) Anaesthesia for Caesarean section with ketamine. *Anaesthesia*, **31**, 883.

Downing, J.W., Houlton, P.C. and Barclay, A. (1979) Extradural analgesia for Caesarean section: a comparison with general anaesthesia. *Br. J. Anaesth.*, **51**, 367.

Dutton, D.A., Moir, D.D., Howie, H.B., Thorburn, J. and Watson, R. (1984) Choice of local anaesthetic drug for extradural caesarean section. *Br. J. Anaesth.*, **56**, 1361.

Dripps, R.D. and Van Dam, L.D. (1954) Long term follow up on patients who received 10 098 spinal anaesthetics. Failure to discover major neurological sequelae. *J. Am. med. Ass.*, **156**, 1486.

Embrey, M.P. (1961) Simultaneous intramuscular injection of oxytocin and ergometrine: a tocographic study. *Br. med. J.*, **i**, 1737.

Eng, M., Bonica, J.J., Akamatsu, T.J., Berges, P.U. and Ueland, K. (1975) Respiratory depression in newborn monkeys at Caesarean section following ketamine administration. *Br. J. Anaesth.*, **47**, 917.

Filshie, G.M. and Sanders, R.R. (1977) Outpatient termination of pregnancy. *Br. J. Obstet. Gynaec.*, **84**, 509.

Filshie, G.M., Sanders, R.R., O'Brien, P.M.S. et al (1977) Evacuation of retained products of conception in a treatment room and without general anaesthesia. *Br. J. Obstet. Gynaec.*, **84**, 514.

Finster, M., Poppers, P.J., Sinclair, J.C., Morishima, H.O. and Daniels, S.S. (1965) Accidental intoxication of the fetus with local anesthetic drug during caudal anesthesia. *Am. J. Obstet. Gynec.*, **92**, 922.

Francis, H.H., Miller, J.M. and Porteous, C.R. (1965) Clinical trial of an oxytocin–ergometrine mixture. *Aust. N.Z. J. Obstet. Gynaec.*, **5**, 47.

Fraser, A.C. and Tatford, E.P.W. (1961) Management of third stage complications in domiciliary obstetrics. *Lancet*, **ii**, 126.

Galbert, M.W. and Gardner, A.E. (1973) Ketamine for obstetrical anesthesia. *Anesth. Analg. curr. Res.*, **52**, 926.

Gate, J.M. and Noel, J.D.O. (1967) Syntocinon and ergometrine in the prevention of postpartum haemorrhage. *J. Obstet. Gynaec. Br. Commonw.*, **74**, 49.

Hicks, J.S., Levinson, G. and Shnider, S.M. (1976) Obstetric anesthesia training centers in the U.S.A.—1975. *Anesth. Analg. curr. Res.*, **55**, 839.

Hodgkinson, R., Bhatt, M., Kim, S.S., Grewal, G. and Marx, G.F. (1978) Neonatal neurobehavioural tests following Cesarean section under general and spinal anesthesia. *Am. J. Obstet. Gynec.*, **132**, 670.

Hollmen, A.I., Jouppila, R., Koivisto, M. et al (1978) Neurologic activity of infants following anesthesia for Cesarean section. *Anesthesiology*, **48**, 350.

Hoult, I.J., MacLennan, A.H. and Carrie, L.E.S. (1977) Lumbar epidural analgesia in labour: relation to fetal malposition and instrumental delivery. *Br. med. J.*, **i**, 14.

Humphrey, M.D., Chang, A., Wood, E.C., Morgan, S. and Hounslow, D. (1974) A decrease in fetal pH during the second stage of labour when conducted in the dorsal position. *J. Obstet. Gynaec. Br. Commonw.*, **81**, 600.

Husemeyer, R.D. and White, D.L. (1980) Topography of the lumbar epidural space, a study in cadavers using injected polyester resin. *Anaesthesia*, **35**, 7.

Ingemarrson, I., Westgren, M. and Svenningesen, N.W. (1978) Long-term follow-up of preterm infants in breech presentation delivered by Caesarean section. *Lancet*, **ii**, 172.

James, C.F., Gibbs, C.P. and Banner, T. (1984) Postpartum perioperative risk of aspiration pneumonia. *Anesthesiology*, **61**, 756.

James, F.M., Crawford, J.S., Davies, P. and Naiem, H. (1977a) Lumbar epidural analgesia for labor and delivery of twins. *Am. J. Obstet. Gynec.*, **127**, 176.

James, F.M., Crawford, J.S., Hopkinson, R., Davies, P. and Naiem, H. (1977b) A comparison of general anesthesia and lumbar epidural analgesia for elective cesarean section. *Anesth. Analg. curr. Res.*, **56**, 228.

Jaschevatzky, O.E., Shalit, A., Levy, Y. and Grunstein, S. (1977) Epidural analgesia during labour in twin pregnancy. *Br. J. Obstet. Gynaec.*, **84**, 327.

Jawalekar, K.S., Jawalekar, S.R. and Mathur, V.P. (1972) Effect of ketamine on isolated murine myometrial activity. *Anesth. Analg. curr. Res.*, **51**, 685.

Johnstone, M. (1972) The cardiovascular effects of oxytocic drugs. *Br. J. Anaesth.*, **44**, 826.

Jouppila, R., Jouppila, P., Kuikka, J. and Hollmen, A. (1978) Placental blood flow during Caesarean section under lumbar extradural analgesia. *Br. J. Anaesth.*, **50**, 275.

Kane, R.E. (1981) Neurological deficits following epidural and spinal anesthesia. *Anesth. Analg.*, **60**, 150.

Knox, J.W.D., Bovill, J.D. and Clarke, R.S. (1970) Clinical studies of induction agents. XXXVI. Ketamine. *Br. J. Anaesth.*, **42**, 875.

Laing, D.Y.S. (1963) The emergency obstetric service Bellshill Maternity Hospital, 1933–1961. *J. Obstet. Gynaec. Br. Commonw.*, **70**, 83.

Lee, W.K., Baggish, M.S. and Lashgari, M. (1978) Acute inversion of the uterus. *Obstet. Gynec.*, **51**, 144.

Leeton, J.F. (1974) Emergency complications of the third stage of labour and early puerperium. In *Obstetric Therapeutics*, ed. Hawkins, D.F., p. 442. London: Baillière Tindall.

Little, W.A. and Friedman, E.A. (1958) Anesthesia for twin delivery. *Anesthesiology*, **19**, 515.

Littlewood, D.G., Scott, D.B., Wilson, J. and Covino, B.G. (1977) Comparative anaesthetic properties of various local anaesthetic agents in extradural block for labour. *Br. J. Anaesth.*, **49**, 75.

Livnat, E.J., Fejgin, M., Scommegna, A., Beiniarz, J. and Burd, L. (1978) Neonatal and acid–base balance in spontaneous and instrumental vaginal deliveries. *Obstet. Gynec.*, **52**, 549.

Lyons, E.R. and Papsin, F.R. (1978) Cesarean section in the management of breech presentation. *Am. J. Obstet. Gynec.*, **130**, 558.

Maresh, M., Choong, K.-H. and Beard, R.W. (1983) Delayed pushing with lumbar epidural in labour. *Br. J. Obstet. Gynaec.*, **90**, 623.

Martin, H.D. and Dumoulin, J.G. (1953) Use of intravenous ergometrine to prevent postpartum haemorrhage. *Br. med. J.*, **i**, 643.

Marx, G.F. (1984) The plot thickens. *Anesthesiology*, **60**, 3.

Marx, G.F., Cosmi, E.V. and Wollman, S.B. (1969) Biochemical status and clinical condition of mother and infant at cesarean section. *Anesth. Analg. curr. Res.*, **48**, 986.

Marx, G.F., Luykx, W.M. and Cohen, S. (1984) Fetal–neonatal status following Caesarean section for fetal distress. *Br. J. Anaesth.*, **56**, 1004.

Mathie, I.W. and Snodgrass, C.A. (1967) The effect of prophylactic oxytocic drugs on blood loss after delivery. *J. Obstet. Gynaec. Br. Commonw.*, **74**, 653.

Matouskova, A., Dottori, O., Forssman, L. and Victorin, L. (1975) An improved method of epidural analgesia with reduced instrumental delivery rate. *Acta obstet. gynec. scand.*, **54**, 231.

McKenzie, R. (1977) Postpartum tubal ligation. In *Pain Control in Obstetrics*, ed. Abouleish, E. Philadelphia: J.B. Lippincott Co.

McKenzie, R. and Shaffer, W.L. (1978) A safer method of paracervical block in therapeutic abortions. *Am. J. Obstet. Gynec.*, **130**, 317.

Milne, M.K. and Murray Lawson, J.I. (1973) Epidural analgesia for caesarean section. *Br. J. Anaesth.*, **45**, 1206.

Moir, D.D. and Thorburn, J. (1980) Epidural analgesia for Caesarean section: evaluation of an improved technique. In *Proceedings of the Second Symposium on Epidural Analgesia in Obstetrics, Coventry*, ed. Doughty, A. London: H.K. Lewis.

Moir, D.D. and Wallace, G. (1967) Blood loss at forceps delivery. *J. Obstet. Gynaec. Br. Commonw.*, **74**, 424.

Moir, D.D., Slater, P. Thorburn, J., McLaren, R. and Moodie, J. (1976) Epidural analgesia in obstetrics: a controlled trial of carbonated lignocaine and bupivacaine HCl solutions. *Br. J. Anaesth.*, **48**, 129.

Moodie, J.E. and Moir, D.D. (1976) Ergometrine, oxytocin and epidural analgesia. *Br. J. Anaesth.*, **48**, 571.

Moore, J., McNabb, T.G. and Dundee, J.W. (1971) Preliminary report on ketamine in obstetrics. *Br. J. Anaesth.*, **43**, 779.

Morgan, M., Loh, L., Singer, !.. and Moore, P.H. (1971) Ketamine as the sole anaesthetic agent for minor procedures. *Anaesthesia*, **26**, 158.

Noble, A.D. (1972) In *Proceedings of a Symposium on Epidural Analgesia in Obstetrics*, ed. Doughty, A., p. 106. London: Lewis.

Noble, A.B. and Murray, J.J. (1971) A review of the complications of spinal anaesthesia with experience in Canadian teaching hospitals from 1959–1969. *Can. Anaesth. Soc. J.*, **18**, 5.

Palahniuk, R.J., Scatliff, J., Biehl, D., Wiebe, H. and Sankaran, K. (1977) Maternal and neonatal effects of methoxyflurane, nitrous oxide and lumbar epidural anaesthesia for Caesarean section. *Can. Anaesth. Soc. J.*, **24**, 586.

Peltz, B. and Sinclair, D.M. (1973) Induction agents for caesarean section: a comparison of thiopentone and ketamine. *Anaesthesia*, **28**, 37.

Penrose, B.H. (1972) Aspiration pneumonitis following ketamine induction for general anesthesia. *Anesth. Analg. curr. Res.*, **51**, 41.

Phillips, O.C., Ebner, J., Nelson, A.T. and Black, M.H. (1969) Neurological complications following spinal anaesthesia with lidocaine. *Anesthesiology*, **30**, 284.

Ranney, B. and Stanage, W.F. (1975) Advantages of local anesthesia for Cesarean section. *Obstet. Gynec.*, **45**, 163.

Rennie, A.L., Richard, J.A., Milne, M.K. and Dalrymple, D.G. (1979) Postpartum sterilisation–an anaesthetic hazard? *Anaesthesia*, **34**, 267.

Roopnarinesingh, S. and Kalipersadsingh, S. (1974) Manual removal of the placenta under ketamine. *Anaesthesia*, **29**, 486.

Rucci, F.S. and Caroli, G. (1974) Ketamine and eclampsia. *Br. J. Anaesth.*, **46**, 546.

Russell, I.F. (1985) High spread after 2 ml of bupivacaine plain solution. *Anaesthesia*, **40**, 199.

Salvatore, C.A., Cicivizzo, E. and Turatti, S. (1965) Breech delivery with saddle-block anaesthesia. *Obstet. Gynec.*, **26**, 261.

Savege, T.M., Blogg, C.E., Foley, E.I. et al (1973) The cardio-respiratory effects of Althesin and ketamine. *Anaesthesia*, **28**, 391.

Schwartz, M.S., Virden, S. and Scott, D.F. (1974) Effects of ketamine on the electroencephalograph. *Anaesthesia*, **29**, 135.

Scudamore, J.H. and Yates, M.J. (1966) Pudendal block—a misnomer? *Lancet*, **i**, 23.

Shnider, S.M. (1970) Anesthesia for elective cesarean section. In *Obstetrical Anesthesia*, ed. Shnider, S.M. Baltimore: Williams and Wilkins.

Sosis, M. and Ahmad, I. (1984) An efficient technique for performing extradural blockade. *Br. J. Anaesth.*, **56**, 928.

Spence, A.A., Moir, D.D. and Finaly, W.E.I. (1967) Observations on intragastric pressure. *Anaesthesia*, **22**, 249.

Stabler, F. (1957) The obstetric flying squad. *Br. med. J.*, **ii**, 217.

Stolp, W., Sangrehr, D. and Sokal, K. (1968) Application of ketamine in obstetric anesthesia. *Geburtsh. Gynäk.*, **169**, 198.

Stonham, J. and Moss, P. (1983) The optimal test dose. *Anesthesiology*, **58**, 389.

Taylor, A.B.W., Abukhalil, S.H., El-Guindi, M.M., Tharian, B. and Watkins, J.A. (1977) Lumbar epidural analgesia in labour: a 24-hour service provided by obstetricians. *Br. med. J.*, **ii**, 370.

Thorburn, J. and Moir, D.D. (1981) Extradural analgesia: the influence of volume and concentration on the mode of delivery, analgesic efficacy and motor block. *Br. J. Anaesth.*, **53**, 933.

Weekes, A.R.L., Cheridjian, V.E. and Mwanje, D.K. (1977) Lumbar epidural analgesia in labour in twin pregnancy. *Br. med. J.*, **ii**, 730.

Whitford, J.H., Cory, C.E. and Beddard, J.B. (1973) A clinical trial of apparatus for anaesthesia for domiciliary midwifery. *Br. J. Anaesth.*, **45**, 1153.

Williams, C.V., Johnson, A. and Ledward, R. (1974) A comparison of central venous pressure changes in the third stage of labour following oxytocic drugs and diazepam. *J. Obstet. Gynaec. Br. Commonw.*, **81**, 596.

9

Some Obstetric, Anaesthetic and Medical Complications

Pre-eclampsia and eclampsia

The cause of pre-eclampsia remains unknown and pre-eclampsia may be viewed as a syndrome with widespread abnormalities resulting from the pregnancy itself. Although many biochemical, haematological and pathological abnormalities occur in pre-eclampsia, they are usually the result of the disease rather than its cause. Intravascular coagulation is certainly a feature and could explain the effects of pre-eclampsia upon organs such as the placenta, kidneys, liver, brain and lungs. Pulmonary blood flow is sometimes reduced in severe pre-eclampsia (Birmingham Study, 1971) and a mild degree of ventilation/perfusion imbalance may occur, but hypoxaemia has not been demonstrated (Templeton and Kelman, 1977). The homeostatic balance between fibrin deposition and fibrinolysis is abnormal, resulting in a reduced platelet count and an increase in fibrin degradation products. The coagulopathy is usually compensated, and it is rare to be sufficiently severe to require factor supplementation (Sharp, 1977). Plasma and whole blood viscosity are increased (Mathews and Mason, 1974; Thorburn et al, 1982), but the changes are complex, reflecting the haematological effects of severe pre-eclampsia and the relative failure to expand the plasma volume. Fibrin may be deposited in placental and renal vessels and thrombosis and atheromatous changes impair placental function (Robertson et al, 1967). It is uncertain whether these haematological changes are the cause or the result of pre-eclampsia. Fetal growth may be impaired and fetal distress in labour is common. Renal plasma flow and glomerular filtration rate are reduced. Plasma volume is diminished, even in the presence of oedema. Severe hypovolaemia is associated with a high prenatal mortality (Arias, 1975; Soffronoff et al, 1977). The responses to blood loss may be exaggerated. Collapse has occurred after diuretic therapy and was attributed to hypovolaemia (Brewer, 1962). An immunological element in the aetiology of pre-eclampsia is postulated (Robertson et al, 1967). It is postulated that there is partial immunological intolerance to the fetus or the placenta. A vasoconstrictor substance is often thought to be implicated but has not been identified. Serum proteins are reduced in concentration, liver function is impaired when measured by the bromsulphthalein test and, in severe cases, pulmonary function may be impaired.

Treatment of pre-eclampsia

The cure for pre-eclampsia is <u>delivery</u> of the placenta. Other treatments are symptomatic and, at best, gain time for further fetal growth while preventing serious maternal complications. The need to treat mild hypertension (blood pressure <170/100 mmHg) is questionable. The value of <u>bed rest is uncertain</u> and the prescribing of barbiturates and other <u>sedatives</u> is probably <u>valueless</u>. The fetal benefits of the treatment of moderate hypertension are not clear. Treatment with a hypotensive agent will effectively reduce the blood pressure, but this is treating a sign, and the underlying disease process continues. <u>Vessel wall damage</u> occurs if the diastolic pressure is in excess of <u>110 mmHg</u>, and hypertension of this severity should be treated in the maternal interest. <u>Methyldopa</u> is the most widely used and investigated agent and is also known to be safe for the baby. Diuretics are not popular, as they are thought to further reduce the plasma volume, and perhaps adversely affect placental function, but a recent statistical review of the various studies of the effects of diuretics on pregnancy hypertension (Collins et al, 1985) concluded that the evidence was insufficient to enable any conclusion to be drawn. β-Blockers and calcium antagonists are widely used to treat non-obstetric hypertension, and preliminary but anecdotal reports of the use of β-blockers in pregnancy hypertension suggested an association with fetal bradycardia and acidosis (Stirrat and Lieberman, 1977). However, more rigorous studies have failed to confirm adverse fetal effects (Rubin et al, 1983). Initial studies of the use of <u>calcium antagonists</u> in pregnancy-induced hypertension have been encouraging (Walter and Redman, 1984). The advantage that these drugs may offer is a simple and effective oral dose regimen with reduced side-effects. The concomitant effects of general anaesthesia and epidural analgesia frequently required for delivery are not known. <u>Hydralazine</u> is often used as second-line drug treatment, and can be administered as an <u>infusion</u> or by <u>bolus injections</u>. It is safe, effective and widely used (Chamberlain et al, 1978).

Severe hypertension (fulminating pre-eclampsia) exists when the blood pressure exceeds <u>180/120 mmHg</u>. There is usually <u>oliguria</u> and <u>proteinuria</u>. <u>Headaches</u> and <u>visual disturbances</u> may occur and eclampsia must be considered imminent. Immediate and effective treatment is essential and the anaesthetist has much to offer in this report (Thorburn and Moir, 1980). <u>Cerebrovascular accident</u>, <u>cardiac failure</u>, <u>renal failure</u>, abruptio placentae, <u>disseminated intravascular coagulation</u> and <u>eclampsia</u> can cause death. Pre-eclampsia was the cause of 18% of maternal deaths in England and Wales between 1973 and 1975 (Department of Health and Social Security, 1979) and <u>cerebral haemorrhage</u> was the leading cause among these deaths.

Treatment should be aimed at control of the dangerous hypertension, prevention of convulsions and the improvement of blood flow to vital organs, including the kidneys and placenta. The severity of hypovolaemia and the benefits of <u>plasma volume expansion</u> by the <u>infusion of colloid</u> are controversial, but volume expansion may be useful if urine output is low. Attempts at treating intravascular coagulation with heparin have been unsuccessful. Diazoxide is the most effective antihypertensive agent for use in severe pre-eclampsia (Morris et al, 1977) and has replaced protoveratrine for intravenous use. Diazoxide dilates the arterioles and increases cardiac output, so that renal and perhaps placental blood flow are increased while the systolic blood pressure drops by a mean of 50 mmHg and the diastolic blood pressure drops by 30 mmHg after an intravenous injection of 300 mg. However, it is currently less popular, and its use should be limited to severe and uncontrolled hypertension. It should be administered in small bolus intravenous doses of 30–60 mg intermittently. The hypotensive effect lasts for 4–6 hours. Although Caritis et al (1976) observed a decrease in uterine blood flow from a rapid injection of diazoxide in sheep, the technique was found to be harmless in humans (Morris et al, 1977). Diazepam and chlormethiazole are the two most widely used anticonvulsants, and are certainly the agents of choice if convulsions have occurred, but their role in prophylaxis is perhaps less clear. In the treatment of epilepsy, which the convulsions of eclampsia resemble, diazepam is not an effective prophylactic and phenytoin is the drug of first choice, although it has not yet been widely used in obstetrics. A major problem is to identify the patients most at risk of eclampsia. Diazepam has the added advantages of ubiquity and familiarity, but doses in excess of 30 mg adversely affect the neonate. The anticonvulsants of choice are diazepam 10 mg by intravenous injection or an infusion of 0.8% chlormethiazole at 60 drops per minute for a few minutes. When moderate sedation is achieved, the rate is slowed to about 20 drops per minute. Chlormethiazole and diazepam are not antihypertensive agents. The depressant action of these drugs on the neonate does not preclude their use in a crisis. Plasma volume expanders are given to correct the hypovolaemia, reduce blood viscosity and improve blood flow. Many different treatment regimens have been advocated for the management of severe hypertension in pregnancy, but the rarity of the condition prohibits satisfactory comparison of the various drugs and treatment methods. Claims of the superiority of one regimen over another have not been validated, nor are they likely to be. The objectives in the management of severe hypertension are to investigate and stabilize the maternal condition, because delivery is likely to be undertaken within a short period of time. The authors' experience is that patients admitted with fulminant hypertension will be delivered within 24 hours of admission. Treatment is that of the signs and symptoms, and has not yet been shown to alter the rate of deterioration of the disorder. Monitoring will identify adverse haematological and biochemical changes which will assist in determining the point at which intervention is mandatory in the maternal or fetal interest.

The regimen now used at the Queen Mother's Hospital, Glasgow, is as follows:

(A)   Establish the following aids to monitoring and treatment:
          Intravenous infusion.

Central venous pressure line.
Bladder catheter (measure urine volume hourly).
Blood pressure recording (Arteriosonde useful).
Fetal heart-rate monitor.
(B)   Obtain the following estimations:
Serum urea, electrolytes, creatinine, proteins, liver function tests.
Haemoglobin, platelet count, coagulation screen.
Urine osmolality and 24-hour urine collection.
(C)   Give the following treatment:
Diazoxide 30–60 mg intravenous bolus.
Diazepam 5–10 mg intravenous bolus.
Salt-poor albumin as a plasma volume expander.
These measures may be repeated.

The above regimen has been successful in controlling blood pressure in critically ill mothers, and urine volume and osmolality have increased. Platelet counts often continue to fall, indicating that intravascular coagulation continues (Thorburn and Moir, 1980). Early delivery is usually indicated and caesarean section is often preferred to the induction of labour. Epidural analgesia will often be contraindicated by the presence of a coagulopathy in these patients. Intravenous therapy has been monitored by central venous pressure recordings. A Swan–Ganz catheter would give more useful information but should only be used by experienced persons.

Eclampsia calls for the intravenous injection of diazepam 10 mg, oxygenation and airway maintenance. Thiopentone 100 mg may be given by an anaesthetist but in inexperienced hands the mortality from thiopentone has been 16% (Menon, 1969). Ketamine 250 mg in 500 ml has controlled eclampsia (Rucci and Caroli, 1974). Recurrent seizures have been managed with intermittent positive pressure ventilation and a muscle relaxant (Mathie, 1966; Chan and Delilkan, 1970). Convulsions are abolished or modified but abnormal electrical activity may persist in the electroencephalograph. Eclampsia now occurs after delivery in 50% of cases (Gordon, 1970).

In North America magnesium sulphate is a mainstay of treatment, but is rarely used in the UK. Magnesium sulphate is a generalized depressant of the central nervous system and is now usually given intravenously. A bolus of 2 g may be followed by an infusion of 2 g/hour. Careful monitoring is essential. Reflex depression, hypotonia, respiratory and cardiovascular depression and coma may occur. The therapeutic concentration in the blood is 6–8 mEq/litre and the toxic concentration is 12–14 mEq/litre. Overdose is treated by the slow intravenous injection of calcium gluconate, 10 ml of a 10% solution. Intramuscular injections are painful and may lead to abscess formation.

Diuretics are currently contraindicated in pre-eclampsia, even if oedema is present. The already low blood volume may be dangerously depleted and collapse has been attributed to this cause (Gordon, 1974).

Where facilities do not permit the type of intensive therapy outlined above, the obstetrician may have to rely upon the use of a 'lytic cocktail' such as pethidine 100 mg, promethazine 50 mg and chlorpromazine 50 mg given by slow intravenous infusion. It should hardly need to be said that there is now no place for deep basal narcosis with bromethol (Dewar and Morris, 1947) or morphine, chloral hydrate, paraldehyde and chloroform (Stroganoff, 1930). A balanced therapeutic regimen of antihypertensive drugs, anticonvulsants and, if the woman is in labour, analgesic drugs is the current approach and is based upon the concept proposed by Duffus et al (1969).

Hypertension in labour

In contrast to the quite rare condition of severe, fulminating pre-eclampsia discussed above, moderately severe hypertension during labour is quite frequently encountered. The requirements in this situation are control of blood pressure, relief of pain and early delivery. Delivery by forceps or vacuum extractor is often indicated. Continuous lumbar epidural analgesia offers good or complete pain relief and prevents the further increase in blood pressure which accompanies painful contractions. In about 90% of hypertensive patients, a reduction in systolic and diastolic blood pressure can be anticipated. Moir et al (1972) noted a mean reduction of 34 mmHg (4.5 kPa) or 20% in systolic blood pressure and 26 mmHg (3.6 kPa) or 23% in diastolic pressure during epidural blockade in patients in labour with severe pre-eclampsia. Elective forceps delivery can be performed under the epidural block, and the administration of sedatives and narcotic analgesics is unnecessary. In the more severely hypertensive mothers an anticonvulsant may be required in the form of intravenous diazepam 5–10 mg or an infusion of 0.8% chlormethiazole. If caval occlusion is avoided and blood volume is maintained, then placental blood flow is not reduced (Jouppila et al, 1978; Husemeyer and Crawley, 1979) and may even be increased as the result of vasodilatation. Epidural analgesia is contraindicated in the presence of the coagulation defect which may occur in severe pre-eclampsia. If control of the blood pressure is unsatisfactory, hydralazine 5–10 mg may be given intravenously. It should be emphasized that there are no universally agreed criteria for treatment, but if epidural analgesia is providing effective pain relief and hypertension continues to cause concern, conventional drug therapy should be given. Increasing the extent of the epidural block is neither desirable nor usually effective. If hypertension persists following delivery, treatment with oral β-blockers should be commenced, the drug of choice currently being atenolol 100 mg orally daily.

Cerebral blood flow falls when mean arterial pressure is reduced by about 25%, and clinical signs of underperfusion occur when the reduction exceeds 45%. Intravenous diazoxide has caused permanent ischaemic brain damage and blindness in patients with malignant hypertension, and it has been recommended that intravenous therapy be restricted to patients with hypertensive left ventricular failure or frank encephalopathy (Cove et al, 1979; Editorial, 1979). Actual or imminent eclampsia justifies intravenous antihypertensive therapy in the writers' view and it should be remembered that cerebrovascular accidents are the major cause of death in pre-eclampsia. Labetalol, an α- and β-blocking agent which reduces peripheral resistance, is effective. Labetalol is injected intravenously in 50 mg doses. The injection should take at least 1 minute and may be repeated every 5 minutes until 200 mg have been given. An intravenous infusion of 200 mg labetalol in 200 ml of saline may also be used.

If general anaesthesia is used, there is likely to be a further substantial rise in systemic and pulmonary arterial pressure in response to tracheal intubation, extubation and suction (Hodgkinson and Husain, 1979). Deep anaesthesia obtunds these responses but is unsuitable for obstetric patients, and the intravenous injection of hydralazine 20 mg shortly before anaesthesia is induced has been recommended. Sodium nitroprusside or nitroglycerine could be used.

Mendelson's (acid-aspiration) syndrome

The importance of antacid prophylaxis has been considered in detail in chapter 6. It cannot be emphasized too strongly that the prevention of acid aspiration is not based on one therapeutic measure but on the rigorous application of all the steps outlined in chapter 6. The number of patients dying from acid aspiration in the UK is known with accuracy and detail; what is not known is the number of patients who aspirate some gastric contents and survive.

In 1946 Mendelson described 66 cases of the syndrome which has come to bear his name in 43 000 pregnancies. This incidence of 1 in 660 pregnancies is, hopefully, not a representative figure for 1980. The present incidence of Mendelson's syndrome is unknown. Hutchinson and Newson (1975) quote an incidence of 1 in 1100 in surgical and obstetric patients in Auckland. The number of mothers who die of Mendelson's syndrome remains constant. In England and Wales, 14 mothers died from this cause in 1970–72 and 9 died in 1973–75 (Department of Health and Social Security, 1975, 1979). Eight of the women who died in 1973–75 were said to have received oral antacid. In Scotland a mother died of Mendelson's syndrome who had received a proprietary aluminium hydroxide antacid (Scottish Home and Health Department, 1978). Depending upon the vigour with which treatment is undertaken, death may occur within minutes, or the patient may survive for several days with artificial ventilation and oxygen. Long-term survival may leave the patient a respiratory cripple (Adams et al, 1969). According to Cameron and Zuidema (1972) massive pulmonary aspiration of stomach contents carries a mortality of 70%. This figure may not apply to the obstetric patient, particularly if she has received prophylactic antacids. Hutchinson and Newson (1975) reported a mortality rate of 10% in obstetrical and non-obstetrical patients, and Crawford and Opit (1976) noted a 15% mortality from aspiration pneumonitis in obstetrical patients who had not received an antacid. It is Scott's (1978) view that the prognosis of Mendelson's syndrome has worsened in recent years. He points out that all of Mendelson's original 66 patients survived, and suggests that the use of muscle relaxants and intermittent positive pressure ventilation may force gastric contents deep into the lungs and that ergometrine may overload the left ventricle. The writers know of instances where obstetric patients who had received magnesium trisilicate later regurgitated and aspirated stomach contents. Although recovery was often stormy, and extensive atelectasis and infection usually occurred, the patients all survived.

It is disturbing that 13 mothers have died in the UK who have reputedly received an antacid. It is recognized that the details of the antacid regimen may vary and that from 8.5–20% of patients may remain at risk (Peskett, 1973; White et al, 1976) and that the giving of a pre-anaesthetic dose is important (Holdsworth et al, 1977). There remains the possibility that food particles, bile salts and possibly the antacid itself may act as pulmonary irritants. The recent evidence that the aspiration of particulate antacid causes severe and sometimes fatal pneumonitis in dogs (Gibbs et al, 1979) has drawn attention to the role which these antacids may have in the pulmonary damage which follows aspiration of gastric contents. Non-particulate antacids like 0.3 M sodium citrate do not produce such severe pulmonary lesions. The introduction of H_2-receptor antagonists has provided a means of effectively reducing the gastric volume and increasing the pH of the gastric contents. Animal work has suggested that the inhalation of a volume of 0.4 ml/kg of aspirate with a pH of <2.5 will produce permanent pulmonary damage. Increasing the pH permits larger volumes to be aspirated before developing a similar degree of pulmonary damage. The evidence, therefore, clearly supports the rigorous application of measures not only to reduce the pH of the gastric contents, but also to reduce the gastric volume.

There is general agreement that the serious and progressive type of aspiration pneumonitis known as Mendelson's syndrome is due to the entry of gastric juice of pH below 2.5 into the alveoli (Teabut, 1952; Bannister and Sattilaro, 1962; Vandam, 1965; Davidson et al, 1974; Downs et al, 1974). Liquids whose pH is above 3.0 may cause a milder reaction from which recovery is rapid. The initial response to the entry of even a liquid such as Hartmann's solution into the lungs is airway closure or alveolar transudation with a resulting decrease in static compliance and arterial Po_2 within 10 minutes. Where the liquid is acid there is parenchymal damage to the lung due to the chemical burn, and hypoxia progressively worsens and severe metabolic acidosis develops. There is some evidence of a localized intrapulmonary consumption coagulopathy (Davidson et al, 1974), and intrapulmonary haemorrhage and gross pulmonary oedema develop. Infection is not usually a prominent feature.

The patient who develops Mendelson's syndrome becomes gravely ill, usually within 30–60 minutes after aspiration. The signs and symptoms may therefore appear during or very shortly after anaesthesia. Regurgitation and aspiration have not always been noted by the anaesthetist in reported cases, although often there was difficulty with intubation. It is probable that a small quantity of acid gastric juice is sufficient to cause Mendelson's syndrome. Roberts and Shirley (1974) consider that 25 ml may be enough and such a small volume may easily go undetected. Cyanosis, tachycardia and gross pulmonary oedema develop early. Bronchospasm is a frequent although not invariable early response to the acid. Bronchospasm is unusual in amniotic fluid embolism and this may be helpful in diagnosis. Hypotension and hypovolaemia with haemoconcentration are the result of the reactive alveolar transudation of fluid. Cardiac failure may supervene. Pulmonary artery pressure is increased and static compliance is greatly reduced. The arterial Po_2 falls at an early stage and a severe metabolic acidosis develops later. The changes in Pco_2 are often slight (Davidson et al, 1974), suggesting lowered ventilation perfusion ratios, right-to-left shunting, or both. Infection is not usually a clinical or a histological feature. The chest X-ray is likely to show evidence of pulmonary oedema and patchy atelectasis, but there is often poor correlation between the extent of pulmonary damage and the radiological appearances (Downs et al, 1974).

Treatment. Treatment is often ineffective in established, progressive acid-aspiration pneumonitis, and deaths from this condition must be prevented by the prophylactic measures already discussed in chapter 6.

The principal therapeutic measures which may be tried in Mendelson's syndrome are: (1) corticosteroid therapy, (2) artificial ventilation of the lungs and (3) supportive measures designed to treat bronchospasm, cardiac failure and infection. The use of bronchial lavage with saline or sodium bicarbonate in attempts to dilute or wash out the acid is not advocated. The efficacy is very doubtful, the irritant liquid may be further disseminated and it is doubtful if the liquid instilled into the trachea reaches the alveoli. In any case the acid within the alveoli is probably diluted rapidly with alveolar transudate.

(1) *Corticosteroid therapy.* It is generally recommended that a large single dose of a corticosteroid should be given whenever gastric juice is thought to have been aspirated and that corticosteroid therapy should be continued for at least 72 hours if signs of acid-aspiration should develop. This therapy is to be instituted immediately after tracheal intubation and tracheal suction. If the pH of the aspirated material can be determined and is below 3.0, then vigorous treatment is recommended.

The choice of corticosteroid, the dosage schedule and the use of the intravenous or the intratracheal route for administration are all matters of some controversy. Most of the available evidence is derived from the installation of hydrochloric acid into the tracheas of experimental animals. Most workers in this field have found that corticosteroid therapy was of usually slight value (Bannister et al, 1961; Hamelberg and Bosomworth, 1964; Lewinski, 1965). Others have found that corticosteroid therapy was of no value (Awe et al, 1966). The mechanism of the beneficial action, if any, of corticosteroid therapy is uncertain.

It has been suggested that corticosteroids inhibit the inflammatory reaction in the bronchial walls and alleviate bronchospasm (Bannister et al, 1961; Lawson et al, 1966).

It appears that some of the conflict may be resolved by taking into consideration the exact pH of the aspirated liquid. If the pH lies between 1.1 and 1.36, then the mortality rate approaches 100% and steroids are of little or no value (Awe et al, 1966; Downs et al, 1974). If the pH of the aspirate is between 1.5 and 1.75 then vigorous treatment with corticosteroids and intermittent positive pressure ventilation can hasten recovery, although at this pH range all animals, treated and untreated, survived (Lawson et al, 1966). If the pH of the aspirated liquid exceeds 2.1 there is no progressive parenchymal damage (Teabut, 1952; Taylor and Prys-Davies, 1966). A mortality rate of 100% has been recorded where the pH of the aspirate was below 1.75 and there were no deaths if the pH exceeded 2.4 (Lewis et al, 1971).

In interpreting the results of these animal experiments, the non-linearity of the pH scale should be kept in mind. In the numerically small pH range of 1.1–2.1 the change in H^+ activity is relatively enormous.

It is the view of Downs et al (1974) that pulmonary damage is greatest where the pH of the aspirate is below 1.5 and that death is then likely to occur in 80% or more of the animals. When the maximal pulmonary response has occurred then corticosteroids are no longer beneficial. Any benefit from steroid therapy is likely to occur when the aspirated material has a pH within the narrow range of 1.5–2.1.

When faced with a patient in whom regurgitation and aspiration are known to have occurred, corticosteroids should be given, even if their effectiveness is open to question. In the emergency situation the first essentials are pharyngeal and tracheal suction, intubation of the trachea with a cuffed tube and ventilation of the lungs with oxygen. Bronchoscopy is not advised. An intravenous injection of a corticosteroid should be given as soon as possible. Intratracheal administration is not recommended. Crawford (1972) recommends hydrocortisone 300 mg, repeated at 6-hourly intervals, for 48 hours. Methylprednisolone 30 mg or 40 mg/kg body weight at intervals of 6 or 8 hours for 72 hours has been used (Downs et al, 1974; Dudley and Marshall, 1974) as has dexamethasone in doses ranging from 0.08 to 8.0 mg/kg body weight at 6-hourly intervals (Dudley and Marshall, 1974). Dexamethasone 10 mg, then 5 mg at 6-hourly intervals is perhaps the treatment of choice because this steroid does not cause sodium retention and will not therefore aggravate pulmonary or cerebral oedema. Corticosteroid doses should be tapered off after the first 48 or 72 hours. If signs of Mendelson's syndrome have not appeared within a few hours of aspiration it is probably safe to discontinue the corticosteroid and, in such cases, it is unnecessary to taper off the doses.

(2) *Artificial ventilation of the lungs.* The need for intermittent positive pressure ventilation (IPPV) will depend on the volume and pH of the aspirate and the effects of contamination with food particles. The patient's respiratory function should be assessed by arterial blood gas analysis at the completion of surgery. If there is evidence of hypoxaemia, increased airway resistance and reduced pulmonary compliance, IPPV should be continued and the patient transferred to an intensive therapy unit. In the absence of symptoms and signs, the trachea may be extubated and the respiratory function monitored carefully. IPPV may be required for many days (Adams et al, 1969) and there may sometimes have been a tendency to cease ventilator therapy prematurely (Scottish Home and Health Department, 1978). In severe cases positive end-expiratory pressure may be tried and continuous positive pressure ventilation has been successful in dogs (Chapman et al, 1974).

(3) *Supportive measures.* Various measures may be indicated to prevent or to treat specific complications as they arise. Bronchodilators should be given if clinically indicated. Digoxin and diuretics may be necessary if cardiac failure develops. Opinions vary on the use of antibiotics. Histologically, infection is usually absent or of minimal extent in the lungs. The administration of high doses of corticosteroids is thought by some to predispose to infection and therefore to indicate the prophylactic administration of an antibiotic. Physiotherapy and intravenous fluids may be indicated and blood gas analyses will be required for the control of IPPV.

Psychological problems may arise. The patient treated by Adams et al (1969) developed a severe depressive illness which later required electroconvulsant therapy.

It will be apparent that the treatment of Mendelson's syndrome is mainly symptomatic, that it is sometimes unsuccessful and that the application of the various preventive measures discussed in chapter 6 is the most effective way of preventing maternal deaths from Mendelson's syndrome. These measures can never be completely certain and there is of course a strong case to be made for the use of regional analgesia whenever possible.

Amniotic fluid embolism

Amniotic fluid embolism occurs approximately once in 80 000 pregnancies (Lewis, 1964), the mortality rate is about 80% and fetal loss is estimated at 40%. It is thus a rare but fatal condition and is now the commonest cause of sudden maternal death in the course of labour and delivery or immediately postpartum, accounting for 6.4% of maternal deaths in England and Wales between 1973 and 1975 (Department of Health and Social Security, 1979). Vigorous treatment has resulted in survival (Willocks et al, 1966; Lumley et al, 1979).

The clinical features are dyspnoea, cyanosis, circulatory failure and coma. Convulsions occur in 10% of cases. Typically the patient is older, is multiparous and has a tumultuous labour. For amniotic fluid to enter the circulation there must be a tear in the membranes. There is a history of injury to the uterus in 50% of cases (Smibert, 1967) and the trauma may range from artificial rupture of membranes to rupture of the uterus. Amniotic fluid embolism can occur at caesarean section, especially if the placenta is incised. Minor injury to the endocervical veins is common at delivery (Shnider and Moya, 1961).

A coagulopathy is always present by the end of the first hour and may cause severe uterine haemorrhage. Occasionally haemorrhage is the presenting symptom. Some authorities believe that disseminated intravascular coagulation is always present (Beller, 1974), and coagulation within the pulmonary vessels accompanied perhaps by blockage by fetal debris is probably a basic lesion (Tuller, 1957; de Bastos and Srinivasan, 1964). Hypofibrinogenaemia is usual and fibrin degradation products may be present.

The chest X-ray may show diffuse mottling or may be normal, and a lung scan may be helpful in the diagnosis (Morgan, 1979). A definite diagnosis can only be made by the detection of fetal squames, lanugo, vernix, mucin or meconium in the lungs. Special staining techniques are required and at post-mortem examinations sections of lung should be taken from widely separated areas (Attwood, 1972). In life, fetal debris has been detected in blood from a central venous pressure line and in the sputum, after staining with Nile Blue (Tuck, 1972; Schaerf et al, 1977), and these measures are recommended by Morgan (1979). Pulmonary artery catheterization has demonstrated high pulmonary wedge and pulmonary artery diastolic pressures associated with a high central venous pressure (Duff et al, 1983), evidence of intense pulmonary vasoconstriction. The associated hypoxia may intensify these effects, which remain for some days.

Amniotic fluid embolism must be distinguished from clot and air embolism, Mendelson's syndrome and acute left ventricular failure and from eclampsia if convulsions occur. An important diagnostic pointer is the coagulopathy and probability of uterine haemorrhage with amniotic fluid embolism.

The mechanism whereby amniotic fluid embolization produces such disastrous results is uncertain. The evidence has been reviewed in depth by Morgan (1979), who considers that the evidence for anaphylactic shock is not very convincing and that pulmonary vascular obstruction is probably an important feature. Pulmonary vasospasm caused by prostaglandins may be a factor. The coagulopathy is probably primarily a consumption coagulopathy as the result of intravascular coagulation.

Initial treatment is rapid resuscitation, to establish a circulation, and adequate oxygenation with endotracheal intubation and IPPV, and subsequent treatment must be based upon the principles of intensive care. The severe hypoxia calls for oxygen therapy, probably with IPPV. Blood volume should be restored. Isoprenaline infusions may be helpful (Lumley et al,

1979). On theoretical grounds pulmonary vasospasm might be relieved by papaverine or aminophylline, and agents such as indomethacin or aspirin, which inhibit prostaglandin synthesis, could be tried (Morgan, 1979). Control of bleeding calls for blood transfusion. The decision to administer fibrinogen, fibrinolysin inhibitors (epsilonaminocaproic acid or aprotinon (Trasylol) calls for delicate judgement and the guidance of a haematologist. Leeton (1974) recommends the continuous infusion of heparin at a rate of 1500 units per hour, and suggests that fibrinogen should only be given if severe haemorrhage occurs from the uterus in association with hypofibrinogenaemia. Fibrinogen 6 g may be infused over 30 minutes or fresh frozen plasma may be substituted.

Uterine haemorrhage may indicate oxytocin infusion, bimanual compression of the uterus or packing of the uterine cavity. Major uterine trauma may call for surgical repair or for emergency hysterectomy.

Pulmonary (clot) embolism

Pulmonary embolism is now the leading cause of maternal death in the UK. The circulatory and coagulation changes of normal pregnancy encourage the formation of deep vein thrombosis (DVT) with the subsequent risk of pulmonary embolism. Risk factors associated with DVT include smoking, obesity, surgery, previous history of DVT and increasing age. The benefits of vertebral blocks in reducing the frequency of DVT (Davis and Quince, 1981; Thorburn et al, 1980; Modig et al, 1983) are not sufficiently well-recognized. Patients thought to be at risk and those undergoing caesarean section should be encouraged to have their delivery undertaken with epidural or spinal blocks.

Pulmonary embolism of blood clot is briefly discussed because diagnosis is difficult and the condition must be distinguished from other causes of post-delivery collapse such as Mendelson's syndrome and amniotic fluid embolism.

Pulmonary emboli usually originate in the veins of the leg or pelvis and most fatal emboli originate in the ileofemoral veins (Gibbs, 1957). Hypercoagulability and venous stasis in the legs and pelvis predispose to venous thrombosis in pregnancy. It is often presumed that reducing the incidence of deep venous thrombosis should reduce the incidence of pulmonary embolism, although this may not always be the case. Low-dose heparin is not usually given to obstetric patients as a routine but may be given to high-risk mothers, and only a few obstetricians routinely give dextran 70 at caesarean section (Bonnar and Walsh, 1972). Intermittent calf compression can be safely used in the course of caesarean section (Hills et al, 1972) and should be used in patients at special risk of deep venous thrombosis.

The diagnosis of pulmonary embolism is often far from easy. Only 28% have the classical triad of dyspnoea, haemoptysis and pleuritic pain. X-ray evidence is present in less than 50% and ECG changes are seen in 10–87% (American Heart Association, 1973). Hypoxia and hypocarbia usually accompany a pulmonary embolism and, if suspected, an arterial blood gas analysis should be obtained. If this confirms the suspicions, treatment with heparin may be commenced while waiting for a confirmatory ventilation/ perfusion lung scan. Heparin therapy is potentially dangerous, and to be effective in preventing further emboli, full heparinization is essential. It is therefore important to obtain objective evidence of a pulmonary embolism if possible.

The acutely ill patient with a suspected or confirmed pulmonary embolism should receive heparin 15 000 units intravenously and a further 60 000 units in the following 24 hours. Oxygen should be given and IPPV may be needed. Vasopressors are of value in shock due to pulmonary embolism (Price, 1976). The gravely ill patient with a massive pulmonary embolism may improve with intravenous digoxin or ouabain 0.5 mg and an isoprenaline infusion. External cardiac massage has been thought to break up a large clot and lead to its dispersal. Streptokinase therapy is especially hazardous in the postpartum patient because it is likely to cause uterine haemorrhage and, according to Price (1976), is contraindicated. Recurrent emboli may call for ligation or plication of the inferior vena cava (Miles and Elsea, 1971).

Abruptio placentae and defibrination

The anaesthetist may be involved in the management of abruptio placentae (accidental haemorrhage) either in the resuscitation of the patient or in the administration of anaesthesia.

In abruptio placentae it is well-recognized that shock is often of a degree greater than would be expected from the external blood loss. This is because there may be extensive, concealed retroplacental haemorrhage and perhaps also because of coagulation within the pulmonary capillaries (Scott, 1968).

Coagulation failure develops in 20% of patients with abruptio placentae (Hibbard and Jeffcoate, 1966). It is emphasized that only 25% of those who develop a coagulation defect exhibit excessive postpartum or intrapartum bleeding and that, when haemorrhage does occur, it is often due to uterine atony rather than to the clotting defect (Leeton, 1974). The two principal explanations proposed for coagulation failure in abruptio placentae are: (1) simple depletion of plasma fibrinogen owing to the deposition of fibrin in the extensive retroplacental clot (Nilsen, 1963) and (2) activation of the fibrinolytic system either locally at the placental site or generally in the blood stream. Hyperplasminaemia breaks down fibrin, and fibrinogen and the degradation products (FDPs) exert a powerful anticoagulant action (Scott, 1968; Bonnar et al, 1969). Disseminated intravascular coagulation is a recognized complication of abruptio placentae.

Treatment includes early delivery, usually per vaginam but sometimes by caesarean section if the infant is alive and mature (Hibbard and Jeffcoate, 1966). Coagulation failure is more likely to develop if delivery is delayed. Blood transfusion is frequently indicated and, because of the difficulty in estimating the fluid requirements, measurements of central venous pressure are often helpful. In general the volume required will substantially exceed the external blood loss. Blood is preferred to blood substitutes and if the blood is reasonably fresh it will be a source of clotting factors. If blood is unavailable then fresh frozen plasma should be used. It is now considered that hypofibrinogenaemia is not in itself an indication for the administration of fibrinogen (Leeton, 1974) because only one-quarter of the patients with hypofibrinogenaemia develop excessive bleeding. Fibrinogen should be given if severe bleeding ensues or if it is decided to perform caesarean section. Similarly the routine administration of epsilonaminocaproic acid or aprotinon (Trasylol) is not indicated merely because FDPs are detected in the blood. The dosage and administration of these products have been detailed in the preceding discussion on amniotic fluid embolism. A serious consequence of abruptio placentae is renal failure and this may result from the intravascular deposition of fibrin following upon the release of thromboplastins. Oliguria is an indication for the infusion of mannitol in the hope of preventing renal cortical necrosis (Stremple et al, 1966).

Other obstetric conditions in which a coagulation defect may develop include septic abortion, hydatidiform mole, eclampsia, saline-induced abortion and profound shock from any cause. If a dead fetus is retained for more than three or four weeks then coagulation failure may result. Epidural and subarachnoid analgesia are contraindicated in the presence of a coagulation defect because damage to an epidural vein may be followed by the formation of a large haematoma.

Heart disease

In the UK heart disease in pregnancy is now much less common, and this is due entirely to the smaller number of patients with rheumatic heart disease. The incidence of heart disease complicating pregnancy was observed to be 0.5% in Ireland (Sugrue et al, 1981), with rheumatic heart disease occurring in 83.5% and congenital heart disease accounting for 13%. Young women with surgically treated congenital heart disease are now surviving in growing numbers to bear children. Heart failure is also relatively uncommon. Barnes (1974) offers several explanations for the reduced incidence and severity of heart disease in pregnancy, including better treatment and prevention of rheumatic fever, smaller families at an earlier age, better ante-natal care, the abandonment of the misleading New York Heart Association classification, mitral valvotomy during pregnancy and the use of epidural analgesia and powerful diuretics in labour. Nevertheless the call for an increase in cardiac output always puts some additional strain on an abnormal heart.

It is customary to emphasize the time of the maximum occurrence of the development of cardiac failure, but experience has shown that failure may occur at any time (Sugrue et al, 1981) and constant vigilance is essential.

Heart failure occurs most frequently immediately after delivery and is then precipitated by the sudden increase in blood volume which accompanies uterine retraction and placental separation. Death from cardiac failure may occur between 14 and 20 weeks as result of the increase in blood volume and the demands of pregnancy but two-thirds of maternal deaths from heart disease occur during or shortly after labour and delivery (Conradsson and Werko, 1974). During labour tachycardia may precipitate cardiac failure, especially in patients with mitral stenosis. Pulmonary oedema may develop at any time during pregnancy if there is a tight mitral stenosis and may indicate mitral valvotomy. The cardiac output in pregnancy is usually lower in patients with heart disease than in normal pregnant women. Patients with mitral stenosis are especially likely to have a relatively low cardiac output when pregnant (Ueland et al, 1973). The normal increase in blood volume occurs and the arteriovenous oxygen difference is greater, indicating greater extraction of oxygen in the tissues.

Caesarean section should not be performed solely on account of heart disease and, when indicated for obstetric reasons, pulmonary embolism is a particular postoperative hazard. Vaginal delivery is usual and labour is frequently induced. Epidural analgesia is indicated (Barnes, 1974) and should be induced early in labour or at the time of amniotomy. Epidural analgesia relieves pain and distress and reduces the likelihood of tachycardia with associated inadequate filling of the heart in diastole. Crawford (1972) stresses that a tranquillizer should also be given for the relief of anxiety. Suitable alterations in posture will allow pooling of blood in the legs and the creation of a 'physiological venesection'. The sympathetic block which accompanies epidural analgesia reduces peripheral resistance and therefore reduces the work of the heart. It is essential that labour be conducted in the lateral position so that caval occlusion is avoided and venous return is maintained. Intravenous fluids should be given with caution. Arterial hypotension is unlikely if these precautions are scrupulously observed. An injection of phenylephrine 0.25 mg or a dilute infusion of the drug may be used if a vasopressor is required (Saka and Marx, 1976). The epidural block should be confined to the lower thoracic and upper lumbar nerve roots in the first stage of labour and extended to the sacral roots for delivery. Alternatively a two-catheter technique may be used. Epidural analgesia should not be used if the patient is currently receiving anticoagulants. When pulmonary oedema has developed in labour, the institution of an epidural block has been followed by a reduction in heart-rate and the resolution of pulmonary oedema (Moir and Willocks, 1968). If caesarean section is to be performed, then general anaesthesia may be selected because the risk of arterial hypotension is high in association with an extensive epidural block.

Other measures which may be indicated during labour include oxygen therapy for dyspnoea and the elevation of the shoulders upon several pillows. Good analgesia and the relief of anxiety are important. The Valsalva manoeuvre associated with expulsive efforts reduces venous return and causes hypoxia, and should be avoided by elective forceps delivery. The second stage should be shortened by forceps delivery or vacuum extraction and epidural analgesia allows these procedures to be performed. Intravenous ergometrine may precipitate cardiac failure by increasing blood volume and central venous pressure. Intravenous oxytocin 5 units is preferred and should be followed by a slow infusion of 20 units in an appropriate vehicle. Some obstetricians give no oxytocic drug to patients with severe heart disease. The prophylactic use of antibiotics may be questioned, although it is standard practice. The incidence of bacterial endocarditis when antibiotics are not used is <0.05%, and it is not clear if their use would reduce this (Sugrue et al, 1980). Digitalization may be advised before the planned induction of labour in patients with signs of cardiac failure. Digoxin has an action on the myometrium and may shorten labour (Weaver and Pearson, 1973). The pharmacodynamics of drug therapy are altered in pregnancy, and digoxin treatment should be monitored by measuring the blood digoxin level occasionally.

If pulmonary oedema develops then oxygen, morphine and intravenous frusemide 40 mg should be given. Aminophylline 0.5 g by slow intravenous injection may relieve the bronchospasm often associated with pulmonary oedema. A bloodless venesection may be performed by the application of sphygmomanometer cuffs to all four limbs. After 15 minutes the cuffs are released one by one at 5-minute intervals. The inflation pressure should be about 40 mmHg (5.0 kPa). Digitalis is usually ineffective in pulmonary oedema if myocardial damage is absent, and diuretics and other measures to reduce blood volume are required. Congestive cardiac failure is less common and rather less serious, occurring mainly in patients with valvular incompetence and myocardial damage. Frusemide is indicated and digitalis (digoxin) should be administered to any patient who has not already received this drug.

Congenital heart disease without cyanosis will usually be associated with a successful and uneventful pregnancy and labour, perhaps because most patients who pass the age of puberty have a relatively mild defect or have already undergone surgical correction of the defect. The myocardium is usually healthy in these patients, whereas those with rheumatic heart disease may suffer from myocarditis. There is a definite risk of bacterial endocarditis, and all patients with congenital heart disease should receive antibiotic cover for labour and delivery (Barnes, 1974). Patients with ventricular septal defect, complete heart block, patent ductus arteriosus and pulmonary stenosis usually do well. Those with an atrial septal defect usually have a trouble-free pregnancy and labour, although reversal of the shunt due to pulmonary hypertension may occur. The risk of thromboembolic complications is greatest in patients who have had cardiac surgery and in patients with pulmonary hypertension.

Cyanotic congenital heart disease carries a poor prognosis for mother and child. In severe cases the fetal loss may be as high as 80% (Neill and Swanson,

1961) and is due to intrauterine hypoxia, prematurity and dysmaturity. Patients with Fallot's tetralogy are liable to develop extreme tachycardia with hypotension during labour. Eisenmenger's syndrome carries a very grave outlook in pregnancy, and the maternal mortality exceeds 25%. It is therefore usual to advise termination of pregnancy in this condition. If pregnancy continues to term, then vaginal delivery under an epidural block may be decided upon and an oxytocic drug should be withheld (Barnes, 1974). It may be safe to administer oxytocin 5 units intravenously, but ergometrine should certainly be avoided. Asling and Fung (1974) used epidural analgesia successfully for tubal ligation in a patient with Eisenmenger's syndrome. Patients with a left-to-right shunt (e.g. patent ductus arteriosus, atrial and ventricular septal defect, Fallot's tetralogy and Eisenmenger's complex) should not be permitted to develop arterial hypotension, because reversal of the shunt may then occur. The risk of thromboembolism is considerable and elective caesarean section should not be performed solely on account of heart disease. The aim, as with patients with rheumatic heart disease, is the planned induction of a short, painless, anxiety-free labour and elective delivery by forceps. Epidural analgesia is ideal provided that anticoagulants have been stopped and caval occlusion is avoided.

Patients with a cardiac valve prosthesis present the problems of the increased cardiac work load of pregnancy and chronic anticoagulant therapy. Warfarin therapy during pregnancy results in a fetal loss of approximately 40% and a warfarin-induced neonatal deformity in <5% of deliveries. Ideally, heparin anticoagulation should be undertaken before pregnancy occurs and continued to term. However, if the patient presents after the first trimester, warfarin therapy should be continued and changed to heparin at week 37 of gestation (O'Neil et al, 1982). Saka and Marx (1976) advise the use of heparin in the later weeks of pregnancy, the discontinuation of the anticoagulant at the onset of labour and its reinstitution 24 hours after delivery. Labour is managed under epidural analgesia, oxytocin is given instead of ergometrine and bearing down is avoided by elective forceps delivery. Fetal wastage is high in women who receive coumarin therapy in early pregnancy (Lutz et al, 1978) owing to the harmful effects of this drug upon the fetus.

During the last two decades the increasing safety of open heart surgery and the increasing number of reports of successful surgery during pregnancy have made cardiac surgery the appropriate and sometimes preferable alternative to medical management, if the underlying cardiac abnormality is severe and correctable. Unanimous opinion is that surgery should be undertaken as early as possible after the first trimester (Eilen et al, 1981).

Cardiomyopathy of pregnancy has been long recognized, but the literature is confusing because most of the conditions described are non-specific and non-diagnostic, and are often rather remotely related to pregnancy. The subject has been extensively reviewed by Veille (1984) who recommends supportive treatment and consideration of the use of steroids and immunosuppressive drugs.

Respiratory disease

Severe respiratory disease is uncommon in pregnancy and will not be discussed in detail.

Chronic bronchitis and emphysema. Patients with obstructive airways disease are usually little affected by pregnancy but may become dyspnoeic during labour and delivery. Narcotic analgesics need not be given if epidural analgesia is employed, and controlled oxygen therapy may be indicated. Labour and delivery have been successfully managed under epidural analgesia in a respiratory cripple who had just recovered from a severe episode of respiratory failure and who died from this cause three months postpartum (Moir and Willocks, 1968). If long-term antibiotic therapy is to be used during pregnancy to control secondary infection then the tetracyclines should be avoided. These antibiotics cause discoloration of the teeth and hypoplasia of the enamel in the child, and bone growth may be depressed. Rupture of an emphysematous bulla has resulted in the development of a tension pneumotherax during labour (Vance, 1968).

Asthma. Asthma is usually unaffected by pregnancy. Steroids may be administered during pregnancy and it has been recommended that labour and delivery should be 'covered' by the administration of 100 mg of hydrocortisone twice daily for three or four days if steroids have been used within the previous year (Barnes, 1974). The inhalation of isoprenaline for brief periods is considered harmless and the relaxant effet on uterine muscle is of very short duration. The action of disodium cromoglycate on the developing embryo is unknown and the evidence that steroid therapy may cause cleft palate is not very convincing in the human embryo.

Pneumomediastinum. This is a rare complication of labour and is due to the performance of violent expulsive efforts against a closed glottis resulting in subpleural or interstitial rupture of alveoli. Air then tracks alongside the pulmonary vessels to the mediastinal tissues. Air may then spread along fascial planes into the neck and axillae. There may be an associated pneumothorax. Although the grossly swollen and crepitant subcutaneous tissues may create an alarming appearance, recovery is usually uneventful. An antibiotic should be given to prevent mediastinitis and the inhalation of oxygen may hasten the absorption of air.

Jaundice in pregnancy

More than 50% of all cases of jaundice in pregnancy are due to infective (viral) hepatitis. In late pregnancy infective hepatitis is often severe and very rarely may be complicated by acute hepatic necrosis. The prognosis for mother and child is then very poor. This form of acute hepatic necrosis is probably the same as the acute yellow atrophy described by old writers who erroneously attributed the condition to pre-eclampsia.

Other causes of jaundice in pregnancy include drugs such as chlorpromazine and other phenothiazines which may be prescribed for vomiting in pregnancy and liver disorders related to pregnancy. Acute fatty liver of pregnancy is a rare and almost always fatal condition and was referred to as acute yellow atrophy by Sheehan. There are epigastric pain, vomiting, high fever, deep jaundice of the obstructive type and spontaneous haemorrhages. Coma and death follow in about 90% of patients, despite intrauterine death of the fetus or termination of the pregnancy. Transaminases are normal, indicating that hepatic necrosis is absent; the liver is small and yellow and there are foamy cells in the centrilobular regions. Intrahepatic cholestasis of pregnancy is another rare cause of jaundice in late pregnancy. Recovery is usual and the obstructive jaundice is usually not severe and may be due to a physicochemical alteration in the bile. The picture is similar to that produced by drugs such as chlorpromazine.

Anaesthesia will not often be required for patients with severe liver damage and a haemorrhagic tendency. Epidural and subarachnoid analgesia may cause extensive bleeding within the epidural space and should be avoided. A technique of anaesthesia based upon a minimal dose of thiopentone, nitrous oxide, oxygen and a muscle relaxant may be selected.

Diabetes mellitus

The extensive hormonal changes accompanying normal pregnancy have a profound influence on carbohydrate metabolism throughout pregnancy. The alterations in the normal pregnant patient of relevance to the management of diabetes are, briefly, lower fasting and higher peak blood glucose levels, increased insulin antagonism in the second half of pregnancy, increased insulin response in the third trimester, and increased glomerular filtration rate with a reduced tubular absorption of glucose resulting in an increased frequency of glycosuria. The hormonal changes of pregnancy demand more insulin production and the majority of mothers can respond. The few unable to do so develop pregnancy-induced diabetes, usually during the second half of pregnancy. Normal pregnancy is therefore associated with a wide range of blood glucose levels, but the range is relatively narrow compared to even well-controlled diabetes.

Pregnancy profoundly affects established diabetes, irrespective of the onset type, and control is, not surprisingly, more difficult than in the non-pregnant state. Little change of insulin requirement is observed during the first trimester; thereafter there is a progressive and unpredictable increase.

The diagnosis of diabetes during pregnancy was formerly based on the presence of glycosuria, but the relationship between blood and urine glucose levels is extremely variable for the reasons outlined above. The diagnosis of diabetes should be based on the results of a glucose tolerance test, which should be performed if:

(1) the patient is obese, >120% of ideal weight.

(2) exhibits glycosuria twice.

(3) has a history of previous congenital abnormality, unexplained stillbirth, neonatal death or large babies.

(4) has a history of gestational diabetes.

Some controversy exists regarding the ideal glucose load for a glucose tolerance test and the interpretation of the results. A normal test (with 50 g glucose) has a fasting and 2-hour glucose level at or below 6.7 mmol/litre (120 mg%) and a 1-hour glucose level at or below 10 mmol/litre (180 mg %). If two or more levels are raised, the test is positive. It must be emphasized that glucose intolerance adversely affects the fetus, irrespective of the type of intolerance, and from the baby's point of view diabetes in pregnancy is never mild.

The object of management is to attempt to maintain maternal blood glucose levels at or as near normal levels as possible. This can only be achieved by dedicated and enthusiastic cooperation between the patient, diabetic physician and obstetrician. Good control demands frequent estimations of maternal blood glucose levels. Urinalysis is too inaccurate and is no longer used. Diabetic patients ideally should attend pre-pregnancy clinics where they are taught to measure their blood glucose levels at home, and the importance of good control, which is not always easy to achieve, is emphasized. The prognosis when management is based on early and effective blood glucose control as outlined is vastly improved. Despite good diabetic control, fetal abnormality and macrosomia continue to be a problem. Routine antenatal use of ultrasound to estimate fetal size and growth should identify macrosomic infants, and the appropriate time and method of delivery can then be selected. For the majority of mothers with good diabetic control and normal fetal growth, the outlook is excellent. Pregnancy should continue to term or near term, intensive fetal monitoring is unnecessary and caesarean section should only be undertaken if there is an obstetric indication.

Diabetic management for delivery. Insulin requirements during labour and delivery are based solely on the maternal blood glucose levels, which are measured before labour (if induced) and monitored at hourly intervals throughout. Impregnated stick testing is sufficiently accurate. One litre of 5% dextrose solution is infused every 8 hours. Insulin is best administered by an infusion pump containing one unit of insulin per ml of normal saline, and the rate of infusion is adjusted to maintain the maternal blood glucose level at 5–7 mmol/litre (90–125 mg%). This management is continued throughout labour and delivery, and should also be used for both elective and emergency caesarean sections.

Epidural analgesia is the technique of choice for both labour and for caesarean section because it reduces the acidosis associated with normal labour and provides excellent conditions for the baby. Intravenous fluids to combat maternal dehydration or for epidural analgesia should consist of balanced electrolyte solutions without dextrose and should be infused through a separate cannula. If general anaesthesia is required, the steps outlined in chapter 6 should be taken, and the diabetes managed as above. Maintaining the maternal blood glucose at the levels described minimizes the neonatal hypoglycaemia associated with maternal hyperglycaemia.

Maternal diabetic control during pregnancy should not be maintained by oral hypoglycaemic agents, as they cross the placenta, but if used they should be stopped at least 48 hours before delivery.

Diseases of the nervous system

Only selected conditions which may concern the anaesthetist are considered here and then only briefly.

Spontaneous subarachnoid haemorrhage. Subarachnoid haemorrhage is not more common in pregnancy or labour, although the hypertension of pre-eclampsia may be a predisposing factor (Walton, 1953). In about 30% of patients, haemorrhage arises from a cerebral angioma (Amias, 1970) and the prognosis is then relatively good. If coma, convulsions and hypertension occur then the condition may mimic eclampsia, but the absence of proteinuria and the presence of neck stiffness and blood in the cerebrospinal fluid should clarify the diagnosis. A subarachnoid haemorrhage during pregnancy necessitates transfer of the patient to a neurosurgical unit. Aneurysm surgery has been successfully performed under hypotensive anaesthesia with nitroprusside (Donchin et al, 1978) and with trimetaphan camsylate (Minielly et al, 1979). Hypotension caused fetal bradycardia but the infants survived, apparently unharmed; if it appears that essential aneurysm surgery should be performed during pregnancy, and if hypotension is necessary for successful surgery, then it should be used. Usually a vaginal delivery is advocated (Fliegner et al, 1969; Amias, 1970) although a forceps delivery or vacuum extraction is advocated because expulsive efforts are avoided. Continuous epidural analgesia is appropriate and intravenous ergometrine should be avoided because it may cause hypertension. Caesarean section is indicated if the haemorrhage is recent and the mother has not undergone surgery, if the mother is moribund or if obstetric indications are present and the fetus is viable.

Cerebral thrombosis. Although cerebral vascular occlusion is rare in young women, it is relatively often associated with childbearing when it does occur (Jennet and Cross, 1967). Cerebral thrombosis occurs most frequently in the puerperium, and then usually two or three weeks postpartum. Drowsiness and headache are often followed by unconsciousness, and hemiplegia or other focal signs may develop. Although a diagnosis of eclampsia may be considered, the onset late in the puerperium and the absence of pre-eclampsia should suggest the correct diagnosis.

Epilepsy. Epilepsy may become better or worse during pregnancy and deterioration if it occurs may be attributable to salt and water retention. The pregnant epileptic should continue treatment with phenobarbitone, phenytoin or primidone. If it is wished to avoid oral medication in labour then an intramuscular injection of 200 mg sodium phenobarbitone may be given. Epilepsy can usually be distinguished from eclampsia by the history and the absence of hypertension and proteinuria. Status epilepticus may occur in the absence of a history of epilepsy and is a rare but sometimes fatal condition. An intravenous injection of 10 mg of diazepam is recommended and this should be followed by further injections or by an infusion of 100 mg of diazepam in 500 ml. Curarization and IPPV may be required.

Polyneuritis of pregnancy. In this rare condition an extensive lower motor neurone lesion develops and there is associated sensory loss. Ventilatory failure may ensue. Polyneuritis of pregnancy may be associated with hyperemesis gravidarum and is then thought to be due to thiamine deficiency.

Poliomyelitis. Poliomyelitis is said to be more severe and to carry a high mortality rate if it occurs during pregnancy. The fetus does not usually develop the disease but abortion and intrauterine death are quite common and fetal hypoxia may result from maternal respiratory inadequacy. Uterine contractions are unaffected but paralysis of the abdominal muscles will necessitate delivery by forceps. Patients have been delivered by forceps while undergoing ventilator therapy.

Multiple sclerosis. Pregnancy has no effect on multiple sclerosis and the disease has no direct effect upon pregnancy. Because remissions and relapses are notoriously unpredictable, it is customary to avoid epidural and subarachnoid analgesia for fear that a relapse might be attributed (probably erroneously) to the technique of analgesia. Crawford (1978) has given epidural analgesia to three patients with multiple sclerosis after discussion and explanation, and reported 'no cause for concern'. Crawford et al (1981) support the use of epidural analgesia in patients with multiple sclerosis, but Warren et al (1982) noted that recovery took from seven days to seven weeks in the same patient receiving epidural analgesia twice. Spinal analgesia may be preferable, as the mass of drug is less, but Bamford et al (1978) have implicated spinal anaesthesia in multiple sclerosis. It may be an example of defensive medicine to withhold epidural analgesia in painful labour for fear of litigation, but it should be said that the effect of epidural analgesia on multiple sclerosis is unknown and a conservative policy should be followed.

Myasthenia gravis

This rare disease is relatively common in young women and is therefore sometimes associated with pregnancy. Although it could be postulated that the increased output of cortisone and ACTH in pregnancy might aggravate the disease, the effect of pregnancy on myasthenia gravis is variable (McNall and Jafarnia, 1965) and, in Osserman's (1958) series, in one-third of the patients the disease became more severe during pregnancy. Deterioration is most frequent in the puerperium (Fraser and Turner, 1963).

Uterine action is unaffected and if adequate anticholinesterase therapy is maintained during pregnancy and labour, then vaginal delivery is likely and caesarean section is not indicated on medical grounds. Neostigmine or pyridostigmine are given by mouth during pregnancy and should be given by intramuscular injection during labour. Forceps delivery is often required and epidural analgesia may be induced during the first stage of labour. General anaesthesia should be avoided by the use of epidural or subarachnoid analgesia whenever possible. Caesarean section can be performed under conduction analgesia. If general anaesthesia is used then non-depolarizing muscle relaxants are contraindicated. The trachea may be intubated under halothane anaesthesia and the halothane should thereafter be eliminated to prevent uterine relaxation and bleeding at delivery. Anaesthesia and adequate relaxation of the abdominal wall can, in the writers' experience, be maintained by IPPV with cyclopropane and oxygen in myasthenic patients.

About 20% of the infants born to myasthenic mothers will develop transient neonatal myasthenia gravis. The infant lies motionless and may have difficulty in breathing and swallowing. Although recovery is usual within two or three weeks, treatment with pyridostigmine 5 mg by mouth or 0.25 mg by injection may be required. Anticholinesterase drugs pass from mother to fetus and their use may delay the onset of neonatal myasthenia gravis. The anaesthetic considerations for myasthenia gravis in pregnancy have been reviewed in detail by Rolbin et al (1978).

Maternal muscle disease and malignant hyperpyrexia

It is important to distinguish these disorders from neurological disorders, and an objective assessment must be made in patients who give a history suggestive of muscle disease. Screening tests should include respiratory function tests, electromyography and muscle biopsy. Muscle enzyme estimations are of no value because the levels are increased in pregnancy. Muscle disease is relatively common but associated problems are relatively unusual. Over 400 conditions have been described, but the majority are very rare. Suxamethonium is used routinely for endotracheal intubation in obstetrics, and its site and mechanism of action increase its association with drug-induced muscle problems. If muscle disease is known before anaesthesia is required, or a suggestive history is obtained, efforts should be directed to making an accurate diagnosis, and general anaesthesia should be avoided if possible. The use of local blocks should be encouraged, and bupivacaine is the local analgesic agent of choice (Willats, 1979).

If an abnormal response to general anaesthesia involving a rise in temperature or muscle spasm is noted during the anaesthetic, then an elective procedure not involving delivery should be abandoned. The airway should be protected, the ECG, heart-rate, respiratory rate and temperature monitored, arterial blood gases tensions estimated and venous blood withdrawn for measurement of the serum potassium. The first voided specimen of urine should be obtained for myoglobin estimation. Dantrolene and dexamethasone should be administered if monitoring confirms an abnormality and the core temperature is rising. A simple and effective protocol for the management of malignant hyperpyrexia must be readily available together with all the equipment and drugs.

Malignant hyperthermia susceptibility

The effect of pregnancy on malignant hyperthermia susceptible patients is uncertain and only one incident of malignant hyperthermia during labour appears to have been reported, although that patient's mother had died of probable malignant hyperthermia during labour 30 years earlier (Wadhwa, 1977). The condition has been reported during caesarean section under halothane anaesthesia in susceptible animals (Lucke, 1977). It is evident that pregnancy does not protect against malignant hyperthermia, and the obstetric anaesthetist may encounter a patient with this rare, familial and potentially fatal disease.

The known triggering agents must be avoided and, if general anaesthesia is considered essential, then halothane and suxamethonium should not be used. Undoubtedly regional analgesia is the better choice for labour, delivery and caesarean section because it does not seem to precipitate malignant hyperthermia. Epidural analgesia is the best choice. Although subarachnoid analgesia was followed by a substantial rise in serum creatine phosphokinase when given for forceps delivery, the body temperature and vital signs were unaltered (Wadhwa, 1977).

Patients who give a history suggestive of malignant hyperthermia, and especially those whose relatives have unexpectedly died during general anaesthesia, should be screened for the disease. Screening tests include muscle biopsy, electromyography and serum creatine phosphokinase estimation. Patients susceptible to malignant hyperthermia should have temperature and vital signs monitored during labour and delivery under epidural analgesia. Arterial blood gas tension and serum electrolytes and enzymes should be estimated. Willats (1979) successfully used continuous epidural analgesia with 0.5% bupivacaine without adrenaline for labour and forceps delivery in a susceptible patient. Dantrolene for infusion and a water mattress for cooling should be available.

Acute porphyria

Pregnancy probably has a deleterious effect on the acute porphyrias (acute intermittent porphyria, variegate porphyria and hereditary coproporphyria) and an acute attack is more likely during pregnancy (Brodie et al, 1977). It is thought that the sex hormones and in particular dehydroepiandrosterone can precipitate an attack. Brodie et al reviewed 50 pregnancies in patients with acute porphyria. Only one mother died but the fetal loss was 13%. Babies born to mothers who had an attack during pregnancy were smaller. Attacks were not usually provoked by known porphyrogenic drugs.

Epidural analgesia is probably safe in acute porphyria, and any neurological sequelae are likely to be due to the disease. If general anaesthesia is required, the inhalational agents and the muscle relaxants may be used. If an inhalational induction is unacceptable, then etomidate and ketamine appear to be free of risk (Parikh and Moore, 1975; Rizk et al, 1977), but the barbiturates should be avoided.

Phaeochromocytoma

The association of pregnancy and a phaeochromocytoma carries a grave prognosis. A maternal mortality rate of 48% was recorded by Leak et al (1977). In Schenker and Chowers' (1971) series the maternal mortality rate was 58% if the diagnosis was not made before delivery and 18% if it was diagnosed during pregnancy. The fetal mortality is about 50%.

If the diagnosis is made in the early weeks of pregnancy, the tumour should be excised. If diagnosed later in pregnancy, then treatment with α- and β-adrenergic blockers should be continued until near term. The patient should then be delivered by elective caesarean section and the phaeochromocytoma should be excised at that time. Burgess et al (1978) describe the management of a combined caesarean section and excision of phaeochromocytoma. They used a thiopentone, nitrous oxide and relaxant technique with a phentolamine infusion and intensive monitoring. A β-blocker was not used.

Haemoglobinopathies

The sickle cell trait exists in about 10% of persons of African descent (Howells et al, 1972), and routine screening of all such patients has been recommended (Konotey-Ahulu, 1969). Although it is usually harmless, death has been recorded in association with anaesthesia in this condition (Konotey-Ahulu, 1969; Jones et al, 1970). Sickle cell disease occurs when the relatively insoluble reduced Hb-S is precipitated out of the cells. Sickling occurs in sickle cell anaemia, sickle cell Hb-C disease and sickle cell thalassaemia. In some types of thalassaemia there is a failure of synthesis of normal haemoglobin and this condition exists quite extensively among Mediterranean, Middle Eastern, Indian and Chinese races.

Patients with sickle cell disease should be considered as high-risk obstetric patients and should attend the antenatal clinics at intervals of not less than 14 days. A careful search for infection, especially of the urinary and respiratory tracts, should be performed and evidence of endometritis should be sought. If infection develops, vigorous treatment should be implemented. The patient must be admitted to hospital for appropriate antibiotic therapy and hydration. The haemoglobin concentration should be maintained, by transfusion if necessary, at 10–12 g/dl (Tuck et al, 1982). In a crisis, as occurs with a serious infection or if the haematocrit is <20%, an isovolumetric partial exchange transfusion should be carried out using a relatively simple formula described by Nagey et al (1984).

Anaesthesia and surgery may be fatal in patients with sickle cell disease and even in sickle cell trait there is a slightly increased risk. Howells et al (1972) recommend the following precautions before and during anaesthesia:

(1) For carriers of the sickle cell trait: preoxygenation with 100% oxygen before induction of anaesthesia and the inhalation of at least 30% oxygen during anaesthesia, the maintenance of hydration and normothermia and the inhalation of oxygen in the postoperative period.

(2) For sickle cell disease: preoperative transfusion of blood for the often severe anaemia is not usually advisable (Howells et al, 1972; Searle, 1973) because stored blood increases oxygen demand. If given, then a small volume of fresh blood is advised. Preoperative alkalinization with oral sodium bicarbonate and the intravenous administration of this agent during surgery is advised, although its value is uncertain. Maintain blood volume with blood substitutes or fresh blood. Use nerve blocks and epidural or subarachnoid analgesia with normotension. If general anaesthesia is used then preoxygenation, hyperventilation and the avoidance of myocardial depressant drugs is advocated. Despite these precautions the patient may die. The experiences of Homi et al 1979) in Jamaica were encouraging. They administered general anaesthesia on 284 occasions to 200 patients with sickle cell disease over a 20-year period, and suggest that if a careful, uneventful general anaesthetic is administered, then a sickling crisis is unlikely to be provoked, and death attributable to anaesthesia did not occur in that series. Routine blood transfusion was not advised.

Pregnancy imposes additional stresses upon the patient with sickle cell disease and may be a serious threat to life among Nigerian women (Fullerton and Watson-Williams, 1962). Anaemia and haemolysis further increase folic acid requirements, and if these are not met, then a megaloblastic anaemia may be added to the existing haemolytic anaemia. The fetal loss is very high in sickle cell anaemia. Crises are common in the last trimester and in prolonged labour or difficult delivery. Consequently, although caesarean section is hazardous, an early delivery by this means may yet be safer than a prolonged labour (Shervington, 1974). It has been suggested that caval occlusion (concealed or revealed) may cause hypoxaemia and acidosis and so precipitate a crisis (Crawford, 1972); this suggestion seems a reasonable one.

For further information on the large and difficult problem of the haemoglobinopathies in relation to anaesthesia the reader is referred to comprehensive reviews by Howells et al (1972), Searle (1973) and Oduro (1973).

REFERENCES

Adams, A.P., Morgan, M., Jones, B.C. and McCormick, P.W. (1969) A case of massive aspiration of gastric contents during obstetric anaesthesia. *Br. J. Anaesth.*, **41**, 176.

American Heart Association (1973) The Urokinase Pulmonary Embolism Trial: a national cooperative study. *Circulation*, **47**, Suppl. 2.

Amias, A.G. (1970) Cerebral vascular disease in pregnancy. I. Haemorrhage. *J. Obstet. Gynaec. Br. Commonw.*, **76**, 912.

Arias, F. (1975) Expansion of intravascular volume and fetal outcome in patients with chronic hypertension and pregnancy. *Am. J. Obstet. Gynec.*, **123**, 610.

Asling, J.H. and Fung, D.L. (1974) Epidural anesthesia in Eisenmenger's syndrome. A case report. *Anesth. Analg. curr. Res.*, **53**, 965.

Attwood, H.D. (1972) Amniotic fluid embolism. *Path. Ann.*, **7**, 145.

Awe, W.C., Fletcher, W.S. and Jacob, S.W. (1966) Pathophysiology of aspiration pneumonitis. *Surgery, St. Louis*, **60**, 232.

Bamford, C., Sibley, W. and Laguna, J. (1978) Anaesthesia in multiple sclerosis. *Can. J. Neurol. Sci.*, **5**, 41.

Bannister, W.K. and Sattilaro, A.J. (1962) Vomiting and aspiration during anesthesia. *Anesthesiology*, **23**, 251.

Bannister, W.K., Sattilaro, A.J. and Otis, R.D. (1961) Therapeutic aspects of aspiration pneumonitis in experimental animals. *Anesthesiology*, **22**, 440.

Barnes, C.G. (1974) *Medical Disorders in Obstetric Practice*, 4th ed. Oxford: Blackwell.

Beller, F.K. (1974) Disseminated intravascular coagulation and consumption coagulopathy in obstetrics. *Obstet. Gynec. Ann.*, **3**, 267.

Birmingham Eclampsia Study Group (1971) *Lancet*, **ii**, 889.

Bonnar, J. and Walsh, J. (1972) Prevention of thrombosis after pelvic surgery by British dextran 70. *Lancet*, **i**, 614.

Bonnar, J., Davidson, J.F., Pidgeon, C.F., McNicol, G.P. and Douglas, A.S. (1969) Fibrin degradation products in normal and abnormal pregnancy and parturition. *Br. med. J.*, **iii**, 137.

Bonnar, J., McNicol, G.P. and Douglas, A.S. (1969) Coagulation defects in obstetrics. In *Modern Trends in Obstetrics*, ed. Kellar, R.J., 4th ed. London: Butterworth.

Brewer, T.H. (1962) The limitations of diuretic therapy in the management of severe toxemia: the significance of hypoalbuminemia. *Am. J. Obstet. Gynec.*, **83**, 1352.

Brodie, M.J., Moore, M.R., Thomson, G.G., Goldberg, A. and Low, R.A.L. (1977) Pregnancy and the acute porphyrias. *Br. J. Obstet. Gynaec.*, **84**, 726.

Burgess, G.E., Cooper, J.R., Marino, R.J. and Peuler, M.J. (1978) Anesthetic management of combined Cesarean section and excision of pheochromocytoma. *Anesth. Analg. curr. Res.*, **57**, 276.

Cameron, J.L. and Zuidema, G.D. (1972) Aspiration pneumonia: magnitude and frequency of the problem. *J. Am. med. Ass.*, **219**, 1194.

Caritis, S., Morishima, H., Stark, R. and James, L.S. (1976) The effect of diazoxide on uterine blood flow in pregnant sheep. *Obstet. Gynec.*, **48**, 464.

Chamberlain, G.V.P., Lewis, P.J., De Sweit, M. and Bulpitt, C.J. (1978) How obstetricians manage hypertension in pregnancy. *Br. med. J.*, **276**, 626.

Chan, W.F. and Delilkan, A.E. (1970) The management of severe postpartum eclampsia with D-tubocurarine and controlled ventilation in the intensive care unit. *Aust. N.Z. J. Obstet. Gynaec.*, **10**, 187.

Chapman, R.L., Modell, J.H., Ruiz, B.C. et al (1974) Effect of continuous positive pressure ventilation and steroids on aspiration of hydrochloric acid (pH 1.8) in dogs. *Anesth. Analg. Curr. Res.*, **53**, 556.

Collins, R., Yusuf, S. and Peto, R. (1985) Overview of randomized trials of diuretics in pregnancy. *Br. med. J.*, **290**, 17.

Conradsson, T.B. and Werko, L. (1974) Management of heart disease in pregnancy. *Prog. cardiovasc. Dis.*, **16**, 407.

Cove, D.H., Seddon, M., Fletcher, R.F. and Dukes, D.C. (1979) Blindness after treatment for malignant hypertension. *Br. med. J.*, **ii**, 245.

Crawford, J.S. (1972) *Principles and Practice of Obstetric Anaesthesia*, 3rd ed. Oxford: Blackwell.

Crawford, J.S. (1978) *Principles and Practice of Obstetric Anaesthesia*, 4th ed. Oxford: Blackwell.

Crawford, J.S. and Opit, L.J. (1976) A survey of the anaesthetic services to obstetrics in the Birmingham Region. *Anaesthesia*, **31**, Suppl. 56.

Crawford, J.S., James, F.M., Nolte, H., Van Steenberg, A. and Shah, J.L. (1981) Regional anaesthesia for patients with chronic neurological disease and similar conditions. *Anaesthesia*, **36**, 821.

Davidson, J.T., Rubin, S., Eyal, Z. and Polliack, A. (1974) A comparison of the pulmonary response to the endotracheal instillation of 0.1N hydrochloric acid and Hartmann's solution in the rabbit. *Br. J. Anaesth.*, **46**, 127.

Davis, F.M. and Quince, M. (1980) Deep vein thrombosis and anaesthetic technique in emergency hip surgery. *Br. med. J.*, **281**, 1528.

de Bastos, M. and Srinivasan, K. (1964) Afibrinogenemia secondary to pulmonary amniotic fluid embolism. *N.Y. St. J. Med.*, **64**, 1119.

Department of Health and Social Security (1975) *Report on Confidential Enquiries into Maternal Deaths in England and Wales, 1970–1972*. London: H.M.S.O.

Department of Health and Social Security (1979) *Report on Confidential Enquiries into Maternal Deaths in England and Wales, 1973–1975*. London: H.M.S.O.

Dewar, J.B. and Morris, W.I.C. (1947) Sedation with rectal tribromethanol (Avertin, bromethol) in the management of eclampsia. *J. Obstet. Gynaec. Br. Emp.*, **54**, 417.

Donchin, Y., Amirav, B., Sahar, A. and Yarkoni, S. (1978) Sodium nitroprusside for aneurysm surgery in pregnancy. *Br. J. Anaesth.*, **50**, 849.

Downs, J.B., Chapman, R.L., jr., Modell, J.H. and Hood, I. (1974) An evaluation of steroid therapy in aspiration pneumonitis. *Anesthesiology*, **40**, 129.

Dudley, W.R. and Marshall, B.E. (1974) Steroid treatment for acid-aspiration pneumonitis. *Anesthesiology*, **40**, 136.

Duff, P., Engelsgjerd, B., Zingery, L., Huff, R. and Montel, M. (1983) Haemodynamic observations in a patient with intrapartum amniotic fluid embolism. *Am. J. Obstet. Gynec.*, **146**, 112.

Duffus, G.M., Tunstall, M.E., Condie, R.G. and MacGillivray, I. (1969) Chlormethiazole in the prevention of eclampsia and the reduction of perinatal mortality. *J. Obstet. Gynaec. Br. Commonw.*, **76**, 645.

Editorial (1979) Dangerous antihypertensive treatment. *Br. med. J.*, **ii**, 228.

Eilen, B., Kaiser, I.H., Becker, R.M. and Cohen, M. (1981) Aortic valve replacement in the third trimester of pregnancy: case report and review of the literature. *Obstet. Gynec.*, **57**, 119.

Ellis, F.R. (1974) Neuromuscular disease and anaesthesia. *Br. J. Anaesth.*, **46**, 603.

Fliegner, J.R.H., Hooper, R.S. and Kloss, M. (1969) Subarachnoid haemorrhage and pregnancy. *J. Obstet. Gynaec. Br. Commonw.*, **76**, 912.

Fraser, D. and Turner, J.W.A. (1963) Myasthenia gravis and pregnancy. *Proc. R. Soc. Med.*, **56**, 379.

Fullerton, W.T. and Watson-Williams, E.J. (1962) Haemoglobin S.C. disease and megaloblastic anaemia of pregnancy. *J. Obstet. Gynaec. Br. Commonw.*, **69**, 729.

Gibbs, N.M. (1957) Venous thrombosis of the lower limbs with particular reference to bed rest. *Br. J. Surg.*, **45**, 209.

Gibbs, C.P., Schwartz, D.J., Wynne, J.W., Hood, C. and Kuck, E.J. (1979) Antacid pulmonary aspiration in the dog. *Anesthesiology*, **51**, 380.

Gordon, H. (1970) The modern management of eclampsia. *Midwife and Health Visitor*, **71**, 260.

Gordon, H. (1974) Toxaemia of pregnancy. In *Obstetric Therapeutics*, ed. Hawkins, D.F. London: Baillière Tindall.

Hamelberg, W. and Bosomworth, P.P. (1964) Aspiration pneumonitis: experimental studies and clinical observations. *Anesth. Analg. curr. Res.*, **43**, 669.

Hibbard, B.M. and Jeffcoate, T.N.A. (1966) Abruptio placentae. *Obstet. Gynec.*, **27**, 155.

Hills, N.H., Pflug, J.J., Jeyasingh, K., Bordman, L. and Calnan, S. (1972) Prevention of deep venous thrombosis by intermittent compression of calf. *Br. med. J.*, **i**, 131.

Hodgkinson, R. and Husain, F.J. (1979) Systemic and pulmonary blood pressure in severe hypertensive parturients undergoing Caesarean section under general and epidural anaesthesia. Obstetric Anaesthetists Association Autumn Meeting. Birmingham, September 1979.

Holdsworth, J.D., Evans, M. and Roulston, R.G. (1977) Efficacy of antacid therapy. *Br. J. Anaesth.*, **49**, 520.

Homi, J., Reynolds, J., Skinner, A.A., Hanna, W. and Sergeant, G. (1979) General anaesthesia in sickle-cell disease. *Br. med. J.*, **ii**, 15.

Howells, T.H., Huntsman, R.G., Boys, J.E. and Mahmood, A. (1972) Anaesthesia and sickle-cell haemoglobin. *Br. J. Anaesth.*, **44**, 975.

Husemeyer, R.P. and Crawley, J.C.W. (1979) Placental intervillous blood flow measured by inhaled ^{133}Xe clearance in relation to induction of epidural analgesia. *Br. J. Obstet. Gynaec.*, **86**, 426.

Hutchinson, B.R. and Newson, A.J. (1975) Pre-operative neutralisation of gastric acidity. *Anaesthesia and Intensive Care*, **3**, 198.

Jennet, W.B. and Cross, J.N. (1967) Influence of pregnancy and oral contraception on the incidence of strokes in women of childbearing age. *Lancet*, **i**, 1019.

Jones, S.R., Binder, R.A. and Donowho, E.H. (1970) Sudden death in sickle-cell trait. *New Engl. J. Med.*, **282**, 323.

Jouppila, R., Jouppila, P., Hollmen, A. and Kuikka, J. (1978) Effect of segmental extradural analgesia on placental blood flow during normal labour. *Br. J. Anaesth.*, **50**, 563.

Konotey-Ahulu, F.I.D. (1969) Anaesthetic deaths and the sickle-cell trait. *Lancet*, **i**, 267.

Lawson, D.W., Defalco, A.J., Phelps, J.A., Bradley, B.E. and McClenathan, J.E. (1966) Corticosteroids as treatment for aspiration of gastric contents: an experimental study. *Surgery, (St Lous)*, **59**, 845.

Leak, D., Carroll, J.J., Robinson, D.C. and Ashworth, E.J. (1977) Management of phaeochromocytoma during pregnancy. *Can. med. Ass. J.*, **116**, 371.

Leeton, J.F. (1974) Emergency complications of the third stage of labour and early puerperium. In *Obstetric Therapeutics*, ed. Hawkins, D.F. London: Baillière Tindall.

Lewinski, A. (1965) Evaluation of methods employed in the treatment of chemical pneumonitis of aspiration. *Anesthesiology*, **26**, 37.

Lewis, T.L.T. (1964) *Progress in Clinical Obstetrics and Gynaecology*, 2nd ed., p. 48. London: Churchill.

Lewis, R.T., Burgess, J.H. and Hampson, L.G. (1971) Cardiorespiratory studies in critical illness. *Archs Surg., Chicago.*, **103**, 335.

Light, I.J., Keenan, W.J. and Sutherland, J.M. (1972) Maternal intravenous glucose administration as a cause of hypoglycaemia in the infant of the diabetic mother. *Am. J. Obstet. Gynec.*, **113**, 345.

Lucke, J.N. (1977) Malignant hyperthermia in a parturient Poland China sow. *Br. J. Anaesth.*, **49**, 1070.

Lumley, J., Owen, R. and Morgan, M. (1979) Amniotic fluid embolism: a report of three cases. *Anaesthesia*, **34**, 33.

Lutz, D.J., Noller, K.L., Spittell, J.A., Danielson, G.K. and Fish, C.R. (1978) Pregnancy and its complications following cardiac valve prostheses. *Am. J. Obstet. Gynec.*, **131**, 460.

Mathie, I.K. (1966) Severe eclampsia treated by total paralysis. *Scott. med. J.*, **4**, 401.

Mathews, J.D. and Mason, T.W. (1974) Plasma viscosity and pre-eclampsia. *Lancet*, **ii**, 409.

McNall, P.G. and Jafarnia, M.R. (1965) Management of myasthenia gravis in the obstetrical patient. *Am. J. Obstet. Gynec.*, **92**, 518.

Mendelson, C.L. (1946) The aspiration of stomach contents into the lungs during obstetric anaesthesia. *Am. J. Obstet. Gynec.*, **52**, 191.

Menon, M.K. (1969) Obstetrics in India. In *Modern Trends in Obstetrics*, 4th ed., ed. Kellar, R.J., p. 301. London: Butterworth.

Miles, R.M. and Elsea, P.W. (1971) Clinical evaluation of the serrated venacaval clip. *Surgery Gynec. Obstet.*, **132**, 581.

Minielly, R., Yuzpe, A.A. and Drake, C.G. (1979) Subarachnoid hemorrhage secondary to ruptured cerebral aneurysm in pregnancy. *Obstet. Gynec.*, **53**, 64.

Modig, J., Borg, T., Karlstrom, G., Maripuu, E. and Salhlstedt, B. (1983) Thromboembolism after total hip replacement: role of epidural and general anaesthesia. *Anesth. Analg.*, **62**, 174.

Moir, D.D. and Willocks, J. (1968) Epidural analgesia in British obstetrics. *Br. J. Anaesth.*, **40**, 129.

Moir, D.D., Victor-Rodrigues, L. and Willocks, J. (1972) Epidural analgesia during labour in patients with pre-eclampsia. *J. Obstet. Gynaec. Br. Commonw.*, **72**, 264.

Morgan, M. (1979) Amniotic fluid embolism. *Anaesthesia*, **34**, 20.

Morris, J.A., Arce, J.J., Hamilton, C.J. et al (1977) The management of severe pre-eclampsia and eclampsia with intravenous diazoxide. *Obstet. Gynec.*, **49**, 675.

Nagey, D.A., Akawade, N.A., Pupkin, M.J. and Crebshaw, C. (1984) Isovolumetric partial exchange transfusion in the management of sickle cell disease in pregnancy. *Am. J. Obstet. Gynec.*, **147**, 693.

Neill, C.A. and Swanson, S. (1961) Outcome of pregnancy in congenital heart disease. *Circulation*, **24**, 1003.

Nilsen, P.A. (1963) The mechanism of hypofibrinogenaemia in premature separation of the normally implanted placenta. *Acta obstet. gynec. scand.*, **42**, Suppl. 2, 1.

Oduro, K.A. (1973) Anaesthesia and sickle-cell haemoglobin. *Br. J. Anaesth.*, **45**, 123.

O'Neil, H., Blake, S., Sugrue, D. and MacDonald, D. (1982) Problems in the management of patients with artificial valves during pregnancy. *Br. J. Obstet. Gynaec.*, **89**, 940.

Osserman, K.E. (1958) *Myasthenia Gravis.* New York: Grune and Stratton.

Parikh, R.K. and Moore, M.R. (1975) Anaesthetics in porphyria: intravenous induction agents. *Br. J. Anaesth.*, **47**, 907.

Peskett, W.G.H. (1973) Antacids before obstetric anaesthesia. A clinical evaluation of the effectiveness of mist. magnesium trisilicate, B.P.C. *Anaesthesia*, **28**, 509.

Price, D.G. (1976) Pulmonary embolism: prophylaxis, diagnosis and treatment. *Anaesthesia*, **31**, 925.

Rizk, S.F., Jacobson, J.H. and Silvay, G. (1977) Ketamine as an induction agent for acute intermittent porphyria. *Anesthesiology*, **46**, 305.

Roberts, R.B. and Shirley, M.A. (1974) Reducing the risk of acid-aspiration during cesarean section. *Anesth. Analg. curr. Res.*, **53**, 859.

Robertson, W.B., Brosens, I. and Dixon, H.G. (1967) The pathological response of the vessels of the placental bed to hypertensive pregnancy. *J. Path. Bact.*, **93**, 581.

Rolbin, S.H., Levinson, G., Shnider, S.M. and Wright, R.G. (1978) Anesthetic considerations for myasthenia gravis and pregnancy. *Anesth. Analg. curr. Res.*, **57**, 441.

Rubin, P.C., Butters, L., Clark, D.M. et al (1983) Placebo controlled trial of atenolol in treatment of pregnancy associated hypertension. *Lancet*, **i**, 431.

Rucci, F.S. and Caroli, G. (1974) Ketamine and eclampsia. *Br. J. Anaesth.*, **46**, 546.

Saka, D.M. and Marx, G.F. (1976) Management of a parturient with cardiac valve prosthesis. *Anesth. Analg. curr. Res.*, **55**, 214.

Schaerf, R.H.H. de Campo, T. and Civetta, J.M. (1977) Hemodynamic alterations and rapid diagnosis in a case of amniotic fluid embolism. *Anesthesiology*, **46**, 155.

Schenker, J.G. and Chowers, I. (1971) Pheochromocytoma and pregnancy: review of 89 cases. *Obstet. Gynec. Survey*, **26**, 739.

Scott, J.S. (1968) Coagulation failure in obstetrics. *Br. med. Bull.*, **24**, 32.

Scott, D.B. (1978) Mendelson's syndrome. *Br. J. Anaesth.*, **50**, 977.

Scottish Home and Health Department (1978) *A Report on an Enquiry into Maternal Deaths in Scotland, 1972–1975.* Edinburgh: H.M.S.O.

Searle, J.F. (1973) Anaesthesia in sickle-cell states: a review. *Anaesthesia*, **28**, 48.

Sharp, A.A. (1977) Diagnosis and management of disseminated intravascular coagulation. *Br. med. Bulletin*, **33**, 265.

Shervington, P.C. (1974) Common pregnancy disorders and infections. In *Obstetric Therapeutics*, ed. Hawkins, D.F. London: Baillière Tindall.

Shnider, S.M. and Moya, F. (1961) Amniotic fluid embolism. *Anesthesiology*, **22**, 108.

Smibert, J. (1967) Amniotic fluid embolism, a clinical review of twenty cases. *Aust. N.Z. J. Obstet. Gynaec.*, **7**, 1.

Soffronoff, E.C., Kaufman, B.M. and Connaughton, J.F. (1977) Intravascular volume determination and fetal outcome in hypertensive diseases of pregnancy. *Am. J. Obstet. Gynec.*, **127**, 4.

Stirrat, G.M. and Lieberman, N.A. (1977) *Therapeutic Problems in Pregnancy*, ed. Lewis, P.J., p. 45. Baltimore University Park Press.

Stremple, J.F., Ellison, E.H. and Carey, L.C. (1966) Osmolar diuresis; success and/or failure. A collective review. *Surgery, St. Lous*, **60**, 924.

Stroganoff, W. (1930) *The Improved Prophylactic Method in the Treatment of Eclampsia.* Edinburgh: Livingstone.

Sugrue, D., Blake, S., Troy, P. and MacDonald, D. (1980) Antibiotic prophylaxis against infective endocarditis after normal delivery—is it necessary? *Br. Heart J.*, **44**, 499.

Sugrue, D., Blake, S. and MacDonald, D. (1981) Pregnancy complicated by maternal heart disease at the National Maternity Hospital, Dublin, Ireland, 1969–78. *Obstet. Gynec.*, **139**, 1.

Taylor, G. and Prys-Davies, J. (1966) The prophylactic use of antacids in the prevention of the acid-pulmonary-aspiration syndrome (Mendelson's syndrome). *Lancet*, **i**, 288.

Teabut, J.R. (1952) Aspiration of gastric contents: an experimental study. *Am. J. Path.*, **28**, 51.

Templeton, A.A. and Kelman, G.R. (1977) Arterial blood gases in pre-eclampsia. *Br. J. Obstet. Gynaec.*, **84**, 290.

Thorburn, J. and Moir, D.D. (1980) The management of severe pre-eclampsia. *Second Symposium on Epidural Analgesia in Obstetrics, Coventry.* London: Lloyd-Luke.

Thorburn, J., Louden, J.R. and Vallance, R. (1980) Spinal and general anaesthesia in total hip replacement: frequency of deep vein thrombosis. *Br. J. Anaesth.*, **52**, 1117.

Thorburn, J., Drummond, M.M., Whigham, K.A. et al (1982) Blood viscosity and haemostatic factors in late pregnancy, pre-eclampsia and fetal growth retardation. *Br. J. Obstet. Gynaec.*, **89**, 117.

Tuck, C.S. (1972) Amniotic fluid embolus. *Proc. R. Soc. Med.*, **65**, 94.

Tuck, S.M., Studd, J.W.W. and White, J.M. (1982) Sickle cell disease in pregnancy complicated by anti U antibody, case report. *Br. J. Obstet. Gynaec.*, **89**, 91.

Tuller, M.A. (1957) Amniotic fluid embolism, afibrinogenemia and disseminated fibrin thrombosis. *Am. J. Obstet. Gynec.*, **73**, 273.

Ueland, K., Novy, M.J. and Metcalf, J. (1973) Cardiorespiratory responses to pregnancy and exercise in normal womenand patients with heart disease. *Am. J. Obstet. Gynec.*, **115**, 4.

Vance, J.P. (1968) Tension pneumothorax in labour. *Anaesthesia*, **23**, 94.

Vandam, L.D. (1965) Aspiration of gastric contents in the operative period. *New Engl. J. Med.*, **273**, 1206.

Veille, J.C. (1984) Peripartum cardiomyopathies: a review. *Am. J. Obstet. Gynec.*, **148**, 805.

Wadhwa, R.K. (1977) Obstetric anesthesia for a patient with malignant hyperthermia susceptibility. *Anesthesiology*, **46**, 63.

Walter, B.N.J. and Redman, C. (1984) Treatment of severe pregnancy-associated hypertension with the calcium antagonist nifedipine. *Br. J. Obstet. Gynaec.*, **91**, 330.

Walton, J.N. (1953) Subarachnoid haemorrhage in pregnancy. *Br. med. J.*, **i**, 869.

Warren, T.M., Datta, D. and Ostheimer, G.W. (1982) Lumbar epidural anesthesia in a patient with multiple sclerosis. *Anesth. Analg.*, **61**, 1022.

Weaver, J.B. and Pearson, J.F. (1973) Influence of digitalis on time of onset and duration of labour in women with cardiac disease. *Br. med. J.*, **iii**, 519.

White, W.D., Clark, J.M. and Stanley-Jones, G.H.M. (1976) The efficacy of antacid therapy. *Br. J. Anaesth.*, **48**, 1117.

Willats, S.M. (1979) Malignant hyperthermia susceptibility: management during pregnancy and labour. *Anaesthesia*, **34**, 41.

Willocks, J. and Moir, D.D. (1968) Epidural analgesia in the management of hypertension in labour. *J. Obstet. Gynaec. Br. Commonw.*, **75**, 225.

Willocks, J., Mone, J.G. and Thomson, W.J. (1966) Amniotic fluid embolism: a case with biochemical findings. *Br. med. J.*, **ii**, 1181.

10

Resuscitation of the Newborn

In many smaller maternity units the anaesthetist must be prepared to resuscitate the asphyxiated neonate. In larger units a junior paediatrician is often present at operative deliveries but, even so, the anaesthetist can often assist in or supervise and teach the techniques of intubation and IPPV. Every anaesthetist, paediatrician and obstetrician should learn these skills; they are now taught to selected midwives who are called upon to resuscitate babies without medical aid. The techniques can be learned on a stillborn infant, or less satisfactorily, on a demonstration model.

The anaesthetist who is unable to intubate the trachea and carry out IPPV with expertise should not be administering obstetric anaesthesia without supervision. The following brief and mainly practical account is intended to give the trainee anaesthetist sufficient information to enable him to apply his technical skills in a rational way to the resuscitation of the newborn. It is in no way intended as an account in depth.

Aetiology of asphyxia neonatorum

There are of course many causes of asphyxia in the newborn and in most instances the technique of resuscitation is little affected by the cause of the asphyxia. The principal categories are as follows:

(1) Antepartum factors: placental insufficiency, pre-eclampsia, post-maturity, antepartum haemorrhage, maternal hypoxaemia, diabetes mellitus and Rhesus incompatibility.

(2) Intrapartum factors: prolonged labour, depressant drugs, caval occlusion, hypotension, prolapsed cord and traumatic delivery.

Asphyxia associated with foaming at the mouth and nostrils in infants delivered by caesarean section was described by Klein (1972) and may be the result of absence of the squeezing of the thorax which occurs during vaginal delivery.

Fetal asphyxia will often have existed for a greater or lesser time before delivery, and an infant may be born profoundly asphyxiated. When asphyxia is experimentally produced in newborn animals, including Rhesus monkeys, (James and Adamson, 1964; Daniel et al, 1966) by delivering the infants into an oxygen-free environment, four stages of asphyxia are recognized:

(1) A brief period of hyperventilation.

(2) A stage of primary apnoea lasting for 3–5 minutes and accompanied by bradycardia and then an increasing heart-rate followed by a further period of bradycardia.

(3) A stage of gasping of a few minutes duration and accompanied by an increasing heart-rate.

(4) A stage of secondary apnoea after the 'last gasp' with marked bradycardia, hypotension and circulatory failure. The infant dies if untreated. There is an associated severe metabolic and respiratory acidosis.

These stages consistently occur in many animal species, and the timing of various stages can be modified by hypothermia and by narcotic analgesics (Moore and Davies, 1966). The same sequence of events probably occurs in the human infant who has not been subjected to hypoxia in utero and who becomes severely hypoxic at birth. In clinical practice, the infant has usually been hypoxic to some degree before delivery and it may be difficult to decide whether apnoea at birth is primary or secondary, unless treatment is unjustifiably delayed. In the relatively benign primary apnoea, most treatments will be effective and the infant will often respond to tactile stimuli and to analeptics. In secondary apnoea, these treatments are ineffective and, unless oxygenation and correction of the associated metabolic acidosis are effected, then death is inevitable in the infant who is asphyxiated 'beyond the last gasp'. The true test of a method of neonatal resuscitation is its efficacy in secondary apnoea and in this circumstance tracheal intubation, IPPV and intravenous sodium bicarbonate are the most effective techniques (James and Adamson, 1964; Campbell et al, 1966; Daniel et al, 1966). The alveoli at birth are filled with liquid and the essential requirement is replacement of this liquid by air or by oxygen so that the liquid is driven back into the capillaries and lymphatics of the lung.

Negative intrathoracic pressures of up to $80 \, cmH_2O$ (7.8 kPa) and swings of $40-100 \, cmH_2O$ (3.9 kPa–9.8 kPa) occur during each respiratory cycle in the first few spontaneous breaths of life (Donald, 1957; Karlberg, 1969). Lung compliance is at first very low, but increases rapidly with aeration of the lungs, reaching the normal value of about $6.5 \, ml/cmH_2O$ (65 ml/kPa) at 8 hours of age (Chu et al, 1964). In practice pressures of up to 30 or $40 \, cmH_2O$ (2.9 or 3.9 kPa) are used during IPPV immediately after birth until the lungs have expanded, and thereafter pressures of $10-20 \, cmH_2O$ (1.0–2.0 kPa) will usually prove adequate. In preventing alveolar rupture the duration of the positive pressure may be as important as its magnitude, and it is suggested that pressures of 30 or $40 \, cmH_2O$ (2.9 or 3.9 kPa) should not be applied for more than 1 second. Transpleural pressure gradients of up to $100 \, cmH_2O$ (9.8 kPa) occur during the initiation of spontaneous ventilation and it may therefore be justifiable to apply pressures in excess of $40 \, cmH_2O$ (3.9 kPa) very briefly if lower pressures fail to expand the lungs. Spontaneous pneumothorax can be detected radiologically in at least 2% of clinically normal infants (Chernick and Avery, 1963) and need not always be attributed to the use of IPPV. The normal mature infant has sufficient alveolar surfactant to maintain alveolar expansion.

The factors which initiate the first breaths of life are not certainly known. Neither hypoxia nor hypercapnia seems to be of primary importance and it is probable that cold and tactile stimulation of the face and feet normally cause the newborn infant to cry and to breathe. Clamping of the umbilical cord is thought to result in sympathetic stimulation and a fall in carotid body perfusion, with consequent stimulation of the respiratory centre (Purves, 1966). IPPV will often initiate spontaneous ventilation after a few inflations in the less severely asphyxiated neonate.

The time at which the cord is clamped is important. If the cord is clamped too early in infants delivered by caesarean section, the neonatal blood volume is small and there may be a predisposition to the respiratory distress syndrome, whereas if clamping is unduly delayed, the neonate may have a smaller functional residual capacity, tachypnoea, grunting respiration, a lower P_aO_2 and a higher P_aCO_2 (Moss and Monset-Couchard, 1967; Usher et al, 1971; Yao and Lind, 1974). It is also important not to cause partial exsanguination of the infant by elevating it above the mother's abdomen before cord clamping.

Assessment of the infant at birth

The Apgar scoring system was introduced by the late Dr Virginia Apgar, an American anaesthetist (Apgar, 1953), and is now very extensively used to evaluate the condition of the infant at birth, to assess the need for active resuscitation and to make comparisons between the groups of infants for research purposes. Each of the five signs in Table 13 is scored from 0 to 2 and the results added together, giving a maximum possible score of 10. Assessments are now commonly made at 1, 2 and 5 minutes according to a clock or timer which is set in motion at delivery.

Although the Apgar score is related to the severity of asphyxia, there are several criticisms of the system. Five dissimilar pieces of information are added together and are given equal weight. However, the loss of one point for colour is usually of minor clinical significance and is compared equally with a bradycardia of 40 beats/min which signifies grave hypoxia. There is therefore much to be said for Crawford's (1972) suggestion that the Apgar minus colour score should be used, with a maximum possible score of 8. In considering the correlation between the individual components of the Apgar score and the pH, P_{CO_2} and base excess of the blood in the umbilical artery, Crawford et al (1973) found that heart-rate, muscle tone and reflex irritability were most closely related to the biochemical status of the infant at birth. Colour was poorly related and the inclusion of colour reduced the discriminatory value of the total score. The best correlation between umbilical pH, P_{O_2}, P_{CO_2} and the Apgar score exists at the moment of delivery, and in this respect the 'birth' score is more informative than the 1-minute score (Marx et al, 1977).

These workers confirmed that the inclusion of a score for colour detracts from the value of the total score. Gupta and Tizard (1967) advocate the recording of the various details as set out in the Apgar method of scoring but suggest that the actual scoring be omitted because of the uneven and unrealistic weighting given to the various observations. The Apgar score is nevertheless likely to continue to be generally used and there is a suggestion that the score at 5 minutes may give some indication of the likelihood of hypoxic brain damage.

Table 13. The Apgar method of scoring

Sign	Score		
	0	1	2
Heart-rate	Absent	<100	>100
Respiratory effort	Absent	Weak cry: hypoventilation	Good strong cry: regular respiration
Muscle tone	Limp	Some flexion of limbs, poor tone	Well flexed, good tone
Reflex irritability (stimulation of soles of feet)	No response	Some motion	Strong withdrawal and crying
Colour	Blue or pale	Body pink, extremities blue	Completely pink

A simple measure of respiratory activity is sometimes obtained from the time to sustained respiration (TSR). This is the time required for the establishment of regular and adequate spontaneous ventilation after delivery, without stimulation, and gives some indication of the extent of drug-induced respiratory depression, although other factors will affect the TSR. Chamberlain and Banks (1974) suggest that the simple recording of the TSR and heart-rate could replace the Apgar score system. Estimations of the pH, P_{CO_2}, base excess and P_{O_2} of umbilical venous and arterial blood from a double-clamped loop of cord are a useful indicator of the degree of hypoxaemia and are now often used in the evaluation of the effects of anaesthetic techniques and drugs on the newborn. There are indications that detailed neurological assessment of the newborn by a trained paediatrician may prove to be the most sensitive indicator of minor differences between various techniques of analgesia and anaesthesia (Brackbill et al, 1974; Scanlon et al, 1974) but such refinements are unnecessary for the detection of infants in need of resuscitation.

In practice the baby who is apnoeic for more than a very brief period requires assistance, and the baby who is obviously severely asphyxiated at birth requires immediate resuscitation. Asphyxia at birth increases the chance of developing the neonatal respiratory distress syndrome in premature infants and it is therefore especially important that such infants be actively and immediately resuscitated at delivery (Hey, 1979).

Techniques of resuscitation

Routine procedures at delivery:

(1) Note the time and start the clock or timer.

(2) Clear mucus and liquor amnii from the nose and mouth by *gentle* aspiration. The neonate is a nose-breather. Overvigorous pharyngeal suction is now regarded as an important cause of apnoea after delivery (Cordero and Hon, 1971). Stimulation of the posterior pharyngeal wall in the newborn causes relaxation of the vocal cords (laryngeal inhibition), apnoea, flaccidity and bradycardia. If pharyngeal suction is indicated, then a laryngoscope should be used to permit gentle suction under direct vision. A Walpole catheter with a flange near the tip will prevent blind insertion to a depth which may initiate laryngeal inhibition.

(3) Administer oxygen in a stream over the face by nasal catheter or by a suitable face mask. This is especially appropriate if the infant is gasping or breathing irregularly and is trying to establish regular respiration. The oxygen flow rate should be 4 or 5 litres per minute. High flow rates of cold, dry gas may promote apnoea, bradycardia and flaccidity (Brown et al, 1976).

(4) Keep the child warm and dry. Dry the infant with a towel and place it under a radiant heater and on a thermostatically controlled heated mattress. A wet infant loses heat much more rapidly than a dry one and even a healthy, cold infant experiences a fall in P_aO_2 and develops a metabolic acidosis (Gandy et al, 1964; Stephenson et al, 1970). Diazepam and chlormethiazole given in labour promote hypothermia. Heat loss can be reduced by swaddling in aluminium foil or a plastic bag in emergency situations.

(5) Assess the Apgar score at 1, 2 and 5 minutes. Record the details of the various components and the total score.

Resuscitation of the asphyxiated infant:

(1) *Ventilation of the lungs.* Infants who are severely asphyxiated when delivered, infants who remain apnoeic at 1 minute of life and infants whose Apgar score is <5 require active resuscitation by IPPV. Severe bradycardia calls for intubation and IPPV. Although techniques which do not involve intubation of the trachea can be successful, it is recommended that anyone who is skilled in intubation should first insert an endotracheal tube.

The infant should be placed on a firm surface about a metre and a half above floor level. Intubation should not be attempted in the depths of a cot. A common fault is hyperextension of the head. The head should be held in the 'sniffing' position and supported in a ring or held by an assistant. A laryngoscope with a straight blade of the Seward type (Seward, 1957) is recommended. Others may prefer to use a small Macintosh blade or the Cardiff blade (Gray and Rosen, 1967). Pharyngeal suction is performed under direct vision if indicated and the trachea is intubated with a sterile, plastic tube of 10 or 12 FG. If necessary, tracheal secretions are aspirated using a very fine catheter and not by applying suction to the tube. IPPV with

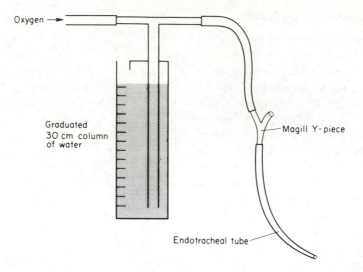

Figure 21. Simple arrangement for IPPV for the newborn including a 30 cmH$_2$O (2.9 kPa) pressure-limiting manometer.

oxygen is now commenced. Inflation pressures should be restricted to 30 cmH$_2$O (2.9 kPa) for 1 second and the respiratory rate should be about 30 or 40 breaths per minute. If this procedure does not inflate the lungs, then a higher pressure may be used briefly. A tidal volume of 20 ml to 40 ml is normal for a resting neonate. A simple water manometer in circuit may prevent the application of excessive pressures, and usually consists of a glass tube 30 cm long set vertically in a water bath (see Figure 21). This arrangement is present in the Resuscitaire apparatus. Although water manometers are extensively used, the delayed response of this type of device could lead to the application of excessive pressure if only for a brief period and the substitution of a mechanical pop-off valve is safer. A simple water manometer with 'safety' blow off at 30 cmH$_2$O (2.9 kPa) can easily generate an inflation pressure of 60 cmH$_2$O (5.9 kPa) if high flow rates are used (Hey and Lenney, 1973). If a Magill Y-piece is inserted into the endotracheal tube, then oxygen can be run into one arm at a flow of 2 or 3 litres/min while IPPV is effected by the intermittent, brief occlusion of the other arm. IPPV should be continued until regular spontaneous ventilation can be maintained and the heart-rate remains over 100 beats/min. The endotracheal tube should be left in place for 1 or 2 minutes after the cessation of IPPV in order to confirm that resuscitation has been successful. If IPPV with oxygen does not result in an increase in heart-rate to at least 100 beats/min within approximately 1 minute, then either the tube is not in the trachea or the circulation is inadequate and external cardiac massage is called for.

It appears that the use of undiluted oxygen is safe (and perhaps more effective) if used only until resuscitation has been successfully accomplished.

Thereafter the inspired oxygen tension is reduced to a concentration that will produce normal arterial blood gas tensions and that will probably avoid the risk of retrolental fibroplasia. In this way the arterial Po_2 of the infant should not remain at high levels. Although it is usual to advocate that inflation pressures be restricted to 30 or $40\,cmH_2O$ (2.9 or 3.9 kPa), the work of Rosen and Laurence (1965) on stillborn infants indicates that considerably higher pressures may be needed for the first few cycles if the lungs are to be inflated. It is therefore conceivable that the desire to avoid alveolar rupture by the use of pressure-limiting devices may occasionally impair the efficacy of resuscitation. In most infants, however, pressures of $30\,cmH_2O$ (2.9 kPa) are sufficient to raise the arterial Po_2, increase heart-rate and, by reducing cerebral hypoxia, to be followed by the onset of spontaneous ventilation.

It is often possible to perform IPPV adequately by the use of a face mask and a device such as the Cardiff inflating bag to which an oxygen reservoir may be attached, and thus to avoid the need to intubate the trachea (Mushin and Hillard, 1967, 1970). Although relatively simple to use, there is a possibility of inflating the stomach if the high pressures which may be needed to inflate the lungs are used or if the upper airway is not patent. An oropharyngeal airway may be helpful in some babies. The Cardiff inflating bag has a pressure limit of $40\,cmH_2O$ (3.9 kPa) but alternative devices such as the Samson–Blease resuscitator have no pressure-limiting device. A suitable paediatric anaesthetic circuit incorporating a bag and expiratory valve may be used and the 'educated hand' of the anaesthetist must then judge the inflation pressure unless a manometer is incorporated in the circuit.

In emergency circumstances mouth-to-mouth breathing may be used and, in that case, the anaesthetist should cover the nose and lips of the infant with his own lips. He should bear in mind the diminutive size of his patient and should expel frequent small puffs of air from his cheeks and not directly from his lungs. If oxygen is available, the puffed-out cheeks may be filled with oxygen. Whichever method of IPPV is used it is important to observe moments of the thorax and to confirm that the stomach is not being inflated.

(2) *External cardiac massage.* If a heart beat cannot be detected, or if the heart-rate is less than 40 beats/min, then external cardiac massage should be performed. The tips of the second and third fingers are placed across the mid-sternum. Compressions at the rate of about 100 beats/min are then gently performed. Some six or eight compressions should be alternated with two or three inflations of the lungs. The single-handed resuscitator should tape the endotracheal tube in position and carry out continuous cardiac massage while oxygen flows, in the hope of providing a pulmonary circulation with alveoli filled with oxygen. If the heart-rate does not increase after performing cardiac massage for 4 minutes, then sodium bicarbonate should be given. Hey (1979) advocates the intracardiac injection of 2–4 mmol in preference to the more usual injection into the umbilical vein.

(3) *Correction of metabolic acidosis.* The severely asphyxiated infant can be assumed to have an associated metabolic acidosis. During apnoea the

arterial blood pH of the neonate falls at a rate of approximately 0.1 unit in each of the first 5 minutes of life and, thereafter, the rate of fall slows to approximately 0.1 unit every 3 minutes (James, 1960).

If the response to resuscitation is delayed, or if bradycardia persists, then the presumed acidosis should certainly be corrected. The administration of alkali and glucose hastens recovery from experimental asphyxia, increases pulmonary blood flow and reduces brain damage (Adamson et al, 1963; Windle, 1963; Dawes et al, 1964). In the probable absence of a knowledge of the base deficit, sodium bicarbonate in 8.4% solution (1 mEq/ml, 1 mmol/litre) should be given in a dose of 3 ml/kg body weight. If the weight is unknown, Crawford's suggestion of giving 7.5 ml of this solution to a small infant and 15 ml to a large infant may be adopted (Crawford, 1972). If the base deficit is known, then the alkali requirements can be calculated from the formula:

Alkali required (mEq or mmol)

$$= \frac{\text{base deficit (mEq or mmol)} \times \text{body weight (kg)}}{3}$$

The sodium bicarbonate solution should be injected slowly into the umbilical vein in order to avoid hepatic damage and the insertion of a fine catheter into the umbilical vein will permit further therapy and blood sampling if this is considered likely to be required. The catheter should be passed 5–10 cm beyond the abdominal wall. Hypoglycaemia is usually a concomitant to severe hypoxaemia in the newborn and the injection of glucose into the umbilical vein may hasten recovery by providing an energy source for the myocardium (Adamson et al, 1963; Windle, 1963). An injection of 5 ml of 20% dextrose solution into the umbilical vein is appropriate.

Sodium bicarbonate should not be given routinely to moderately asphyxiated, but otherwise normal, full-term infants, but should be given as a single intravenous injection to all asphyxiated preterm infants and to full-term infants whose condition remains unsatisfactory 5 minutes after delivery. Continuous infusions of sodium bicarbonate are not recommended after the initial injection (Hey, 1979).

(4) *Narcotic analgesic antagonists.* Narcotic-induced neonatal respiratory depression is likely to be at its greatest between 2 and 3 hours after a maternal intramuscular injection and within a few minutes of an intravenous injection. A consideration of the quantity and timing of maternal narcotic analgesic therapy when an infant fails to establish spontaneous ventilation, despite apparently effective resuscitation, should lead the resuscitator to suspect that there is central depression of respiration by drugs.

The narcotic analgesic antagonist of choice is naloxone because it is apparently free of an intrinsic depressant action and so should be relatively harmless if the diagnosis is in error. Naloxone is effective against respiratory depression caused by pentazocine, whereas levallorphan and nalorphine are ineffective. An injection of 0.04 mg naloxone should be given into the umbilical vein. Alternatively 0.025 mg levallorphan or 0.5 mg nalorphine may be substituted. In appropriate circumstances the response to the injection is rapid and impressive. The action of naloxone is shorter-lived than the action of pethidine and morphine, and it is possible for the depressant action of the opiate analgesic to return after 45 minutes.

(5) *Analeptics*. The use of analeptics in the treatment of asphyxia neonatorum can no longer be justified. In mild asphyxia (primary apnoea and stage of gasping), analeptics are as effective as flicking the soles of the feet (Daniel et al, 1966). In severe asphyxia (secondary apnoea) analeptics may increase the oxygen requirements of the already hypoxic brain and aggravate existing myocardial inadequacy (Cross, 1968; Godfrey et al, 1970). Under experimental conditions the administration of analeptics may accelerate death in secondary apnoea (Godfrey et al, 1970).

(6) *Abandoning resuscitation*. The decision to terminate resuscitative efforts is usually difficult and, to some extent, a personal one. The following guidelines may be helpful to the individual faced with this unhappy decision.

Certainly IPPV and external cardiac massage should be maintained for up to 20 minutes and sodium bicarbonate should have been given into the heart or the umbilical vein before resuscitation is abandoned. If a neonate does not breathe regularly and spontaneously, as distinct from gasping, within 30 minutes of an episode of cardiac arrest or acute circulatory failure, then severe damage with spastic quadriplegia and mental subnormality is probable in about 90% of survivors (Steiner and Neligan, 1975), and many would withdraw resuscitative measures at this point. Nevertheless the neonate seems to withstand acute circulatory arrest for longer than the adult. Where resuscitation of the severely asphyxiated infant is apparently successful, the outlook may be guardedly encouraging. Scott (1976) found that 17 out of 23 surviving infants born with Apgar scores of 0–2 at 1 minute were neurologically normal several years later. A delay of up to 5 minutes in establishing spontaneous ventilation in a mature infant does not affect the outcome (Neligan et al, 1974).

Meconium aspiration syndrome. Unless preventive measures are taken, about 20% of infants born with meconium-stained liquor amnii develop an aspiration pneumonitis and/or pneumothorax. These infants become hypoxic and require oxygen therapy. The mortality rate may be about 11% (Carson et al, 1976) to 23% (Marshall et al, 1978). The syndrome is diagnosed by the presence of meconium-staining of the infant, a chest X-ray consistent with aspiration pneumonitis and clinical respiratory distress and hypoxia within 24 hours of birth.

The importance of careful suction at the moment of delivery has been stressed in the prevention of the meconium aspiration syndrome by Gregory et al (1974). Impressive results have been claimed by Carson et al (1976) by immediate nasal and pharyngeal suction when the head is on the perineum and by subsequent laryngoscopic inspection of the pharynx and larynx, with tracheal suction if meconium is seen. This routine was performed in 661 infants delivered with meconium-stained liquor amnii. Only 23 infants developed the meconium aspiration syndrome and there were no deaths.

REFERENCES

Adamson, K., Behrman, R., Dawes, G.S., James, L.S. and Ross, B.B. (1963) Treatment of acidosis with alkali and glucose during asphyxia in fetal Rhesus monkeys. *J. Physiol., Lond.*, **169**, 679.

Apgar, V. (1953) A proposal for a new method of evaluation of the newborn infant. *Anesth. Analg. curr. Res.*, **32**, 260.

Brackbill, Y., Kane, J., Manniello, R.L. and Abramson, D. (1974) Obstetric meperidine usage and assessment of neonatal status. *Anesthesiology*, **40**, 116.

Brown, W.U., Ostheimer, G.W., Bell, G.C. and Datta, S. (1976) Newborn response to oxygen blown over the face. *Anesthesiology*, **44**, 535.

Campbell, A.G.M., Cross, K.W., Dawes, G.S. and Hyman, A.I. (1966) Comparison of air and O_2 in a hyperbaric chamber or by positive pressure ventilation in the resuscitation of newborn rabbits. *J. Pediat.*, **68**, 153.

Carson, B., Losey, R., Bowers, W. and Simmons, M. (1976) Combined obstetrical and pediatric management of meconium staining. *Pediat. Res.*, **10**, 459.

Chamberlain, G. and Banks, J. (1974) Assessment of the Apgar score. *Lancet*, **ii**, 1225.

Chernick, V. and Avery, M.E. (1963) Spontaneous alveolar rupture at birth. *Pediatrics, Springfield*, **32**, 816.

Chu, J.S., Dawson, P., Klaus, M. and Sweet, A.Y. (1964) Lung compliance and lung volume measured concurrently in normal full-term and premature infants. *Pediatrics, Springfield*, **34**, 525.

Cordero, L. and Hon, E.H. (1971) Neonatal bradycardia following nasopharyngeal stimulation. *J. Pediat.*, **78**, 441.

Crawford, J.S. (1972) *Principles and Practice of Obstetric Anaesthesia*, 3rd ed., p. 253. Oxford: Blackwell.

Crawford, J.S., Davies, P. and Pearson, J.F. (1973) Significance of the individual components of the Apgar score. *Br. J. Anaesth.*, **45**, 148.

Cross, K.W. (1968) Aspects of applied physiology of neonatal circulation. *Br. Heart J.*, **30**, 483.

Daniel, S.S., Dawes, G.S., James, L.S. and Ross, B.B. (1966) Analeptics and the resuscitation of asphyxiated monkeys. *Br. med. J.*, **ii**, 562.

Dawes, G.S., Hibbard, E. and Windle, W.F. (1964) Effect of alkali and glucose infusion on permanent brain damage in rhesus monkeys asphyxiated at birth. *J. Pediat.*, **65**, 801.

Donald, I. (1957) Neonatal respiration and hyaline membrane. *Br. J. Anaesth.*, **29**, 533.

Gandy, G.M., Adamson, K., Cunningham, N., Silverman, W.A. and James, L.S. (1964) Thermal environment and acid–base homeostasis in human infants during the first few hours of life. *J. clin. Invest.*, **43**, 751.

Godfrey, S., Bolton, D.P.G. and Cross, K.W. (1970) Respiratory stimulants in treatment of perinatal asphyxia. *Br. med. J.*, **i**, 475.

Gray, O.P. and Rosen, M. (1967) Cardiff laryngoscope for infants. *Br. med. J.*, **iv**, 48.

Gregory, G., Gooding, C., Phibbs, R. and Tooley, W. (1974) Meconium aspiration in infants: a prospective study. *J. Pediat.*, **85**, 848.

Gupta, J.S. and Tizard, J.P.M. (1967) The sequence of events in neonatal apnoea. *Lancet*, **ii**, 55.

Hey, E. (1979) Resuscitation at birth. *Br. J. Anaesth.*, **49**, 25.

Hey, E. and Lenney, W. (1973) Safe resuscitation at birth. *Lancet*, **ii**, 103.

James, L.S. (1960) Acidosis of the newborn and its relation to birth asphyxia. *Acta paediat., Stockh.*, **49**, Suppl. 122, 17.

James, L.S. and Adamson, K. (1964) Respiratory physiology of the fetus and newborn infant. *New Engl. J. Med.*, **271**, 1352.

Karlberg, P. (1969) Adaptive changes in the immediate post-natal period with particular reference to respiration. *J. Pediat.*, **56**, 585.
Klein, M. (1972) Asphyxia neonatorum caused by foaming. *Lancet*, **i**, 1089.
Marshall, R., Tyrala, E., McAlister, W. and Sheehan, M. (1978) Meconium aspiration syndrome: neonatal follow-up study. *Am. J. Obstet. Gynec.*, **131**, 672.
Marx, G.F., Mahajan, S. and Miclat, M.N. (1977) Correlation of biochemical data with Apgar scores at birth and at one minute. *Br. J. Anaesth.*, **49**, 831.
Moore, W.M.O. and Davies, J.A. (1966) Response of the newborn rabbit to acute anoxia and variations due to narcotic agents. *Br. J. Anaesth.*, **38**, 787.
Moss, A.J. and Monset-Couchard, M. (1967) Placental transfusion: early versus late clamping of the umbilical cord. *Pediatrics, Springfield*, **40**, 109.
Mushin, W.W. and Hillard, E.K. (1967) A neonatal inflating bag. *Br. med. J.*, **i**, 416.
Mushin, W.W. and Hillard, E.K. (1970) Cardiff infant inflating bag. *Br. med. J.*, **iv**, 622.
Neligan, G., Prudham, D. and Steiner, H. (1974) *The Formative Years: Birth, Family and Development in Newcastle-upon-Tyne*. Oxford: Oxford University Press and Nuffield Provincial Hospital Trust.
Purves, M.J. (1966) The respiratory response of the newborn lamb to inhaled CO with and without accompanying hypoxia. *J. Physiol., Lond.*, **185**, 78.
Rosen, M. and Laurence, K.M. (1965) Expansion pressures and rupture pressures in the newborn lung. *Lancet*, **ii**, 721.
Scanlon, J.W., Brown, W.U. jr., Weiss, J.B. and Alper, M.H. (1974) Neuro-behavioral responses of newborn infants after maternal epidural anesthesia. *Anesthesiology*, **40**, 121.
Scott, H. (1976) Outcome of very severe birth asphyxia. *Archs Dis. Childh.*, **51**, 712.
Seward, E.H. (1957) Laryngoscope for resuscitation of the newborn. *Lancet*, **ii**, 1041.
Steiner, H. and Neligan, G. (1975) Perinatal cardiac arrest. Quality of survivors. *Archs Dis. Childh.*, **50**, 696.
Stephenson, J.M., Du, J.N. and Oliver, T.K. (1970) The effect of cooling on blood gas tensions in newborn infants. *J. Pediat.*, **76**, 848.
Usher, R., Saigal, S., O'Neill, A., Chua, L. and Surainder, Y. (1971) Red cell volume in respiratory distress syndrome. *Pediat. Res.*, **5**, 415.
Windle, W.F. (1963) Selective vulnerability of the C.N.S. of rhesus monkeys to asphyxia during birth. In *Selective Vulnerability of the Brain in Hypoxaemia*, eds. Schade, J.P. and McMenemy, W.H., p. 251. Oxford: Blackwell.
Yao, A.C. and Lind, J. (1974) Placental transfusion. *Am. J. Dis. Childh.*, **127**, 128.

Index

Keeping Up With Magda

Keeping Up With Magda

Isla Dewar

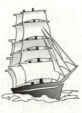

W F HOWES LTD

This large print edition published in 2005 by
W F Howes Ltd
Units 6/7, Victoria Mills, Fowke Street
Rothley, Leicester LE7 7PJ

1 3 5 7 9 10 8 6 4 2

First published in 1995
by Headline Book Publishing

A CIP catalogue record for this book is available
from the British Library

ISBN 1 84505 814 3

Typeset by Palimpsest Book Production Limited,
Polmont, Stirlingshire
Printed and bound in Great Britain
by Antony Rowe Ltd, Chippenham, Wilts.

With love and thanks to Nadia Carlotto
who taught me to cook.

CHAPTER 1

When she first came to Mareth it seemed to Jessie that she had come to live in Toy Town. Toy Town with sex. Nothing, absolutely nothing could break the air of frenetic unreality. It was a huddled place on the edge of the world, only the ancient harbour wall between it and the grubby grey and swelling sea. Next stop – who knew where? The streets were kitchen clean. It had that languid air of permanent pro-crastination. Tourists and other strangers thought that nothing ever went on there. But they were wrong. There was more to life in Mareth than a resigned journey from birth to menopause then death. It seethed. Everything that ever could happen happened there.

Every morning, seven-thirty, regular as clock-work, Jessie was woken by the solid click click clicking of Magda Horn's six-inch stilettos storming up the pavement. Lying in bed, hand between her thighs – a solitary indulgence to check she was really real – unwillingly awake, Jessie would curse the woman in the street below for her noisy footwear. A tangle-haired forty-something hooligan

1

with the brattish way of someone half her age. Oh yes, Jessie had the mark of Magda Horn.

Mareth dawns were exquisite; the sun slid up over the horizon and hung, a glowing red globe, above the harbour. Gulls woke and rose in shrieking, tumbling squalls to claim their space in the day. The first people of the morning, the workers at the quay, the bin men, Magda Horn appeared. Everyone swore. Not a curse, more a rude awakening. Junk language, highly seasoned, quick and easy to use for people who were glad to find the world the way they left it, and who were claiming their space in the day.

Rattling a great clutch of keys and cursing, Magda opened the Ocean Café just below Jessie's window and daily exchanged raw morning banter with the men working on the quay across the road. She swore. And, swift as a nod and a wink, back would come their merry quips, 'Fuck. Fuck. Fucky. Fuck.'

Jessie, moaning on her pillow, reached for her first cigarette of the day, lit it, coughed and complained to the empty room, 'These people can communicate volumes using only one word. What are they all on about? Is that all they can think of to say?'

Granny Moran, known in her heyday as Greasy Mae, came out from the house next door, voluminous tartan dressing gown drawn round her as she shuffled swollen-footed in worn and ancient pink slippers over the road to the harbour's edge

2

to spread breadcrumbs and bacon rinds on the ground. Seagulls took hysterics, came squabbling and crying, fighting each other and the wind, to swoop for food.

'Hey Mae,' a swearer on the quay called, 'cold enough for you?'

'Fine healthy weather,' Jessie heard Granny Moran's cracked and over-used voice reply. 'Kills all them bloody germs. An' watch yer bloody tongue when you bloody speak. I hear you swearing every morning. I've heard enough of that language to do me all ma days. Besides I knew yer granny.'

'I thought you *were* his granny,' another swearer joined in. 'The way you carried on, thought you were everybody's granny.' Granny Moran would never escape her raunchy past. The old lady sucked her gums and stared through the freezing January fog at the thickly anoraked gathering on the quay. Muttering fiercely, she turned back to her front door. It seemed to Jessie that when Granny Moran spoke to herself, her language was as monstrous and vivid as everyone else's.

The swearers, who always enjoyed their own jokes hugely, roared and laughed. A seagull screeching wildly soared past Jessie's window, splattering shit on her little white Peugeot parked below. And she swore. This language was catching.

In the café below, the first rock'n'roll of the day started. The Rolling Stones; bass thudded through the ceiling, rattling the windows. 'Soul Survivor', Jessie heard Jagger holler, and stiffened. The din worsened. Pots clattered, crockery crunched, cutlery rattled. Magda made the same thunderous noises every morning. Jessie wondered vaguely if she knew she was still in bed and made a din deliberately to irritate her. The life's philosophy of such a strident personality could only be: I am up therefore everybody should be up. Then she started on the children.

Every day she brought trailing behind her a brood of six or seven luminous infants, assorted sizes in multi-coloured shell-suits and back to front baseball caps, like pick'n'mix kids. Jessie could never decide if morning to morning it was the same six or seven straggling along the harbour swinging schoolbags, kicking stones and discarded coke tins, yelling taunts and laughing insults. Once inside the café, Magda fed them breakfast and a stream of abuse. 'Are you going to eat that or are you going to sit there doing your junior James Dean act?' Clatter of pots, bang of door, rattle and crunch of crockery, babble of voices and laughter. And Jagger's howl.

'Well, I'm not havin' any adolescent crap here. Bugger off and be moody somewhere else. Come back when your hormones have settled down.'

Slam, blam, crash. The smell of bacon wafted from the outlet ducts at the back of the café. Cereal rattled into bowls. Jessie lay tense with the strain of listening to other people's lives. She imagined

4

everyone down there in the cheery warm café busy eating cornflakes and being young.

'The bloody noise and mess, a bit of child abuse would do the lot of you some good,' Magda's voice cut through the din.

'Oh God,' a communal groan. 'That old threat.'

Despite herself, Jessie smiled.

Seeking solace after the life she had sought to make perfect had taken a vicious turn, Jessie had come to the noisiest, rudest place in the world.

The first time Magda Horn ever spoke to Jessie Tate, Jessie was standing at the harbour's edge staring out to sea. The wind was whipping her hair about her face and she had tears in her eyes. From her window she had seen porpoises swimming by and had rushed out clutching her binoculars to get closer to them. There they were sloping and dipping, effortlessly through the freezing grey swell only yards from the pier end. Oh God.

Jessie spent hours at the window of her flat above the Ocean Café looking through her binoculars. It was addictive. Sometimes it hurt. She spent so long staring into the dazzle, sun on water, that when she turned back into the room the light had blinded her and it was a while before she could see properly again. She watched gulls squalling and bickering. Eiders busying by, dowdy ladies, gaudy males. Boats came and went, churning trails of frothing water behind them. Mostly, however, she watched the sea. The hugeness, bulk and constancy of it fascinated her.

That day a strange shape loomed, grey against the light. Just a small triangle in the midst of all that sea. Then it was gone. She watched. It loomed again. And again. More and more of them. She gasped. Porpoises. Her heart tumbled. Crying in triumph at her find she ran out of her flat, down the stairs and over the road to the harbour's edge. She had to get closer to them. They were so beautiful. It was an effort stopping herself diving in and swimming after them. Foolish in March.

'What's that you're seeing then?'

Magda stood behind her, looking quizzically out to sea. She had seen Jessie standing shivering in T-shirt and jeans as close to the water as a person could get and, fearing the loony woman upstairs was about to do something silly, had rushed out of the café to stop her.

'Porpoises,' Jessie's voice cracked; she couldn't contain her joy. 'Have you seen them out there?'

Magda smiled. 'They sometimes come by. Means good weather. So they say. Haven't noticed it myself.'

Jessie pointed to where she had seen the porpoises. Tears streamed down her face. 'They're beautiful,' she said, 'so incredibly beautiful.'

'Yes,' said Magda flatly. She had lived here all her life, had seen porpoises before. But then, these days Magda felt she had seen everything before.

'No,' Jessie insisted, barely able to focus. She was weeping openly, tears streaming damply down her face, nose running, upper lip quite out of control, 'you don't understand. The porpoises. They're wonderful.' Her face crumpled into full hormonal blubbering.

Magda nodded, 'Of course they are.' She shivered. In skimpy black skirt and gaudy pink shirt, she too was inadequately dressed. Also she felt undermined by Jessie's sophisticated thinness. And could hate her for it. One of Magda's many many theories was that a woman's life was written on her hips and stomach. Hers told a tale of surfeits: alcohol, food, sex and children. Hers were hips of excesses. Jessie's said control. One swift eye flick and Magda knew she was in the company of a woman who could casually refuse pudding or place an abstemious hand over the top of her glass before it was refilled. Here was a woman who could say no and think nothing of it. Magda recognised the mixture of envy, respect and loathing she felt when she met someone like Jessie. Though, that same swift eyeflick had also registered a certain slackness round the belly. A recent indulgence, Magda thought. Life has caught up with her. She returned to the café, picked up a cloth and feverishly wiped the bar.

'See that new woman upstairs?' she said to Edie. 'Well I thought I was bad come the time of the month. But by God she's totally off her head. There's a woman seriously in need of a cup of hot

7

chocolate and a whipped cream doughnut. She's awash with hormones.'

It was their first meeting though they had been watching each other for months.

CHAPTER 2

The baby died. Jessie lay back in the delivery room eyes fixed on the ceiling. She was aware of mumbling white-coated strangers moving near her. An embarrassed rustle, nobody spoke. Dr Davies stood at the end of the delivery table, 'I'm so sorry, Mrs Tate,' he said, smiling apologetically. 'We'll have an autopsy, find out what went wrong. Now we'll get you to the ward so you can rest.' He patted her. Professionally sad. 'Never mind. You're young. In a few weeks you can try again. Think of all the fun you'll have.' In shock, sweat-drenched, hair matted after thirteen hours in labour, Jessie stared at him dumbly and nodded. 'My baby,' she thought, 'baby boy. He would have been mine.'

Four months, two weeks, six days later it came to Jessie what she should have said. 'Piss off.'

She had risen from her sleep screaming, 'You bastard. How dare you?' Alex had only momentarily opened his eyes to look at her. He'd got used to her rantings. Loony time, he told himself mildly, pulling a pillow over his head to obliterate the ravings.

9

'Piss off, Dr Davies. I'm coming to get you, Dr Davies. Think of all the fun I'll have.'

It had been going on for some time, Jessie's insanity. It was a hum in her head, a tunnel she was in. Alone. She had been going to have a baby. Death had not occurred to her. 'Dead,' she would say. 'Dead. Dead,' trying to imagine the numbness of it. The finality. Her baby, tiny corpse, white and perfect, lifeless alone in the depth of the earth. She kept conjuring up images, torturing herself. Couldn't help it. A million avenging hormones coursing through her urged her on. Equipped and ready to nurture, she didn't know how to handle grief. 'Dead. Dead. Dead.' A mournful monotone.

'Stop it.' Alex spoke from the depths of irritation. Tired and lonely, he wanted some comfort. He wished the demented recluse he was currently sharing his bed with would go away and his real wife would come back. His real wife, the one with pale painted toenails, who wore a silk ivory teddy in bed and shared Sunday morning champagne picnics under the duvet, warm bagels filled with scrambled eggs and smoked salmon, Nina Simone being sultry on the bedroom CD player. Of course all he had to do was shop for bagels, eggs and smoked salmon and do it. But shopping had been Jessie's part of the deal. He loved that life. This is how we live, he often said. This is who we are. So, he ached for Jessie's return, and if this one didn't come soon, he was sorely tempted to find her elsewhere.

'I think you're enjoying the pain.' She considered this. Perhaps he was right. Perhaps she had to have pain. Needed the hurt. It was, after all, her fault. Guilt consumed her. Nights she lay awake staring into the dark, reliving the pregnancy minute by minute, trying to pinpoint the actual moment of blame. She hadn't taken her iron tablets. Had she? She couldn't remember. She'd drunk too much. She should not have worked past the sixth month. She should have stopped as soon as she knew a baby was on the way. She'd developed a passion for tomatoes, too much acidity. It was all her fault. She had walked too much. Stayed up too late. Not drunk enough milk. Worn too tight clothing when she saw how huge she was getting. Stopped the proper circulation getting to the infant. Nights she tossed and turned, rolled her head on the pillow trying to stop the ache. The guilt. The guilt. The guilt.

She was haunted by the child she was sure she had killed. She imagined him, a dark-haired, sombre little one, staring at her, wide brown eyes. She stood in the nursery they'd prepared for him, gently fingering the clothes he'd never wear. She thought about him as he might have been. A toddler stumbling after her in the park, laughing, hair blown behind him, chubby fingers stretched out to reach her. Would he have been bright? Her child? Of course he would have been.

She recalled the little life she had plotted for him as she stroked her swollen belly, felt him kick

11

and move within her. Now he wouldn't learn to play the piano. Wouldn't ride a bike. Wouldn't go on holiday to Cornwall every year as she'd done. Wouldn't sit on his grandfather's knee listening to the stories she listened to before him. Wouldn't. Wouldn't. Wouldn't. The wouldn'ts went on and on. She listed them, brought them out to heighten her hurt. The pain got too much to bear. She was alone in her tunnel of grief, beyond the comfort that Alex or her friends offered.

It was a long slow sink into the black. When she first got back from hospital she seemed to be coping. Her doctor called, his young face creased with concern. 'I'm so sorry, Mrs Tate. How are you?' She sat palely, legs curled, on her sofa smiling slightly. 'I'm fine,' she said. Absurdly, he believed her. The local health visitor called in several times during Jessie's first fortnight at home. Jessie would see her car drawing up outside and swiftly add some blusher and lipstick to her brave face. She hated the bustling intrusion. The health visitor, however, didn't intrude for long. There were people who were actually sick or old to tend, and mothers who had actual babies; besides, Jessie seemed so sane.

When her chums and late-night drinking companions, Trish and Lou, called to see her bringing vodka, white chrysanthemums and sympathy, Jessie cracked a few weak jokes and mustered some enthusiasm for Lou's new car.

'She seems all right,' Trish said as they drove away.

But Lou said, 'Hmmm. You never know with Jessie.'

After five weeks, Jessie went back to the office, far too soon. She worked as an editor in a small publishing firm. She sat at her desk desperately trying to concentrate. Tears flowed down her cheeks and fell on the typescript she was reading. 'What's the point?' she said. 'What's the point?' It was all she could say, all she could think. Someone called Alex who came, wrapped his coat round her, and led her out to his car. She never went back.

She gave up her job, and lay in her bed late in the mornings, television on. She watched it glumly, her face rarely registering an expression. She stopped cooking, stopped dressing. Roamed the house all day in jeans and a torn sweatshirt. A slow sticky mess gathered in the kitchen, in the bathroom, dishes in the sink, dust and crumbs on the floor, scum in the bath, brown stains in the lavatory, bins overflowed. There were damp towels, the laundry smelled, the grill-pan reeked of stale fat. She didn't change the bed. Newspapers piled in the living room. Ashtrays overflowed. Alex found some willing comfort in a girl at work called Annie, a replica Jessie. He came home late, sometimes not at all. Jessie hardly noticed. She did not deserve a husband. Her body had failed him. She had killed his child, her child.

She walked to the corner shop every morning, bought a pack of Marlboro and five bars of

13

chocolate. She ate, smoked, drank coffee, no milk, no sugar. Numb, cocooned in guilt, she would stand at the window for hours, staring out at the garden eating peanut butter straight from the jar, letting the silence and her shame roar inside her head. She fooled herself she was enduring. But she was in hell.

She did not emerge suddenly. It just occurred to her one morning that her car had been lying neglected for weeks. She rammed her spoon into her Sunpat jar, put it down on the windowsill and went to the garage. She did not expect the car to start. But it did. Perhaps, then, she thought, she ought to go somewhere.

She went back into the house to fetch a jacket, her chequebook, some loose change, and was filled with a rush of urgency. Her heart thudded, panic moved wildly within her. She must go now. She must get out of the house this minute swiftly before the phone rang, Alex turned up unexpectedly, before something – anything – happened to stop her. She ran out of the door. She drove blinking at the world. Everything was still there as it had been before she renounced it. Traffic rumbled. Cars jostled from lane to lane. Billboards jarred, slick and gaudy messages. Skinny-faced youths leant on traffic barricades, meanly watching her go. Watching everybody go. Radios blared. Life was so noisy. Overhead a crane heaved. She leaned down on the steering wheel, watching it, flooded with fear. What if it fell? I do not want to die, she whispered. On

pavements people ratted to and fro carrying brief-
cases, bags, books. On a whim, it seemed, they left
their safe runs to dash free-fall through the cars.
Women pushed prams. An old man in a brown hat
waited by a tree, patient whilst his dog sniffed and
peed. Bikes weaved through the traffic lanes.
Everything was moving. Everything was busy. All
that life out here, minutes from her front door. And
she had forgotten about it. She clacked through the
pile of tapes beside the gearstick, selected Van
Morrison, found her sunglasses then, signalling,
shifted down to three, put her foot flat to the floor
and shot forward through the traffic, weaving in
front of less decisive cars and into the fast lane and
down the Queensferry Road and out of Edinburgh.
She didn't know where she was going. Just out of
town.

She headed north. At the Forth Bridge she paid
her toll and came out from the barrier at speed.
She was with other cars doing the get-into-the-
fast-lane-first dash. She hated bridges. She always
gripped the wheel and stared grimly ahead in a
headlong rush to make it to land again. What if
it broke in two whilst she was driving across it?
She'd plummet into the sea. But today she felt
jubilant to be so high above the water. She allowed
herself swift sidelong glances at the river weaving
and widely gleaming.

The rhythm of driving returned to her. Once
learned, like riding a bike or making love, never
forgotten. She hummed along in top gear, easily

overtaking everything that appeared before her. Van sang, she joined in. Badly. She hammered up the motorway, then on a whim signalled into a slip road and headed for the coast. The scenery changed. More sky. Light and cloud. She drove and didn't think, didn't contemplate her loss, didn't wonder what might have been if . . . and if . . . and if; even Alex didn't occur to her. The tape ended and a sign loomed before her. Tourist Trail. She took it. The road twisted and looped, seemed to turn back on itself. She couldn't decide what to play next. Mozart, *The Marriage of Figaro*. Chorus, orchestra, tenor, soprano eased exquisitely from her speakers. She passed fields and, poised at the foot of little hills, little houses like children's drawings with perfect smoke curling from perfect little chimneys. All those weeks, days, hours she had been tucked away this had been out here carrying on as if tragedy never happened. She crested a hill, and gasped. The sea was before her, glistening and moving, spreading to the horizon and beyond. She snapped the cassette out of the player.

The road along the coast was straight and flat. She found her favourite Billie Holiday. That still and mournful voice slid out: 'April in Paris'. She made it seem like the saddest place on earth. Villages were strung out a mile or so apart. Little places, cobbled streets, pantiled roofs. They were built sloping up from the sea. The old houses clustered round the harbour, moving up through the

16

centuries to the Victorian houses at the top of the hill, and modern bungalows on the main road. She stopped at Mareth on the road between Largo and Shell Bay. She had not until now known this place existed.

It seemed to Jessie that this was the place to be. Nothing could happen to you here. It was sleepy and slow. The air smelled of coal fires and sea. There were seventeenth-century, teeny-windowed houses on one side of the road, on the other the shore and a small harbour. Buildings were painted different colours: blue, pink, dark red. This place sparkled. A row of well-spaced, ancient trees lined the narrow pavement.

Even then Jessie noticed the Ocean Café. It was small, windows steamed, temptingly seedy. She heard some blues playing inside. People would be having fun in there.

The terraces were separated at intervals by a series of tiny, cobbled, evocatively-named lanes: Tolbooth Wynd, Peep'o'Day Lane, Water Wynd, that sloped steeply to the High Street. Jessie chose Peep'o'Day Lane, couldn't resist it. It was so narrow that she could touch each side with arms outstretched. The stones on the walls were old, old, worn, touched by three hundred years of passers-by.

The High Street was also painted, shops and more houses. A pub, fronted with tubs overflowing ivy, a betting shop, an ironmonger's, a butcher's and a Spar grocery store. There was a car park hidden behind a row of giant trees, probably more ancient than the village. Jessie wandered about, staring into shop windows. Children played in the street, trundling up and down on trikes. Jessie stared: when had she last seen that? This place was safe.

Young and Neil, Solicitors and Estate Agents, were set back off the High Street, down a steep wynd that led back to the harbour. Jessie read the properties for sale advertised in the window. Immaculate residence, must be seen, spacious, open outlook, well-stocked garden – estate-agent-speak broke all colloquial boundaries. Wherever you were you understood exactly what they were on about. On impulse she went in. She stood nervously at the desk.

'Yes?' a young blonde receptionist smiled at her. She wore pink, everything pink.

'I was wondering . . .' Jessie spoke softly, un-certain. Until this moment she hadn't known she was going to do this.' . . . If you had anything to rent about here.'

'I'll get Mr Young.'

Pretty in Pink disappeared, came back seconds later with a Suit wringing his hands, smiling weakly. Striped shirt, polka-dot tie, hair waved back, he peered at her through wire specs. This could be Alex. Alexes were everywhere, smitten with style, aching for wealth.

Thinking of him now she realised that Alex didn't have a life, he had a masterplan. He mapped out his days like an old campaigner spending time each evening putting the final touches to the blue-print of the day ahead. He rose each morning, showered, shaved, moisturised his skin and scented the body he worked hard to preserve in peak condition. He spent some time laying out clothes on the bed: shirt, tie, jacket, trousers, choosing the right combination to suit both his mood and the world he was about to face. He would leave the house before eight and come home some time after nine. He was a resources manager with a video company that produced films for advertising agencies. He was a busy busy man.

'I have to be there,' he said. But that wasn't it. He had to be seen to be there. Jessie sighed. 'You are present at the job from seven in the morning, till seven at night, and the job is present in you all the bloody time.'

Looking at this man in front of her now, noting a small stain on his tie and the way he ran his fingers over his chin, she realised that beneath the veneer there was a certain uncertainty. 'This man is as insecure as I am,' she thought then, realising the truth behind her husband's meticulous routine and design for living, 'as Alex is.'

'Something to rent?' said the Suit. There was The Steadings. A converted stable block just out of town. Five bdrms, gym, kitchen with Aga, two baths, spacious living rm, dining with french windows to patio. He smiled at Jessie, scrutinising

19

her. Old jeans, baseball boots, torn sweatshirt, no make-up; when had that hair last seen a comb? Ah, no. He didn't think so.

'I'm sorry,' he said, 'not at the moment. If you'd like to leave your name—'

'There's that flat on the shore. Above Magda's . . .' Pretty in Pink chipped in.

Derek Young paused.

'The shore,' Jessie brightened. That sounded just right.

'It's a bit of a mess, I'm afraid.'

Jessie shrugged. So what was a mess to her? A mess? She could take this man home, show him a real mess if he wanted messes.

'It sounds perfect,' she said. Regretted right away that she sounded so keen. 'How much is it?'

'Ah . . .' Derek Young had had enough time to reconsider his initial judgement. The hair – beneath that tangle – was very expensively cut. The filthy jeans had cost a bit too. He couldn't see the label on the jacket, but the sunglasses were Armani. He knew, he had the same pair.

'Four hundred . . . and –' dared he risk it? – 'fort . . . um . . . fifty a month.'

'I'll take it.'

'You should see it first.'

'Fine. I'll see it. Then I'll take it.'

CHAPTER 3

Jessie moved to Mareth. She bought food at the local Spar, posted mail at the post office, and went for daily walks round the harbour, stepping over heaped nets and ropes. She stood at the pier end staring at the horizon. Several times a week she walked along the shore, past the last few houses on West Way that led down to the sand. Jumping from rock to rock, carefully keeping the salt water from her precious Timberlands, she would make her way to the foot of the cliff path. Puffing, she'd climb the over-grown muddied way to the top. The wind would push her hair from her face, whip her breath away. She would stare down to where the grassy slope turned sheer. Far below the sea churned and frothed white over jagged rocks. Fulmars gath-ered noisily, clumsily on the cliff face. She would stand for hours watching them career absurdly in, making sometimes two or three runs before they managed a landing. It surprised her. She always thought birds and animals managed their lives perfectly. There was something cheering about these birds and their duff attempts at coming in to land. 'It isn't just me that screws up, then.'

The aloneness exhilarated her one day, saddened her the next. But she could not find the deepening silence she sought. The rattle and hum from the Ocean Café downstairs reminded her constantly that there were other people in the world, all of them having a better time than she was.

She had thought that if she could spend some time speaking to nobody, a stranger in a strange place, the turmoil in her head might cease. She might find some peace. But after only a short time in Mareth she stopped being a stranger. She became 'that funny woman that lives above the Ocean Café. Who is she anyway? And what's she doing moving into a place like that, this time of the year?'

Here in Mareth everyone knew everyone. They knew everything there was to know about each other. And what they didn't know they assumed. Their assumptions were passed on in conversations and gossip in shops, kitchens, living rooms and bars until distorted by time, speculation and rumour, the assumptions became facts. And who would meddle with facts? Certainly nobody in Mareth, where the crack was so beloved it was the stuff of life itself. There was nothing better than a good rumour. People here were prepared to believe and in time heartily narrate the assumptions even about themselves that had passed into local folklore. They were their own myths and legends. And proud of it.

People started to nod to her when they met her in the street. It was a curt, uncomfortable nod, with a 'ynumph' sort of a greeting. A shy acknowledgement that she was in the same world, country, village, street as the nodder and it didn't seem right not to say something about it. Ynumph fitted the bill, or sometimes nyoink. Jessie hadn't mastered the sound effects and said a crisp and distant g'morning, or gd'afternoon. They nodded because she had been discussed, dissected and decided upon. So now the nodders felt that they knew all about her and were therefore obliged to say hello, or as near to hello as they could get.

Jessica Tate was thirty-four years old and living separately from her husband. Everyone knew that. Derek Young had extracted the information whilst preparing the lease on No. 38 The Shore, the flat Jessie rented from his partnership, and Pretty in Pink, Shona Kerr, who was now into powder blue, had passed it on. Jessie was tallish, thinnish, had dark hair and no visible bloke to replace her husband. In whispered discussions in the Anchor and Crown it was being speculated that the broken marriage left her bitter and hating all men; likely, perhaps, even to be turning into a lesbian. But the Ocean Café rejected this notion. It was the café opinion that she was just recovering from some sort of break-up and in no need of a new relationship.

Jessie had a lot of books. What did she want with all them books? Ruby at the Spar mini-market

23

wanted to know. Had she a lot of reading to do? Or had she read them all? If so, why bother carting about a lot of books you've already read? They'd just clutter up the shelves when you could have a few nice ornaments and a pot plant. Jessie bought macaroni and spaghetti, which she called pasta, tins of tomatoes, onions, whole-meal bread, Alta Rica coffee and bars of fruit and nut chocolate when she shopped. Everybody knew that. Ruby told them.

Jessie had red knickers, black knickers and silky green camiknickers. They'd been spotted on her washing line. But so far no bra. She'd not need a bra with them wee tits, Woody at the Anchor and Crown said. Jack, his barman, agreed. Besides, them bull dykes don't wear bras. Do they?

Jessie wore 501 jeans and boots and a soft, all-enveloping jersey. The boots were tan leather and cost a bomb, everyone thought. But they didn't cost as much as the dark burgundy jersey which came from one of them designer shops and was probably cashmere. And though it had come from Benetton and cost twenty-five pounds, the guessing on its price was two hundred pounds and rising. Of course Jessie had other clothes: striped silk pyjamas, a patterned robe, a navy nightdress which wasn't as nice as the pyjamas but probably warmer these cold nights. Especially for someone who slept alone. Jessie wore a leather jacket sometimes, and sometimes a long black coat. When she wore her long black coat, Mareth decided she was mourning her long-lost lover. Mareth had a romantic heart.

Jessie drove a three-year-old Peugeot that needed a new exhaust. Freddie Kilpatrick who owned the local garage knew this because one night on the way home from the Ocean Café he had lain on the road and slid under it. Ah, he had smiled, knew it. When he got home his wife looked at his back and said scathingly, 'Have you been looking under cars again?'

Lying under Jessie's Peugeot, he'd figured out his business plan. Didn't Crumbly Al have just such an exhaust lying in his scrapyard. He could swap the Fiat gearbox he had in the back of his workshop for a couple of central-heating radiators Joe Roberts the plumber had lying in his yard. And swap Crumbly Al the radiators for his exhaust. He could have it ready when Jessie brought the car down to him in about a couple of weeks. She'd not get much more out of that thing, he reckoned. He fished some string from his pocket and tied Jessie's ailing exhaust up. He couldn't risk her breaking down somewhere else after all the trouble and bartering he'd have to do to get the right part for her motor.

Jessie didn't get much mail. 'Only stuff about her credit card, and bank statements,' Duncan the postie said. And though her phone rang a fair bit she rarely answered it. Granny Moran knew this. She mentioned it when she was at the post office picking up her pension. 'She's avoiding somebody,' she said. Could it be she was on the run from the police?

Magda at the Ocean Café laughed out loud. 'That one,' she said squeakily, rubbing a peephole in the café's steamy window to watch Jessie stump round the harbour, 'is only on the run from herself.' Remembering a couple of mornings ago when she had come face to face with a tearstained Jessie at the café door, added knowingly, 'Look at her go. Striding about all hours speaking to nobody, leaving the phone ringing, all weepy and eating chocolate. It can only be one thing . . .' The café held its breath. When Magda spoke, an opinion worth hearing and discussing was on the go.

'It's hormones,' she said, nodding at her own wisdom. 'It's purely hormonal.' Several faces joined Magda's peering through the peephole at the hormonally stricken Jessie. Word spread. And so when men met Jessie in the street they said ynumph or nyoink, making a wide berth. Hormones, especially female ones, were to be avoided. Women, however, stared at her piercingly, trying to fathom the depth of Jessie's woes. Hormones; they knew about hormones.

The flat was miserable. Even Jessie in her doldrums could see that. It smelt not just of damp but as if dozens of unwashed agoraphobics had lived here, cramped and refusing to go out. It had two rooms, a bedroom and a living room with cupboard-size kitchen off. It has potential, Jessie told herself as she unpacked. I can make something of this. I can make a statement about me. Just me and nobody else. This is a wonderful opportunity. I can be happy.

As the little world outside speculated about her she painted the bedroom a pale smoky blue, the living room and kitchen white, and the bathroom a sagey green. She put up pictures, installed a small sofa, but left the carpet which was so vile she found something comforting about it. She liked to imagine the cosy mores of the person who would choose such a thing.

This is me, she thought. In the blue and sweary chilly mornings she lay listening to the ribaldry outside and felt almost at home. In the evenings young bloods would come duding out of the Ocean Café, hollering. Their raw voices cut through the night, and if Jessie was foolish enough to come to the window to watch the goings-on they would shout up to her.

'Hello darlin',' drunken voices, 'show us yer tits.' They'd wiggle their hips at her, uninhibited sexual motion, 'C'mon down. Look at this,' and someone would moon at her. White bottom gleaming under the streetlights. 'Let's see *your* arse, darlin'.'

Jessie would gaze sadly down. 'Not a bad bum,' she'd think. 'Seen better.' Then she'd go back to her fireside, turn up her Mahler and try to read.

The streetlamp mooners started to come by every Saturday night. They would call her name. 'Hey, Long Coat, come an' see this.' Mareth's fascination with Jessie's manic strides round the harbour in her long black coat had gained her the nickname. Foolishly she would go to the window to look at them. After one particularly raucous evening there was a whole row of bums shining in the night for her to view.

'Good heavens,' she breathed, staring down mesmerised. She hadn't the gumption to pull her curtains and declare her disinterest. There were fat bums and medium bums and tight little nubby bums with cute little side indents that a person could certainly consider giving a second glance. Jessie did. And as she did, Magda Horn came out, keys in hand, to lock up for the night. She did not shriek; scarcely noticed the row of exposed cheeks. Jessie was impressed.

Magda looked up at her. 'So what do you think,' she called, pointing to the first bum. 'A five probably. And this,' she indicated the next arse, 'a two. A seven. A three, an eight. Oh Lipless, you're only a one: you'll have to start some serious bum workouts.'

Lipless rose indignantly, heaving up his pants. 'It's not that bad, Magda. You'll go a long way before you see an arse as magnificent as mine.'

Magda hooted. 'As long as you think so, Lipless. I'd hate you to get some sort of complex about what you've been bringing along behind you all these years.'

Lipless slapped his rear, 'Me and my arse get along just fine, Magda.'

'I have the same thing going with mine,' Magda said, bustling past them.

'Ah Magda,' Lipless said, shaking his head in admiration, 'you've a great arse on you.'

'I know,' she said, walking off down the street, well aware the mooners were now all upright and staring at her bum.

'Enjoy,' she called. 'This is as close as any of youse will get to it.'

The mooners below moved off mumbling. And Jessie, returning to her sofa, hurt her back trying to look over her shoulder at her own backside. It was the first time she had thought about herself, her appearance in months. Perhaps she was getting better.

CHAPTER 4

The bum incident happened only a couple of days after the porpoise incident. Jessie now considered she just about knew Magda Horn and could therefore go into the Ocean Café. She had been under its steamy spell ever since she'd arrived. Mornings the thick aroma of coffee spread through the chill air, evenings the boozy wafts and babble were almost irresistible. But only almost. Jessie was astute enough to know that Mareth was not the sort of place that welcomed unaccompanied female strangers into its drinking establishments.

The first time she went into the Ocean Café she stood nervously at the door. Was this the right thing to do? To come in here? Conversation slowed, stopped. Heads turned. What does she want? It was a horrible moment. Magda broke it.

'What can I get you?'

'Coffee,' Jessie spoke weakly, taking a seat by the window, far from where the in-crowd sat. The chair scraped loudly on the floor as she pulled it back, wood against wood, a long farty noise. 'Sorry,' she said, mostly to the chair.

'Black? White? What sort of coffee?'

'Black, please. Strong.'

Magda brought it. She smelled of musk. She laid Jessie's coffee on the table and alongside it a chocolate croissant.

'I didn't ask for that,' Jessie pointed at the plate.

'You didn't have to.' Magda sounded snippy. If she decided you wanted a chocolate croissant, you wanted a chocolate croissant. And, staring in surprise at the delicacy in front of her, Jessie found that she wanted it. She started to eat slowly, picking bits off and putting them carefully into her mouth. Conversation started up again as the bar accustomed itself to her sudden presence.

There were four men at the bar, workmen from the quay. Jessie recognised them. Three were drinking coffee and eating bacon rolls. The fourth thumped the bar with his fist, demanding whisky.

'Not from me you'll not get that at this time in the morning,' Magda shook her head. 'Not you anyway.'

'Why not me?'

'You and your liver are shrivelling visibly, Lipless. If you want whisky, go and shrivel your liver somewhere else. You can have soup.'

'Soup, Christ. Soup. I hate soup. Soup's just a cheap way of disguising mushed-up vegetables. There's something sneaky about that.'

Magda stared at him stonily. Lipless continued, 'What's this you have about feeding people anyway?

31

Offering me soup. Giving her,' he jerked his thumb towards Jessie, 'that chocolate thing.'

'That's hormones,' Magda explained.

'Christ, Lipless,' another of the workmen whined, 'now look what you've done. She's going to start on about hormones. Can't you just eat some soup?'

'No. I hate soup.'

'See,' said Magda, 'some people say love or money makes the world go round. Rubbish. It's hormones.'

'Eat your fucking soup.' One of the workmen yanked the plate in front of Lipless.

'It only just came to me the other day that hormones were at the root of all our triumphs and tragedies. I mean, a hormoneless person is one of those bland sorts. You know, beige cardy harmless. If everyone was like that there'd be no wars. No passion. But where does that get you?'

Nobody answered. Lipless sucked at his soup. His work-mates shifted uneasily, chewing their food. They had a gnawing feeling that any moment Magda was going to start talking about periods and other female atrocities. 'Don't start, Magda. Please,' one of them pleaded.

'Oh, but I've started. So I'll finish,' Magda grinned. There was nothing more enjoyable than making men squirm. Once in full flow she was unstoppable. 'Us women can get all hot and bothered. We start stroking our men saying we want a baby.'

'That happens to me all the time,' said Lipless sadly. 'Every night.' He continued eating his soup.

'It's nuts. Babies. I ask you, who wants them?'

'Wimmin,' said someone. 'Babies are not a man's idea.'

'It's nothing to do with women. It's hormones. Women say they want a baby but in the depth of them they know it's the end of them. Once you've had a baby that's it, you'll never go out again. You'll be in for the next ten – fifteen years. And what are you to a baby anyway? The face behind the spoon till you become the face behind the cheque-book. They start needing money to sate the demands of their own leaping hormones.' She leant on the bar, holding her coffee cup, addressing nobody in particular. Not caring that everybody was pretending not to listen. She was working out her thoughts. Jessie watched, intrigued.

'Don't you agree?' Magda suddenly asked her.

She shrugged, 'I suppose if I could have a hormonectomy, I would.'

'Time for us to get back to work,' Lipless shoved his empty soup bowl across the bar. 'Look, I ate it.'

'And wasn't it good?' Magda demanded.

'Yes. As a matter of fact it was. Don't tell me what it was. I'd rather not know. There was garlic and funny stuff in it. And I don't eat that kind of thing. And now I have to go back to work and it's all your fault, Magda Horn.'

'My fault?' Magda pointed at herself, eyes wide. Innocence.

'Yes, your fault. If you didn't keep feeding me instead of letting me drink I'd've died long ago and I wouldn't have to go out in the cold and work.'

'Oh, blame me,' Magda said mildly. 'Everything's my fault.'

He left, heaving himself into his faded navy jacket, rasping insults and self-loathing.

'You know you're really alone when you don't have someone to blame,' Magda shrugged to Jessie. Crumbling slow pieces from her croissant and carefully placing them into her mouth, Jessie considered this. She must be truly alone then. For who had she to blame? Herself and only herself. Magda, however, knew who she had to blame for the absurd path her life had taken. Her mother. Every so often Magda was consumed with rage against her mother. Calling her by her full name, Mary Lomax, as if she was miscalling her best school-chum and not the woman who gave birth to her, she would throw cutlery and plates the length of the Ocean Café shouting, 'Bugger you, Mary Lomax.'

Everyone near to her knew of this rage and hatred: Little Jim Horn, whose name she had taken, father of her four children, her four children and Edie who worked beside her in the café. The only person it seemed who did not know about Magda's fury was Mary Lomax.

The rages completely swamped Magda, seeming to well up within her from nowhere. A thought, a song, a smell; anything that brought back past times could set it off. Once it had been more than that. Once the rage had been constantly with her. That it had now been reduced to sudden maddening outbursts, steaming blood pressure and a few bits of broken crockery pleased Magda. She considered she was getting better. She was coming to terms with her inadequacies. And, in particular, that one inadequacy that loomed large every single day of her life. Magda Horn could neither read nor write. She had been a difficult child. That one has always been a trial, her mother would say, shaking her head. She remembered those years before Magda started school as being the worst, noisiest in her life. She remembered spending them rushing around bent double, arms outstretched, trying to keep up with her exuberant daughter. 'Children are fine right up until they can move about on their own,' she expounded over gin and tonic at the Anchor and Crown. 'After that it's hell. The best thing you could say about our Magda was that she left me so shagged out I was too knackered to do anything about having another baby. She was the most effective contraceptive ever.'

At Mareth Academy it was decided that Magda had limited learning capabilities. She couldn't concentrate. Her books were a mess. They were actually so filthy that disgusted teachers held them in horror between thumb and forefinger at arm's length, as if they could catch something nasty from them. Her handwriting scrawled illegibly. Erratic, her reports said. And, work this year has proved once again beyond Magda's comprehension. And, this child is uncontrollable. The more she was criticised, the wilder she got. During her first seven or eight years in school Magda sat in front of the sort of teachers who thought the way to reach Magda's brain was up through her backside. She was beaten daily.

In time she discovered that teachers are cowards. Or at least the ones who taught her were. They had an inbuilt loathing of violence when it was turned against them. Magda bit and kicked and scratched and howled and they stopped hitting her. The headmaster, a quiet man called Harvey Scott, suggested she be sent to a special school, but Mareth looked after its own. When Granny Moran took to wandering round the harbour in her nightgown looking for her long-dead husband, whoever found her took her home, put her to bed and locked the door. When Gordon Masters drowned, the whole village went quiet for weeks, curtains were kept drawn, children told not to shout in the streets till it was decided by some silent mutual agreement that the period of mourning was over. When Freda Bishop, after watching one too many dismaying documentaries on the gruelling miseries of post-holocaust life, and convincing herself that the day of reckoning was nigh and the bomb about to be dropped, decided to camp on her roof so that she would see the plane coming in over the sea, nobody minded, really. They took her thermos flasks of soup and cheese sandwiches and called soothingly from the street below that the bomb wasn't coming and if it did they'd all go together and wasn't that the best way?

The suggestion, then, to send Magda to a special school wasn't favoured. She was Mareth born and bred. In Mareth she would stay. Stay she did, in a constant state of outrage. Taking tantrums, shouting, swearing, banging her desk lid, jumping on her seat, chattering to her friends in class – when she went to class.

Magda was fourteen when Alice Barnes came to Mareth to teach English. The girl interested her. Here was a highly intelligent, outstandingly outrageous pupil who could barely read. Dyslexia occurred to her.

'What,' Mary Lomax had sighed when Magda's condition was finally diagnosed, 'in the name is that?'

'Word blindness,' Alice Barnes said slowly. She was used to incensed parents. 'And more than that. They think it's to do with both sides of the brain being the same size.'

Mary Lomax had eagerly seized upon this piece of information. 'I always knew she was loony.' She pointed dismissively at Magda, 'Typical of you to have a weird brain.'

'On the contrary,' Miss Barnes remained calm. 'I'd say your daughter was very remarkable. It's hardly surprising she behaves the way she does. She's had years of frustration. But she has got through school scarcely able to read, using only her memory. She seems to be able to commit great tracts of information to her mind after only one hearing. It's amazing.'

Magda's young heart had leapt. She wasn't the silly stupid erratic worthless child she was constantly being told she was. She was amazing. She had always suspected that. Mary Lomax, however, was not one to praise children. It didn't do to tell them they were amazing. They'd get above themselves.

'Well, she isn't all that amazing to me,' she said harshly. 'Is this dyslexia thing hereditary?'

Miss Barnes nodded, 'Can be.'

'Ah.' All was clear to Magda's mum. 'In that case she got it from her father.'

Alice Barnes ignored this remark. 'Thing is, most dyslexics are highly intelligent. Talented one way or another.'

This professional declaration that she was not vastly stupid came in time, just, to save Magda's sanity, but was too late for her self-esteem. The humiliation of being permanently bottom of the class, of having her school-mates snigger when her marks were read out, left its mark. Atrocious, despicable, try harder, unreadable, you are a thoroughly stupid child, see me: phrases from her education that Magda would run through her head, torturing herself. Everybody else looked at a page of print and read stories. She looked and saw rivers of white running through black type. Enlightenment, the things that people knew, would never be hers. She had stumbled through her school years bedevilled by bewilderment. She was alone, looking in on life, never taking part. The rage started.

She discovered rock'n'roll. There was a beat to her fury, a rhythm. And when it wasn't actually playing, it was playing in her head. The Stones, Dylan, Lou Reed, Aretha Franklin, The Who. She never switched them off. She woke to them, cooked to them, fucked to them. Sometimes it seemed that there were folks out there who were even angrier than she was. Maybe she wasn't quite as alone as she thought.

On her truant afternoons, Magda would sit out on the point, letting rip the rhythms in her head. Thinking. She wasn't part of the world. Nobody would let her join in. Things were a mystery to her. What were people on about? She couldn't understand anything. It seemed to her that there was a smug society of women who understood the mysteries of life: knitting patterns, how to bake scones, why it was necessary to put white cloths over the back of sofas and chairs, how to change a baby, how to put rollers in your hair, how to arrange flowers, the correct way to wipe a sink, all that and oh, a whole load of other stuff that she didn't understand. For some reason women who joined the smug society, the society of always being right, didn't like her. She worried them.

Furthermore, she was scared stiff of becoming one of them. Alice Barnes spoke to the Mastertons, owners of the Captain's Table, a four-star restaurant along the coast where she and her husband often ate. They gave Magda a job waiting tables. It didn't work. She was slow, could barely write down the orders, could not contain her rage. When customers laughed at her obvious failings, she tossed down cutlery before them. She whipped menus away before diners had finished reading them, tutted and sighed at those who took too long to choose what they wanted to eat. She was out of her depth. These glossy diners who knew a Beaune from a Margaux and what was a good year for Chardonnay, who knew without asking what fillet of sole veronique was and how monkfish should be roasted and how to serve crêpes more than scared her. They chipped away at the edges of her already low self-esteem. Her inadequacies reached howling point. She knew herself well. She was a slow, shiny-faced, shovel-handed, large-hipped waitress whose stupidity was written all over her face. She knew nothing of the gleamy candlelit world of gourmet dining. She was hurting and it showed. How it showed when a long established customer crisply demanded bisque homard with a decently chilled Sancerre and, as Magda struggled to wind her uneducated tongue round the order, raised an amused eyebrow to his co-diners who all sniggered. Oh it showed then.

Magda, unable to contain any more humiliation,

threw her order pad across the dining room, picked up a fork and held it threateningly under the eyebrow-raiser's nose calling him a 'Bastard . . . bastard –' she struggled here for the ultimate insult – 'man,' she screamed. The room silenced. The discreet clatter of upmarket cutlery, the chink of plush crockery, the dulcet babble of mock élitist conversation stopped, all stopped. Well, well, well. This was hardly the stuff of a civilised evening out. Secretly though, the only thing everybody in the room felt was relief that this hadn't happened to them. They were, after all, the bourgeoisie. Every eyebrow in the room was raised. By rights Magda should have been fired for her outburst. But George the chef pleaded her case. He had been watching her. Magda had been hanging about in the kitchen even on her days off. Food intrigued her. It was George's idea to move the absurd and gawky girl to the kitchen, a stroke of genius. Magda's salvation. Magda could cook. She was a natural. Those large hands that could not properly grip a pen could slice and chop and mix with ease. The girl that had turned in filthy and illegible schoolwork could turn out the most delicate of pastries, the most exquisite of sauces. Outside in the world, Magda was still Magda: enraged, unmanageable. In the kitchen she was turning into a queen. A goddess.

And oh, the thirst for knowledge. Every day a new culinary term. One day Madga came home and asked her mother what a marinade was. George

41

had mentioned making one and she hadn't a clue what it was.

'A whatinade?' Mary Lomax said, instantly dismissing anything that was new to her. 'Never heard of such a thing.'

Next day, Mary asked Granny Moran, who sucked her gums, shook her head, and doubted there was such a thing.

'Have you ever heard of a marinade?' Granny Moran asked Lipless, who worked on the pier. Lipless curled his lip. 'If y' can't drink it I won't know about it.' Still, he asked Ruby at the Spar mini-market who didn't know but at lunchtime asked Woody at the Anchor and Crown but he didn't know either. After a couple of days it was established that nobody in Mareth knew what a marinade was. But Magda came home and told her mother it was just a mixture – oil and wine maybe with some herbs and garlic – that you soaked meat in.

'Why would you do that?' Mary wanted to know.

'So it'll taste better.'

'Doesn't it already taste fine? Don't they buy quality meat at the Captain's Table?'

'Yes, of course they do. Just a marinade sort of changes the taste. Makes it more complex, deeper.'

'What's wrong with meat tasting of meat? Good plain food, that's what you want.'

Sighing, Magda realised there was nothing she could say on the subject of marinades, or anything else really. But the word went round Mareth that the oh so posh Captain's Table bought meat that was so bad they had to doctor it with garlic and herbs and such like fancy stuff to make it edible. Local custom at the restaurant dipped for a while. But picked up again as there was nowhere else to go that was special for anniversaries and birthdays and well, it was agreed that if they did marinade their meat it certainly made it tasty. An interest in wines and olive oil began to slowly spread through the village. At the mini-market Ruby added a couple of bottles of Beaujolais to the three bottles of sherry, half-dozen cans of lager and two bottles of whisky that made up her booze section. She also put a small packet of mixed herbs next to the salt and pepper, her seasonings section and some garlic appeared alongside the fruit and veg. Though Ruby folded her arms disapprovingly and expounded on the subject of garlic. 'I can't be workin' with the likes of that,' she said.

Magda meantime was gaining a reputation as something of a cook. People would come to her door, or stop her in the street and ask for culinary advice. What should they make for tea tonight? Tagliatelle was all very well, but how did you actually cook it? Were there any quick puddings you didn't need to actually cook, you could just, well, sort of make? What was an interesting thing to do with haddock?

'Put it in a cheese sauce. Smoked haddock and fresh makes it better. Y'know, tasty. Just slice up the fish and put it in. It'll do in no time in the oven. I dunno, maybe one side of "Exile on Main Street". Or maybe the whole of "Sad-Eyed Lady of the Lowlands". And you can mix cheeses as well. For a spot of piquancy. Know what I mean?' She would have mentioned adding grapes or a splash of white wine or scattering some pine nuts over the top, but was well aware of her neighbours' culinary limits. Some folks bought a jar of mixed herbs and it did them for ten years, maybe more. At the word piquancy, Magda would make a small circle with her middle finger and thumb. But nobody in Mareth really minded this little flash of gourmet upmanship. They knew she wasn't getting above herself. She was just getting her act together. Surviving.

Magda worked at the Captain's Table for ten years. Tears and tantrums, rage and flying cutlery. But something started to happen, to slowly happen. There was a drift of new faces appearing mostly at the weekends. They would sit in quiet raptures over the food that was placed before them, leaning towards each other exchanging forkfuls.

'Taste this, carrots and mushrooms sort of sliced up and cooked together.'

'No, look. Have some of these little potatoey things. What's in them, d'you think?'

People would ask for recipes and would send their compliments to the cook. But the Mastertons knew better than to bring Magda out to meet her fans. Her loathing of the people she fed still showed. 'Posh fucks,' she would say as she poured an apricot and brandy sauce over pork fillets. 'And why do they have to eat in French? They don't fart in French, they don't snore in sodding French, or belch in French.' She would steam about the kitchen waving her hands in the air, smacking her forehead, nutting the air, imagining no doubt that some snotty diner was the victim of her assault. 'Prats oohing and aahing over some food, as if they ate anything other than instant chips all week. Sitting in their catalogue clothes out for the evening talking shite, pretending to be nice people.'

Hands on hips, she would gaze witheringly through the screen door at the diners. 'Nice,' she would say, 'who wants to be nice? Where did nice ever get you?' She held the concept of nice in contempt. She loathed nice. It seemed to her that her mother had squandered her whole life pursuing the notion of nice. 'That's not a very nice thing to say, Magda.' 'Don't do that, Magda, that's not nice.' 'Nice people don't go out dressed like tramps, Magda. Cover yourself up.'

'Nice, nice, nice, nice. To hell with nice,' was Magda's conclusion. Nice got you nowhere.

Mary Lomax's ambition to live the nice life faded every Friday night when she would go down to the Anchor and Crown. She would without fail drink too many vodka and cokes and end up imitating Elvis. She would pull her hair down over her eyes, deepen her voice and run through her repertoire of The King's greatest hits. Her cronies would root for her, clap and shriek as she strutted across the floor, wiggling stiffly her sixty-four-year-old bum, thrusting her groin. She would wave her arms above her head and holler 'Jailhouse Rock' and 'Heartbreak Hotel' in her sandpaper voice. Sometimes she would abandon Elvis for Roy Orbison but it wasn't the same with Roy, too much angst.

But oh the reckoning from her conscience on Saturday morning. Sitting in a heap of pink velour dressing gown, she would clutch her sex'n'chocolate mug, swigging hot tea, chastising herself, 'Oh, I don't think I was very nice last night. Never again. Remind me to stay away from the vodka in future.'

But of course she never did. Come next Friday she was in need of another bout of sleaze. Magda could never decide if she preferred her mother when she was living her neat and tidy behind-net-curtains nice life or when she was out pubbing, being bawdy. Either way she was embarrassing.

CHAPTER 5

Money had never really occurred to Jessie. She had always had it. Until today when she'd put her card in the cash machine and found her account empty. Panic prickled and flushed through her. What to do?

This was a new dilemma. For the first time in her life there were no incoming funds to replace the break in her cash-flow. Her parents had supported her through her lean student years, but no way could she contact them for help now. This escape was hers, and she would see it through on her own, her way.

She walked slowly back down the cobbled wynd to her flat, reviewing her situation. Her bastard husband must have cleaned out their account. Another move in their game of marital chess. Checkmate, she thought. She had very little cash left, but enough food to do for the rest of the week. And then what? Starvation? According to Freddie Kilpatrick at the garage, her car needed a new exhaust. How was she to pay for it? Also the rent was due in a couple of weeks. She'd be cold, hungry, homeless and without transport. Life sucked. She wearily climbed the stairs to her flat. She shut the door behind her and threw herself on the sofa.

Below, the Ocean Café was operating full throttle. Rock'n'roll, songs of freedom that people had been writing and singing and jumping up and down to whilst she was tucked away, cocooned in her perfect life. She heard Magda join in, and knew she'd be in the kitchen moving in time, hips swaying, jiving on the spot as she chopped onions and celery. She was making pasta, the smell came up through the vent. It smelled more desirable than ever to Jessie now she couldn't afford it. She sighed. Moved into a depression. A deepening thoughtless black, a mood that started, it seemed, in the pit of her stomach and spread through her. There was no logic involved. She lay back and let the despair roll.

Late afternoon, as the room darkened, she reached for the phone and dialled Alex's number. He'd be at the office. Better to get him with eaves-droppers around, then he couldn't swear back at her.

'Alex, you bastard,' she said as soon as she heard his voice on the other end.

'Jessie? Is that you?' It was strange to hear him. He sounded unsure of himself. Guilt, no doubt.

'Yes it's me, you bastard. Who else do you think it would be? Are you such a bastard everybody who phones you calls you a bastard?'

'No,' he said flatly.

'You shit, you emptied our account. I've no money.'

'What else was I to do? How else was I to find out where you were? Jessie, I've been worried sick. Where are you anyway?'

'Mind your own business.'

He heaved a tired sigh. 'Grow up, Jessie. We've things to sort out. Tell me where you are.'

'Mareth,' she told him. This wasn't right. This wasn't what she wanted to do. She wanted to scream and shout at him. She wanted to hurt him. She wanted him down where she was.

'Mareth? Where's that and what are you doing there?'

'Up the coast. And just living . . .' Then, an after-thought. 'In poverty.'

Downstairs, Magda's cooking shifted gear. The Stones started up. Jessie imagined Magda boogying round, tossing chillies into a pot from across the kitchen as she had once seen her do when she'd been having coffee and her now regular morning chocolate croissant. Magda and Edie had been jiving about, chopping, singing along, slapping each other's hands high in the air, moving in natural harmony, having a good time. Jessie had watched sadly. Life and friendships had never been like that for her. Of course there was Trish and Lou and others, but all they did was speak.

Alex had always been jealous of her women friends. Especially Trish and Lou. 'They'll lead you astray,' he said.

'If anyone is going to lead me anywhere, astray is where I choose,' Jessie told him.

'When are you coming back?' he asked her now.

'I'm not,' she said surprising herself. 'I'm never coming back.'

'For Christ's sake, Jessie. What are you doing there?'

'The hell's it got to do with you. And some of that money you emptied out of our account is mine. Put it back.'

He hung up. She lay listening to the dialling tone till its hum and the darkness filled the room. She had a horrible feeling that no good was going to come of that call. 'I should not have told him where I am.'

The rock'n'roll din had stopped. It was so easy now to let her depression flow. She could slip effortlessly into it. A hollowness. God, she could almost hear it. She stretched out to feel the full benefit of this gloom. Her hand fell to the floor. She could feel the rough of the patterned fireside rug against it. The room smelled of yesterday's coal fire, and her perfume. There was no noise, only her breathing. Outside a slow car rolled carefully along the shore, engine humming. Someone called, 'Hey,' a raw and primal call, deeply male, it cut through the evening. 'He-eey pal.' Boys should get voice licences before their balls are allowed to drop, Jessie thought. The Ocean Café was coming to life, that meandering drone of alcoholic conversation.

'I am enduring,' she said. The words hung in the air.

'I . . . AM . . . ENDURING,' she said again, listening carefully to herself. She sounded sad, addicted to sadness. 'Oh, no. I'm not.' She rose. Took the last of her cash from the table where she'd spread it before her to despondently consider. And went downstairs.

She slapped her hand on the café counter and demanded a large whisky. 'A single malt,' she said. 'A double.'

Magda waved her arm towards the large selection of malts on her upper shelf. 'What'll it be?'

'Lagavulin. A huge Lagavulin with very little water and no ice.'

Magda placed it in front of her. She lifted the glass and breathed in the fumes. A deep whiff of Scottish gorgeousness, the whole of life caught in glass. Peat and earth, sweetness and wind. Fire to the throat. If she listened to it she'd hear eagles call and if she could look into the depth of it she'd see hills purpling into the distance and mountain streams, perfect water. The longing it set up in her, she was intoxicated already.

'Are you going to drink it, then?' This prolonged savouring was beginning to irritate Magda.

'In a minute,' Jessie said. 'I want to enjoy this. I can't afford it. Booze you can't afford is the best booze.'

'Thought you had plenty of money.'

Jessie smiled, 'So did I. But there you go . . .'

51

She didn't feel like giving out explanations right now.

'So what are you going to do?'

'Dunno. Find work, I suppose.' Jessie took her first fiery sip. And coughed.

'What do you do?' This is what Magda had always wanted to know.

'After I graduated I worked in PR for a while – a couple of years, I think. Then I switched to publishing. I headed a department that did literary textbooks. We were working on a series where we invited critics to write concise, accessible books on the works of renowned writers.'

'You'll not get a lot of call for that here,' Magda said.

'No. I didn't think so,' Jessie readily agreed with her. 'I also used to freelance, writing occasional articles for women's magazines.'

Across the bar, Lipless stopped eavesdropping to remark that he'd read an article in a woman's magazine in the dentist's waiting room and it was all about orgasms. 'What a thing to write about. Who'd want to read that?'

'You did,' Magda scarcely interrupted speaking to Jessie to tell him.

'Yes, me. But that was only because I was having root canal work.'

Jessie and Magda stared at him.

'I needed something to take my mind off it.' He pursed his mouth, raised his eyebrows. What fools wimmen were that they did not see that.

'We were just bringing out a book about Virginia Woolf when I left,' Jessie spoke slowly. She didn't know whether or not she missed work. 'Then we were talking about expanding our range to music, critics writing about musicians. Not just, you know, Wagner and Mahler, but Bessie Smith and Charlie Parker. Maybe even Zappa and Van Morrison . . . it could be fascinating . . .'

'Yes,' said Magda. Bessie Smith, Van Morrison, she'd heard of them. Now they had a mutual point of reference, Jessie was slightly less different. The distance between her and Magda narrowed. Perhaps she was just a person after all.

'Y'know young Shona works up at Young's the solicitors?' Lipless asked.

Magda nodded and asked Jessie if she was going to go back to finish her musician project thing. Jessie shook her head. 'No. No.'

Till this moment she hadn't realised how distasteful returning to her old life had become to her. She really wanted to hear about Shona who worked up at Young's the solicitors. She remembered Shona, Pretty in Pink, who had suggested the grotty flat above the Ocean Café. She remembered well the day she'd been so desperate she'd accepted the flat unseen, and agreed to the ludicrous rent.

'Well . . .' Unconcerned with Jessie's conversation with Magda, Lipless continued his gossip. 'Shona stole a magazine that she'd been reading in the dentist when he called her in. She was getting one of her back teeth filled. And did a competition in it. And she won a car.'

'Did she?' said Magda. 'I never knew that. That red car she drives about in?'

Lipless nodded, 'A boxy thing with brown seats. I never liked it.'

'No,' said Jessie, 'I think I'd like to stay here.'

'It was the brown seats,' said Lipless. 'They were pale, the colour of sick.'

'You're just jealous. You've never had a new car in your life.'

'Rubbish. It was a crisps competition. Some crisp company, and along with the magazine entry form she had to send in six empty packets and a slogan on why she liked chilli'n'cheese potato snax.'

'Well, there you go. She worked for it.'

'Did she buggery.' Lipless was incensed. 'It was her wee brother said they were cheesily the chilliest potato snax ever. And she got the bags from us one lunchtime. And the dentist provided the magazine. What did she do?'

'Had the gumption to put it all together?' suggested Magda.

'She bought the stamp to send it all in?' suggested Jessie.

'That car should've been sold and the money divided equally between us all. If you ask me. Fair's fair after all.' Lipless drove his finger into the bar, emphasising his point.

'Here is a bitter man,' Magda said to Jessie.

'Well, the dentist could have got something. At least we all got the crisps.'

'How bloody trivial can you get?' Magda wanted to know.

'Oh, a lot more trivial. It takes years. Years and years. A truly trivial mind is a wonder to behold,' Lipless boasted.

'So it is,' said Jessie.

'Is it triviality you're after?' Magda asked.

'Yes. I think, perhaps, it is. Why not?'

'I can give you that. I'll be needing help for the summer. Some hard mindless waitressing, graft.'

'And the pay?'

'The pay!' Magda roared. 'The pay sucks. You're in Mareth, baby. But we'll feed you.'

'Oh, righto.' Unused to such directness, Jessie succumbed.

Lipless suddenly confessed that he supposed he really did like reading about women's orgasms. Orgasms, he said the word gruffly. Plainly he did not trust pleasure. It would take its toll of you in the end.

'I suppose women fascinate me more than anything. I mean, who the hell are they? And what do they think about? And why don't they let me into their secret?'

'What secret?' asked Jessie.

'Exactly,' said Lipless. 'What secret.'

'You wouldn't think,' said Magda watching him go, 'that man had a degree in philosophy.'

'My God,' Jessie gasped. 'No, you wouldn't.'

'That's because he hasn't,' said Magda. 'Jessie, you've got to stop believing all you're told. In fact, I'd advise you not to believe anything you're told. But that's just me.'

Outside, Lipless was moving slowly through a gathering guffawing throng of women.

'Actually,' said Magda, 'it's sad really. Since his wife died, Lipless doesn't live life. He just copes.'

'What happened to his face?'

'He was standing on his boat going out to check his creels. As he went out someone fishing off the harbour wall cast out and the hook caught his upper lip and pulled it off.'

Jessie's hands flew to her face. 'Oh horrible. Oh ghastly.' Then, gazing up from her squeamishness, 'Is that true?'

'Oh yes,' said Magda.

'Isn't it a bit cruel to call him Lipless?'

'Yes. I suppose. Ain't life a bitch? It just sort of started. He's used to it. Signs his Christmas cards Lipless.'

Outside, the throng got noisier, a rising shriek.

'What's going on out there?'

'The lady regulars at the Anchor and Crown have hired a coach. They're off to London to see *Cats*.'

Through the hazed window – early evening the café hadn't hit full steam – Magda pointed at a small, thin woman with tightly permed hair who was loudly supervising the loading of a vast amount of alcohol on to the bus. She was pointing and waving and hooting with bawdy laughter. A deep howl, the throaty ravages of booze and fags.

'That's my mother,' said Magda.

But Jessie did not look where Magda directed. She was watching with horror a man pushing his way through the crowd. He was clutching his jacket, painfully protecting its perfect cut from the jostle and throng.

'Oh God no,' Jessie wept. 'That's my husband.'

CHAPTER 6

Ginny Howard was one of the élite. It wasn't hard for her. Some are born to it, she said, and some have to strive for it. She was born to it. It came naturally. Though, as she always said, she had a deal of respect for those who set about civilising themselves. 'Always a worthwhile pursuit,' she maintained, nodding vigorously at her unquestionable rightness.

She was committed and committeed. 'There are people who turn up everywhere,' Magda said. Ginny Howard turned up everywhere. She was the insistent and highly vocal chairwoman of MIG, Mareth Improvement Group. She was once seen striding the length of Mareth counting the litter bins. 'There are not nearly enough of them,' she complained to the council, writing crisply on MIG headed notepaper. 'No wonder our streets are plagued by crisp bags and cola tins.'

The doings of the MIG were despicably worthy. Ginny Howard's sudden appearance on the street made people duck into doorways, dive for cover. She had a vile knack of making people do what she wished them to do: bake pancakes for Children

58

in Need, collect money for the local lifeboat, take a stall at the church fête, no matter how they felt about it themselves. She had a look that defied resistance, an emotional bully. She would thrust out her bosom, heave herself up to her full and electrifying five foot three and glare. It was generally felt she was wasted chairing the Mareth Improvement Group; such a woman could sort out the Middle East, or at least get the ozone layer patched up. Though considering her two pressed and shiny children, Judith and Brian – their cowed please and thank-you ways and shrill, sanctimoniously weepy passion for whales and tigers, and their embarrassing clothes (their gloves were sewn to their sleeves) – it was unanimously agreed that the Middle East would be more content with its turmoil than anything Ginny Howard might inflict on it.

Her success was, of course, in knowing her limitations. She never, at least publicly, took on someone who would get the better of her. From that simple rule had grown her reputation for invincibility. Only Magda had seen her off. And at that it hadn't been the confrontation the villagers had hoped for. It was a simple exchange of opinions. Magda's had been the riper.

At a wedding where the bride had been deliciously pregnant, bulging in eight months' bloom out of her bridal gown as she waddled down the aisle, Ginny Howard had bristled disapproval. She looked Magda grimly in the eye. 'I can't say I like today's modern relationships. Call me old-fashioned, but I simply don't believe in sex before marriage. Do you?'

To the surprise of surrounding eavesdroppers, Magda agreed. 'Absolutely,' she said. 'It rumples your wedding frock and your veil goes all askew.'

Lovely. Ginny Howard nil, Magda one. It was a score Ginny secretly vowed to settle.

Alex looked round Jessie's flat. He did not bother to conceal his horror. 'You live here?'

Perhaps there was some mistake. She was joking, surely. Any moment she would remove him from this small place with its dubious smells and reveal to him her real home. But she didn't. Instead she spread her arms and smiled. 'Isn't it wonderful? Don't you just love it?'

'No.'

Jessie wasn't undermined by his lack of enthusiasm. 'I love the smallness of it. Cosy, don't you think?'

'No.' He twitched. She had him. A glimmer of triumph sparked within her. She went for the kill. 'Yes, cosy.'

'Cosy?' The word came icily to his lips. Cosy, he loathed cosy. Detested its cloying ethos.

'Cosy and comfy,' she crowed. Ha ha, the glee of it.

'God's sake, Jessie.'

'What?' She turned her gaze on him. Innocence. This was the man who loved space, Nordic

60

sparseness. He was driven to distraction by anything – a discarded training shoe, an abandoned half-read newspaper, a jacket yanked off and left over the back of a chair – anything that disrupted the flow of light and space of his perfect décor. He loved the home they shared. Its polished floors, matching sofas, Persian rugs filled him with pride every time he came back to it. On days off he would pad through it barefoot, listening to Maria Callas.

He bought the right paperbacks and CDs. He drank the right wines. He was a man who worked hard at his lifestyle. A zeitgeist kind of guy, who would always be right about everything, because he kept redefining the meaning of right. He made sure his definition of right was always ahead of the game. When, for example, he noticed that the local supermarket stocked his favourite green and gold hexagonal coffee cups, he knew they had to go. He dropped them off at Oxfam the next day and bought something plain, Parisian and café-style to suit his mood of the moment.

'What?' she said again.

He turned on her, 'You know perfectly well what. How could you live like this? In this rathole. Jessie, I hate to see you in a place like this.'

'Rathole.' A shrill protest. 'Rathole!' Even shriller. 'This is my home.'

'I thought your home was our home.' A sincerely delivered and effective sermonette. She felt the regulation rush of guilt, almost said sorry.

'Leave me alone, Alex. This is what I want.'

'Why?'

'I don't know. Don't ask me that.'

'What can I ask you?'

'I don't know. Leave me alone.'

She couldn't collect her thoughts, didn't want to collect her thoughts. For the last few weeks since leaving Alex she had been cruising on instinct and was, she considered, doing fine. But plainly he was not going to leave her alone. He stood before her, hands thrust into his pockets, head slightly bowed. She could read this man, she knew his every gesture. Language? This body was a book she'd read over and over. He was going to make a pass. He wanted to fuck.

'Don't,' she said before he even moved to touch her. His hands were still deep in his pockets.'

'Don't what?'

'You know what.'

'No I don't. What?'

'You want to go to bed, don't you?'

'No.'

'Of course you do. I know you, Alex. That's your answer to everything. We have a baby and it dies and you want to get into my knickers as if that would've made it all better.'

'It might have helped. It might have kept us together.'

'Sod off,' she dismissed him. 'I have never felt so bad. I realise now that nothing bad had ever happened to me before that. I got into the

62

university I wanted, the course I wanted, the degree I wanted, the job I wanted. I had never failed at anything. Failure just never crossed my mind.'

'You didn't fail.'

'Tell my body that. I feel like I failed, Alex. I couldn't come to terms with it.'

'So you left.'

She shrugged. Surely that was obvious. 'I rather think you left long before me.'

'What do you mean by that?'

'You were never there. You went back to work as soon as I got back from hospital. I needed somebody, Alex. I needed you.'

He looked at his feet and sighed. Jessie waited for an answer, an explanation. 'I didn't know what to say,' he said. He was no more used to failure than she was.

'Listen to us,' said Jessie. 'How could such a brittle relationship have survived tragedy and trauma?'

'When are you coming back?' He didn't want an analysis of his marriage, he wanted everything back the way it was. He was fighting for the life he'd worked hard to construct.

'What happened to your girlfriend? Has she dumped you, too?' Jessie only now realised how deeply she was hurt by his affair.

He shook his head. 'You don't understand. It was just a fling. It didn't mean anything. I needed somebody, Jessie. I needed someone to hold me.

I was hurting too, you know. I shouldn't have done it. I'm sorry.' He looked repentant. He loved Jessie and though he'd strayed often enough in his head, he'd only actually physically been unfaithful once before. With Trish, Jessie's friend. He just didn't rate monogamy as highly as she did. He wanted this to be over, and was irritated that Jessie wasn't responding in the way he imagined she would when he worked through this scene on his drive to Mareth.

'Are you coming back?'

'I don't know.'

'Don't know. Don't know. That's all you say. Do you know anything? Let's work on what you do know.'

'I don't know what I know any more.' Jessie was tired of all this. His arguments were so clinical. He made logic of everything. And she was beyond logic. She existed now on feelings. Her actions were based on messages from her gut. She no longer trusted clear thinking. She knew he would push her and push her till he got the answer he wanted. Why didn't he leave her alone?

'Oh God,' she burst out, 'it's over Alex. I'm not coming back. I don't miss you. And I don't miss your tired little dick pressing against me at night.'

Alex hadn't till this moment realised how much he loved her, how deeply she could hurt him. Even when he'd discovered her gone he hadn't acknowledged his pain. He could fix this. He could talk her into coming back to him. He had been always

64

able to talk Jessie into doing whatever he wanted her to do. She was his. He was stunned by this vile blow. There were tears in his eyes.

Jessie hadn't really meant to hurt him. She just wanted him down where she was. She felt suddenly awful, suddenly shamed and suddenly, and for the first time in her life, utterly utterly powerful.

Magda got out of bed, 'You should sleep on the damp side.'

'Sorry,' Jim had arranged his body ready for sleep but rolled over to look at her.

'It should be part of the wedding vows. Stuff all this love, honour and cherish rubbish. It ought to be, do you James Migilvary Horn take this Magda for your lawful wedded wife and promise always to sleep on the damp side, never to toss your dirty socks under the bed, and to hang up the towels properly after you've used them? That'd half the divorce rate.'

'Christ, Magda, will you shut up?'

'No.' She was striding out of the room now. Jim raised himself on one elbow, 'Anyway, we're not married. Is this a proposal?'

'No. But when I do get married that's the ceremony I want. But I don't want a husband. You're just a sex object to me.'

'Suits me.' Jim heaved himself back into his favourite sleeping position.

Magda went downstairs to the kitchen. Lately

sleeping had been a problem. She made some tea and sat at the table.

'Darkly whining,' she muttered to herself. 'I spend my nights darkly whining.' She liked the phrase. She liked words. Her inability to decipher them written down meant that they came to her aurally, and each time they came to her they came afresh. In her head she strung them together in her own way. At the moment darkly and whining were her two favourite words. She turned them over and over, muttered them during the day as she stirred her sauces and made incisions in chicken breasts ready to insert slivers of garlic and ginger.

Darkly whining. Darkly whining. Darkly whining. Forever darkly whining. She had been aware recently that repeating darkly whining was beginning to replace her rages.

For the last few days she had been filled with foreboding about her mother's trip to London. She couldn't fathom why. Her mother had been away on coach trips before and had come home safely. Even if she didn't come home safely, Magda didn't know what degree of concern she could muster. But there it was: a flutter of nerves in her stomach whenever she thought of her mother. Jim had come to dread Magda's feelings. He who scoffed at religion and superstition had come to respect, even dread, the flutterings in the pit of his lady's stomach.

With virtually no education, instincts were all

she had. She paid them heed. Sitting now at her kitchen table, doing nothing to counter the early spring splintered chill, she let her feelings roll.

Here she was, forty-three years old, a man in her bed, four children all healthy and reasonably sane; she owned – well, sort of owned – a café; she made money, had her own house – well Jim's house, car, television, stereo, everything she could want she had. And yet. Big sigh, Yes but.

'Life's yes-buts, are a bitch. Yes but. Yeah but. Yeah but. Yeahbut. Yeabut. Yeabut. Yeabut. Yeabut. What we have to contend with is the yeabut factor.'

Her tea was cold. She drank it anyway. So what was her yeabut factor? Magda was used to the night. A long-time insomniac, she knew it well. Could tell the time by the shade of grey filtering past the edges of her curtains. She knew the rhythms of her home as it creaked and shifted through the dark. The kitchen looked out on to the sea and she could hear the surf heaving on to the shore not far from her front door. She pulled the curtains. The world outside was exquisite. Too beautiful by far, she thought. She did not trust beauty. A huge moon lit the bay and spread a path rippling over the water. A fishing boat chugged out to sea, masts lit.

'You don't fool me pretty picture postcard scene,' Magda said. 'There's shit in these waters. And that's the Johnston brothers going out. They'll be below with a crate of lager watching skin-flicks on their video.'

She was a cynic. Her constant refusal to commit depressed Jim. She gave him and their children her furious love, but considered nothing else merited it. A beautiful landscape was a beautiful landscape, yeabut. Yeabut there would be no doubt stray used condoms lying just out of view, and noisy jets screaming overhead. It was the same with everything. There was always a yeabut. 'Couldn't you just relax and like something?' Jim would sigh.

But Magda said nope. She couldn't. Wouldn't. If she just relaxed she felt she would lose her edge, the diabolical lippiness would go. And that would be the end of her.

Lately, though, when she wasn't expounding life's yeabuts, Magda would fall profoundly silent. She would sink deep into her own quietness, her mobile face falling into a sulk. Sometimes she would say nothing for hours. She might bite her lower lip or twist the silver snake ring on her left hand, but she would say nothing.

'God, you're so silent. Are you in mourning or what?' Jim, unable to bear her silence, let loose his frustration. And Magda stared at him in surprise, still saying nothing. Jim threw his newspaper at her before storming from the room.

'I think you're right,' Magda said to him in bed. 'I think I am in mourning.'

'Who's died?'

'Me.'

'What sort of garbage is that?'

'Not garbage. I don't actually think I've died. I just haven't lived.'

'Oh, don't give me that. I can't stand that stuff. Have you been reading the Californian dictionary of Clichéd Crap?'

'No,' Magda told him stiffly. 'I haven't been reading anything, have I? That's what I'm in mourning for. What might have been. If things had been different.'

Jim said nothing. He wasn't going to pursue this conversation. Why didn't people just accept what was? He lay waiting for one of Magda's smart remarks and when it didn't come put his hand on her back. She turned to him. He pulled her head down to kiss her and ran his fingers across her tits. Twenty-odd years together, she should be used to this. He shouldn't still excite her. But he did. She loved the soft just inside his mouth, would trace it with her tongue. And his face, steady calculating eyes, cherubic lips firmly pursed beneath his cropped dark beard.

And when she went down on him. The taste of him was always the same. An indefinable mix of salt, always salt, the sea, oil and Palmolive he lathered himself with every night before he came to bed. She would stroke the inside of his thighs, then draw her nails round his bum, and down to where it set him moaning. Far away above her she would hear him. He would be fraying at the edges, losing control, giving in to her. She would hear him gasp and would stop to watch him. Oh don't, he'd say, don't stop, holding her head, pushing it back down. Don't. Stop. She would look at his face folding, unfolding with pleasure. She would purse her lips and grin. She could get him, every time she could get him.

She never tired of him and sometimes she resented it. She wished there was a cure for him, a potion she could take that would make her immune to him and his moods. She would no longer try to assess from the way he came down the stairs in the morning, and the way he slammed the door when he came home at night, how he was feeling on a day-to-day basis. She wished he didn't have such an effect on her. With Jim she wasn't in control and that unnerved and annoyed her.

In her direst moments she cursed the debt she thought she owed him. He had rescued her from herself. When she was at full teenage wildness he had taken her in. One night at the Anchor and Crown, after he had finished drinking, he put his empty glass down on the bar, walked across to where Magda was making a lot of noise drinking with her friends, looked directly at her, extended an inviting hand and said, 'Coming?'

She got up from her seat leaving a half-drunk vodka and coke – she always remembered that vodka and coke – and went with him. Just like that, like a scene from a bad B-movie. She'd gone to his house and had lived there ever since. After a year she ceased to be Magda Lomax and became Magda Horn. At the time it surprised nobody really, and was only a topic of gossip in Mareth for a couple of days. There was something natural and right about it, the tempestuous girl and the self-possessed fisherman. He was a match for her. At last Magda was removed from Mareth's conscience. Nobody worried that an outrageous and uncontrolled intelligence had been left ignored. And Magda? Life, Magda told Jim, would be a synch if it wasn't for feelings.

Downstairs she made tea and sat, as she did most nights, staring out of her kitchen window. She ran through the people she'd been to school with. Most of them had long left Mareth. Where were those little people with their bony knees and scrubby hair and the seething squabbling playground life they'd led.

'Where are you, little zoo?'

Gone to become photocopy-machine salesmen, a florist, a marine, a dental mechanic and what else? Wasn't that nose picky smelly Carstairs boy an art historian? Little fart. And where could she go? She laid her cheek on her hand. If only she could cry, that would help. But crying was a treat she'd long grown out of.

'Oh, bugger this,' she said, 'where does wondering get you?'

But wondering was part of Magda's life. It's my hobby, she said, wondering about other folks, women especially. Magda mentally divided women into groups. There was the divine sisterhood of rightness who belonged to the holy church of

71

Tupperware. There was the group of incomers in trendy clothes who all had some connection with the university ten miles up the coast. They wore long skirts and big boots, jeans and baggy shirts, waved their arms about and said um and ah a lot when they spoke. They came to the Ocean Café and drank wine or pints of beer. They spoke about books and films and relationships. What so-and-so did with so-and-so and who was sleeping with whom. What did whossname really meant when he said such and such. It was a complex, judgemental world of intense friendships and, as far as Magda could tell, faked orgasms.

Did all women fake it? Did they tell each other about faking it, how to do it? Ostracised at school except for Edie, Magda had never had a close female friend. And her mother had never discussed anything with her, from the keeping of a bank account to coping with her periods. They had come as a complete surprise to her. A boyfriend had told her about sanitary towels. The same boy had told her about sex. Chat with her mother, then, about faking orgasms had been out.

Orgasms. Magda had been having them for years before she knew that's what they were called.

She wondered if individual women stumbled across making mock moans of delight, lying on their backs waiting soullessly for the humping to be over. Did the divine sisters of rightness from the holy church of Tupperware fake orgasms? Did they ever have sex? If so, would they remove their sensible shoes, cosy anoraks and neat little strings of pearls? Magda doubted it.

'Magda,' small voice wailed from upstairs. 'Magda. I can't sleep.' All her children called her by name.

'OK, Rosie,' she said, 'I'm coming.'

The child was already halfway down the stairs. 'Back to bed,' Magda ordered. 'School tomorrow.'

'I hate school.'

'No you don't, you love it. And you're going tomorrow.' She took Rosie's hand and led her back towards her bedroom.

'Tell me a story, then,' the child wheedled.

Magda looked down at her daughter. Rosie, seven years old, her youngest child, with her sallow complexion and mane of unmanageable hair was a replica Magda. When she looked at her other children, Magda saw Jim; when she looked at Rosie she saw herself. And her heart went out to her. Poor little bugger, she thought.

'All right.' She watched Rosie clamber back into bed and pulled the covers over her.

'Twice upon a time there was a frog . . .' she said, gently moving the hair from the child's forehead.

'Twice. You only get upon a time once.'

'Not if you're reincarnated. Then you get twice.'

'If you're reincarnated,' Rossie crisply corrected, 'you don't get to be a frog twice. Only once, then you move on.'

'Yeabut,' said Magda. 'This was a bad frog. He had to do his frog time over to get it right.'

73

'Ah,' said Rosie. 'It'd be like you. Darkly whining. That's what you're always saying.'

'There you go,' Magda grinned in surprise. She had no idea she said the thing out loud.

'You'll have to be Magda twice upon a time, just like the frog.'

'Oh goodness,' Magda said. 'There's something to darkly whine about.'

Mary Lomax didn't trust London. There were too many people. Looking each one in the eye in passing exhausted her. Furthermore, nobody said hello. In Mareth people always said hello if you knew them or not. It was just manners, wasn't it? It was gritty here, smelly. She had London in her eyes, and London up her nose.

'Oh,' she declared to her friends in the bar of their hotel, 'I wouldn't live here if you paid me.' She sipped her sherry and heartily agreed with herself. Sherry because she didn't trust herself with her usual vodka. It didn't do to get legless and sing old Elvis numbers when there were strangers about. She hunched herself against the city. Held her stomach in, kept her face straight and tried not to think about the red dress.

But it was there. It had wormed its way into her soul. And she could not sleep or eat for thinking about it. She had given her heart to it.

She had arrived in London at six o'clock in the morning, crumpled and sweaty. All the others on the coach had gone into their hotel to bathe, or

74

snooze till breakfast, but Mary had been too excited to do that. She wanted to sightsee right away. Urgently now in case this wasn't really happening, in case all the sights to see suddenly disappeared. She walked through empty streets, listening to the lonely clicking of her high heels and was overwhelmed.

As the morning went on, the city gathered speed. By eight it was going full hurtle. Thrumming traffic, a rush of people, people wearing breathing-masks riding mountain bikes, blank faces, weird hairdos, fabulous clothes, dreadful clothes. She was swimming against the tide here. All those people, and everybody looked at her, a swift eyeflick, but nobody registered recognition. Not a nod to let her know she was alive and in the same world as they were. She didn't know what was going on, had the urge to find a back street café to hide in. She was engulfed by her smallness, thinness and the cheapness of her clothes. She wanted desperately to apologise to someone, everyone. Everybody that walked down these streets had somewhere to go, and she hadn't. She felt lost. All these people around here knew some sophisticated secret about living she didn't. She was an open-faced fool, the hurtling crowds could all, she was sure, at a swift, dismissive glance see that.

But she was really overwhelmed by the shops. The shops, the shops, so many shops. Turn a corner, a new street full of shops; walk the street, turn a corner – another street, another long line of shops. In Mareth there was one street with six shops in it. There you could buy almost anything and be home in time for the four o'clock soap. You would never have thought there was so much to spend your money on. No wonder people got into debt. That was what was so good about Mareth, you couldn't really overspend there. There was nothing you really really wanted. A loaf of bread, a tin of beans, you wouldn't lose your soul to anything like that.

She saw the dress in a window tucked in the heart of Kensington. One look and the desire to own it consumed her. For her entire London trip, Mary thought of nothing else. All through the performance of *Cats* she dreamed of the red dress. What would she look like in it? Where could she wear a frock like that? Could she even put it in her wardrobe? All her other clothes seemed suddenly tawdry. Oh, what was the matter with her? She couldn't afford it. Couldn't afford it, pah, what difference did that make? She couldn't go into a shop like that. Posh folks went there, rich folks; they'd spot her for the bumpkin she was right away. No, it was not for the likes of her.

Still she lusted. It wasn't red exactly. Not obviously red like your ordinary cheap catalogue red dress. This red was deep and rich and lasting; reds in her life so far had been innocent paintbox colours. This red you could bury your face in. You'd have to put moisturising cream on your shoulders and shave your armpits for a red like this. Oh, she wanted that dress.

Looking at it she was a child again, living on the outside, nose pressed against the window. And looking at it she knew what the city was about. It was about having the savvy to buy the right thing and go to the right places. It was about thinking on your feet. Worrying what Ruby at the Spar was saying about you behind your back had nothing to do with it.

The shop was expensive. Everything about it said expensive: the dark green paintwork and gold lettering, the striped canopy, the swirling gold leaf that wound round the doorpost. Everything. Mary could not enter. She was sixty-four years old and worked three mornings a week cleaning Dr MacKintyre's surgery. She had only been to London once before. What did she know? All the words to 'Jailhouse Rock' and 'Hound Dog' for goodness sake. People who wore a dress like that never admitted to knowing such songs. And yet. Why shouldn't she have it? Her money was as good as any. 'I'm gonna have it. I'm gonna have it,' she promised herself over and over. Over and over. I am going to have that red dress.

The bus home was leaving at three in the afternoon. At twenty to two, Mary found herself walking to the shop. She hummed 'Blue Suede Shoes', a belligerent sort of a song, as she walked. Concentrating on it took her mind off her fear. She walked into the shop and imagined a hush. People were looking at her.

A woman stepped forward. 'Can I help?' Rounded, educated vowels. Mary felt as if she was gasping for breath, she was swamped by her inadequacy. This woman was thin, as Mary was. But anyone could see it was a different kind of thin. Mary's was natural. It came from lack of food when she was young. This woman's was acquired. This was the proper kind of thin.

'How much is that dress in the window?' Mary wanted this over as quickly as possible. She wanted out.

'The red one? Nine hundred and twenty-seven pounds.'

Mary flinched. What? Nine hundred and twenty-seven pounds. Her car cost less than that. She fought to hide her astonishment.

'Do you take credit cards?'

'Yes. I'll have to phone.'

'I'll take it,' Mary said.

'Don't you want to try it on? It may need altering.'

'No,' Mary waved her arms in dismay. No. No changing rooms, no fuss. Just let her out of here.

'No, I have to catch a bus. I have to get home to Mareth. I'll take the dress.' She instantly regretted admitting to the bus and Mareth. Now they had verbal evidence that she was not one of them.

She handed over her card and hoped to sink

unnoticed into a corner whilst all the fussing, phoning and wrapping went on. She hoped to be unnoticed lest they shoo her out, as she shooed schoolboys and old men from the surgery with a flap of her duster when they trod on her clean shiny floor. She wanted out of here. She didn't know what to do. Did she stand back, arms folded? Or did she stay at the counter and chat? No chatting was out. She wanted to tell them she liked the paint outside. It looked velvety. But thought if she mentioned this they would laugh at her. I am a fool, she thought. These people can see I'm a fool.

In silence she watched the dress being spread on the counter, then folded, wrapped in tissue paper. Not white tissue paper, but dark navy pulled from a drawer in perfect sheets. When she got home she would iron that tissue. She would keep everything perfect.

Still she was scared. What if they decided she was not good enough to buy the dress? Not quite the sort of person they wanted to sell it to?

The saleswoman put down the phone and smiled at her. 'That's fine,' she said.

Still Mary panicked. Maybe her money wasn't good enough. Maybe they wanted rich money, not cleaning-lady money. There was a difference.

When she finally got the dress it was swathed in tissue and placed in a thick cardboard bag with two long dark red cord handles. She wanted to thank the saleswoman profusely, invite her to look in should she ever find herself in Mareth. But refrained. She humbly took her parcel and walked back to her hotel and the bus home. Her heart pounded, she was flushed with triumph. I have seen the other side, she breathed. She felt like a stormtrooper who, armed only with a red patent handbag and a plastic rainhat, had accomplished a successful raid on the enemy. If they'd spotted her they hadn't let on.

'I've got it. I've got it. I've got it.'

Triumph buzzed through her. As she walked from the shop her mincing, high-heeled steps quickened. She had to be away before they discovered the mistake, before they rushed after her, demanding the dress be returned to them. They could not possibly have meant to sell such a frock to the likes of her.

CHAPTER 7

Jessie never knew if she was shocked or delighted at Magda's OC scheme. It was cheeky, rude even, utterly wrong, and, she had to admit, very satisfying. When she first saw the special red-bordered OC bills she had thought the initials stood for Ocean Café. But they didn't. They were for Over Charge. Magda vented the rage certain customers brought out in her by bumping up their bills. The amount varied according to how much she had been irritated. It hadn't been an organised decision, this OCing of people. It had just happened. Magda drifted into it.

When she first took over the Ocean Café she was filled with a mix of enthusiasm and rage. She loved the place. Had always loved it. From the first time she had ever come to it as a child she loved it. The old mahogany counter, the sturdy wooden tables and solidly comforting ladder-back chairs with intricate flower patterns on faded velvet cushions. The walls were wood-panelled halfway up, then there was a layer of dark-red deco tiling and after that some ancient faded wallpaper. And on the far wall, ridiculously out of place, an Alpine

81

scene. She had moved silently about the bar, stroking it, whispering, 'Mine. Mine. Mine.' Then, a realist always added, 'Well, not actually mine. Mine and Edie's and Jim's. But mostly mine . . .'

The Ocean Café brought her joy. The customers caused her rage. She tried to get along with most of them but finally settled into a role of bawdy, bossy cook and barkeeper. She discovered that people accepted being bossed, even liked it. She chipped people for their dietary deficiencies. Made grown seafaring men eat their greens. Involved the unlikeliest people in culinary debates. But she never could come to terms with serving people she didn't like.

Her old primary school teacher, Miss Clarkson, had come in for some lunch and had beamed at her, patronisingly remarking, 'Well, Magda, who'd have thought it? You've made something of yourself. The girl least likely . . .' And she'd laughed heartily. Magda seethed. She'd hated this woman for years, remembered with biting bitterness the beatings she'd received for her constant inability to master basic literacy. The humiliation haunted her yet.

'You, Magda, come out here. Look at this work. Messy, messy, messy. You're such a grubby child.' That fiendish face would be thrust close to hers. Magda could see the wiry hairs sprouting untamed on her chin. 'Your work's atrocious. Do you know what you are, Magda? Lazy.' On an authoritarian high, she would whirl Magda round, lift her skirt and, taking her ruler from her desk, whack her backside. 'Lazy. Lazy. Lazy.' Whack. Whack. Whack. The watching rows of children, unable to control their fear that this horror might happen to them, dissolved into alarmed sniggers.

This had been an almost daily occurrence in Magda's early school days. For her education had not been an enlightening of her spirit or opening of her mind. Education had been a sore bum. Keen to keep her pupils in a state of fear, when there had been no naughty children to chastise, Miss Clarkson would give her desk a sound thrashing, 'This is what I do to those who don't work.'

Her teaching methods had a profound effect on her pupils. She would point at a child and demand, 'You there, six sevens. NOW.' Her stubby finger, the finger from hell, jabbed with such ferocity that little minds numbed, throats seized, the blood chilled. The only functioning organ was the lower bowel. Her classroom reeked constantly with the farty smell of fear.

Standing in the Ocean Café years later, confronted by that same ogre, Magda realised how little she had recovered from the humiliation. She flushed deeply, couldn't meet the old lady's watery eye and dropped the cup she was holding.

'Ha ha,' her teacher scolded triumphantly. 'The same old Magda.' She pointed across the room, 'I'll have the chicken in ginger and honey and I'll have it over here.' She sat down by the window.

Magda disappeared into the kitchen. For some minutes she stood staring out into the restaurant. Then she turned and slowly started to wash some dishes. She would never serve that old cow. Never. Never. Never.

'Christ, Edie,' she hissed. 'When you meet one of your old teachers, pacifism flies out the window, you realise what violence is for. Nut the bastards. Do some damage to the arseholes who damaged you.'

The dragon sat for some time before she realised she was not going to be served. Other people arrived, ordered, ate and left. Still she sat.

'What's happened to the service around here?' she called. 'I've been waiting for hours. A person could starve.' Nothing happened. In the kitchen nothing stirred.

'I will not serve that old bag,' Magda said, tears in her eyes. 'I will not carry food out to her. I will not.'

'Spell school for me, child,' the beast had demanded, shoving her crumpled ancient face close to Magda's. Terror. No six-year-old bladder could cope. There was a sudden hot pool at Magda's feet, her shoes were horribly damp. Magda never forgave that degradation. Never forgave. She hid in the kitchen, skulked by the sink. Tutting, sighing and muttering, typical and, what else could you expect from a girl like that, Miss Clarkson left.

Magda regularly refused to serve people she did not like. To the embarrassment of other customers the hated ones were left sitting looking sheepish, or howling dissatisfaction at the service.

'For heaven's sake,' Jim told her, 'you're in business. You can't choose who's going to eat your pasta and who isn't. You're not here to judge personalities. You're out to make money.' He emphasised this last by jabbing at her chest with his blackened oily finger. Magda watched it, cross-eyed. He was right, of course. Wasn't he always? God she could hate him for that.

'But I hate these people,' she protested as her latest bunch of rejected lunchers walked, baffled, across the road to their car. They had committed the unpardonable sin of being patronising. Had spoken to Magda in ringing, rounded tones, expressing disbelief in the likelihood of anyone in such an unsophisticated part of the world having heard of balsamic vinegar.

'They're such wankers.'

'Wankers with cash. When they go they take their cash with them instead of leaving it in your till.'

Their voices drifted back. 'Extraordinary.' 'I can't believe it.'

'Take their cash, Mags. Take it for the poor and the meek. Strike a blow for the misunderstood. Avenge the child you were, the infant with the constantly sore bum. And if you don't take it for any other reason, take it so you can pay the lease on your café.'

Not long after that, Magda had devised her OC method of charging. She put extra money on the bills of those customers she found hateful, patronising, or who had wronged her in her turbulent youth.

When the dreaded Miss Clarkson returned for a second attempt at sampling Magda's chicken with ginger and honey sauce, she had been OC'd. And how. The meal had been excellent and, expressing some surprise at Magda's ability to do anything well, she had paid up willingly. The excess money had been put aside in a jar. With Edie's help, Magda had in time found a home for it that she was convinced Miss Clarkson would find distasteful. The Lesbians in Wheelchairs Encounter Group had received the money.

A woman with Magda's rage soon accumulated quite a bit of OC money. The rule was that the charity must truly horrify the OC'd one. Dishonest though it was, OCing people did a lot to soothe Magda's childhood humiliations. And it made wiping up after and serving obnoxious people almost pleasurable.

'It's better than therapy,' she confessed to Jim. 'And it isn't costing a thing.' She was delighted with herself.

At first Jessie had protested. OCing people she said was immoral. You couldn't charge people some phenomenal sum just because you didn't like them. You couldn't send other people's hard-earned money off to outré causes. It wasn't on. Magda stared at her. She was wondering what outré meant but knew this wasn't the moment to ask.

But that was before Jessie had her first hateful encounter. A bulky boozy-faced man had summonsed her across the room with an officious flick of his hand, complaining loudly that there were only six croutons on his soup. Jessie had fetched some more and, as she turned to go he said, thanks girlie and patted her bum. Oh, the rush of loathing. Jessie's eyes glowed momentarily red. She'd a swift flash of herself crashing her tray down on the arse-patter's head whilst shoving his soup-hot spoon up his nose. She swallowed. And returned to the kitchen.

'Did you see that?' she fumed. 'That arsehole. The shit . . . Jesus, who does he think he is? My bum's mine.'

Magda went to the kitchen door and peered out. 'Oh, look at him. Right-wing hetero with macho problems. I think he could send a little contribution to Gay Poets for Socialism, a wee something to help fund their next leaflet. What d'you think, Edie?'

'Oh yes. Poor old sod. Give him an extra potato with his duck. Keep his strength up.'

It was some time before Magda saw the dress. She knew it was in her mother's house, she had seen the carrier bag and the beloved tissue wrapping. But Mary was reluctant to take it out. Several times a day she went through to her bedroom to examine and cherish her purchase. She would run her hand over the bag and peer into it. She had bought an entry into a new world. This was the sort of thing real people had in their wardrobes.

John Lomax, her husband, sighed every time he came across the bag in the bedroom. 'I'm tripping over that thing,' he complained. Though he wasn't. The dress hadn't been two days in the house and he hated it already. It was dresses like this that made husbands disappear into sheds at bottom of the garden, or hide behind newspapers. He knew his life was about to be disrupted. This dress gave him indigestion.

'When are we actually going to see it?' Magda asked. 'You can't keep it wrapped up for ever.'

Mary knew this. It wasn't that she didn't want to unwrap the dress. She just wanted to preserve the whole package. Besides, if she removed the dress from its bag she would have to face the challenge of wearing it. Eventually, though, she did carefully ease it out of the bag more tenderly than she ever treated any infant. She unfolded the precious tissue wrapping and, breathless with awe, lifted the dress and held it to her face. It was wonderful. The smell of it. The unsullied newness of it. No sags at the bum or creasing round the thighs. No stains.

'Oh, I love you,' she told it, putting it on her special padded green velvet hangar and hooking it on to the back of the door. Then she gently smoothed out the tissue and laid it in a drawer. The knowledge that the dress was here in the house filled her heart, she did not want to leave it. Took regular trips through to the bedroom to say hello to it.

'Hello, frock. How are you hanging there?' For heaven's sake, she cursed herself, she was talking to a dress. She couldn't help it.

She hadn't felt like this since she'd been fifteen and wildly and totally in love with Lawrence Kemp who sat across from her in the French class. She had forgotten this thrill. Now it came flooding back. The way her heart pounded when he leaned over and asked if he could borrow her pencil. And how she held it close after he handed it back; it was still warm where he'd held it. Her fingers curled round the very spot his fingers had curled round. Was there ever a thrill like that? Secretly, in bed that night, she had put it to her lips. Lawrence, she whispered his name. He never found out about the crush she had on him.

The suddenness of this memory shook her. She sank on to the bed. She felt as if she held her life before her. It was clear, she could see everything. She had wanted to be a nurse but her parents had considered her too young to leave Mareth.

'I could have gone,' she said. 'I was not too young.'

She had stayed home. Worked at the fish shed filleting cod and haddock before she met and married John. Lawrence had become a surveyor.

'I didn't know,' she said again, surprised at the sound of her voice in the empty room. 'I didn't know.' She stared sadly at the floor, red and gold patterned carpet. 'I didn't know I was going to get old.' A tear slid down her cheek. 'It's over, all over. I won't ever be a nurse. My God,' an almost violent revelation, 'I'm going to die one day.'

Jessie enjoyed waiting tables. When she got home after a night's work she would flop exhausted on to her bed. There was something virtuous about the ache, the stiffness in every muscle and every bone she felt when she tried to get up in the morning. For a while she contemplated a change of image: glossier lipstick, dramatic layerings of mascara, more cleavage – though she didn't actually have any cleavage – jaws in nonchalant motion with gum, a teetering, stilettoed walk; but could she ever power-mince like Magda? She decided she couldn't keep it up. She was just beginning to realise how exhausting the business of being female could be.

Mareth was waiting, little village poised and still, for the visitors to arrive. They came every year, droves of them, to wander round the harbour, lick ice-creams, chatter and stare. At last a first few hardy souls in Barbours braved the spring storms, high tides, driving winds to walk, bent horizontal, faces scrunged against the weather, coats flapping, along the shore. They watched the waves, white horses, galloping in, ran backwards as the surf chased their shoes. They wondered at the ancientness of it all: timeless stones, cobbled streets, houses with steps up to the front door, lace curtains hanging on twelve-paned windows.

'It's all so dinky,' they would say. They were wrong, of course.

They came into the café bringing in the cold clinging to their clothes. They would order Magda's tiny onion soup, tiny onions glazed and golden in a thick tomatoey stock with pasta and ham, topped with freshly grated parmesan. It was garlicky and filling. It made diners aglow with such well-being they wanted to go on and on eating. And they usually did. They oozed anticipation at Magda's duckling with baby turnips, or smoked fish omelettes or pesto-topped baked salmon. And they ended with Magda's bread-and-butter pudding, buttered brioche spread with bitter marmalade dipped in fresh orange juice and baked in a creamy vanilla custard. Flushed and replete, the eaters would go smiling into the soft Mareth night watched by Magda and Edie.

'I think the shellfish and courgette risotto and the lamb stew are definitely on tonight. Fact, I don't think they're going to make it home. Look at them. Look at his hands.'

'Ooooh.' Edie craned up to watch the lovers' progress to the BMW they'd parked on the harbour. 'More fun than I'm going to have when I get home.'

'Do you ever get lonely, Edie?' Magda asked.

'Oh, I used to. But after you've lived alone for a while you come to quite like it. I get home after midnight most nights and I don't feel like talking to anybody. After a day in here all I want to do is lie down. I have a bath, pour a wee whisky . . .' she indicated with two abstemious fingers the size of the whisky.

Magda made the same gesture, indicating a much larger measure. 'A wee whisky,' she mocked. Then, 'Still, you do get a bed to yourself. I'd love that.'

'Magda Horn,' Edie scoffed. 'You'd hate to have a bed to yourself. You wouldn't know where to put yourself.'

Then an afterthought, Magda said, 'Have you ever faked it, Edie?'

Edie looked at her. Every time she told herself that Magda could never again surprise her, Magda surprised her.

'Well,' she shrugged, shook her head, flustered. 'As a matter of fact. Yes. Yes, I have.' Jessie, carrying a couple of truffle tortes, stopped to listen, fascinated. She found it hard to imagine thin little, shy little Edie doing it, far less faking it.

'Have you?' Magda turned to her.

Jessie reddened, 'Um, well, yes. Yes. Me too. I have.'

'How did you know to do that? Who told you about faking it?'

Jessie and Edie exchanged baffled looks. 'Just came to me one night when I was with Fred. He was taking ages. You know,' Edie shrugged, embarrassed at this confession.

'No, I don't know,' Magda looked hurt. 'Nobody tells me anything.'

Lipless, leaning on the bar clutching a pint, bent forward. 'I'll tell you something, Magda. I've never faked it.'

Magda stared at him bitterly, 'Well, you wouldn't would you? Don't have to. You'd only be fooling yourself.'

The dining room silenced, everyone stopped eating and looked at Lipless. 'There was no need for that,' he said. 'That was a bit rude.'

'So it was,' said Magda. 'Never mind.' She went into the kitchen and put on James Brown.

'Very rude indeed,' Lipless complained into his beer. 'Even if it is true. How did she know.'

The silence evaporated. Cutlery began to chink again. The eating started up. Life went on.

Jessie loved her new life. This work was restorative. It was, she told herself, honest. She served tables. She mastered new skills, carrying half a dozen plates at a time whilst kicking open the kitchen door. She ironed tablecloths and napkins, laid table, wiped, shouted orders, joined the steamy clamour in the kitchen and went home to bed. She didn't fret about what other people said or what they might be doing behind her back. She did not lie awake at night worrying about the long-term implications of remarks she had not properly registered when they were made to her.

She carried food to hungry people and, as she laid their plates before them, she could eavesdrop. She had fascinating fleeting glimpses of other people's lives. Best of all, she could watch Magda.

All her life she had fought for what she thought she wanted: a degree, a job, a relationship. Now she wanted none of that. She wanted to be able to cook like Magda, wear absurd shoes like Magda, move around the kitchen like Magda.

'Hey boogie,' Magda would shout, waving her spoon in a moment of culinary joy. 'Don't take three steps when fifteen and a wiggle of the hips will do.' And The Rolling Stones would play. And Jessie wanted to be able to make rude remarks like Magda. She wanted to be Magda.

Billing and ordering at the Ocean Café were intriguing. The menu, small and daily handwritten by Edie, consisted of three choices of starter, main course and pudding. Each item was given a colour. On the kitchen wall was a diagram of the table layout. Orders were taken and, instead of writing them down, magnetised coloured tokens matching the colours of the daily dishes were stuck on the diagram. As dishes were taken to the tables the tokens were removed. Jessie found it very confusing.

'Why can't I just give you a note?' she wanted to know.

Edie shifted her feet uneasily. Magda sniffed. 'I have my methods. They work for me.' She turned back to the carrots she was noisily shoving into her food processor.

'But,' ignoring the restrained atmosphere, Jessie persisted, 'yesterday I served someone a tarragon chicken that had a yellow token in it.'

'Yellow for chicken, that's right,' Magda nodded. Her scheme obviously worked. She vigorously scraped her mass of grated carrots into a dark blue bowl and started on the dressing.

'This restaurant is run oddly if you ask me,' said Jessie.

'Well nobody's asking you.' Magda turned her back on her and poured some runny honey into a mixing bowl.

'Well,' Jessie only wanted to make things more organised and remove the worry of small metal tokens finding their way into the food, 'also last week there was a white token in the brown bread ice-cream.'

'Oh,' Edie shrugged.

'Shouldn't that be brown? I mean in the brown bread ice-cream?' Magda looked quizzically at Edie.

'No,' Edie raised a soothing hand to calm the rising angst. Angst that Jessie seemed unaware of. Magda spooned balsamic vinegar into the honey.

'How much of that do you add?' Jessie had recently become keen to learn some of Magda's recipes. And her carrot salad seemed a good place to start. Everyone liked it.

'It is my aim,' Magda confided, 'to make every-one in Mareth eat this. I'll make the bastards healthy. And that old shite optician Carter'll go out of business.'

'So how much honey and how much vinegar do you add?' Jessie loomed over her shoulder.

Magda looked slightly alarmed at the question, 'Just some. You can feel it. I mean, sometimes the carrots are drier, woodier. It all depends.' She waved her hands. Precision irritated her. 'You can just tell,' she said. 'Then there's the olive oil and some salt and pepper. Then you can drop in a spot of walnut oil, and coriander. It's not always the same. See,' returning to her original theme, 'carrots. They're good for the eyes, aren't they?'

'No,' said Edie. 'I think that's just a bad joke about never seeing a rabbit wearing glasses.'

'Why isn't it always the same?' Jessie said. 'Surely people want the carrot salad to be the same every time they order it.'

Magda found it hard to pass on her skills. Many had asked and were usually sent scurrying from the kitchen. 'Questions, questions, questions. Don't ask. Just look. Take it in. Breathe it. Be it. Do it. That's how to learn.'

'Ah,' Jessie nodded. 'Only I seem to need some point of reference.'

'Rubbish. You just make it.'

'But how do you make it the same if you don't have a recipe?'

'It isn't the same. Is anything that's worth knowing the same every time? Is sex the same?' She started vigorously mixing her dressing. 'No. Sometimes it's wild, or passionate or cruel or comforting. Well . . .' she spread her hands. Jessie was tempted to point out that it was only a carrot salad and was it really likely to be cruel or

96

passionate or wild? But she could see Magda's temper rising. Something was bothering her. She returned to the tokens.

'Yes. I see,' she said. 'I just thought writing the orders down would speed things up. Would make things easier. Cleaner . . .' She tailed off.

Magda turned suddenly furious. 'Can't you see I don't want a new method? I don't want efficiency. I want my tokens. I like my tokens. They're my tokens and they work for me.'

'I just . . .' Jessie spread her arms weakly.

Magda glared at her. Jessie wilted. Angry, Magda was more than formidable. She was terrifying. She seemed to fill the kitchen. Edie looked to be getting smaller. She was backing towards the door.

'God dammit,' Magda yelled. 'Can't you tell? Can't you sense there's something wrong. Isn't it obvious that I have to have the tokens because I can't fucking read or write. I'm illiterate. I'm a great big illiterate fool. That's what. That's me. Sod it . . . and dammit . . . and . . .'

She took her bowl of carrots and threw them across the kitchen. It smashed fabulously against the wall, splattering gratings everywhere. It was surprising how far they flew.

'Now look what you've done,' Edie tutted.

'And I really liked that bowl.' Magda kicked a stray bit of broken crockery. Jessie didn't know what to do. 'I would never have guessed,' she said quietly. 'You're such a good cook.'

'That's it for me,' Magda said. 'Cooking's what

I do. Cooking. Fucking and having babies. That's all.'

Jessie stared at her. All? By God it was more than she could do. She couldn't even decently lose her temper. Well, not like that anyway. Common sense would have prevailed. She would have had the bowl in her hand, then at the last minute, considering the consequences, put it down. She wished she could throw things about like that.

'Well,' Magda relieved the tension, 'peel some more carrots.'

CHAPTER 8

June. The full gaudy parade was on. Jessie could hardly push her way along the street. It was a time of ice-cream lickers and starers. Multi-coloured shell-suits on the move, shuffling slowly along the shore filling the litter bins, dragging vast bulging bags of beach stuff – rugs, buckets, spades, hats, balls, inflatable dinghies, booze, food, stuff – along the West Way to Mareth's small scrap of sandy beach. Locals knew the best swimming beaches along the coast but rarely told tourists about them.

Magda got ready to make the bulk of her annual income. The café filled. Days crowded in one against the other. Jessie moved into an exhausted haze. Even when she was away from the café she could smell chips. The backs of her legs ached. Someone asked if they could have tomato ketchup to put on their chicken with button mushrooms and Jessie whirled round and snapped, 'No. No you can't.' And had been shocked at herself. But not shocked enough to apologise.

The kitchen hit hyper-steam. Bunty, who came in at weekends to wash dishes and had a hygiene problem, came in every evening and had a heightened hygiene problem. Even when she wasn't at the café, when she was at the end of the harbour breathing in huge gulps of fresh air, Jessie thought she could smell her. She would discreetly try to sniff her own armpits, checking that the problems weren't catching. Odours from Magda's kitchen clung to all her clothes. When she stared in the mirror she saw a strange face looming back. Hair dishevelled, pores opening round new wrinkles on her face. She had bags under her eyes. Sometimes, lying on her bed, she would remember fondly the office she had once inhabited. Plants on the windowsill, constant fresh coffee, the soothing whir of her Apple Mac, pleasant voices, accents she understood. Why was she doing this? She was aware that sometimes a whole week would pass without her once thinking of her little son, Dr Davies and her guilt. She knew though that this was no real way to cure the blues. She soothed herself body and soul, listening to Mozart. She thought she must by now know a lot of things she didn't know before. If only she could put her finger on what they might be.

'I see Non-existent Dave's back,' Magda said, nodding towards the bar.

Edie coyly stuck her head through the kitchen door and greeted him, 'Hi Dave.'

'Edie,' he acknowledged her. She ducked back.

Of course Magda had affairs. These affairs were mostly with people passing through. She didn't want complications. But of all her illicit lovers, Non-existent Dave was the one she couldn't put out of her mind. It had the tingle factor, she supposed. The swiftness, wildness, wrongness of what they did, mostly in the kitchen, was thrilling. She caught her breath remembering.

'You serve him, Jessie,' she said.

'Non-existent Dave?' Jessie couldn't believe some of the nick-names. 'Sounds existential.'

'Existential,' Magda silently mouthed the word to Edie behind her back. And they both went, ooooh. And laughed.

'What the hell is existential?' Magda asked.

'It's a philosophy,' Jessie told her. 'Um . . .' she waved her hands about, '. . . um . . . to do with existence. Jean Paul Sartre. Um . . . it's like the future doesn't exist . . . and . . .'

Edie was carrying the big soup pot into the kitchen, through from the dishwashing area. It seemed to make her even smaller. Magda had her hands in a sinkful of cold water scrubbing mussels.

'Well . . .' Jessie wished she hadn't started this, since she was beginning to realise she didn't properly understand it herself. 'See, he questioned things like existence . . . or he questioned our view of existence, our experience of it . . .' Edie and Magda watched her.

'This Sartre bloke,' Magda said, 'he got paid for this?'

Edie heaved the soup pot on to the stove. Magda wiped her chilled hands on her apron.

'So he said we couldn't be sure things existed or not? Is that not just like a man,' Magda roared. 'Christ, don't tell Jim about that. Take the bins out, will you? No. How can I? We can't be sure they exist.' She nudged Edie. 'That's the best one yet.'

'And he got paid for it,' Edie reminded her. 'What are we doing slaving here?'

Jessie went to serve Non-existent Dave.

The name came from his great scheme. A computer ace, whilst working with the district council he'd wiped himself and his house from their records thereby freeing himself from local taxes. He had also removed all evidence of himself from the filing system. He'd emptied and closed his bank account. The council wanted to fire him for not coming to work. But there was nothing to fire. His plan was to hack into the computers of his credit card companies and remove himself from their records. He wondered if it was possible to wipe himself from the Inland Revenue records.

His great scheme had been that for a fee he would, using his home computer, hack into any system necessary to remove his clients from the face of the earth. He'd even offered to remove all evidence of Mareth itself. But discussions in the Spar and the post office supported the notion that someone would notice. There was hardly anyone in the village that hadn't been tempted. In the end all Dave did was fix the records that the harbour constantly needed repair. They'd been repairing the same bit of harbour wall for the past two years. It was good for Lipless and his work gang. And it was good for Lipless's liver. Magda kept him fed and refused him alcohol before noon. But they all knew that in the end someone would notice.

Dave's fate since he became non-existent confirmed Magda's passionate belief in irony. She believed in little else. She still prayed the same prayer she had been offering to whoever was up there since she was ten years old, hiding in her head from the sick slap-on-the-side-of-the-head philosophy of her Sunday school teachers, 'God help me please, and bless me. Keep me sane and safe from the Church of Scotland. Amen.'

Magda believed there was irony and only irony. People would all get what was coming to them in the end. And Non-existent Dave's fate proved her point. Not long after his wiping himself from the face of the earth, his wife left him for an ostentatiously rich builder. Then his nineteen-year-old son disappeared. He'd set off along the beach after drinking a vodka laced with acid one fabulously hot summer afternoon wearing only cut-offs and canvas deck shoes, walking walking past the shimmer till he was gone. He'd never been seen again. Searches found nothing. No washed-up body, no clothing nothing. Dave even became briefly existent again, registering his son as a missing person. But nothing. After that Dave started drifting. He disappeared from Mareth sometimes for months at a time, sometimes years.

'There,' Magda said when Dave first disappeared. 'Told you so. It's irony, that's what it is. Everybody gets what's coming to them in the end.'

'Oh boy. It really is a religion with you. I can just see you,' Jim amused himself, 'standing in the pulpit belting out your hymns, gospel style. You got what was comin' to ya babe. You had it comin' all along. Oh lordy lord.'

Magda didn't reply. What was coming to her then? Considering her relationship with Non-existent Dave? Her best affair ever. The heated rush and whispered urgency of it. The freedom when he slipped off her bra and the air hit her tits. His hands on her, his skin, skin on skin. It was like being teenage again. That first fuck when you first discover the wonders of fucking. Magda had been on the table and all she could say was, 'Do it. Do it. Do it.'

She plunged her hands back in the icy water, started feverishly scraping a mussel. 'It's been a while,' she said. That familiar longing started deep deep inside her. 'I have to go,' she said, a sudden urgent statement. She threw the mussel she was working on back into the water and left. Wiping her hands on her apron, ridiculous heels echoing on the cobbles, she hurried along the shore to Jim's yard, just past the harbour.

It was empty, silent and empty. The office was locked up. She looked round. She never felt she belonged here. She knew, standing amidst the bits of engine leaning on the *Sad-Eyed Lady*, his boat, she was out of place. She was wearing a short skirt and denim shirt tied around the waist, and her shoes were patent and pointy. In the evening when cooking she would dress like a cook, as the environmental health regulations demanded. A cook in a baseball cap, the only thing she could bear to wear on her head. But in the afternoons when she had also to wait tables she didn't bother. A breeze came in from the sea and above her swallows shrilled and cried. Something was wrong.

She hurried back along the shore past the Ocean Café to their house on the West Way. Jim, sitting at the kitchen table, was surprised to see her. Magda looked at him and knew this was not the moment to say she got horny scraping mussels and had come to find him, you know, just in case he might be persuaded to share her mood. Something was wrong.

'What is it?' she asked.

He shrugged. Spread his palms. 'That's it,' he said.

'What's it?'

'My yard. It's over. Isn't it?'

She watched him. His face was grey. 'Bank's called in the loan. And I can't pay my taxes. I'm bust, Magda. Bankrupt.'

'You can't be,' she protested. 'How can you be?' Which really meant how can you be when I know nothing about it? She sank into a chair opposite him. How could she have missed this? Something as big as this. She opened her mouth to ask all the questions crowding into her mind, but not a sound came out.

Jim shrugged and sniffed, 'There you go,' he said. 'The house is safe, I think. They'll take the yard. Sell off everything.' He did not look at her, did not meet her eyes. 'Bastards,' he said.

'Why. How could this happen?'

'Somebody didn't pay me so I couldn't pay somebody else. In my case the somebody elses I couldn't pay were the bank and the Inland Revenue. That'll do it every time. They'll see you off.'

'How long has this been going on? You didn't tell me.' Magda couldn't grasp what she was being told.

'Months. Months and months.' He put his hand over his eyes. He didn't want to look at her. 'I know I didn't tell you. I thought I could handle it. I thought.' He took a deep breath, adjusting his nerves. 'I think I thought if I ignored it, it would go away. I couldn't face it. I didn't tell anybody.'

She came to him. Took his head in her hands and held him against her. He clung to her. He was falling. He sank his face deep into her, breathing her. She smelled fishy. Her hands were cold. Still he clung and she touched the top of his head with her lips. He pushed up her skirt, ripped at her knickers, 'Wait,' she pulled them off. And he brought her down on top of him.

'No. No. This isn't right.' He shoved her off.

Gripping his trousers he shoved her towards the bedroom. But they only made the stairs. Uncomfortable love. The edge of a step at the base of her spine cut into her. She wanted him to stop and didn't want him to stop. But he was far away, he was working out his ache. Pounding and crying. And when he came it was the nearest to screaming Magda had ever heard him.

She went to wash herself. When she came back and he was still lying spread out on the stairs, 'This is me then. Lying on my back with my trousers at my ankles,' he said.

Magda scarcely looked at him, 'Always liked you best like that,' she said. 'Defenceless.' She stepped over him and through into the kitchen.

Jim rose, slowly heaved his trousers up as if they were extraordinarily heavy, and followed her. 'I don't know why men wear trousers,' he said. 'The only good part of any day is when you take them off.'

'Life isn't that bad,' Magda assured him crisply as she made coffee.

'Yes it is. It's worse.'

She was rumpled when she returned to her kitchen. Her skirt was tellingly wrinkled round her arse, and she hadn't buttoned herself up properly.

'Where have you been?' Edie wanted to know. Though she knew very well.

'Just out,' said Magda. 'I had to see Jim about something.'

Edie turned to Jessie and they both mouthed, oooooh, behind her back.

'I see you,' Magda grunted. 'I see you both.'

And out at the bar, Non-existent Dave yelled that there was no service here and what did a man have to do to get a drink?

'Oh piss off,' Magda called back. Damn staircase. She was going to have a hell of a bruise on her bum tomorrow, and as far as she was concerned it was all Dave's fault.

The frock hung on the back of the bedroom door. Mary hadn't faced the trauma of trying it on. As yet it was enough to look at it, to own it. Mary would lie in bed at night and admire it. Even in the dark she knew it was there. And was thrilled.

'That thing's been there weeks now,' John said, yanking at it. 'Are you going to wear it or what?'

'Mind your own business,' Mary said. 'And take yer grubby hands off my dress.'

John belched. That frock did terrible things to his digestive system. He went out to his car and drove to the cliff. He had to get away. His heart burned with badly digested food. He could still taste the hamburger and chips he'd had for lunch. It'd be with him for a couple of days yet. Why did he eat that stuff? Warm from the sun streaming through his windscreen, safely away from his wife's neurosis, he would sleep. Everyone in Mareth knew this was his habit, nobody disturbed him. Locals out taking the air or walking their dogs tiptoed by. Ssssh . . . John was sleeping. And he needed his sleep. They all knew why, Mary snored something awful. Had done ever since her menopause.

Back in her bedroom, Mary pulled the curtains and stood a moment in the soothing dark. Then she slipped out of her frilly blue afternoon blouse and dark brown skirt. In stockinged soles she padded through to the bathroom and washed. She put on fresh make-up, carefully lining her eyelids and taking off the excess lipstick on a bit of toilet paper. Back in her bedroom she took her Christmas bottle of Chanel from her underwear drawer and scented her wrists and behind her ears.

'Now. The dress,' she muttered, plucking up her courage. This was the moment. It had come.

Nervously she removed the dress from the green velvet hanger and laid it on the bed. She slid down the zip. Then at last she stepped into it and gently gently pulled it up. It fitted. It fitted perfectly. She smoothed her hands over her hips. Not a sag, not a bulge. Over the shoulders, perfect. Under the arms, perfect. She could hardly breathe for the pleasure of it. Tears misted her eyes. 'Oh my. Thank you, God.'

She walked stiffly across to the mirror and looked at herself. The dress was wonderful, she could see that. There was nothing wrong with the dress. Oh no. It was her that was wrong. Her face was old and wrinkled and had a slightly surprised look on it. How had that happened to it? Her face was letting the frock down.

★　　★　　★

Four Harrys lived in the yard at the back of the Ocean Café. There was Black Harry, White Harry, Orange Harry and Stripy Harry, assorted cats, assorted sexes all called Harry because one name was enough. Harry, Magda would call out the back door, and the cats would appear rushing through the dark. They were gourmet beasts, no tinned cat food for them. And though Magda had them all neutered so that they wouldn't stray, there was no chance any of them would move away. Life outside the Ocean Café was too sweet.

'Still,' Magda said. 'It'll stop them breeding. There's too much breeding going on around here anyway.' Harrys would drape themselves on her windowsill and Harrys would lie along the yard wall idly watching, waiting for tasty bits. They all knew better than to follow Magda home.

'You're not worming your way to my fireside,' she told them firmly as they lined up for their trout-in-red-wine leftovers. Sleek and glossy, weaving through her legs, purring.

Recently, however, Black Harry had taken to sitting mournfully on Jessie's doorstep, yowling plaintively to be let in.

'He knows a sucker when he sees one,' Magda said. The betting in the café was three to one that the cat would be on Jessie's bed by the end of the week.

'Nuts.' Magda knew a sucker when she saw one, too. 'She's desperate for a cuddle, that one. She

110

won't hold out past tomorrow.' She was right. Black Harry's desperate pleas were too much for Jessie to bear. She let him in. Magda pocketed her winnings, ten pounds.

'He'll see you all right,' Magda said, nodding at the cat. 'He'll help cure whatever it is that ails you that you're not telling anybody about.'

'What ails me?' Jessie looked at her.

'What ails you.' Magda gave her a serious bit of eye contact.

'What makes you think something ails me?' Jessie said slowly.

'When people are all you read, you read them very well,' Magda told her.

So Black Harry moved in, spent nights purring on Jessie's bed and days draped on the windowsill beside the geraniums.

Geraniums. Geraniums in the window by the sea, that's for me, Jessie thought. She had been passing Frankie's Ironmongery at the time. A shop that defied every modern sales technique. The window displays were so messy, they could have been a definitive piece of anti-design. There was a lavatory and three clay pots in one, and a scattering of ancient boxes of nails in the other. Locals knew that the windows had been like that for years and years. Occasionally tourists would stop and wonder. Did this mean something? Was this some kind of minimalist statement?

It was one of Mareth's long-standing rumours that Frankie was a millionaire. But Jessie doubted it. Though he did have a unique method of pricing his goods.

The clay pots reminded Jessie of trips to Provence and Italy. She would buy a couple and have them in the window overflowing with geraniums.

'I'll have a couple of clay pots,' she pointed to the leaning tower of various-sized pots precariously placed in the corner. Frankie moved stiffly over to it.

'Size?' he asked. The conversation here was minimalist also.

'Oh, medium.'

He moved stiffly back with two pots and charged her eight pounds.

'That's a terrible price for two pots,' Jessie complained.

Frankie readily agreed, 'It is that.'

The customer standing behind her joined in, 'I'll have a couple of them too, Frankie.'

'That'll be three pounds,' Frankie said.

Jessie was incensed. 'How come it's eight pounds for me and only three for him?'

The question seemed so absurd Frankie almost didn't answer. He leaned forward, pointed to the other customer. 'He's local,' he said.

'So am I,' Jessie told him.

'You live here?'

'Yes.'

'You're not just on holiday?'

'No.'

'Where do you live?'

'On the shore just above the Ocean Café.'

Frankie put his face close to hers, 'And are you renting or buying?'

'Renting.'

'And what are you going to be doing with the pots?'

'Planting geraniums,' Jessie replied, surprised that she was actually putting up with this.

Hmm, a scraping sound – Frankie rubbing his unshaven chin. 'All right. That'll be five pounds then.'

'That's still two pounds more than him.'

'Ah yes,' Frankie nodded. 'But I haven't known you all my life.'

CHAPTER 9

'It's my face,' Mary whined, 'it's ruining my new dress.'

John didn't quite know what to say. 'Why don't you go down the pub?' he countered. 'It's been weeks since you went. A few drinks and a spot of Elvis'll fix you.'

'Don't be silly,' Mary cried. 'I can't afford any of that. I have to get my hair done. I have to buy new shoes. I have to get new face cream and pluck my eyebrows. And . . . oh . . . you don't know what a dress like that needs. I mean, even the bedroom looks drab with it hanging there. I was thinking we could get some new wallpaper at the weekend, and you . . .'

She didn't need to finish. John sank into his chair and stared glumly down at the criss-cross pattern on his jersey. He felt his face crumple. His discontent and bewilderment showed constantly. He was lonely. A better man than me, he thought, would go through and cut that frock to shreds. A piece of clothing had got the better of him. A strident bit of cloth that glowed triumphantly at him as he lay in bed. Oh, he hated that dress.

*   *   *

Mareth youth was wild. Always had been. Shore boys and their cars along the harbour, screech of wheels, handbrake swiftly on and they would spin. Even in the direst weather they wore only T-shirts, Marlboro packs tucked into the sleeve. They leaned out of their car windows, banging the roof with the flat of their hands and yelling. Yeeha. Yeeha.

They were the yeeha generation. And their music would play. Howling through the night, thudding from deep inside their motors. In summer they took to the water. They skidded speed-boats round and round the bay, still hollering.

Granny Moran sometimes came slowly to the front of the building to watch them and shake her head, sadly. 'Too much wildness,' she'd say. 'They've got more life in them than they know what to do with. It's the fishing. They're brought up wild to go out to the fishing. But now it's all gone. They've nothing to do with their wildness.' And she'd shuffle back indoors.

There were casualties. Tom Bailey drank fifteen cans of Becks and a bottle of vodka and spun his car right off the harbour and drowned. Emily Brown got raped at a party. Woody at the Anchor and Crown refused to serve Little Weasel on account of he looked fourteen and had done since he turned twenty. Before that he looked twelve. Weasel, in a fury, had put on a balaclava and returned to the pub waving his father's gun. He'd shot the chandelier and his own left leg. 'Always hated that thing anyway,' said Woody, sweeping up the shattered glass. He claimed two thousand pounds damage from his insurance company and happily settled for eight hundred. It had only cost him a tenner in a car-boot sale.

Younger yeehas emptied half the contents from a two-litre coke bottle and refilled it with vodka or cider, sometimes vodka and cider. They would drink at the end of the harbour till reeling with alcohol and angst they would come yelling and vomiting back into the world where they'd unleash their yearnings and rage upon litter bins, parked cars and the bus shelter. And when Jessie passed, moving swiftly from the Ocean Café to her own front door they'd yell, 'Fancy shagging that?' Or, 'Great tits on that thing.' More like no tits on that thing, she thought. But she didn't know how to cope. Magda would get the better of them. They seemed like subterraneans lost in their own little world of hopelessness and anger.

'There's not many insurance men and accountants in the making yelling out there,' Magda said.

'They're so wild,' Jessie complained. 'So full of wildness.'

Magda nodded. 'Still,' she said. 'Best time for it. Get all the vomiting and howling over with when your digestive system is young enough to cope.'

Her own two older children, Janis and Joe, were among the shouters and vomiters.

'It's our own fault,' she told Jim. 'We shouldn't

have given them these silly names. They went through their young childhood sounding like something from a sickly kiddie's television programme.'

'We had to give them something to rebel against,' Jim decided. 'They'll thank us for it yet.'

The naming of children was always a problem in Mareth. Jim came from a long succession of Jims. It was something of a scandal, though a small scandal by Mareth standards, that he'd broken the mould and called his own son Joe. But, as he said, 'How many Jims can you take?' His father had been Jim, his grandfather therefore had been Big Jim, making him Little Jim. When his own son was born he would have become plain Jim had he not been called Joe. In the complex system of Jims it seemed to Jim that if you were born plain Jim you were all right. But if you were born to be a Little Jim you remained a Little Jim all your days, no matter how big you actually grew.

And the Jim-ing of Mareth went further than that. There were more families of Jims than just the Horns. Jims became known for their jobs – Postie Jim – or nicknames – Haddock Jim – or after the boats they had sailed on – Bountiful Jim; and when they had sons there was Big Bountiful Jim and Little Bountiful Jim. It was an intricate business that was just the nature of things in Mareth. But Jim had had enough of it.

'This pecking order of Jims has to stop,' he decreed. The naming of Joe caused a storm in his family. His mother hadn't spoken to him for two years. Magda was the same. She came from a long line of Marys. Her mother had broken the line because her husband John was not Magda's real father.

Though she had never mentioned this to either Magda or John. Magda after Mary Magdalene seemed more than appropriate. And Magda didn't mind. In fact she often said, 'My name's the only thing I really like about me.'

Joe's break from tradition did nothing to stop the wildness though. He had done the full drunken thing: stolen a car, driven foot to the floor beyond its capabilities, crashed it out on the coast road and walked footsore and sorry for himself fourteen miles home, where Magda and Jim were sitting at the kitchen table waiting for him.

They knew all about it. The whole village knew all about it. But nobody called the police. They didn't use police in Mareth if they could help it. Best to sort out your troubles yourself.

'What did we do wrong, Magda?' Jim asked, running his fingers through his hair.

'Had children,' Magda said. 'It could've been worse. He could've taken up religion.'

In fact she found it easy to forgive Joe. He had her heart. And he had been so filled with guilt and shame he'd put his head in his hands and wept. 'Will you stop that?' Magda said, tears streaming down her face. Didn't matter what her child had done, she couldn't bear to see him hurting. 'How can I do dreadful things to you when you cry?' Which made him cry harder.

Joe sorted out, they now had Janis to keep them awake at nights. She had stopped eating. Daily, before her mother's eyes, she was getting thinner and thinner. Magda knew better than to nag, except nagging was what she was best at.

'Will you please eat. Just something. A tomato. Some melon. It doesn't have to be fattening. Just eat.'

Janis had stared at her palely and slowly put a sliver of melon into her mouth, and let it lie there. She would not chew. She glared at her mother with passionate defiance.

'God dammit child, will you eat? What's wrong with you?'

Janis spat out the melon. 'It's you. It's fucking you, you fat slag. I don't want to look like you.'

Shocked and deeply hurt, Magda put her hand to her face. 'Well, congratulations, Janis. At last we agree on something. I don't want to look like me either.'

Lying in bed Saturday morning, Jessie saw the seagulls come yammering in. They swirled and jostled outside her window and she heard the loud splat, splat, splat as they shat all over her car. It was too much. Too much.

'That's it. Damn birds,' she swore and leapt from bed. Time to do something about this. She pulled on a T-shirt and a pair of knickers and swiftly ran out of her flat. She had to catch Granny Moran in the act of actually feeding the birds to get her to stop. Confrontation, that's what any decent therapist would tell her to do.

'Confrontation. Confrontation. Confrontation,' she muttered as she hurtled down the stairs to the main door. And there, just as she suspected, was Granny Moran in the tartan dressing gown spreading bread crusts, old sponge cake and bits of bacon for the birds. Sparrows hopped eagerly and seagulls swooped.

'I wish you wouldn't do that,' Jessie said shrilly.

'Do what?' Granny Moran sourly replied. She knew very well what Jessie was talking about.

'Feed the gulls. Look. They shit all over my car.'

The old lady looked over at Jessie's splattered car and sucked her gums the way she did, making time, gathering her thoughts. 'Have you ever thought that they just plain don't like your car?'

'No,' said Jessie. 'I'm not getting neurotic about this. They'd shit on any car. They don't just single out mine.'

'Are you sure about that? They don't like foreign motors. That's a fact.'

'They're seagulls, for Christ's sake. They can't tell where a car is manufactured.'

'But they weren't always seagulls,' Granny Moran looked at her and laughed. Didn't she know that? This strange city woman was a fool.

'Oh no.' Jessie's protest had been stopped in its

tracks. 'What did they used to be before they were seagulls?'

'Well,' Granny Moran sniffed deeply. 'I don't know about your seagulls. But mine, the ones that fly over every morning, are all my friends and relatives come by to see me. The ones that've died, like.'

'Ah,' said Jessie.

'That'll be why they shit on your car. They don't know you. You're not kin. Your kin'll be back where you came from. City sparrows, chattering starlings and the like.'

You've certainly got the measure of my chums, Jessie thought.

'You're young, though,' Granny Moran patted her arm. 'You'll not know many dead folk.'

'Now you come to mention it,' Jessie shook her head. Though she knew one, and if he could be a bird – the purest bird – the whitest bird – her grief was almost bearable.

'There you go,' Granny Moran said almost cheerily. 'Nothing to fear about dying, though. Peace and freedom. First you become a bird. Flying round to see all your friends and family. See they're all right without you and letting them know you're fine, chirping a wee song for them.' She flapped her ancient arms and lifted herself on to her toes. She who longed to be up and away looked grimly down at her puffed, deformed arthritic feet swelling inside their grubby slippers. For a moment Jessie caught a glimpse of the woman who sixty years ago

121

had driven men wild. 'Then when you've done with your goodbyes you're off to the other side where everyone who has gone before is waiting. Waiting and waving and calling your name. Ah yes,' she smiled, watery-eyed with longing, 'death's a fine thing. The time of your life.'

Then there was Annie, Magda's third child. She was a joy.

'That girl is no problem at all,' Magda said to Jim. 'She's a worry. And she's so clever. She speaks French and wins prizes at school. Where did she come from? Do you suppose they gave us the wrong baby? Look at Joe. If they had exams in training shoes and rap artists he'd get A's. And Rosie. Rosie's wild.'

It was true. Annie was popular at school with her friends and her teachers, a pleasure to teach, they said. Annie worked about the house. Helped Rosie with her homework. Annie smiled and joked a lot. Annie worried Magda to bits.

'It's not right. How can she be so constant? I actually like the child. But I don't understand her. I understand the others – stealing cars, not wanting to look like your mother. That's all teenage stuff. But she's so calm. So nice. I tell you, Jim, no good'll come of it.'

The last customer had gone, Jessie and Magda sat at the bar drinking. Nirvana's slow angst howled from a car parked outside the café.

'Listen to that,' Magda said. 'Oh, don't you remember being like that? Raw and misunderstood. God. Sometimes I still feel like that. Don't you?'

'I was never like that. Looking back I realise I was the perfect daughter and perfect pupil. I spent my adolescence sitting in my bedroom studying.'

It was probably true. Whilst Magda had spent her late teenage out on the point, enthusiastically discovering sex, smoking dope in a fug of rock-'n'roll, Jessie had been busy doing what she was told.

'Ha,' cried Magda. 'Don't boast to me. And don't go thinking you've escaped being raw and misunderstood. You don't have to be sixteen to be adolescent. It can strike at any time. It's one of life's recurrent phases.'

'You've seemed pretty mature to me,' Jessie swallowed some whisky.

'Oh, it'll be back. I'm not cured of teenage tantrums. I'm just in remission.'

'What are we going to do?'

Jim shook his head, 'There's nothing to do. It's over. They'll sell off my stuff. Pay some debts. That'll be that.' He put his face in his hands, rubbed the bridge of his nose with his fingertips. 'There you go.'

Magda stared at him. Hello, Jim. How are you feeling in there? Are you coping? He rarely showed emotions. She said nothing.

123

'It was just a knock-on sort of thing. This bastard owed me money and another bastard owed him and another bastard owed him and so on. And when one went, we all went.'

He had signed on today. Unemployed. He had sat for three hours in the Social Security office listening to piped music, surrounded by welfare families. Children had run around squealing, desperate mothers tried to control them vocally, yelling deranged orders, anything rather than actually get up out of the safety of the plastic seat and move centre stage to the middle of the waiting area. They felt vulnerable enough without doing anything that might get them noticed.

It was another world there. He'd hardly spoken since he got home. Magda dreaded this silence. He came and he went, he moved about the house and he said nothing. He sighed.

'Oh shut up,' Magda said.

'What d'you mean shut up? I didn't say anything.'

'You didn't have to. What you're not saying is enough.'

He rose, sighed again and left the room. Magda ran after him, beat his retreating back with her fists. 'Will you shut up being silent and say something?' And for the first time he did not knock her back, did not even grab hold of her arms and stop the blows. He stood, slightly bent. Taking it.

Magda stepped back. 'Oh don't be like that. Don't.' She ran from the house. Her children watched, shocked.

'What's going to happen?' Rosie asked. Janis bit her nails, didn't reply. Joe's mind temporarily flooded with horror stories to horrify her. He loved to watch her face fill with fear. They'll take the house and we'll have to live in a cardboard box at Shore's End. They'll sell off all your stuff, your Lego and Game Boy and send you to a children's home. But no. He said nothing.

Annie put her arm round her. 'Everything's going to be fine,' she said. 'You'll see.'

Magda, watching guiltily through the window, chastised herself. 'God,' she thought. 'My daughter's a nicer person than me.' She kicked the wall, hurt her toe and stumped off back to the café.

CHAPTER 10

'So,' said Non-existent Dave, 'do I have to go through all the motions to get into your bed?'

Jessie almost said no. But that would mean he would get into her bed without going through any motions. And if she said yes, it would mean motions then bed.

'What do you mean motions?' she asked as she put a whisky before him.

'I mean a date. Dinner, stuff, whatever. Then bed.'

Jessie smiled. She wasn't going to get involved in this conversation. 'Only Black Harry gets into my bed.'

'A cat. Probably more reliable than me anyway.' He sipped his drink and smiled at her. He was going to have her.

Before coming to work, Jessie had phoned Alex and told him she wanted a divorce. 'And I want my share of the money you emptied out of our account.'

'Why. Can't you hack it as a waitress?'

'It's mine. I earned it. You have no right to it. You bastard.'

126

'You're getting coarse, Jessie. This is a side of you I never knew existed.'

'It's my adolescence. I'm having it late. Best time, you enjoy it more.' She heard his exasperation steaming down the line and laughed as she hung up.

Looking at Non-existent Dave, she let her new-found adolescence roll. He had all the qualifications to be on the receiving end of a teenage crush. He was intriguing and quite nice-looking. And, if she was going for full brainless superficiality – he wore the right sort of clothes: 501s, boots, a leather jacket and white shirt. He had what Magda's Janis would call a serious haircut. Cool was the word she would use if she were sixteen.

Somewhere in the depth of me a sixteen-year-old is wildly waving, trying to get out, she thought.

'Yes,' she said suddenly. 'You have to go through all the motions. Dinner, gifts, flowers whatever. Flash car if you can work it. All the motions you can think of, as many motions as you can get.'

'Then . . .' Dave raised his eyebrows – hopefully.

'Then nothing. I'm fickle and unreliable,' Jessie folded her arms.

'Come on, Jessie. Gimme something.'

'Then maybe. Maybe's it with me now.'

'Maybe's fine.'

Dave smiled. He could work on maybe. He rarely failed.

★   ★   ★

The bedroom had been redone. Mary tried to make it look like the shop. 'The dress'll feel at home,' she said.

'It's a dress,' John told her, no emotion in his voice. None left. 'It doesn't notice where it is.' He was deeply perturbed. This dress was more than a dress. It was the enemy. It brought discontent. His wife was no longer happy with the life they had, the life they worked for – she wanted more. She was abandoning her very roots looking for a life she couldn't have.

Still they redecorated. Deep green walls, pale gold wood-work. Suddenly the bed seemed inadequate, then the wardrobe and the dressing table. Mary replaced them both, along with the bedcovers and the curtains. At last she felt the dress had a proper setting. Now it needed a worthy owner.

'I'll need to get my hair done,' she said. 'Something special.' She patted her chest. This frock was giving her indigestion too.

'We can't afford it,' John said. 'And if you do get your hair done. Then what? When are you going to put the damn thing on? And where can we go? We've no money left.'

Annie discovered the letters. They lay wedged and crumpled at the bottom of Rosie's schoolbag, along with a collection of chewed crayons, pencils, a ruler, half a cheese sandwich, banana skins, an apple core, empty crisp bags and sweet wrappers. Annie's face distorted in horror each time she dipped her hand into the bag. What was it going to bring out next? The letters.

She smoothed them out, decrumbed them, and through the stains of melted chocolate and coke, read. Deeply concerned about Rosie. Behavioural problems. Unable to cope with the set work. Worryingly behind. Disruptive in class. She showed them to Jim.

'Have you ever seen the like?' he said. 'Some of these are months old. Who does little Rosie remind you of?'

Annie nodded.

'Does the world need two Magdas?' Jim asked.

Annie shook her head.

Still, next day it was Magda who went to see Rosie's teacher, though the very smell of school still filled her heart with horror and fear.

When Jim told her about the letters she had summoned little Rosie to the kitchen to explain. 'Why didn't you show them to us?' she asked.

Rosie shrugged, 'Dunno.'

'Dunno,' Magda chastised. 'Dunno. Where would children be without dunno?'

'Dunno,' Rosie said. Magda glared at her.

'Also,' Rosie squeakily complained. 'I have the Lego scheme to work on. It takes me all my time.'

'The Lego scheme?' Magda asked. 'Is this something you're doing at school.'

'Yes. See,' Rosie folded her little arms and

explained. 'Every time you do something good with the Lego, Miss Frazer puts it in the cupboard. So . . .' Her eyes brightened. Plainly the Lego scheme was filling her with enthusiasm. 'I'm really good at Lego and every time I make something it gets into the cupboard. Well if everything I make gets put in the cupboard, there'll be none left. It'll be the end of the damn Lego. And if we don't have the Lego there'll be nothing to do at the end of the day and we'll get sent home and I can watch the afternoon soaps with Gran in her red dress.'

'No,' said Jim slowly. 'She's not like you. She's worse. She's got brains. That's a smart plan. Good on ya, Rosie.'

Joe sneered, 'God, you're thick, Rosie. They'll just buy more Lego. Or else they'll take everything apart and you'll have to build it all up again.'

'Your Grandma sits in her living room watching soaps in that bloody red dress?' Magda found the news hard to bear. 'That's so sad.'

'But,' Rosie was devastated, 'if they buy more Lego, it'll take for ever to get it all in the cupboard and I'll never get to sit with Gran in her red dress. And I want to specially when they do up the living room so it's special just like a palace. The sort of place a red dress needs. I want to go there.'

'They just did up the bedroom,' Magda said. 'What do they want to go doing their living room? God I hate that red dress.'

'It's lovely,' Rosie protested. 'It's beautiful. Gran

is saving it for good. When good comes she'll have something to wear.'

'How do you know good when it comes?' asked Jim.

'You just know it,' Rosie overflowed enthusiastic naïveté. 'Everything is shiny and you put your red dress on.'

Magda was playing her old Blondie records full blast. She was trying hard to blot out her thoughts. Life was closing in on her. A terrible silence was hemming her in and she didn't know what to do about it. Jim rarely spoke and her children had long-since disappeared to some private place in their heads. The Ocean Café did not bring in nearly enough money to support them all. In fact if it wasn't for Edie she doubted the café would make any profit at all. Edie saw to it that Magda kept her flamboyant cooking methods under control. Edie did all of the buying and all of the pricing. Edie knew what was in the freezer and what was in the cellar.

Magda confronted herself with a set of what-ifs? What if Jim couldn't get work? What if he lost his beloved *Sad-Eyed Lady* and never set sail in her? What if Rosie never learned to read and write and ended up like her? What if Edie died – the café would go down hill. No boatyard, no café – it would be the end of them all.

Magda didn't worry constructively. She presented herself with a series of potential dire events and let her feelings roll. Magda worried with her gut, nerves constantly shifting in her stomach. She bit her nails, clattered pots, threw ladles and lifters into the sink. She picked fights.

Edie knew to keep a low profile. She hid in the office, out of Magda's way.

Jessie still had things to learn about people who lacked the kiss on the cheek and how-are-you-darling veneer. 'I'm going out with Dave,' she said. 'I'm taking your advice. Doing the teenage thing. Listening to my instincts, going with my heart.' She was proud of herself.

'If you must,' growled Magda. 'If it works for you. It's not the bit most folks go by. The heart is the second most important organ.'

Jessie said that she wouldn't ask what the most important organ was, but presumed Magda didn't reckon the brain.

'Go with the groin, baby,' Magda started shaking her pan on the burner. 'This omelette pan isn't working. Someone's been using my omelette pan. Do you hear me, Edie, somebody's been touching my omelette pan. And when I find out who . . .' she banged and raged. 'I'll kill them. No I won't. No killing's for wimps. I'll cut off their most important organ.'

Magda in the schoolroom, Rosie's hand in hers. Schoolrooms still smelt of schoolrooms. After all those years seeking enlightenment in education, they hadn't sorted that out.

'Your daughter has learning difficulties,' Miss Frazer said, leafing glumly through Rosie's maths jotter.

'You don't have to tell me. I know all about it. She's dyslexic.'

'We haven't ascertained that as yet.'

Magda felt a sudden rush of childish defiance. She was a big girl now, she could be rude to teacher.

'Surely it crossed your mind that something of the sort must be wrong. She gets all her numbers the wrong way round for a start,' Magda said.

'It could be carelessness.'

'It could be. But it isn't. She's a bright wee thing. She deserves a chance. She should be seeing a specialist.' Magda didn't want to get angry. Getting angry didn't help. But the blood was starting to hurtle through her veins. She was clenching, unclenching her fist. It wasn't this teacher. It wasn't this school. It was her past visiting her. The mis-understanding she'd suffered, the bullying. She now knew it would always be there. She didn't want that for Rosie. She gripped Rosie's hand so tightly that she whined and tried to pull it free. 'Why haven't you arranged for her to see a specialist? Why didn't you phone when you got no reply to your letters?'

It hadn't been a good day for Miss Frazer. A child had been sick on the floor in the morning, another had taken the class scissors and cut off her best friend's hair – trouble brewing there. Someone else had lost her packed lunch and another had gone home in the wrong shoes. Miss Frazer was dreaming of a hot bath and a huge gin and tonic. Magda Horn was the last person in the world she wanted to see. But then, even on a good day, Magda Horn was the last person in the world she wanted to see.

'I want to know,' Magda's voice cut insistently through her end-of-the-day mental and emotional fuzz, 'why Rosie hasn't been sent to a specialist?'

This time Miss Frazer got the rush of childish defiance. 'I don't know,' she countered shrilly. 'She just hasn't. So sue me.'

'Sue you,' Magda fumed. 'Sue you! Who do you think I am? This is the lower classes you are dealing with, pal. You won't find yourself in a pleasant, sunny little courtroom with some LA lawyer looking after you. Oh no. We don't do nice things like sue. We put shit through your letterbox. We pour sand in your petrol tank. We're nasty.'

Rosie's teacher looked amazed. She knew teaching had been a mistake. She should have gone into computers. 'Are you threatening me?'

Magda sank awkwardly into one of the tiny kiddie's desks. 'No,' she said. 'No, I'm not. I'm just still shouting at the old bag that stood in front of me all those years ago, trying to teach me. I think I've been shouting at her all my life.'

The room was silent. The silence getting thicker all the time.

'See,' Rosie, too young to recognise the nuances of quiet, turned to her teacher. 'See, that's why I'm the way I am. My mother's really embarrassing.'

CHAPTER 11

Ginny Howard was the Mareth Improvement Group. She bustled daily up and down the narrow village wynds, thinking only of improving and maintaining Mareth. She moved, bent double, along the shore in the evening glow, moving between the trees as the dying sun spread light on the water and eiders gently cooed and warbled, a gentle gossipy call, scooping up rubbish. Tutting loudly about litter-bugs she would pick up empty crisp bags and chocolate wrappers and pop them into the plastic bag she carried everywhere, for proper disposal later.

It was Ginny Howard who had organised the planting of a thousand daffodils either side of the village. The Mareth Improvement Group had eagerly waited for the fabulous drift of yellow that spring would bring to its roadside. But the fabulous yellow had appeared not at the roadside but in most of the gardens. There had been a deal of midnight trowelling of bulbs.

'Well,' said Ruby at the Spar, arms crossed in indignation. 'Why should all the visitors get the good of the daffs? It's those that live here should get the pleasure of them.' This seemed very plausible. More midnight trowelling till all that was left of Ginny's Wordsworthian vision was a few scrawny blooms blowing feebly.

It was Ginny Howard who had organised the Mareth Outdoor Music Festival when Edith Howell the local music teacher had trundled her piano out on to the harbour that had for the occasion been garlanded with bunting. But the heavens had opened and the Steinway ruined. Edith had stoically tried to play some Schubert, her favourite. But really, above the wind and the rain, nobody could hear a thing. She was still trying to get the Improvements Group to stump up for the damage to the piano. Solicitors letters were being exchanged, but no money was forthcoming.

It was Ginny Howard who decided that Mareth could easily win the Prettiest Village competition, if only they had hanging baskets. She had organised baskets overflowing with geraniums, lobelia and nasturtiums to be placed strategically throughout the village, high on lampposts and shopfronts. 'Keep these plants safe from vandalistic hands,' she warned.

Her improvements group had been hugely excited by this. Until the watering detail came to be organised. Suddenly people had urgent things to do – such busy lives. Walter, a retired librarian, had obtained at a substantial discount, he told the group, a piece of rather special watering

137

equipment. It was a tank that was strapped to the waterer's back. On one side of the tank was a hand pump, on the other a hose. By cranking the pump, the waterer could create enough pressure to send a formidable spray upwards through the hose.

'And thus,' said Walter, 'water the plants without actually having to carry ladder and watering can about the village.'

The group nodded approval, then spent time considering their shoes. Actual eye contact with Ginny somehow always ended in having to perform some vile chore. In public.

In the end, Ginny strapped the horrendously heavy tank on her own back and went lumbering through the village at dawn, looking like a Martian from a kitsch fifties B-movie. She set off at dawn because she didn't want anybody to see her. But of course they did. And they remarked upon it joyfully to her husband Jarvis, the local bank manager. There were no secrets in Mareth.

Feeling his standing in the community was at risk, Jarvis forbade Ginny to do any more watering. 'The plants can die,' he said. 'Stuff the Prettiest Village competition. You have become a laughing stock.' So Ginny caught Walter with some viciously piercing eye contact at the next Mareth Improvements Group meeting, and he found himself unwillingly appointed official waterer of the hanging baskets of Mareth. Ginny didn't think he was up to it, and spent mornings leaning out of her upstairs bedroom window with a pair of binoculars watching Walter's laboured progress through the streets with the tank of water on his back.

'Never thought water was so heavy,' he groaned, wheezing in dismay.

And Ginny, looming dangerously from her window, could be heard to cry, 'He's not doing it. He's missing the flowers. The spray is going right over the top of them on to the milk van. Good heavens, he's watering a cat on a windowsill now.' Hanging precariously from her window she yelled, 'Don't pump so much. Easy. It's an art.'

Recently Ginny had been composing a letter to the council pointing out that the harbour wall seemed to be constantly under repair. And why was that so? And was it some danger to the public? And if it was shouldn't they be told about it? But her concern about the harbour wall had been put on hold by the news sweeping through the village that Jim Horn's boatyard had gone into liquidation.

There could be a way here to get rid of that dreadful Ocean Café. She had to think about it carefully.

'Who owns the actual yard?' she asked her husband. 'Did Jim Horn lease it?' And more subtly she hoped, 'Does that Magda actually own the Ocean Café? Will she have to sell to pay Jim's debts?'

'Doubt it,' Jarvis said. 'She rents the place.'

Ginny said hmmm. Jarvis didn't want anything to happen to the café. He ate Magda's crêpes there most days. He was Mareth born and bred. The Ocean Café was part of his youth. He could remember being five years high, sitting on the dark red and chrome stools at the bar, little legs swinging. He had stared deep into the Alpine scene painted on the wall, imagining himself standing on the highest mountain top. He had stared so long, imagined so hard, he could smell the icy air. In his dream he spread his arms, stepped from the mountain top and flew into the deep deep blue, high above the peaks. He didn't want anything to happen to Magda's café. If it did he might even have to deal with Magda. And nothing, nobody terrified him more than Magda Horn. The woman had hairs on her armpits.

So, the living room wasn't up to snuff. John was past protesting. He mildly hoped that, if he complied, the strange malaise, the discontent would leave his wife and the old singalong lady would return.

They choose a red wallpaper with a gold fleur-de-lys pattern.

'Not the sort of thing you usually associate with small bungalow rooms,' the sales lady said breezily. The doors, skirting and ceiling were all white. The turquoise and pink swirling patterned carpet seemed suddenly inadequate. It was replaced and a leather chesterfield replaced the pink three-piece suite. Mary looked at it thoughtfully. Yes, she thought, the lady who sold her the frock wouldn't mind it here. It would do.

Mary had long stopped going to the pub. It was lonely, yes, and she missed her old pals. But singing in the pub wasn't on any more. It was cheap and she knew the lady who sold her the red dress was not the sort to drink half a dozen vodkas, link arms with her mates and sing 'Bye Bye Blackbird'. She had reached out to a new world with her red dress. It had no sequins, no frills, no buttons or buckles – none of the usual fripperies Mary demanded of party frocks. This was a dress for fierce social climbing. It would not take to Mary's old hearty round. Conga lines and karaoke were beneath it.

They had dipped deep into their savings to accommodate the frock into their household, but still John thought that if Mary wore it for at least one evening, she might get it out of her system.

'Why don't we book at the Captain's Table and have a really good night out? Dinner, wine, the works. You can wear your dress,' he said.

Mary nodded. 'Perhaps,' she said, knocking her chest with the side of her fist, wondering what the lady in the dress shop did for indigestion. She had considered phoning to ask but knew they'd think she was insane.

She was looking a bit better. Her hair was done and she was plastering her face with liposomes and vitamin E, hoping that a miracle might happen. 'Soon. We'll go soon.'

'When's soon?' John asked.

'Just soon,' Mary said. Soon was when the liposomes fulfilled the promise on the side of the little jar and some of her wrinkles smoothed out. She worried about actually wearing the dress on an outing. It would mean a trip in John's car. And could she be seen getting out of a ten-year-old rusting Ford with fluffy dice hanging in the back window? True, she conceded, the dice had come with the car and John just hadn't bothered to remove them. In fact they'd been a family joke. But still, fluffy dice and her in her red dress? She didn't know how to tell him. So she sat in her newly palatial living room with her red dress on, watching soaps.

'Why did you buy it?' Magda demanded when she came round to view the new living room.

Her mother had opened her arms, adoring the revered garment. 'All my life, all my bloody life I have never had what I wanted. Then I saw this. And I wanted it. I got it. And now it's mine. And now nothing can hurt me. I have this dress and I'm ready for anything.'

It wasn't easy stripping off. Jessie doubted her body. It had been over a year since she had let anyone see it. She had stretchmarks and her breasts sagged since her pregnancy. Back in her other world she had visited the gym twice a week. But here in Mareth she thought she had achieved a new understanding with her metabolism. She thought that the weight she put on eating Magda's cooking she took off again rushing around waiting tables. Recently, though, woefully considering her thighs, she'd come to the conclusion that Magda's cooking was making more inroads on her body than the rushing around serving tables could cope with.

Dave picked her up just after eleven when she finished work. The night was still and warm.

'I don't like the looks of this date,' Jessie complained. 'I wanted a posh dinner, wine. That sort of thing.'

'You're in Mareth and when in Mareth . . .' Dave said.

They drove along the coast beyond the village and turned down a rutted track leading to the sea and came out at Ardro Bay. Huge cliffs black in the night, white sand and a glassy sea. Jessie was stunned.

'This place is beautiful. I never knew it was here.'

'You have to be local,' Dave told her. They left the car and walked over the grass, rabbits scudding away as they passed. He carried a couple of Tupperware boxes.

'Is that dinner?' Jessie eyed it suspiciously. 'I was hoping for something grander.'

'Grander than what?'

'Grander than anything that can be carried in a plastic box.'

'Ah, the things that can go in a plastic box.'

He spread a rug on the sand. They sat together,

leaning against a rock. The breeze softly hit her face. His presence almost overwhelmed her. She played with the neck of her T-shirt. She knew she had a nervous rash on her throat. 'This is where I used to come in my youth,' Dave told her. 'We all did. Magda too. Did our courting here.' He smiled to himself, remembering. Jessie slipped off her espadrilles and dug her toes in the sand. She started playing with it, lifting soft handfuls, watching it run through her fingers.

'We were a tortured lot, except Magda. We were going to change the world. We played guitars and wrote poetry. Crap. All crap. Only Magda got it right.'

'But she wouldn't have written poetry,' Jessie said.

'No. She just said her thoughts out loud and some of them were in verse. Nothing written down, ever.'

A boat chugged out to sea, masts lit; the sound of its engine echoed and reverberated round the bay. A seagull cried. Dave picked up a pebble and threw it into the sea. It hit the water with a hollow plop.

'We all went on to university. Magda stayed. We were all Bob Dylan or Jim Morrison or Joni Mitchell. Only Magda was Magda. She didn't know who else to be.' He sighed. 'God I envy that woman. Take off your clothes.'

'What?'

'We'll swim. Skinny dipping at Ardro Bay. I'm a boy again.'

Jessie pulled off her T-shirt. Felt vulnerable.

'What sort of thoughts in verse did Magda have?'

Dave stood up and undid his belt. 'We wrote all that jingle jangle tumblin' twistin' leavin' in the mornin' farewell to the man who stands alone on the hill stuff and congratulated each other on how wonderful we were. Long-haired girls in flowy dresses, skinny boys in blue jeans, all aching to escape. And Magda'd come mincing by, the way she does in her tiny skirt, wiggling her hips and laughing at us. Arty farty arses, she'd say.'

Jessie took off her jeans. Sat in her knickers.

'Then she'd start. She did these absurd little verses to irritate us.'

He took off his jeans. No boxers, nothing. Jessie tried not to stare. This was cool. She did this all the time. She was cool. No she wasn't. The nervous rash on her throat was spreading.

'I bet,' Dave said, 'that every one of these people have forgotten the pretentious crap they wrote and I bet every single one of them remembers Magda's poems.'

'Tell me then,' Jessie cried. 'I need to know. I need to know everything about Magda.'

Dave put his arms round her. Strange, a new man. A person, thought Jessie, gets too used to one lover. Different skin, a new smell. A new routine. He ran his hands down her, slowly pulled off her knickers.

'I'll tell you one of Magda's more memorable

poems,' he whispered. He put his hands on her bum. She shivered. A poem by young Magda the rebel. Little boats out on the water, late gulls calling and the sounds of the sea, the earth was about to move.

'Tell me now, tell me now,
What do you see
When the Invisible Man goes for a pee?'

He laughed, 'Isn't that great? Doesn't it just slay you?'

Jessie was never so surprised. She laughed – but only at Dave laughing. Somehow she'd expected some rage, some emotional turbulence from somebody who had something to be angry about.

Dave couldn't stop smiling. 'I haven't thought about that for years. Did she up us all or what? She'd be down at the shore throwing off her clothes, yelling that stuff at us. Oh, she was always the best.'

'Tell me now. Tell me now. What do you see when the Invisible Man goes for a pee,' Jessie repeated it. And thought about it. And laughed. 'Were there any more?'

'Lots. Tell you later.'

They went together into the water. The cold hit their chests and the breath rushed from their lungs.

'It's all right once you get used to it. It's not that cold at all,' Dave gasped.

From the rocks jutting into the sea, a seal cried. A long low lonely howl drifted into the dark. A baby crying? Someone lost?

'Just a horny old seal,' said Dave. 'Oh God gimme some action. Howl howl. Got de blues.'

'It's beautiful,' said Jessie. A fulmar, always curious, came by swooping low. Who's this swimming in my sea? The chill eased. Jessie let go, sank into the water and moved with it. Let it wash over her, through her. She soaked her hair, and swam through the dark. The seal called again. They swam together. Said nothing. If she even mentioned how perfect this was she would spoil it. He did not touch her. They floated side by side, watching stars. He left her, ran back up over the sand and came back with his box.

'Food,' he said. He handed her a cheese sandwich.

'Is this it?' A hunk of cheese in huge slices of bread.

'Plain cheese, clean and strong. Not mascarpone with tomatoes or brie with bacon. Magda is spoiling you.'

Dave floated the picnic in a plastic box between them. Her fingers were wet and salty and nothing ever tasted so good.

'And now, this,' Dave said. From his second floating box he brought out six more boxes, each fitting into the one before, and a dozen candles. 'You can only do this when the sea's like this, glassy calm and friendly.' One by one he lit the candles, melted the end, dripped wax to make a hot pool in one of the boxes and stood the candle in it. He floated the boxes, flickering light, dancing on the water, round them. Their circle of lights in the water. The horny old seal slid off his rock to swim by and watch. Huge gleamy head, silky eyes.

Dave opened a small round silver flask and handed it to Jessie. Whisky burned down her throat, she coughed and wiped her mouth with the back of her damp hand.

'Lagavulin. Your favourite.'

'How did you know?'

'I know.'

They paddled the water, handing the flask back and forward. And when he kissed her, whiskied lips on hers, it was almost too much to bear. She curled her legs round his waist and held on to him. Whisky. Cheese. Mouthfuls of sea. His hands moved down to her bum and he slid into her. They sank. Underwater kissing. On each other, in each other and still not close enough. Breathless they broke apart and struggled up to the surface. Rose foaming and gasping. They shook the water from their faces, pulled air into their bursting lungs and started over.

Afterwards, they sat together watching the night, saying nothing. He pulled the rug round them.

'Ah well,' Dave was miffed, 'I used to be able to do it in water. I must be getting old.'

Jessie, busy desanding herself, didn't answer.

'That's the problem with beach sex.' Dave lent a wiping hand. 'Bloody stuff gets everywhere.'

'Everywhere,' Jessie agreed.

'Everywhere,' Dave said softly. Turned her to him. Started over.

Magda had drowning times of the day. Times when she would be doing chores she had done a million times before, that had become automatic enough to no longer need any thought. It was then her mind would drift and her past would flash before her and she would look up suddenly, gasping for air and furious.

She would be stirring a béchamel gazing soulfully into the pot, waiting for the slow white mass to turn glossy and her reasoning and logic would wilt; she'd only have her memories and instincts. She'd be drowning in the béchamel. Why did she have a mother who dressed in a hideous gold shirt with shiny sequins in a butterfly pattern across the tits and who sang 'Jailhouse Rock' in the pub? And why was that mother now sitting in a depressed heap in the living room she considered to be palatial waiting for life to catch up with the absurd promise of a red dress?

Stirring furiously, Magda would look up, 'Bloody cow,' she would yell. 'Arse.' And she would throw her wooden spoon across the kitchen. If the fury was especially bad she would hurl her pot of sauce too. The far wall was pock-marked with Magda's drowning times. Environmental Health Visitors eyed it suspiciously, 'There may be germs.'

'Stuff germs,' Magda told them. 'My life's on that wall.'

CHAPTER 12

Granny Moran waved her ancient arm in the direction of the harbour.

'Used to be a forest of masts,' she said. 'A forest.'

Jessie said oh and did it? And sipped her tea.

'See now,' Granny went on. 'Only four boats. Five if you count Jim's *Sad-Eyed Lady*. But that'll never see the water now. Will it?'

Jessie sipped her tea. She was shagged out. Could hardly walk and still had sand where she didn't want sand to be. She shifted itchily.

'Y'can't sit still, can you?' Granny said. They were side by side on the doorstep. 'Of course in them days there were fish. Now look, the fish've gone. In them days a man was away at the fishing four maybe five days. They'd be home for the weekend. Now look, they've got to go further and further to find the fish. They're gone weeks at a time. It's not right. Look at them young ones . . .'

Jessie stared at her mildly.

'They're all noise and running around getting into trouble. That's 'cos the men are away. Then the young ones won't stay. They'll leave Mareth

151

looking for work. The fish go then the folk go.'
She sighed.

'I remember the herring used to come by. The
sea turned silver. Silver. Used to be someone
waiting out on the point there by Ardro Bay and
when he saw them come he'd ride along the
coast ringing a bell. And we all knew the herring
were here. Course there were boats then. Proper
fishing. That was over seventy years ago. I've
seen the changes. That harbour was a forest of
masts.'

'Was it?' said Jessie. 'Must've been a sight.'

'That it was. And I'll tell you people weren't the
same. There was more caring. If a captain knew
one of his crew was drinking all his money, he'd
see the wife got the pay. Young Jim Horn, his
dad was an awful man,' Granny Moran shook her
head. 'Ooooh an awful man. Drinking! He could
drink. Well, his mother used to send young Jim
down to the harbour when the boats came in and
Captain Bowman used to give him the money to
take home. See you wouldn't get that now. It was
different then. A forest of masts it was. There wasn't
a family in Mareth didn't make a living from the
boats. When the fishing prospered everyone prospered. And if it didn't, everybody felt it. Folks stuck
together then. Freddie Kilpatrick has the garage
now. But he used to do the engines. Wasn't a thing
he didn't know about engines. Taught Jim Horn
all he knows.'

'Yes,' said Jessie, discreetly slipping her hand

down the back of her jeans to scratch and ease her sandy bits, Granny Moran put her liver-spotted hand on Jessie's knee.

'He's a fine boy, Jim Horn. A fine boy. Magda's fine too. A wee bit wild. But her heart's in the right place.'

Her heart is not the bit she's interested in, thought Jessie.

'Even if she can't do batter,' Granny Moran said.

'Batter?' said Jessie.

'Yes batter. She can't do batter. Oh, she can make them pancaky things, but she can't make a good battered fish like me. Like I used to make when I had the café.'

'You had the Ocean Café?'

'Oh yes,' said Granny Moran. 'Still do. It's mine. Just let Magda cook in it. She rents it. But she can't do batter.'

Well fancy that, thought Jessie. It took her mind off her sandy bits.

'When I had it, all folks wanted was fish and chips. Came for miles. Things were simple. But then I could do batter.'

'Right,' said Jessie. 'Batter matters.'

'Yes. Now I bought the café from an Italian couple. They had it first – did fish and chips like me. And it was them gave me the secret of batter. But I had to promise not to give it away. And I haven't. It's with me yet.'

Magda had pleaded for the secret of batter. But Granny Moran considered her promise to be sacred and wasn't letting go of it. Batter bothered Magda, but then she knew that most cooks were bedevilled by something. George at the Captain's Table for example couldn't do sponges. They never rose for him. And George told her that the chef who taught him couldn't do omelettes. Still she worked on her batter and her failures contributed many a mark on her drowning wall.

'Oh yes,' mused Granny Moran, 'in them days I just crossed the road and bought the fish straight from the boats. Filleted it and gutted it myself out the back and you never tasted better. Then –' she drifted into her own musings – 'when the herring came they laid them out on the harbour wall and it turned silver. Silver with the scales. It was different then . . .' she waved her ancient arm towards the harbour. '. . . It was—'

'A forest of masts?' suggested Jessie, looking wistfully out at the horizon.

'Yes,' Granny looked at her in surprise. Now how did she know that?

Jim didn't know what to do. It's over, it's over, my life's over, over and over, the words spun through his head. It came out of nowhere and haunted him. When nobody was looking he shook his head wildly to get rid of it. But it kept coming back.

'It's over.'

At first he walked. He walked through Mareth round the harbour right out to the end to stare at the sea, watch seals passing. When he was done staring he walked back into the village along the shore out the other side past the new clifftop bungalows that only incomers were daft enough to buy – the gales hit them full-blast come winter – and for miles along the beach till he was exhausted. Striding, striding. It's over. It's over. It's over. He recognised a dementia creeping within him. He was facing emotional collapse. He stopped striding.

He stayed home and watched daytime television and only stopped when he caught himself and Lipless seriously discussing the sleazy ethics of the bitch in the afternoon soap who replaced her wheelchair-bound husband with a blond dude with perfect pecs. He might have cooked had not Magda's prowess overawed him. He read but he wasn't an indoors sort and headaches plagued him. He was alone, moving by day through a nervy nightmare and couldn't wait to get to bed at night to get away from it. He slept deeply, dreamlessly. But in the morning there it was again, the ache.

'It's over. It's over. My life is over.'

It was a slow time for rumours in Mareth. The new fancy waitress at the Ocean Café was seeing Non-existent Dave. But since, according to the rumour anyway, she was going to go away with him and become non-existent herself there wasn't a lot to gossip about. So for the moment people settled for the supermarket rumour. Jim's boatyard was to be bought by an international supermarket chain who were going to build a hypermarket. The hypermarket had started as a small supermarket but as the rumour spread the size and quality of the building had grown.

Frankie in his ironmonger's had welcomed the prospect at first. Then, upon reflection, gazing at his window display of lavatories and clay pots, thought not. He didn't think the sort of folks that would come flooding into Mareth to a hyper-market would be likely to come buying lavatories or clay pots. And furthermore he didn't want to sell any to them. He did not like dealing with strangers, not in droves anyway. One at a time was fine: you could look at them closely and make up a life for them, which helped you know if you liked them or not. Trouble with strangers – you just decided they might be an OK sort of person, someone to have a beer with at the Ocean Café – then you never saw them again. Strangers were queer folk.

Freddie Kilpatrick at the garage didn't see much profit coming his way either. Unless of course he could see his way to helping some of the incoming cars to break down in the huge car park they were going to be building. Or he could build a car wash for motorists to use on their way home. He could install new self-service petrol pumps, sell sweets and flowers and sandwiches. Get his wife to make them. Perhaps serve hot coffee and teas. Sell souvenirs of Mareth, little mugs and key rings with

A Present from Mareth on them. He'd be rich. Holidays in Florida. He looked out at the rubble and bits of engine cluttering his forecourt. Plans, water rates, surveyors, then after everything was built he'd have to stay open till nine maybe ten at night to pay for it. He'd end up with a heart attack. He clutched his chest imagining the huge pain that would hit suddenly. He'd read about such things in his wife's *Woman's Own*. No. Better not bother.

Ruby at the Spar was incensed. What was wrong with your own local grocery shop? Service with a smile she yelled, thumping her fat fist on the counter. 'I even sell garlic and funny peppers for those that use them. Look,' she waved grandly at her shelves. 'Toilet rolls, light bulbs, frozen peas. There is nothing for sale at a hypermarket that you couldn't buy here.'

Jim meantime found Joe's old mountain bike abandoned and rusting in the back yard. He oiled it, tightened the chain, raised the saddle, pumped up the tyres and set off with no destination in mind. He just wanted to go. He cycled round the coast to Ardro Bay and stood for a while looking at the water, ripples. He tried not to think. Thinking did you no good at all. There was only the movement of water, the sun on his face and the shrill cry of summering terns. The air was warm, smelled salty, sea fresh. On a whim he took off his clothes and waded into the waves.

He moved strongly out to the far rocks. He'd

been swimming these waters since he was a boy. A small wind ruffled the surface, cool on his face. The effort shortened his breath. To hell with it all, he thought. Moving further and further out. It got deeper, movement easier. He swam out of the bay. Away, away and away, he said, spitting out a mouthful of water.

He stopped, treading water, looked ahead. Eyes at surface level. There was only water ahead. Miles and miles of moving water. A gull circled above and he could die now. It would be all right. If he looked down he couldn't see his legs moving in the depth. He let go and sank. Soundless in the deep, shafts of light could hardly penetrate more than a couple of feet. He kicked and shot up, burst back into the world surging out of the water. The shore was miles away. Christ, I've swum further than I thought. He could see the bike lying and his clothes, two tiny misshapen heaps far far away, and in a mild panic started swimming back towards them.

Suddenly, sun on his face, sea on his skin, he was smiling. Songs from distant times in his life started humming, uninvited, through his head. Guitar riffs that played and sang through the days when he grew from boy to man. He remembered. He remembered the summer of his last year at school, his seventeenth summer. They had come here, a whole crowd of people, to skinny-dip and drink cider. They'd snuck off into the rocks and made love, first salty tasting sex and never to be

158

so sweet again. They'd built huge bonfires and dreamed. They were going to leave Mareth and be great. Great musicians, great writers, great doctors. They were seventeen, mediocrity wasn't written into their plans. He had never wanted to leave. Even then he loved the place. It was comfortable, it fitted him. Now the great doctors and great musicians and great writers were drifting back. They were insurance men and they were salesmen and they were school teachers. They were all ordinary. When they looked at him he could see a certain envy behind the 'Great to see you again' greeting. You are the one who should be ordinary, they were thinking. What was that all about?

He remembered his mother and father. His father drank and his mother cleaned up after him. His father had not been a bawdy drunk. He drank and sang a little and apologised for being drunk and said he'd never drink again. Next day he would be drunk again and apologising again.

His mother would bundle him out, overly wrapped against the chill. He had waddled up the same wynd, little bear of the morning, to the same school his children now went to, and they sat in the same classrooms he had once sat in. But they were not sitting rigid with fear as he'd been. His teacher wielded his belt and called for the class to chant their times tables. Every single child in a sweat of fear and prickly heat from the layers of fierce clothing. Mistakes were beaten out of you, glories rewarded with a grunt. He remembered teachers incandescent with rage at the smallest misdemeanour. If they just spoke they were dragged to the front of the class and beaten.

'We were seven or eight years old,' Jim said out loud. 'We were tiny.'

What was that all about?

Now here he was. About to lose everything, when all he'd done was graft. What was that all about?

When he at last reached the shore he ran wildly through the surf waving his arms, yelling and screaming at the top of his voice. 'What was that all about. What was that all about . . . ?'

Back home hours later, awakened muscles aching, he put the bike back in the yard and looked about. The children's old sandpit still there, neglected, weed-strewn after they'd grown and left it behind. The Horns' back yard was disgracefully cluttered: bits of things, toys, a rusting pair of shears, Magda's old washing machine that they'd been meaning to throw out for three years. There was a scrubby lawn, and blowing on the washing line the checked blue and white tablecloths from the Ocean Café, brought home and laundered every night. 'God we're messy,' he said out loud.

When Magda came home and asked him what he'd been doing all day he told her he'd been out in the yard and thought he might plant some potatoes.

★   ★   ★

160

It was ten o'clock on Saturday night. Shore boys were out in force. They sat in the bus shelter hollering. Their cries, a loud raw and primal noise, were incomprehensible. They passed cider around, threw the empty bottles at passing cars. They drank more and played a ghetto-blaster. Full volume, there was only noise, obliterating brain cells, obliterating thought. Songs about people being hung by their dicks and getting their arses sewn up seriously rapped out, ricocheted and boomed round the bay.

'That's not very nice,' Jessie said.

Magda looked weary, 'There you go with that N word again. Keep telling you no good comes of nice.'

'It seems to be some sort of sound trap.' Jessie pulled back the curtain to look out.

Magda nodded. 'Yes,' she said wistfully, 'good acoustics for when you're needing a sound track to your life. We used to do that. Same life. Different sound track.' She shoved aside the curtain to look out. A single shore boy had broken away from the pack and was leaping ritually on a car roof. 'But we didn't do that.'

She banged on the window, 'Cut that out,' she yelled. Shore boys didn't scare her. She knew all their mothers and their grandmothers. She lost enough money through her own rage and swearing and didn't intend to lose more through young bloods leaping on her customers' cars. She stepped out of the café, stood at the door, 'Bugger off the lot of you,' she shouted, waving them off with a sweep of her arm. They laughed at her. She steamed over to them, grabbed the car roof trampoliner by the arm, then by the collar of his Adidas sweatshirt.

'I said bugger off you little arsehole. One swift movement of my knee and I'll render you a virgin for ever, you little shit.'

Windows flew up, Shore residents hung out, bawling encouragement. 'Tell him, Magda.' 'Nut him for me, Magda.' A car moved slowly by. Inside, sitting removed from reality on velour seats, Kiri Te Kanawa soaring on the in-car CD obliterating all street sounds, Ginny and Jarvis Howard watched. 'That Magda Horn is so gross,' Ginny shuddered, but could not stop watching. Inside Kiri sang. Outside Magda raged in what seemed like silence.

The boy sniggered. They all sniggered. There was something. A movement of the eyes, a leaning of skinny teenage bodies towards the men's lavatory on the quay. Magda shoved her captive away. Without thinking she shouldn't she stormed through the door marked Gents. Inside was covered with graffiti. She recognised one word – Janis. She didn't have to be able to read, the walls spoke. They spoke dirty. She returned to the café.

'Jessie, come with me. Come see this.'

Jessie followed her. 'I can't go in here. It's the men's loo.'

162

'Just come,' Magda said. 'You have to read this and tell me. I need to know . . .' Jessie followed her in.

Janis is a hole, was sprayed large and red over one wall. The place smelled foul. Water ran, a tank gurgled. Janis is a great fuck was sprawled on another wall. She turned. I've shagged Janis Horn written hugely on the wall opposite the Janis is a hole wall. Underneath the shagging boast someone else had written so have I and another had added me too. And someone else asked, who hasn't?

'I don't think you need to tell me,' Magda said. 'I may be stupid but I'm not that stupid. I know these words. You don't have to be able to read to know these words.'

Jessie apologetically read the walls out loud. Magda felt sick. Her knees were weak. She could hardly breathe. Her hand flew to her mouth. 'Oh, Janis,' then, covering her face with her hands, shook her head. 'Oh no, Janis.'

Slowly they went outside. Shore boys scattered, laughing. Magda stood, arms by her side, breathing deeply. 'I need to go home,' she said.

Janis was slumped on the sofa watching a video, cars overturned in flames, guns roared and beefy men shouted muthafucka. Magda stormed over to her and slapped her hard. Her head reeled. It was a vicious blow. She gasped. 'What was that for?' she cried. Her hand flew to the battered, swiftly reddening cheek.

'You know,' Magda shouted. 'You know damn fine what it's for.'

'No I don't,' Janis shouted back.

Magda put her face close to her daughter's. 'Yes you do,' she hissed. 'You can't hide it from me. I know everything. I've seen it.'

Janis went quiet.

'You slut,' Magda yelled. 'You slut.'

Janis sulked, 'If I am I got it from you.'

Magda lifted her hand again. Janis didn't flinch, stared defiantly at her mother, 'Didn't I?' she said.

Magda lowered her hand. Her rage had lost its edge.

'What have you seen?' Jim wanted to know.

'The filth written about this one in the men's on the shore.'

Janis winced.

'Janis Horn's a great shag. I've shagged Janis. Janis is a hole.' Magda threw up her arms in despair. Janis flushed scarlet.

'For Christ's sake, girl, what have you been up to? You know what people are like round here. You'll be a slag for ever.'

Janis no longer met her gaze.

'You can't go by what you read on toilet walls,' Jim protested.

Magda rounded on him. 'Oh yes you can. It's the truth isn't it? You've been shagging all these blokes, haven't you?'

Janis shrugged and nodded.

164

'See,' said Magda. 'I knew it. People write the truth on toilet walls. If you're ever going to write any sort of truth, where else are you going to write it?'

CHAPTER 13

It was inevitable that Jessie's old friends would seek her out. It seemed to Magda that they came in batches. They did not venture to places as far flung as Mareth alone. They needed support. But curiosity gripped them. They were compelled to see where Jessie was living and find out why she had abandoned them.

Trish and Lou arrived in Lou's Beetle convertible. They slammed the car doors and gazed about them, blinking. Such light, such space – hard to deal with. Staring out to sea they could almost feel their pupils shrink, coping with the dazzle. So this was the place. It was stark and simple, a row of houses facing the sea, a café, and they led such complex lives. Mystified, they looked around.

'What do people do here?' Trish said to Lou. They shook their heads, mutually baffled. Tentatively they climbed the stairs to Jessie's flat and knocked at the door. She let them in. She wasn't sure if she wanted them here. Her old life would not easily overlap and blend in with her new one. She didn't like her flat when she saw it through their eyes and shrank from their unspoken criticism. Plainly they were working hard at not commenting on the smell – unwashed agoraphobics – gosh, she'd forgotten about that. She'd got used to it.

'Oh yes,' Trish said. There was a long silence and she raked through her mind for something reasonable to say. At last she came up with, 'Cosy.' Jessie knew they would talk about her when they went away. She tortured herself imagining what they'd say. She opened a bottle of Australian Chardonnay. Lou was surprised that you got such a thing here.

'What did you expect, Newcastle Brown and Irn Bru?' Jessie snapped. 'Actually, Magda has quite a good cellar.'

'Ah, Magda,' Trish smiled secretively. She'd heard from Alex about Magda, was planning to meet her, to look her over and report back. Jessie knew that when she left the room to fetch glasses from the kitchen they'd exchange looks, mouth surprise. She hated that. They'd be raising their eyebrows at her sideboard, hideously large, darkly wooden, filling the room. And her carpet, Jessie grinned. Yes her carpet was truly loathsome. You could work up a lather hating it. She'd come to terms with it months ago, in fact was developing a fondness for it.

'So you're working as a waitress?' Trish asked as Jessie came back into the room. There was a stiffness in her tone. They were concerned for Jessie and the turn she'd let her life take. It seemed to them that Jessie hadn't forsaken her old life, she had forsaken them, their friendship. Jessie nodded.

'Why on earth?' Trish wanted to know.

'Need the money,' Jessie said. 'And there's not a lot of call for book editors round here.'

'I could believe it,' Trish agreed. 'You could of course go back to your old job.' She crossed the room and kissed Jessie on the cheek the way she would have if they were meeting in some city bar. She'd been so surprised at the flat she'd forgotten to do it when she arrived.

'We miss you, Jessie. When you left we phoned and phoned. But you didn't answer. Where were you?'

Jessie sat down, stuck her hands in her pockets, leaned back. 'Somewhere inside my head or striding maniacally round the harbour,' she said. 'I can't come back yet. Can't face it? Need a change? Too far to travel from here? Pick your answer. Actually I quite enjoy waiting on tables. There's something totally physical about it. And mindless. There's a freedom . . .' She drifted off, explaining her decision more to herself then either of her friends. 'But why travel? Why live here anyway? I mean, what do people do here?' Lou needed to know.

'They eat. They watch television. They drink. They think about things. They chat. Mostly I suspect they gossip and . . . what do people do anywhere?' Jessie asked.

'Well darling,' Trish smiled. 'If you don't know . . .'

'They have relationships,' Lou interrupted.

'Oh that,' Jessie curled her lip. 'Been there. Done that. Read the book. Saw the film. Didn't buy the T-shirt. Got pregnant. It didn't fit.' She pulled up her knees, heaved her sweater over them and stared morosely ahead.

She had thought she was over it. It was weeks since she had been swamped with sudden rage, or found herself motionless in a torpor of overwhelming sadness. She thought her grieving was over. She no longer mourned the child she knew so well and hadn't got to meet. She now realised that she would never stop grieving. Maybe it wouldn't hurt so much.

'Oh bugger it all,' she said. 'Bugger everything.'

'Alex is well,' Trish said, pointedly refilling her glass.

'Oh him,' Jessie sneered.

'You know, of course, that he's seeing somebody?' Lou said.

Jessie nodded.

'She's a lot like you,' Lou went on.

Jessie nodded again. 'That figures. Every shirt Alex buys is blue. Every pair of shoes is brown. Every suit is charcoal grey. He had a rackful of polka-dot ties. If this woman looks like Jessie, you can bet the woman before me looked like Jessie too.'

Lou considered this a moment and considered Jessie a moment. Was she up to any sort of banter? Then she said, 'You probably all look like his mother.'

Jessie grinned widely then pulled the neck of her sweater over her head, hiding herself, the shame and disgrace of being a nice, respectable person in a torridly self-seeking world.

'Oh God,' muffled cry. 'I do believe you're right.'

'Yes,' Trish joined in. 'Every time we went out you always complained that men thought you were nice.'

Jessie grinned, remembering nights they'd had, bars they haunted, conversations and confessions. She thought they mattered more to each other than their husbands or lovers did. They worked up huge phone bills swapping tales. Even when there was nothing to say they could talk for hours. Every upset, every embarrassing moment was drawn out and discussed. Jessie sometimes thought that she lived her life not for the moment but for the pleasure of talking about the moment afterwards with her friends. She missed them, and she forgave them in advance for the horrible things they would say later about the sideboard and carpet that were, after all, not her fault.

'You were always complaining you were a failed hussy. All the men you ever met wanted to take you home to meet their mother,' Trish said.

'And they always liked you,' Lou grinned.

'True. True,' Jessie smiled amiably. 'But now I'm working on it. I'm working at being a cow. It's hard, but someone's got to do it.'

Jessie took them downstairs to the Ocean Café. They stared in disbelief at Magda. Trish smiled triumphantly and remarked that she thought people stopped looking like that in 1966. 'Before I was born,' she added, smirking even more triumphantly. She lit a Marlboro and watched the door Magda had disappeared through. Magda served them monkfish with olives, tomatoes, and a side dish of spaghetti with courgettes. Afterwards she brought them strawberries with a jug of ice-cold vanilla cream. She would have flavoured them with balsamic vinegar, but had peered into Lou's car and seen the mess. Twix wrappers, Marlboro packs, a gin bottle, a chequebook, three coats and a jacket and umpteen folders heaped on the back seat. There was even a coffee cup on the floor by the driver's seat. Clear evidence of a ludicrous life. 'Coarse, bottom feeders,' she said to Granny Moran. 'Secret chocolate eaters, stress and not enough good sex.'

'Right enough,' the old lady agreed. 'A bit like yourself these days.' Magda said something like hymph and shrugged. But she refused Trish's money. 'Friends of Jessie's,' she said, 'and the eavesdropping was too good to charge you. All that relationship stuff. And speaking about other people's problems.'

'A glimpse of our busy city lives,' Trish patronised. Magda, who had heard the 1966 remark, waved her off. 'Oh, I think I know your life. Didn't it used to be a movie with Jacqueline Bisset?'

'Hardly,' Trish said. Lou watched. Watching was

Lou's forte. She was a skinny skinny bottle blonde with a serious Marlboro habit. She looked out of place on her brief self-conscious walk through Mareth, from car to Jessie's door. But then she looked out of place anywhere but in a darkened bar, drink in hand. She didn't engage in conversation much, spent her socialising time looking round making sure there was nobody skinnier, more weirdly dressed than her. She was expert at the city bar game of dismissive glances and instant judgements. She could do little else.

They drove several miles in silence. Then Lou said to Trish, 'God that woman can cook. And in such a place. Waste really.'

And Trish replied, 'Jacqueline Bisset. Cheek. I'd have thought early Katharine Hepburn or Jeanne Moreau at least.'

It had been a while since the Horns had gone out as a family. But here they were in force, scrubbing the walls of the men's lavatory on the shore. Rosie stayed with Edie in the café.

'I don't want to answer any awkward questions,' Magda said.

Rosie, however, told Edie she knew what shagging was. 'I'm special,' she said. 'I've got a special teacher. And now I can read some bits of the magazines under Joe's bed.'

'I'll bet you can,' Edie said. 'You'll have to bring me one.'

Janis hung her head and muttered darkly to

herself. She vowed to leave Mareth. When scrubbing with Vim and bleach didn't remove Janis's disgrace, Jim and Lipless started to paint over it, cursing about the match on television they were missing.

It was too humiliating for Janis. She took off, running out of the small utilitarian building fast as her Doc Martens could carry her, her crochet jacket flapping behind her. She was crying so much she could hardly see. There was a bus waiting at the stop. She jumped on it. She would leave Mareth now. She would never come back. Ever. She didn't care what happened to her, she just wanted away. She sat shivering on the back seat. Mascara'd tears streaked her cheeks, her nose ran. She could hardly breathe.

Magda, stepping out for a minute, leaning on the wall, saw the bus leave, saw Janis cowering in the back, and opened her throat, 'STOP THAT BUS!' When the bus didn't stop, Magda took off after it, running full tilt along the road, ignoring cars coming towards her.

'Don't you think you can get away from me,' she bellowed. The bus gathered speed. And so did Magda.

Lipless and Jim came out to watch, paintbrushes dripping. Jessie stepped out of the café and Granny Moran leaned out of her window.

Magda caught up with the bus and began to batter on the back with her fists. 'Stop this bus.' It lumbered slowly on, ignoring her. Magda at full steam, ran alongside banging furiously on it. 'You are not going to run away. You are not.' Janis sunk low in her seat, sniffing and choking, wiping her nose with the back of her hand. Oh please let this not be happening. Oh please bus gather speed and leave this dreadful woman behind.

'GET OFF THIS BUS,' Magda screamed. 'Get off. I won't let you leave. There's too much to do.' The driver, at last realising something was happening, slowed down. Magda didn't. She carried on running beating the side as she went.

'What about me?' she yelled. 'What about me?'

The bus stopped. Janis emerged slowly, sheepishly, looking round, checking that none of her friends had been witness to this bizarre event. She walked up to her mother. 'What do you mean? What about you? This is about me, who cares about you?'

Magda stared hard at her daughter. 'I bloody care about me. And so do you.'

The pubs in Mareth rarely closed. They pulled the curtains so that no chink of light showed to any patrolling late-night lawman. By midnight the place looked lifeless, but behind closed doors the bars were lit and busy. It wasn't really that important to hide illicit drinking from the police. Off duty they joined the secret drinkers behind the curtains. But hiding the goings-on was a mark of respect; local police did not want to arrest people they'd gone to school with, and perhaps see them heavily fined. People had to live and let live.

Over the years Magda had curbed her drinking habits. 'There is a time in your life,' she said, 'when you realise that even though you're still young, your digestive system isn't. Know what I mean?' She slugged her vodka and coke thoughtfully. 'You're out late, drinking. And you get this slow shrivelling feeling in your stomach. It's like once you pass forty your digestive system becomes unionised. It demands regular hours, won't function before seven in the morning and after eight at night. "You can do what you like," it says. "But I'm knocking off. Drink what you want, eat what you will. But you're on your own, pal."'

Tonight Magda was on her own. Life was getting gruelling, something tangible to darkly whine about, and a huge amount of vodka might ease the ache. Edie and Lipless were drinking at the bar. Magda and Jessie sat at a table, a bottle between them. Magda poured.

'I used to drink whisky. But I thought I was going to die from it.' She raised her eyebrows. It was the nearest to shame she ever got. Considering drunken moments past she brushed some crumbs from her skirt stretched taut round her stomach bulges. Then played with the collar of her pink denim shirt un-buttoned to mid-cleavage, a little distracting fidget to take her mind off the atrocious moments that were flooding back to her. The sweat of her evening's cooking had left her with little make-up. There was no concealing the lines round her eyes, or the unkindnesses time and life had done to her skin.

'Malt. Drink it and it's like drinking silk. You don't get drunk, you slip into a world where you are invincible and understand everything. Know what I mean?'

Jessie looked at her. 'Why did you give it up if it's so wonderful?'

'Open pores. Foul breath. Decaying liver. Loss of brain cells. Black holes in my memory. Waking up in the morning wondering how did I get here into this morning and knowing from the feeling in the back of my throat that I've been snoring loudly, mouth wide open, saliva dripping. Looking across the pillow, seeing someone sleeping beside me and thinking who the hell is that? Know what I mean?'

Jessie looked appalled. Couldn't hide it. Magda's heart swelled. There was nothing so gratifying as shocking someone, especially someone so extravagantly full of her own rightness as Jessie.

'No,' Magda continued. 'I don't expect you do know. Too much control.'

Jessie put her feet up on a chair and said that she didn't think she had too much control. And anyway what was wrong with control? 'I mean I try to plan my life to get the most out of it. Don't you?'

Magda spread her arms. 'I'd like to. But my planning usually comes to nothing. My life has to be elastic-sided to allow room for the unexpected.'

'Elastic-sided life,' Jessie said flatly.

'You know what I mean. When life smacks you

in the face and your plans disintegrate . . .' She held out her hand, fingers spread open. Her planned life disintegrating through them.

Jessie sniffed.

'Things just happen,' Magda went on. 'Look at all these people here. Do you think they were planned? Most of them just happened. Right now Jessie Tate, in some council bedroom on some divan bed some teenage girl is getting screwed for the first time, looking up at the posters of her nonsensical heroes and thinking "is this what it's all about? – I don't reckon this much." And in nine months' time another little unplanned person will come into the world. Right now some old lady is lumping up some long road carrying a bag full of Safeway fast food and she's thinking, "How did this happen to me? This isn't what I wanted." Don't get me started. Planning, what good does planning do?'

'It's just after midnight, Magda,' Jessie scoffed. 'I don't think any old lady is lumping anywhere with a bag of fast food from Safeway.'

Magda refilled her glass. 'So c'mon. What just happened to you?'

'When my life stopped going as planned? I had a stillborn baby. I needed a little bit more than an elastic mentality to cope. I fell apart. Now, though, I wonder if it hadn't been that, would it have been something else? I was due to fall apart.'

'Me,' said Magda, 'I fall apart a little more every day.' She swigged her vodka, looking over the rim of her glass at Lipless and Edie. She could tell they were talking about her.

'She's getting worse,' Edie said.

'I've noticed,' said Lipless. They both whispered.

Magda poured another drink. She shut her eyes and let Aretha Franklin drift through her. If she got it right, every corner of her mind would be taken up with that voice and . . . And she would not worry about her mother hiding from the world in her newly palatial living room. Or her daughter who seemed to be screwing just about every male in Mareth. Though recently Janis had seemed to be returning to the world. Yesterday she had actually smiled and this morning . . .

'Janis ate a bit toast this morning,' Magda said suddenly. And Jessie nodded.

'Yes,' Magda nodded. 'With honey. I think she even kept it down.'

Jessie nodded again. And reached for the bottle. She was past feeling good. The room wasn't yet reeling, but she didn't trust her legs. 'Honey,' she said. 'Honey's good.'

Then there was Jim. Magda snorted, Jim. He had been seized by some sort of hyper-activity which unnerved her. He had planted their back yard with potatoes and other vegetables. Magda was sure it was too late in the year to get a crop and had told him so.

'Rubbish,' he sweepingly dismissed her. After the great planting he'd started on the house, polishing, scrubbing, wiping, cleaning out cupboards. It was hell. Magda no longer knew where anything was. Not that it mattered. She spent so little time at home anyway.

'There's not a lot of sex going on in this house these days,' she complained to him. Then, wondering where exactly Janis got up to whatever she was getting up to, 'At least if there is I'm not getting any of it.' Jim told her to bugger off and did she think he should paint the hallway white again or would she like a colour this time?

'Why are you painting when you could be in bed with me having sexual intercourse?' Magda wanted to know. 'Stuff painting.'

Jim burst out laughing. Formal language didn't suit Magda; when she said sexual intercourse it sounded like some polite afternoon activity to be accompanied with tea and scones. Magda was offended. After that they stopped speaking. After that they avoided eye contact. After that they moved aside when they met in the hall, in the living room, in bed no touching. No contact at all.

Magda was horny. Life without sex wasn't easy. The less sex she had the more she thought about sex. She shifted from foot to foot whilst she cooked, she crossed and uncrossed her legs when she sat. She sighed. She snorted. She snapped. When Jim had been away at the fishing before he opened the boatyard, she had relieved her ache. Men were easy. There was always one at the café interesting enough to take home. Only now her children were old enough to see what was going on. Besides, Jim was home all day. Damn the man, she muttered icily. And across the room they were still discussing her.

'Her omelette pan,' Edie raised her eyes. 'If I hear any more about that bloody omelette pan . . .' She didn't finish, couldn't conjure up anything dire enough.

'She hasn't thrown it, though?' Lipless asked.

'Oh no,' Edie shook her head. 'She loves that pan. Says she had it perfect and someone's been meddling.'

'God help whoever it is if she finds out . . .'

'She throws other things, though. And argue.' Edie leaned forward and dropped her voice even lower. She watched, checking Magda wasn't watching her. 'Argue. I've never seen her so bad. The other day we had this really loud bloke in. He was shouting, waving his arms about, annoying everybody. Proper prick. And Magda comes storming from the kitchen, tells him to shut up. And he says no. And she calls him a rude, stupid fart and he says, what did you say? And she says he's a stupid fart. And he says he's never been spoken to like that in his life. She says you mean nobody's ever told you what a stupid fart you are? And he says no. So she says well, ain't life full of surprises? Then he refused to pay his bill. And he'd had lobster.' Money mattered to Edie. Her father, a newsagent, had instilled sound business sense in her. She'd put money into Magda's business planning a twelve-year burst of hard graft then

180

retirement. Fifteen years on, retirement was drifting further and further away.

Aretha sang. Magda thought about sex, imagined kissing, being kissed. She ripped open some faceless man's shirt, licked his chest. Slid her hands round his bum. His tongue moved in her mouth and his hand pushed up her pink shirt.

'Oh . . .' she said. Told herself to stop. In a minute she'd break up the little discussion between Lipless and Edie at the bar. She turned to Jessie who was lying back now, resting her glass on her forehead, singing softly, 'What was wrong with your baby anyway?' Magda asked. 'Why did it die?'

'Die?' said Jessie. 'Why?' She looked alarmed. Nobody had ever asked that. 'He just died,' she said sadly.

'Nothing just dies,' Magda disagreed. 'Everything dies of something. Flu, a broken heart . . . something.'

'It was his kidneys, they said. And there was something wrong with his heart and lungs,' she spoke flatly. For a second she was back in the ward with the doctor poised at the end of her bed, ready to waft off, white coat floating behind him. He spoke loudly. Everyone could hear what was wrong with her baby. Everybody knew it had died. Everybody knew she had failed.

'It would have been a sickly child,' Magda said.
'So the doctor said,' Jessie agreed.
'But it's your fault. The heart and lungs and

that? You did it, somehow you did something wrong?' Magda smiled slightly. Jessie winced. How did she know that? She didn't reply. She could deal with everything except sympathy.

'Never mind,' she stared into the alcoholic distance. 'There's nothing wrong with death. Time of your life.' She flapped her arms. And flew. Lying in her chair, tears in her eyes.

'Guess who you've been talking to.' Magda gently patted her arm and got up to change the tape, leaving Jessie to rearrange her face and wipe her eyes. 'We'll have to get you a huge tartan dressing gown and a bag of bread to feed the gulls every morning.'

She put on 'Let It Bleed'. Started to sing along, swaying. Outside a boat chugged noisily into the harbour. Gulls cried. Fisherman shouted as they tied up at the quay. They floodlit the deck so that they could sort out the catch. Inside Magda sang along with Mick. Lipless and Edie watched her, silenced at last. Lipless swigged a bottle of Bud.

Magda loosened up more, spread her arms, writhed. 'Oh I used to love this. Things I've done to this. Ceilings in my life and this song playing.'

Lipless stared down into his beer, feigned dis-interest. Magda shook her body at him. 'I love to dance. Don't you love to dance? I could boogie the night away. Couldn't you Jessie?'

Jessie struggled to sit upright. 'No. I'm past it. Too old to dance.'

'You're never that. Besides you're not old.'

'OK. I'm too middle-aged to dance. Too sad to dance.'

'You'll do fine, Jessie. Dance if you want to. Nobody's looking. Only them.' Magda nodded to Edie and Lipless. The music roared, tumbled frenetically. Lipless, on account of his missing lip, was having trouble drinking from the bottle. Lager dripped down his chin on to his sweatshirt.

'D'you miss kissing, then, Lipless?'

Lipless snorted. He wasn't admitting to missing anything. He watched Magda dance, hip-swaying round the room. She was alone, alone with the Stones and her memories. Her head was filled with the rattle of guitars and the howl of harmonicas. Nothing else.

'She's still got a great body,' Lipless said to Edie. And sighed. 'Indeed. Ah indeed. Pity she's such a cow.' He swigged more. Dribbled more. 'I mean I wouldn't have her for my woman. Actually I pity Jim.' Drunkenly he pointed his bottle at Magda. 'Great arse. But she speaks too much. Things she says. She's not very—'

Magda, still dancing, was listening eagerly. Vibrantly amused. 'I'm not very what?' she demanded. Lipless looked at his feet. Didn't answer.

'Well?' Magda wasn't letting go. 'What . . . ?'

Lipless considered his drink.

'Oh you don't need to tell me,' Magda taunted. 'I know. Magda's not very nice. That's it, isn't it? You're right. I'm not nice. Nice! Nice! I'll never be nice. I refuse to be nice. Nice sucks.' She waggled her body at him. 'Where did nice ever get you? Answer me that.'

She picked up Lipless's leather jacket, ran to the door, and threw it furiously into the night.

'Get out. Both of you talking about me. Discussing me. Get out with your nice.'

Silently Edie picked up her jacket and handbag, and moved to the door. She needed air. Lipless followed.

'Away you go,' Magda screeched, standing in the open doorway. 'You bastard needing women to be nice. Nice!' She spat the word as if she hated having it in her mouth. 'Nice!' She heaved off her shirt, tossed it down. Then her bra. She threw it into the street after the jacket. Her tits tumbled out. 'Bugger nice.'

Enjoying her fury, Magda moved back into the room, danced round the tables. Cradling her breasts, she drifted off. She remembered skinny-dipping, oh summers ago, that feeling when the water smoothed over her, icy. Jim would pull her to him. Even now she could feel the hardness of him, muscles down his neck and back. Mouth so soft, touching him, kissing him, slowly biting his lower lip. She curled her legs round him. It had been Jim, hadn't it? She stretched her hand out through her reverie to touch his face. Was it shaven or not? Not. She chose Jim for her bed and he made it into her fantasies too.

'Magda,' Jessie's scolding voice cut into her dream. 'That wasn't very . . .'

'Nice?' Magda pointed accusingly. 'You were going to say nice.'

'Yes I was,' Jessie admitted. 'But it wasn't, was it?'

'Well,' Magda was indignant. 'Fuck are they wanting folk to be nice to them? Whatever did they do to deserve that?'

She danced. Put her hand down between her legs, candidly confessed, 'I'm not nice. I'm a shit. I'm a bitch from hell. I refuse to be nice. Stuff nice.'

Turning to Jessie she stretched out her hands. 'C'mon, be nasty with me.'

John in his living room alone staring at the fire-place. He'd just noticed the quiet. How long had that been going on? Time was Mary would be in the kitchen raw-voiced and roaring out golden oldies from her rock'n'roll days, and from upstairs the thumping bass of Magda's records. Always voices, always noise and always movement, people coming and going, doors banging. It scared him this quiet.

He remembered Magda. Little wilful child in his life, where had she come from? Nobody in his family looked like that: wild hair, extravagant nature. The madam she'd been. He smiled. The tantrums she'd taken. Magda came to mind, six years old, returning from Sunday school, feeling the heat. As she walked she'd ripped off her clothes bit by bit, layer by layer till she arrived home naked, clothes strewn in a long trail behind her. She was seeking relief from more than the August sun. Religion, discipline, sitting in neat rows with other children, tight shoes – all that enraged and stifled her. John looked up suddenly. Magda had been an extraordinary child, full of mischief, full of life. Why hadn't he realised it at the time?

Mary worked hard, yelling at Magda, smacking her, locking her in her room, trying to turn her into something she wasn't. Boring and safe. Like him. Mary had dragged Magda screaming and kicking to school, still the girl would lie in front of the gate, drumming her feet, howling. Then she'd tear off her clothes and throw them about the playground. Naked and screaming, young Magda had been willing to go to any length to escape the classroom.

All that time, through all the screaming and all the beatings he'd turned his back. Left the room. Gone to the pub. Driven out to the cliffs to sit in the car and stare at the sea. He'd done anything rather than join the confrontation. He told himself now that he should have spoken out, done something. 'Even though she wasn't mine.'

He knew that. Had always known that. Once he challenged Mary, 'That girl isn't mine, is she?'

'How could you say that to me?' Mary was shocked and hurt. 'How could you accuse me of such a thing?'

'Because it's true,' John said softly. And Mary said

186

nothing. Walked from the room. What he should have said, he now realised, was that he didn't care. It didn't matter to him. He loved Magda more than anybody else in the world.

Magda missed Jim. Feeling he had let her down he removed himself from her. He'd turned into some stranger and she didn't know what to do to bring the man she knew he was back to her.

Jim knew Magda, every curve of her. He could tell just by touching, spreading his fingers on her shoulders, the mood she was in. Only he, in the quiet of their night-time bedroom, knew how to take Magda apart. When he loved her she would grip his back, dig her nails into his bum and swear and swoon. Oh you bastard, you bastard. Sometimes she would laugh with the joy of it. And sometimes, only sometimes, he could make her cry.

He would take her to him, and kiss her. He would run his hand over her thighs and slip them between her legs, two gentle fingers into the dark of her. Soothing her, touching her. Kissing her. And after she'd come, he'd kiss her longingly as he had done on the first night they'd met. It was the first time Magda had been kissed. Everything before that had been mindless necking.

Magda would put her head on his shoulder. 'Oh don't do that. I can't stand it. Don't be kind to me.'

She always found kindness unbearable. It made her weep. So, he'd kiss her again. Out on the bay a heron would call, a deep rasping cry. And in the deep of their house their babes would be sleeping.

That was the Jim Magda wanted to come back to her. She wanted to say, 'Be kind to me. I hate it when you're kind to me.'

CHAPTER 14

Stepping into a Mareth morning was like stepping into a radio soap.

'Good morning, Lipless.'

'Morning, Granny M.'

'G'morning, Jarvis. Off to rob the bank. Ha. Ha. Ha.'

'Morning, Edie. No, I'm off to look at your overdraft. Ha. Ha. Ha.'

The soft rush of bicycle tyres on tarmac. Jim Horn pedalling by on his way to Ardro Bay for his swim. 'Morning, folks.'

'Morning, Jim.'

The click clicking of Magda's heels as she came along the quay, still trailing behind her a clutch of children to feed.

Jessie lay above it, listening. She knew everything now. The scream of gulls when Granny Moran scattered her crusts and bacon rinds. The council lorry rumbling to a halt, Lipless and his work gang tumbling out, then the clatter of their tools being tossed down to them. Walter lumbering by, bent double with his watering device on his back. The squeak of his pump, the hiss of spraying water.

Jessie lay above it, listening to it, head in the crook of Dave's tattooed arm, smoking a Marlboro. A dog barked. The postman called good morning to Magda and rattled the café's letterbox. 'A gas bill for you. And that looks like another steamer from the bank.'

Jessie lay with Dave, her body curved round his. 'Do you know any more of Magda's poems?'

'They weren't poems. They were childish chants against her arty-farty peers. Considering that they're going for shocks, why do flashers bother with socks? That sort of thing. They were taunts aimed at us. She didn't mind us being pretentious and shutting her out, she minded us shoving her separateness in her face.'

Jessie wrestled with this vision of young Magda. She imagined her standing alone, never accepted and never seeking acceptance.

'Magda's Magda, just that.' Dave sighed. He was sick of Jessie's constant questions about her new heroine. 'She doesn't let anybody away with anything. That's why she likes you. She trusts you. She thinks you're nice.'

'Nice?' Jessie was horrified.

'Yes, Jessie. Face it, you're nice.' He took Jessie's cigarette and stubbed it out and pulled her on top of him.

'You like it best on top.'

'Absolutely.'

'Why?'

'I like to see what's going on.'

The eight o'clock bus rattled by. Dave moved into her. The milkman stopped his van at the door of the café and called out, asking how many pints today?

'Christ knows,' Magda answered. 'Ten? I'd ask Edie but I'm not speaking to her. She's been discussing me with Lipless.'

The bed creaked. Dave watched her face, did not touch her. Did not put his fingers on her nipples or on her bum, underneath it, centre of it. No. He watched as Jessie moved against him, and as she slipped off on her own, pursuing her moment.

The children in the café laughed and ate and threw bits of bacon sandwich at each other. They were not Magda's. They came because she offered food in the morning. She believed in breakfast. At first she offered cornflakes to kids who took to the streets early because their mothers worked at the canning factory or the fish shed. Then it was eggs and bacon, now favourite was scrambled eggs with ham, peppers, tomatoes and garlic: piperade, though none of them called it that. The multi-coloured morning children sat round the table discussing soap plots, football, videos, and if oak-smoked bacon was tastier than old-fashioned thick cut and the fluffiness of the perfect omelette. Jessie breathed and whispered and moved. And lost control.

'Oh God.' And, 'Yes.' And, 'Touch me . . .' She beat him, little ineffectual fists flying.

The bed groaned and shuddered. It was not up to all this activity. Dave laughed at her, was tempted to leave her till she was screaming at him, swearing at him, letting go at last. But he put his arms round her and moved into her harder. Jessie cried out. Magda leaned against the café door drinking coffee.

'Grand day,' Lipless called.

'Grand indeed,' she agreed.

The bed moved into the wall. Banged and thumped against it. Bomp bomp bomp. Jessie howled and Dave laughed. Magda got a broom and banged its handle on the ceiling. Jessie heard it.

'There are children down here,' Magda called. Jessie knew the life's philosophy of such a woman could only be – if I'm not getting any, nobody gets any. She came. She came like she hadn't in years, let go and yelled. A cry from the deepest hollows of her. Just pleasure, just instinct. Felt that shudder move up through her entire body and oh she cried out more.

Later, when she went down to work, Dave, bare-chested, leaned out of the window watching her go. The crew on the quay clapped and cheered at her. Good one, Jessie. She blushed. Dave lit a cigarette and laughed. In Mareth everybody knew everything about everybody. Sometimes Jessie found that hard to cope with.

Thirty-four years ago when Edie McCormack was eight and standing in the school playground, her best friend Isobel Hargreaves turned to her and said, 'You know, Edie McCormack, if you don't mind my saying so, you'll never amount to anything in life. You're too quiet, my daddy says.'

It had been a turning point in the life of young Edie. Until that moment it had never occurred to her that she had to amount to anything. Her *Girls Bumper Book of Nature*, cuddly stuffed dog Willie, her wooden-handled skipping rope and her dreams of riding the range with Calamity Jane had been enough. She had thrown her skipping rope down, walked slowly to the bench inside the wooden shelter and sat, legs stretched straight out before her, staring, at her black lace-up school shoes. Life had never been the same again. She worried a great deal about amounting to something.

If she only knew what it was she should amount to. Her gym mistress had once solemnly told her that all girls should have a heroine, someone they could secretly look up to, someone they wanted to be like. For years, when finding herself embroiled in life's little situations – the first sweaty twelve-year-old hand to clumsily reach for her breast, the delicious illicit pleasure of it; coming to school with no PE kit; starting to menstruate; being caught smoking in the school lavatories – Edie had coped by sweeping her fine straight hair from her forehead, whispering to herself, thin lips moving as if in prayer, 'What would Doris Day do now?'

Then her father had bought the newsagent's business in Mareth and moved his family there.

Then Edie had met Magda. One swift glimpse of the wild one moving through Mareth High tossing her hair, and Edie had abandoned Doris for ever. Here was a real heroine. The things she could learn from Magda. That night in front of the mirror she had held a tight fist in front of her and slowly she had let her middle finger stand up alone. 'Fuck off,' she said slowly, lovely lovely new word. 'Fuck,' jerking the defiant finger up and down. It was the first thing she'd learned from watching Magda from afar. Edie knew there would be more. Magda knew everything that school wouldn't teach her.

When the family sold up their business and moved on, Edie stayed in Mareth. She did the accounts and was receptionist at the Captain's Table. She watched Magda. There was not a day passed when she did not wish she had the courage to do the things Magda did, say the things Magda said.

In time Edie married. Her husband Fred had been killed in a car crash. He'd been with another woman at the time. Edie bowed her head, the shame of it. But there had been a few thousand insurance money. For months Edie had considered her new bank account, weighing up her new situation. At last she'd worked up enough courage to go to Jim Horn and tell him that word in Mareth was Granny Moran was giving up the Ocean Café. If she leased it, could he get Magda to come cook?

Jim had stared at her. Magda in her own café?

No way. But the proposition plagued him. If Magda was in Mareth and away from the Captain's Table, her secret sexual doings would be curtailed. He could keep an eye on her. He matched Edie's money, signed the lease with her and took out a loan to revamp the kitchen.

'Edie?' Magda said. 'Little wimpy Edie? Her?' She couldn't believe it. But her own café? It was more than she'd dared hope for. She couldn't help smiling. 'And it's still got the Alpine scene?'

'Oh yes,' Jim nodded. 'Would we dare get rid of that?'

So Magda took over the Ocean Café. First time she went there she stroked the bar and the tables and the chairs. 'Mine,' she said. 'All mine. Well, mine and Edie's and Jim's. But mostly mine.'

Now Edie knew that it wouldn't be Magda's for long. And Magda wasn't even speaking to her. Though of course that absurd hostility wouldn't last long. Magda's sulks never did. But now that Jim was bankrupt the bank was about to turn nasty. Edie could not meet the loan payments without Jim's help. It was likely the café would go bust too. She moved her thin and innocent lips as if in prayer. 'Now,' she whispered, 'what would Doris do about this?'

'So,' said Magda suddenly, 'how are things with Dave?'

As if she didn't know. But other people's sex lives were always interesting.

'Fine,' Jessie said. Silence, thinking about the fineness of it. Then, 'Yes fine. But we don't actually talk much. We do other things. But we don't talk. He isn't the sort you could confide in.'

'Confide.' Edie and Magda looked at each other, shared shock. Without any negotiations or retributions they were speaking again. Hallelujah.

'You can't confide in men,' said Magda. 'They're not for that.'

Jessie stopped laying the tables – blue and white check cloth, knives, forks, salt and pepper and daisies in blue jars – to think about this.

'What are they for then?' she wanted to know.

'Making babies,' Edie told her. 'And doing jobs that need going up a ladder.'

'Rubbish.' Such . . . such . . . She was stuck for a definition. Such sexism. Yes, that was it sexism.

'If you were honest with yourself,' Edie said, giving Jessie her best serious gaze, 'you'd admit men aren't for telling your troubles to. They're just not for that.'

Jessie shook her head in dismay. She wasn't admitting to this. Though a small voice somewhere in the back of her head reminded her that she thought men were for carrying heavy luggage and telling bad jokes to. However, she told them indignantly that what one should look for was a full relationship. When she, Lou and Trish had discussed the perfect man, they all agreed he'd be, 'A friend and a lover. He'd listen, and talk – discuss stuff. You'd be able to tell him your troubles.' She repeated the notion to Edie and Magda now.

'You can't tell men your troubles.' Magda hooted derision. Did this woman know nothing? 'You can't confide in them and you can't tell them your troubles. You tell your troubles to a woman. She'll listen and sympathise. She'll let you get it all out. If you tell a man he'll *do* something about them. Men are like that. They *deal* with situations. Women watch them marinate, wait whilst they stew. They keep an eye.'

Jessie shook her head. No, this wasn't right. 'You think men and women should lead separate lives, then?' Jessie asked.

'They do in Mareth,' Edie said. 'Here we have three sorts of human being: men, women and incomers.'

'Oh yes,' Magda nodded. 'Incomers can be men or women. Mind you, I like men. They're one of my favourite sorts of human being. I'd let my daughter marry one. But I wouldn't want to be one. A woman's the best thing in the world to be.'

On Thursdays Magda took her mother's shopping list to Ruby at the Spar. 'That's an awful lot of indigestion powder Mary's buying these days.' Ruby scanned the list critically. Magda agreed, and added that Mary had changed since her trip to London.

'Don't know what to do with her,' she worried. Lately Mary had sunk deeper into herself. She daily cleaned her bungalow, wiped the sink unit, dusted the mantelpiece, vacuumed the floor, made the bed. She did it all the way her mother had taught her years and years ago. Dust your surfaces before you do the floor, then vacuum up the fallen dirt. Carry clean cloths and polish with you. Put polish on with a circular movement, take off same way. Living room and laundry Mondays, bedroom and ironing Tuesdays, lavatory and change bed Wednesdays, kitchen Thursday. Friday would be hallway and shopping, but she didn't like going out these days. People looked at her. And recently she felt uncomfortable with that.

She drank tea. She watched soaps and went through to the bedroom to look at the red dress. It was still wonderful, but its presence hanging on the back of the door no longer thrilled her. She did not know where to go with it on. So she saved it for good. Good would come along one day, something really special and she'd be glad she'd waited. Sometimes, though, thinking about it, her heart hurt and she couldn't breathe. She'd sink on to the bed, banging her chest with her fist, cursing herself for eating too many digestive biscuits instead of proper food.

John came home from work every day at six-thirty and they'd have something hot properly at the table, not on their knees in front of the television which was how people who didn't know better ate. Poor things. John would clear the dishes and she'd wash up wearing pink rubber gloves to protect her hands.

198

Sometimes little Rosie would come by and they'd get the best china out and drink tea together. On Thursdays Magda brought in the shopping. Usually she'd pop something special she'd made in the fridge, saying, 'Try this tonight.'

There'd be chicken cooked in red wine with tiny onions and mushrooms, or sea bass rubbed with sea salt and green peppercorns, olive oil and lemon, a grape tart shiny and perfect, gâteau plithviers – melty almond paste, noisettes of lamb in a redcurrant coulis.

'Noisettes,' Mary said to John across the table. 'What a funny word. Noisettes. Fancy our Magda knowing a word like that. Fancy her being able to cook a noisette.' Their Magda who lay naked and drumming her heels at the school gate. 'How did she learn that? Noisettes. Noisettes. Noisettes.'

She would run the word over her tongue, marvelling at the wonder of it. Oh life was lovely. Full and lovely, waiting for good.

'Ah, ladies,' said Jarvis, waving an arm towards Magda and Edie. 'Come in and sit down.'

The two stepped cautiously into his office and slowly and in unison lowered their bums on to the seats on the customer side of his desk. They were, Magda noticed, slightly lower than his. There was something horribly headmasterish about this. Magda refused to acknowledge the tremor in the pit of her stomach. This man was not going to frighten her.

'Well,' Jarvis smiled at them. 'I thought it time we had a chat. Um, certainly before things go too far.'

He played nervously with his pen, tapping it on his desk as he spoke. Jim Horn had taken out a substantial loan to refurbish the kitchen of the Ocean Café. There hadn't been a repayment in six months, more. Head office was badgering him for action. Some movement on the account. Ginny was more than hinting at him closing the café down. Why, for heaven's sake, did she so loathe the place? Maybe she knew she'd lost her husband to it. He was addicted to Magda's crêpes and to daydreams whilst gazing at the Alpine scene.

'Thing is,' Jarvis said, trying to bring to mind the tricks he'd learned on his customer relations course. Body language, eye contact, what was all that? Now, when he needed it, it seemed to have vanished from his brain. 'We have to have some movement on your account.'

'Seems to me,' Magda interrupted. 'That there is a lot of movement on it. All of it in your favour. I mean your interest charges . . .'

Jarvis had tried desperately to get hold of Jim Horn. He had written, phoned and even knocked on his door. But Jim had opted out of the world. He would not open letters or pick up the phone and whenever someone came to the door he hid.

'The Ocean Café's overdraft isn't all that healthy, I'll admit. But I'm prepared to let that go for the moment. No. It's the loan we're worried about.'

'Loan?' Magda knew nothing about a loan.

'Ah, yes,' said Edie quietly. 'Jim took out a loan to cover costs when we took over the café.'

'Loan?' said Magda again.

'Yes,' said Jarvis. 'I have actually tried to get in touch with Jim. But he seems to be constantly unavailable.'

'You can say that again,' Magda agreed heartily. She looked around. What a boring office. Polished wooden desk, phone, green carpet.

'You should get a few pictures up,' she waved at the walls, 'brighten up the place. A nice Alpine scene,' she grinned. She'd noticed.

Jarvis sucked in his breath. 'I don't know if you are aware, M . . . M . . .' did he call her Mrs Horn or Magda? He always avoided names when addressing her, 'Um. But Jim used your house as collateral.'

'So?' Magda took some gum from her pocket, unwrapped it and put it into her mouth. Edie watched in horror.

Jarvis tightened his lips. Nobody made him uncomfortable the way Magda did. Her presence on the other side of his desk irritated him greatly. There was something uncompromisingly female about her. She was all woman, and he didn't know how to handle her. Thus far in his life his dealings with women had been primal. Primal and nothing but. Women had bedded him, fed him, schooled him, scolded him, bathed him, tucked him up at night, kept him in his childhood place,

201

spanked his bottom for being naughty. He couldn't cope with them.

Looking for some minor activity to distract him from the rage he felt gathering within him against this particular member of the female species, he raked about in his mouth with his tongue for bits of leftover lunch caught between his teeth. It didn't work. He grabbed a pencil and pointed it at Magda.

'We are going to have to see some sign of movement in your account,' he barked. 'You don't seem to understand. Unless we get, and get soon, some repayment on this loan, we could have your house.'

Edie reached over to pat Magda's arm. 'Please, Magda,' she was pleading for Magda to keep her mouth shut. But never in her life had Magda held her tongue. She was not about to start now. She looked at him coolly. How dare he try to scare her? Him with his suit and tie and manicured nails. And her with four children to clothe, feed and house. 'So who are you?' she said. 'The testosterone kid?'

CHAPTER 15

There are pictures in Magda's head. They are of other people's lifestyles. They come from magazines. Houses, rooms with white carpets and long sofas, rooms with stripped pine floors and tumbling plants, women with perfect haircuts, wearing suits and high heels sitting in bars, climbing into cars. The pictures are of the life Magda imagines people live in the huge world beyond Mareth.

Sitting at her kitchen table three o'clock in the morning, drinking tea, she flicks through these pictures saying yeabut. 'Yeabut, I'll never see any of it.' It seems to Magda that nobody notices she rarely leaves Mareth. Where could she go? How would she get there? She had failed her driving test eight times. Each time with more bile and venom than the time before. She couldn't master the Highway Code. Rules of any kind mystify her.

With Jim's help she had memorised the registration number of every car in the street outside the testing office so that she would pass her eyesight test. Oh there was nothing wrong with Magda's eyes. She could see for miles and miles.

She just made unexpected sense of what she saw. It made no difference, still she failed. This last time because she'd turned into the wrong street and when this was pointed out to her she'd done a U-turn and headed back the way she'd come.

'Why can't I do a U-turn?' she asked. 'What's wrong with that? I didn't hit anybody. There was nobody around.'

'It's against the rules,' the inspector told her. 'It's not part of the Highway Code.'

Back at the café she raged and stamped. 'God dammit. It was perfectly safe. Bloody man with his bloody rules. If a woman wrote the Highway Code it'd just be take care and don't bang into anything or run over any children. Everyone understands that. But men. Men have to have rules. Rule number so-and-so don't do a U-turn. And don't say nasty things to the test inspector and don't play any Rolling Stones tapes during the driving test. Keep a clean nose. Watch the plain clothes. You don't need a weatherman. To know which way the wind blows. Stuff it. Who wants to drive anyway?'

'Actually,' Jim carefully pointed out, 'that was written by a man. Um, Magda, you didn't play the Rolling Stones during your driving test, did you?'

'There's a problem with that?'

Jim shook his head. There was no arguing with Magda. Still, she'd failed and that was that. She was stuck. She could get the bus. But, what if she got on the wrong one? And besides, so profound was her dyslexia she couldn't read street names. She feared getting lost. Whilst taunting others about the tight control they kept on their lives, she hated losing the grip she kept on her own.

Lack of a licence did not totally stop Magda driving. She shot about Mareth in Jim's fifteen-year-old BMW collecting veg, delivering her mother's shopping, on the four days of the week the local police station was unmanned. The three days it was manned she walked. She was kept informed of unscheduled visits by the policemen who drank at the café after their shift was done.

'What's on the menu for lunch tomorrow?' one would ask, stretching. 'Might look in.' And Magda would know not to let them see her driving illicitly. They knew she did it of course. She knew they knew. They knew she knew they knew. It was a situation she was accustomed to, could deal with. Life went on.

At five, cursing and whining and saying yeabut, Magda returns to bed. She lies listening. Jim breathes noisily and outside the swallows are already swooping and crying. At six-thirty she wakes. Seven, she drags herself from bed. She showers. Clothes are never a problem. She always wears whatever is cleanest. She knows Jim is not sleeping. She knows he knows she knows. She lets him pretend and wakes her children. Seven-thirty she is on her way to the Ocean Café. The familiar click of her stilettos sounds up the empty street.

'Hey Magda,' the bin men call leaning from their

lorry. They come every morning to the shore where they clean up the mess, the huge greasy spreading of carryout bags and wrappings stuffed into the litter bins by tourists during the day and dragged out by seagulls scavenging in the night. 'Who are you feeding today?'

'Who knows?' Magda calls. 'They all look the same to me.'

There are always children to feed. They appear, it seems, from nowhere, a small drift of hopeful hungrys. Sometimes her own join them, sometimes not. Schoolchildren get free breakfast at the Ocean Café, everybody knows that. Billy the egg man leaves extra most days, and the milk van puts free pints on the doorstep. After all, their own children have in their time eaten Magda's bacon sandwiches. In school it is obvious who has been to the café and who hasn't. Well-fed children do not wriggle and yawn and chatter in class. Well, not so much as hungry ones.

'Nobody ever learned anything on an empty belly,' Magda says as she moves through the kitchen, full bustle. 'And don't think any of you will get away with just eating. I'll be asking questions soon enough. I want to know how you're all doing.'

Lipless and his crew arrive as she opens up. 'Great day, Magda.'

'For some,' she shouts back.

In the back yard the Harrys sit patiently waiting for food. Now there are five; two more have turned up since Black Harry left the back yard for Jessie's bed. Ginger Harry and One-Eyed Harry. 'The hell have you been up to?' Magda asks One-Eyed Harry as she puts out the bowl of scraps: trout, salmon, lamb and chicken with wholemeal breadcrumbs and a side order of milk. 'Too much tom-catting around. What does it get you? One eye and a bashed ear. Now I've had your balls cut off. Life's a bitch.' The cat arches his back and purrs furiously.

Outside on the shore, the dustcart returns to empty the litter bins and reline them with black polythene bags. Magda hears the banter, the junk language. Then the shrill shriek of seagulls as Granny Moran shuffles across to the edge of the quay to spread, with aching, gnarled hand, crusts and other leftovers. The eight-twenty bus rumbles by, sleepy workers on their way to the fish sheds.

Magda pours coffee and takes it to the front door. She leans, clutching her cup, drinking slowly. Her stillness only shows on her morning face. As the day gathers steam, her rage takes over. This is the best time of the day. She has the world to herself – apart from Duncan the postie cycling by, and Lipless and his crew on the quay, and the ladies of the fish sheds knocking on the window of the bus, waving wildly. Everybody calls her name. But apart from all that she has the world to herself.

Nine o'clock, Edie arrives, breezing smally in. She hangs up her coat and bag through the back.

In the office she phones the fish man, checking today's prices. Behind her Magda complains, 'Tell him I don't want any of that effing stringy monk. I want the good stuff, same as he sends to the Captain's Table. And,' raising her voice so that she can be heard over the phone, 'if that lemon sole was fresh yesterday, I'm a virgin.'

She returns to the kitchen. She has to make thirty little pots of chocolate for the lunchtime and dinner menus. And strawberries are past it, but the raspberries Edie bought yesterday were good. 'Get some for freezing,' she says. 'Rasps freeze. And when Jessie finally climbs out of her bed, tell her to go up to the house for the tablecloths. I forgot them.' Magda always forgets them. She bangs the ceiling with a broom. 'Get up. Are you out of bed? What are you doing up there?'

Edie pokes her head out of the office and tuts. 'Leave her alone.'

'Why should I?'

'You just don't want anybody to have fun, Magda Horn. If you're not getting any, nobody gets any.'

Magda goes grumpily to the kitchen. 'What'll it be?' she calls. 'The Stones. Great day for it.' She puts on 'Beggar's Banquet'. Jumps around. Edie holds her head and disappears. How can someone play that stuff first thing in the morning? It's like eating chocolate first thing. Or drinking whisky first thing. But then, she has often seen Magda do both. Will she ever grow up?

Jessie passes the window. The men on the quay

cheer and yell. 'Ho Jessie, how're you doin'? Who're you doin'? Come over here darlin' we've got something to show you. Ha. Ha. Ha.'

Dave hangs out of the window. 'Filthy bastards.'

Jessie does not come into the café. She's off to collect the tablecloths from Magda's house. Magda always forgets them.

She knocks gently on the back door. Jim is in the kitchen drinking coffee. He hands her a cup. He knew she was coming. Magda always forgets the tablecloths.

'Potatoes look good,' says Jessie, peering into the garden.

Jim nods. 'Yes. Good,' he agrees. Then, 'What do you think of the hall? It's a pale greeny colour.' Jessie follows him through.

'It's taupe,' she says.

'Taupe,' Jim looks baffled. 'What sort of a colour is that? I've never heard of it.'

Jessie shrugs. Jim complains, 'You turn your back for a minute and they invent a new colour. Taupe. Nobody ever mentioned it to me. There wasn't any taupe in my school paintbox.' He dips his brush and wildly starts on the wall, brushing away his indignation. Colour it taupe, which is no colour at all for indignation. Jessie takes the tablecloths and leaves.

By eleven the tables are set. Lipless and his crew come in for coffee. Magda refuses Lipless alcohol. 'You can have coffee and a croissant with bacon,' she says.

Lipless shifts bulkily from foot to foot. 'I hate fancy food. I just want a wee whisky with a wee pint of beer to follow. That's all.'

'You'll get some food before your liver goes the same way as your dick and stops working. Eat or I'll start talking about periods and my mother's hysterectomy.' Magda points firmly at the plate in front of Lipless. He eats. Across in the corner the first customers of the day, trippers in woolly jerseys and jeans with ironed seams look alarmed and ask Jessie for the bill. Edie comes out of the office. She has the menu which she writes every day in careful, perfect calligraphy. Thick strokes up, thin strokes down. Or is it the other way round? She doesn't know, she just does it.

Starters
Soup of the day: Lentil and tomato. Garlicky and good for you.
Mussels in curried cream sauce. Comforting if you're a wee bit glum.
Melon with Parma ham. Just plain tasty. There's always melon for folks who find soup too heavy and don't like mussels.

Main course
[Edie always writes main course. Magda hates fancy names, like entrée.]
Roast monkfish in fresh tomato sauce. Lots of Vitamin C, chippers you up.

Smoked fish omelette. An Ocean Café regular, our golden oldie.
Noisettes of lamb in redcurrant coulis. Eat it and weep, white boy.
All served with today's selection of fresh veg, or salad. Or chips if you must.

Puddings
Little pot of chocolate. Thick and rich, clings to the throat all the way down.
Grape tart. Shiny grapes, cream sauce, sugar almond pastry. It's wicked, it isn't good for you – it's everything a pudding should be.
Melon stuffed with raspberries and kirsh. Fresh fruit, Vitamin C, again disguised by booze.
Coffee with mints.

Jessie looks at it.
'Isn't kirsch spelt wrong?' She no longer knows. She thinks recently her brain has been replaced with a small bit of chewed bubblegum.
Edie frowns. 'Kirsh,' she says. 'I always spelled it that way.'
'Ah,' says Jessie. Edie's writing is so positive, she makes spelling errors with such panache it's hard to spot them. 'I'm sure it's got a c in it.'
Edie stares hard at the menu. 'Do you know,' she admits at last. 'I do believe you're right.' She bustles back to the office. Reappears seconds later with the amended menu.

'Yes, definitely.' She is pleased. 'Thanks for that. I'd have looked so stupid.' She shows Jessie the new menu. Melon with raspberries and Ckirsh. Jessie stares at it. Doesn't dare mention the misplaced c.

'Great,' she hands it back, smiling. Edie puts on her coat and goes off to Neil and Young solicitor's where Shona, Pretty in Pink now into pale green, taupe?, will photocopy it. One copy for each table. Jessie serves an American tourist coffee and a chocolate croissant then goes to help Magda prepare the veg and salads.

Outside, Weasel the street-sweeper trundles his cart along the shore. He stops to pick up some crisp bags and coke tins. Trundles wearily on. In an hour he will come slowly down the other side of the street and Magda will hand him out a chicken mayonnaise sandwich.

Jessie scrubs new potatoes and tops and tails green beans. Magda will steam them to make a warm salad: beans, tomatoes, almonds, mustardy French dressing. In the evening she will serve this with pieces of chicken tossed in sesame seeds. Edie returns with the menus, puts them in their red folders. Tourist cars line the harbour. A few drift over to read the menu Edie sticks to the café window. They register surprise at such a selection in such a place.

'I mean,' a voice floats in, 'look at that Alpine scene.'

Magda peers out at them. 'There's a couple of

monkfish and a little pot of chocolate if ever I saw them.'

'There's something funny about the menu,' Edie squints at the monkfish and little pot of chocolate. 'I can tell. They're laughing at it.'

'Folks laugh at anything,' Magda flaps her hand dismissively. She puts her thumb over her wine bottle, controls the flow on to her pan. Sizzles. The smells drift out. Two monkfish and little pot of chocolate come in. Can't resist it.

Jessie takes their order. She comes back, arranges the coloured tokens on the board. 'Two monk-fish, one omelette. No starters. Puddings are two grape tarts and a little pot of chocolate.' She calls out the order anyway. 'Table two.'

'Told you,' Magda prides herself on always knowing what customers will choose to eat before they know themselves. 'I wish you'd discussed the omelettes with me. I wasn't wanting to do omelettes today. I've redone my pan several times, soaked it in olive oil. Dunno.'

'We always do smoked fish omelettes,' Edie hotly defends the omelette inclusion.

Lipless lumbers in. Magda puts extra virgin olive oil in a pan, adds garlic, waits till the aroma hits her, adds a couple of ladlefuls of soup. She empties the contents of the pot into a bowl, parsley on top. Jessie takes it to him with a basket of bread. He tucks a white napkin into his collar. Eats slowly. Staring ahead.

'Hey Magda,' he bawls suddenly, terrifying the

213

monkfish and pot of chocolate. 'This soup's got garlic.'

Magda appears from the kitchen. 'Of course it hasn't Lipless. You're imagining it. And don't you go eating just the white bread. Wholemeal keeps you regular.' She smacks his wrist.

'Everybody says my breath smells,' Lipless sulks.

'Get some toothpaste from Ruby,' Magda turns to go.

'It certainly smells very garlicky.' The little pot of chocolate joins in, sniffing the wafts of soup floating across the restaurant. Magda gives her a long withering stare.

Jessie nudges Edie, 'The little pot of chocolate got the Look.'

'Don't say anything,' Magda hisses returning to the kitchen. 'It's good for him.'

Other diners come in. Jessie moves tokens on to the board. Table five: two monkfish with salad. One melon with ckirsh. One little pot of chocolate.

Table three: Soup. Lamb. Grape tart.

Jarvis arrives. Magda gets her crêpe batter out. Heats the pan, smokily hot. Lets a thin film spread over the surface, waits till it bubbles and firms, flicks it over, lets it brown, removes some mussels from their shells, takes some creamy curried sauce from the pot, adds mussels, folds them, with an extra dash of white wine, into the crêpe.

'Help him dream about flying off the mountain,' she grins.

She takes it out personally. Leans over him. Cheek close to his, boobs on show. 'There you are. Your favourite,' she speaks huskily. Laughs. Walks back slowly. She knows he's watching her arse. Laughs again. The three crowd in the door watching him. He eats. Jaws moving almost mournfully, he looks longingly at the scene. Magda brings him a glass of wine. Soon he will stop eating and only stare. Then he will be up in the chill mountain air, moving, arms spread, through the pristine cloudless sky. Edie sniggers.

'It's lack of sex,' Magda nods knowingly. 'He's not getting any.'

'You'd know,' Edie moves to the till as a monk-fish comes over to pay. He raves. But points at Jarvis. 'Why is he getting something different?'

'He's the bank manager,' Edie says. The monk-fish nods. Tells the other monkfish and little pot of chocolate. They all nod. Jessie collects plates. She has to wash them. There is not enough crockery to have it out of commission whilst a dishwasher goes through its cycle. They wash as they go, working in perfect harmony. Saying little, feeling slightly neurotic today, they listen to Jackson Browne.

Lipless leaves. He doesn't pay.

'Poor bugger,' says Madga. By the end of the evening she will have made enough profit from his drinking to cover the soup. Jessie clears the monk-fish table. Removes the cloth. Shakes it. Reverses it. Puts it back on. By two-thirty the lunchers have gone.

'Not a lot today,' says Edie.

'Midweek,' says Magda. 'What d'you expect?'

Mrs Lawrence, who makes the chocolates at home, brings in a fresh batch. Magda pays her from the till. Gives her extra.

'Why did you do that?' Edie is enraged.

'Her man's not working. She needs it. Five children . . .' Magda is unrepentant. Edie shakes her head. The café will be in overdraft for ever. They clean up the kitchen.

'You know who I hate?' Magda says, apropos of nothing.

'Who?' says Jessie.

'George Bernard Shaw,' says Magda.

'But he's dead.'

'Just as well. I really hate him.' Jessie and Edie exchange baffled looks. Jessie eats mussels for lunch. Magda drinks coffee. Edie has grape tart and some cheese. She wants a pot of chocolate but pots of chocolate are popular with customers and they don't want to run out. Besides, Magda always knows what's missing.

At half-past three Dave stops his car outside the café. Jessie gets in beside him. They're off swimming to Ardro Bay.

'Ha,' mocks Magda. 'She'll get sand up her arse and worse. She'll suffer later.'

'Jealous,' says Edie. Magda makes to hit her. Edie laughs. Outside a bus shudders to a stop. Magda rushes to the door with her no coach parties sign. She sees Jim cycling by, going home. Jessie and Dave will have disturbed his swim.

'He doesn't like to share a beach. Likes it all to himself. I think he'd like the bloody world to himself,' she says. Edie says it must be hard for him. Magda sniffs. They are not going to change the menu for dinner, except to add the chicken. Magda pours a drink. Lately, Edie thinks, she has been drinking too much. She sees gannets flying far out past the harbour, sun glinting on them. Such white birds, whiter than the rest. What powder do they use? She goes off to make the chicken changes to the menu.

A couple, chilled after walking the length of the beach and back, come in for a coffee and a glass of brandy.

'A wind's got up.' They clutch their cups, warming their hands.

'Jessie'll be back soon then,' Magda looks out to see if Dave's car is back. She lays out lamb noisettes on a tray. Brushes them with oil, scatters rosemary on top. Rubs cooked sweetened redcurrants through a conical sieve. Puts on another tape. Seagulls screech. Granny Moran spreads out their afternoon feed.

'Ah, Freddie McGregor,' she calls. She's been reading the obituaries. 'Thought you'd be round today. Some bits of fruit cake. You always liked that.'

Lipless comes in for afternoon coffee. Magda

gives him a slice of yesterday's apple cake. Notices Jessie and Dave clambering out of the car. From here she can see Jessie's chilled complexion, red and goosepimply. Her jaw is chattering.

'Stupid cow,' thinks Magda. 'That's what you get.'

'Just a wee drink,' Lipless whines.

'No,' Magda snaps. Soon the bed upstairs will start. God, that woman's insatiable. Other customers look up in mild surprise. Glad really that they didn't ask for a drink too. The whole building suddenly chunters and rumbles as ancient plumbing springs into action.

'Bastards are having a bath,' Magda says indignantly to Edie.

'They're allowed.'

Annie and Rosie come to see her. They drink coke and sit at the bar.

'Has Janis eaten today?' Magda asks.

'Yes, she ate a couple of spoonfuls of cornflakes and took a banana to school,' Rosie watches everything. 'And I got my special teacher today, too.'

'Not bad,' says Annie.

'Not bad at all.'

'Joe's got a hangover. Drinking again. And Jim's still painting the hall.'

'Life goes on,' Magda muses. Upstairs the bed slowly creaks. She casts her eye at the ceiling. To hell with them.

'I'll be home at half-past four for an hour,' she tells them.

Robert from the market garden brings in fresh veg. Edie takes him into the office to settle his account. Magda considers the cherry tomatoes. Smells them. Fabulous. She takes them into the kitchen, washes them and reduces them to fresh pulp in her food processor, rubs them through her sieve. Fresh uncooked tomato sauce with just a touch of ginger and maybe some sugar. She starts preparing the monkfish.

Her father comes carefully in, head round the door, checking his welcome before the rest of his body follows. Magda pours olive oil into a pan, adds garlic and chillies some tomato pulp, basil, sugar and wine. As it heats and reduces she puts in fresh prawns. Waiting for them to turn opaque she puts pasta into a pot of boiling water. When it's ready she fills two carryout trays.

'How is she anyway?' She sprinkles parmesan on each before sealing them.

'Worse,' says her father. 'Won't go out at all. Complains about her indigestion. Sits in front of the telly all day.'

'Won't she see a doctor, then?'

'She says doctors know nothing about the human digestive system. She can cope with it herself. Bicarb.'

'You know,' says Magda. 'I think she's getting smaller.' She gives him the food. He leaves shaking his head. She's right, Mary is shrinking.

A bus squeals to a stop outside. Ladies of the fish shed dismount, cackling laughter, heated gossip. A couple come into the café for a drink. Magda serves them. 'How're you?' 'Fine. And what'll we do for tea tonight?'

'What've you got?'

'Guess,' they shout, a fish shed habit, it's so noisy there. 'Fish,' they yell, holding out their opened bags. 'Haddock.'

'Put it in the oven with some soy sauce over and lemon. Do you have garlic?'

'Garlic salt.'

'That and a touch of ginger. And a spot of water. Not much, a splash. It'll take about four or five songs on the radio in a medium oven, as long as the disc jockey's not wittering on about something.'

She returns to the kitchen. The ladies of the fish shed agree, Magda's looking tired. 'Pale and tired,' they nod. 'Not herself at all.'

The council lorry comes by, Lipless and his crew leave the harbour. Lipless will wash and shave and come back wearing his blue evening polo shirt. Magda will feed him and then he will get a drink, 'The woman's a cow.'

Magda goes home. She kicks off her shoes and lies on the sofa. Annie brings her coffee. 'I've brought lamb for you,' Magda tells her. Annie nods. She will cook it later. Magda drifts into a sleepy distance. She can hear sounds of her household but they are far away. Joe goes out. Jim comes in from the yard with potatoes. Rosie puts the television on and weaves herself round her on the sofa to watch.

Janis is saying, 'Meat. Disgusting. I'm not eating that. I'm a vegetarian. I don't eat dead animals.'

Annie is indignant, 'When did you become a vegetarian?'

Janis, 'Ten minutes ago. I just decided.'

'Shut up. Oh please,' Magda moans.

She returns to the café. Gives the Harrys their evening feed. Last meal of the day for them. She will not leave food out at night. Rats.

Edie does not go home at all during the day. There is nobody there. The Ocean Café is home. She takes a walk along to the postbox. Bills to pay. The phone rings three times when she's away. Three reservations. Magda remembers them all. Edie will write them up when she comes back.

'You can't turn your back for a second,' she says. Then, remembering Magda's lunchtime outburst, 'How come you know George Bernard Shaw, then?'

'There was a big picture of him in school. Remember? In the hall?'

Edie shakes her head. Jessie comes in and the evening starts. There are drinkers at the bar and five tables to serve. She serves the drinkers and carries food to and empty plates from tables, arranges tokens on the board. Edie does the bills. Magda cooks. Someone orders the smoked fish omelette. Magda swears, 'Sod this pan,' everyone hears. Jaws stop chewing, forks are poised between plate and lips. Magda crashes and bangs. 'This

221

should slide off. It should be fluffy and perfect. Golden and softly fishy inside. Sod this pan.'

At nine she stops and comes out for a drink at the bar. She has not eaten properly all day. She nibbles as she goes, a bad habit. Jessie serves Lipless, 'A man has to go through hell to get a drink here,' he says.

'I can't imagine why you've got it in for George Bernard Shaw,' Jessie wants an explanation to Magda's surprising lunchtime remark.

Edie says, 'We'll have to go through the cellar tomorrow. We're running short on Australian Chardonnay and it's really popular with these August people.'

'Yes,' says Magda. 'July folk like Riesling. Riesling and Vimto. Not together, though.'

'And you get a lot of Sancerre and Chablis folk in September,' she nods at her own wisdom. Then, 'Actually, I got pregnant by George Bernard Shaw.' She turns her little eager face to Jessie. Edie has a tiny body and a huge voice. The restaurant has hushed. Jessie doesn't know what to say.

'Oh?' says Magda, adding more vodka to her coke.

'Well,' Edie draws her breath. This is a big story, 'I used to eat all these health foods, y'know. And in the health shop there was these packets of burgers made up to an original recipe by George Bernard Shaw.'

'George Bernard Shaw burgers,' says Magda. 'Who'd've thought it?'

'Exactly,' says Edie. 'So I thought, that'll do me.' She raises her eyes, flaps her hand in dismay. 'Well. Roughage did you say? No human being needs roughage like that. And if George Bernard Shaw needed roughage like that, no wonder he looked so grim. Wonder he had time to write all them plays.' All conversation has ceased. Diners eavesdrop blatantly.

'I only had one, maybe two, George Bernard Shawburgers and my goodness – diarrhoea did you say? DIA-RR-HOEA. You never saw the like. So much so my pill went right through me. And I got pregnant. It was George Bernard Shaw did it. No doubt about that.'

'See,' says Magda. 'Told you I hated him. I'll probably do a stew with parsley dumplings when it gets colder. And some steamed puddings. What happened to the baby, then?'

'Miscarried. I cried and cried,' says Edie.

'I didn't know that,' says Magda.

'No,' says Edie. 'That was twenty years ago. More. God knows what the child would've been like.'

'George Bernard Shaw,' hoots Magda.

'Mightn't have been that bad. You don't know what he was really like,' Edie says. 'You only ever see his face. And I like to see a man's bum. I like a good bum.'

'The good thing about a stew is it improves with time. And you're not in a constant lather. It's there doing on its own, like,' Magda has nothing more to say about George Bernard Shaw.

Jessie clears a table. Edie does the bill. Diners have stopped eavesdropping, the hum of conversation resumes. But departing gentlemen are aware of Edie watching their bums. They don't know what to do about it. Magda laughs. Edie sighs. More folk who won't be back. Jessie clears the tables. Magda drinks some more.

Joe, who has been pubbing, brings some friends back to the café. 'I'll cook,' he says.

Magda hates people in her kitchen. She twitches, eyes Joe evilly. 'Don't,' she says.

'Don't what?' He spreads his hands. Innocence.

'I don't know. Just don't.'

'Can I cook?' Joe folds his arms. And Magda says yes, but don't mess up and don't use everything. And she can't think of another don't so stares at him witheringly.

'Oh the Look,' Jessie points. 'That's twice today.'

Magda doesn't know what to do. She does not want anybody using her pans in her space. But she wants to be her child's friend. In a month he will be out of her life, off to college. She shrugs.

'The thing to remember about being a parent is you can't win. You'll never win with children. In the end they'll leave you and you'll cry for the life they'll have and for yourself for missing them.'

'But,' says Edie. 'They might not leave. Some children don't.'

'Ah,' says Magda 'Then, you'll cry for the life they'll not have and for yourself for being stuck with the little buggers. You can't win with children.'

The last diners leave. Edie takes their money. Clears the restaurant till. Puts the money in the safe in the office till morning. Magda pours another drink. Joe and his friends leave. Magda takes a look round the kitchen. She picks up a tomato, smells it. Puts it in the fridge.

'It's been a tomatoey sort of a day.'

At midnight the Ocean Café closes. Magda locks the door. Jessie goes upstairs to Non-existent Dave. Magda heads home. Edie, bag banging on her leg, coat buttoned, walks tiny steps, amazing speed, in the opposite direction. She stops mid-stride, turns suddenly. Opens her throat and bawls, a street stopper of a voice. Walking backwards she yells, 'MAGDA. That wasn't George Bernard Shaw. That was Captain Mareth. He founded the school.'

Magda is surprised. Fancy that. I always thought it was George Bernard Shaw. 'I still hate him,' she roars back. Seagulls gathering on the quay, hovering ready to scavenge the bins, rise in unison. Like a wave.

Home, Jim has finished the hall.

'Yes,' Magda nods. 'It's good. Good colour.'

'Taupe,' says Jim.

'Taupe!' Magda looks disbelieving. 'Never heard of it. You sure? D'you think they saw you coming?'

'Taupe,' says Jim. 'Definitely taupe.'

Magda has a bath. Soaks away the day. Then walks naked down the hall to bed. Jim is already there pretending to sleep. It's the familiar knowing routine, the silent lie. He knows Magda knows he is pretending. She leaves him to it. And sleeps. At ten past three, always ten past three she will wake. She will get up, go downstairs and make tea. Sitting at the kitchen table she will unfold the pictures in her head, and, darkly whining say, 'Yeabut. What about me?'

CHAPTER 16

When the baby died, Jessie was taken to the maternity ward. She lay in a small side room with three other mothers and their babies acclimatising herself to the rhythms of motherhood. Every four hours bottles of formula were brought round, and every four hours Jessie said, 'I don't need it. My baby died.' Every four hours her grieving started anew. The other three mothers, all much younger than her, formed a mum's vigilante group. They had an anti-Jessie rota. Armed with gaudy tabloid information about the insanity of childless mothers, they decided their infants were not safe if left alone with Jessie. They took it in turns to stay behind on watch whilst the others ate, went to the lavatory or phoned home. Jessie felt like more than a failure, she was a person to be loathed and feared. All she wanted was someone to love her. All she wanted was Alex to put his arms round her.

When she got home he hovered round her, bringing her tea and asking if she was all right.

'Fine,' she said, sometimes six or seven times a day.

'Alex, I'm fine.' He seemed to need to hear her say it though. Her reassurances released him from guilt. They allowed him to run away back to work because the sadness at home was too much for him to bear. They should have clung to each other and cried together. They should have shared their grief, then maybe Jessie would not have felt isolated in guilt.

She remembered desperately wanting her mother. She longed for her to be there to talk to, stroke her head, touch the sore bit, make it better, tuck her up and tell her to never mind. But her mother didn't come. She found life difficult when it did not move seamlessly, smoothly from one day to the next. Upsets upset her. If a spilled jug of milk caused her to flap her dishcloth and fuss, a dead baby was more than she could bear. Besides, confronting it meant confronting, in some measure, her daughter's sex life. How could she do that when Jessie was in her mind always, six years old in a pretty blue dress, bow at the back, ribbons in hair running across the lawn – a butterfly cupped in her hands?

Jessie was a precious child. She spent her perfect suburban childhood being doted on by two people who thought they would never be parents. She had everything – and a rocking horse too. Her father, a quiet balding man, came and went. When she was ten she wrote a poem about him: Here comes Jack in his hat and mac, he says good evening every day and good morning when he goes away. Her teacher had written 'a nice concise poem, Jessie.' But her mother didn't like it at all.

'I don't think this is very nice, Jessie. Not at all what we should be letting your teacher see. And we do not call our fathers Jack.' Jessie, however, was proud of her poem.

She couldn't remember much about her childhood. Other children came round to play and looked at her things with envy. She had almost every toy imaginable, but the thing that caused most resentment was her Mickey Mouse luminous alarm clock. She remembered crowding with several others into her parents' wardrobe and shutting the door so that they could marvel at the glowing green face and hands. Her mother discovered them.

'Jessie, we do not go into wardrobes with these children, boys especially. It is not done.' Jessie had asked why but no satisfactory explanation was forthcoming.

Now Jessie puzzled over her childhood. She tried to bring to mind specific events, but couldn't. Something must have happened. They had a colour television set, but she couldn't remember it coming into the house. Where had the Mickey Mouse luminous alarm clock come from? Who had given her it? She couldn't remember. Her mother and father must have argued from time to time, but she couldn't remember a single cross word ever being uttered. All she remembered was the politeness. They said dear a lot. Yes dear. No dear. Dear dear. Oh dear.

Her father left the house every morning at seven-thirty and returned at half-past six. Good morning and good evening. She left for school at eight and returned at four-thirty. Bye Mummy and I'm back, Mummy. Homework, supper then bed. Was that it? No arguments, no dirt, no sex, no laughter? Had they come as a family to the Ocean Café they would have been August people, Chardonnay or a nice Burgundy.

'Shall we have a nice Burgundy, dear?'

And had Magda misbehaved, shouting and swearing, they would all have stared deep into their lemon sole and pretended it was not happening. That's the sort of folks they were.

Jessie remembered seasons. Building a snowman in winter. Borrowing coal from the bucket by the fire for eyes and a carrot from the vegetable basket in the kitchen for a nose. And the summers of her childhood were sudden. That escape from school and there it was, warm weather. All she could remember of them were small things: squatting low in the flowerbeds, the brown smell of earth, watching a worm, putting captive caterpillars in a jar and thinking they'd take for ever to turn into butterflies, sitting on the back doorstep shelling peas. But there must have been more to her life than that, surely there must.

In Mareth there was that same childish joy in summer's arrival. She woke one morning in May and there it was, summer. August and it was still there. It seemed to lie in the bay. It turned the air soft and silky. Every day Jessie walked through it, felt it on her arms and bare legs. She felt strong. So strong, so different she sometimes forgot her old life. But it was there in her head and it wasn't going to go away.

It came back to her in a series of flashbacks. A moment from her past would be with her, vividly with her. Every colour, every movement, every word spoken was so much more clear than they had been when they actually happened.

When Alex went back to work she watched him painfully going through his shower, shave and clothes routine. He moved stiffly, his suffering spread through his whole body. They exchanged silent distress signals, saying nothing about their pain.

'I have to go now. Will you be all right?'

'Yes. I'm fine.'

'Do you want me to bring you anything when I get back?'

'No, Alex. I'm fine.'

She wanted her mother to come with armfuls of flowers. But of course she hadn't. She hadn't even phoned. When Jessie phoned her she said, 'Well, dear, how are you?'

'Fine,' Jessie lied.

'I thought you'd cope. You always muddle through, even when you were little you muddled through.' There was a long silence. Neither knew what to say. Jessie didn't want to ring off; by hanging on she still had her mother there in some sort of contact. But that was that, the tragedy had been discussed, Jessie's mother moved on to talking about the weather and their new car. When she rang off, Jessie sank deeper into her tunnel. Now she was really alone.

She thought she had come to Mareth and left her despair behind. These past days, however, she felt the blackness returning. She was beginning to stare again. She would come home from work, sit in her chair by the window and gaze out to sea, saying nothing. If Dave asked her what was wrong she would wanly reply, 'I'm scared.'

'What are you scared of?' Dave asked.

'If I knew that, I wouldn't be scared.'

Dave told Magda. 'Jessie's gone all funny. You couldn't speak to her, could you?'

Magda looked at him witheringly. 'Speak to her. Make her better. Bring back the woman you first fancied.'

Dave shrugged. 'I don't know what to say.'

Magda went upstairs to Jessie's flat. The door wasn't locked. Locking doors was not the Mareth way. She found Jessie lying curled on top of her bed.

'What's wrong with you?' she asked. As if she needed to ask.

'There's nothing wrong,' Jessie lied. 'I'm fine.'

'Here we go, thundering into your middle class politeness. Of course you're not fine . . . Look at you. Look at your face, it's crumpled like an old potato. You've been crying.'

'I don't know.' Her sigh shook her entire body. 'I thought I was getting better. But I keep thinking about the baby. It would have been ten months now. Would it have been walking and talking?'

Magda shook her head, 'Not quite. He'd have been on his way, though.'

'I can't stop thinking about it. It keeps creeping up on me.'

'You thought it was going to just go away? It comes back and back and back and it hurts a little less each time.' She sat on the bed, stroked Jessie's hand.

'The wound never goes away?' Jessie was surprised.

'You don't see much, do you?' said Magda. Jessie looked at her sharply.

'Most of the world,' Magda said, 'has been poleaxed at some time or other. You see it in the café, everyday people who've been hurt. You can see it in the way they drink too much too quickly or the way they drift away from the conversation around them and sink into themselves, or stare out to sea, or laugh too loudly at some pathetic joke. Now you've been poleaxed too. You've joined the walking wounded. Welcome to the human race.'

Jessie didn't know what to say.

'You're building up some emotional immunity. Life won't hurt so badly next time it hits.' Magda was matter of fact about poleaxing.

'Is this why you're the way you are?'

Magda didn't let go her hand. Reached out to gently push the hair from Jessie's eyes. Sometimes, though she fought hard not to be, Magda was momma to the world.

'And how am I?' she asked.

Jessie searched for the appropriate words, 'I dunno. Loud. Brash . . .'

Magda laughed.

'See me? When I was at school and I couldn't read or write, everybody used to laugh at me. The teacher hit me. Every single day she would call me out to the front of the class and hit me. My mother beat me. My father hardly spoke to me. Jessie, when I grew up I thought so little of myself, I was the town bike. Know what I mean? I had two miscarriages when I was still in my teens, before Jim took me in. Oh, I've always had a mouth on me. But one day when I was working at the Captain's Table, the boss started on me. I was useless, I was this. I was that. And he would. He would what? What could he do to me? I'd had so much pain I couldn't hurt any more. I was invincible. Know what I mean?'

Jessie gazed at her. Tears still streaming from her.

'Wash your face,' Magda bossed. 'Come to work. Have a drink. Join the walking wounded at the bar. You'll get better this time and next time you'll get better quicker. And maybe one day you'll be invincible, too.'

Jessie heard Magda going off down the stairs,

shouting back at her, 'Oh yes. Invincible. I don't cry. I don't hurt. Not me. I am woman. I am invincible.'

She heard Magda enter the Ocean Café. 'Invincible,' she shouted. 'I am Invincible Woman.'

There were moans and groans and grumbles of disbelief, snorts of derision. 'Here she goes. Will you listen to that? Invincible. Ha. Ha. Ha.'

'Invincible,' Jessie whispered. And joined in the laughing. 'That'll be right.'

It was true. Mary Lomax was getting smaller. She was moving into herself. Shoulders hunched, head bent and looking thinner and thinner as the weeks went by. The red dress hung loose on her. But Mary didn't think so. This was natural thin, proper thin. The same sort of thin as the woman with the lovely accent and soft eyes in the dress shop. She admired herself in the mirror. Yes the red did something for her, lit her face. She moved stiffly down the hall and into the living room. John was sitting watching football. He did not turn as she came. He did not like to look at her these days.

'Look at me, John,' Mary commanded. 'Look at me.'

John turned. The room was dark but for the light from the television. It was unbearable to look at her, this small shrivelled woman he had loved, drowned by the dress that had driven her crazy. The crowd roared. 'Oooh,' the commentator snapped 'surely that was a penalty. But the ref hasn't seen it.'

'Look at me,' she said again. 'I'm gorgeous.'

It wasn't that Ginny Howard was frigid exactly. She just forgot about sex. Day to day there was so much to do, by the time she lay down in bed at night it didn't occur to her. Jarvis didn't like to remind her. He thought he might get used to it. But knew he wouldn't. He dreamed of someone charming and, well, nice, who'd be like Magda, or like he imagined Magda to be, in bed. He was fascinated by Magda, and terrified of her.

He had one abiding memory of her. She had been in his class at school. Once, in a chemistry class, after the teacher had been horribly scathing about her work, Magda had stepped to the front of the rows of desks.

'Get back to your seat, girl,' her teacher demanded.

Magda shook her head. 'What sort of way is that to speak to somebody?' she asked.

'I'm tired of you and your messy attitude.'

Magda shrugged. 'I just don't understand,' she said.

'Well, I can't explain it any better.'

'Do you always speak to people like that? Does it make you feel better? Do you feel good making people feel terrible about themselves? Is it 'cos you're a man? But you're such a bully I don't think you're a man at all. I think you're a coward.'

And before the hushed schoolchildren she had reached forward and gripped the poor fellow right between the legs. The surprise and shock on his

236

face was something none of them would ever forget. 'Just as I thought girls,' she said. 'Nothing there.'

For days the class had waited to see what retribution Magda would suffer. Nothing happened, but the mockery stopped. Jarvis had been misty-eyed in admiration for the girl – just so long as she kept her distance and didn't come near him.

It wasn't just sex he missed. He wanted someone to chat to. Someone who wouldn't clear the table the instant he stopped eating. Someone who didn't think it wicked to leave a coffee cup on the floor beside the sofa. Who would sleep naked, go to bed Sunday afternoon when the kids were out, who would make love outside the bedroom.

Last week Ginny had risen at five-thirty to clean the house, and this week she had told him she was thinking of doing it in the evening before she went to bed to save her doing it in the morning. He winced. How had this happened to them? And where was the nubile, willing woman he'd married? The one who'd willingly wriggled beneath him in the back of his Ford Cortina all those years ago after the golf club Christmas party.

The silence woke Jessie. It took her a while lying staring at the ceiling to realise why she felt alarmed. Eight in the morning already and there were no gulls crying outside.

'Granny Moran,' she said, urgently getting out of bed. In T-shirt and knickers she stood on the landing, banging on the old lady's door. No reply. Trembling Jessie tried the handle. The door was open. Only incomers with their city fear and loathing locked their doors.

Inside the flat was dark, smelled musty. Jessie moved slowly down the hall. The thick chenille door curtain swished behind her. She tiptoed and gently called on Granny Moran. 'Hello-o.' Spindly, uncertain voice moving through the awful silence.

The living room was dark, thick red curtains drawn. Jessie heaved them back and stepped back as light flooded the room. She looked round: several overpoweringly large pieces of dark mahogany furniture, a table with a bowl of wrinkled fruit dead centre, a beige velvet straight-backed chair in front of the biggest television she'd ever seen, but no Granny Moran. Heart pounding, oh God please don't let me find a dead body, she crept through to the bedroom.

Granny Moran was in bed. Her head lolled on the pillow, long grey hair spread out, mouth open, she stared wordlessly at Jessie. She was pale, pale, grey pale. Her glasses, false teeth and gold bracelet watch lay on the dresser beside the bed. Jessie fetched Magda.

Magda took Granny Moran's cold hand in hers and reached out to touch her cheek. 'Fetch Dr MacKintyre,' she said. 'Edie'll have the number.'

Jessie ran downstairs to the café. The workers on the quay watched her go and did not whistle and stamp. They knew when something was wrong. The morning children eating their breakfasts cried 'woooooo' then stopped. The air today was different, foreboding. Somebody was dying.

Dr MacKintyre came and went. He listened to Granny Moran's failing heart, took her pulse and shook his head. 'There's not a lot I can do. I don't think I even know how old she is,' he said.

Magda rubbed her eyes, 'I don't think she knows herself.' They looked at the old lady.

'You're not moving her. She'd want to go here at home. It'd kill her to die in hospital,' Magda insisted.

'You must think me more insensitive than I do myself,' the doctor said stiffly. He'd had recent dealings with Magda. Last year she'd found a lump on her left breast. It turned out to be a benign cyst. He'd looked at her over his half glasses and asked what she expected at her age? Magda's survival depended on never letting anyone get away with anything.

'At my age I expect to get patronised by doctors who look at me dismissively over the top of their specs reminding me of my age.'

He left, promising to look in later. Meantime, was there anybody who could sit with the old lady? They took it in turns. Magda, Edie, Ruby from the Spar and her oldest daughter, then Jessie after lunches were finished. She felt privileged and terrified. What if the old lady actually died when she was there? She didn't think she could cope.

Granny Moran's bedroom was dark and cool.

The old lady's laboured breathing scarcely touched the silence that spread outward beyond the airless, stuffed room to the street. Cars crawled past and the workmen on the quay whispered when they swore. At four the old lady stirred, her rattling chest eased. Moving her hands painfully, she signalled Jessie over.

'Magda,' she croaked, the word barely coming out of her throat. Jessie ran downstairs, knocked on the café window. In baseball cap and apron, Magda sat on the bed, leaning her ear close to Granny Moran's lips. Jessie hovered in the doorway. She didn't know what to do. She shouldn't be here, turned to go.

Magda stepped back, shaking her head. 'No, stay. It's all right,' she grinned hugely.

Granny Moran sighed, lifted her worn translucent, liver-spotted hand and waved. Did Jessie hear her say, 'Bye, Bye'? There was a gleam in her watery eyes. She was off. Time of her life.

Magda put her arm round Jessie when she cried. Stroked her hair, kissed the top of her head. And Jessie loved the smell of Magda, sweat and raspberries and garlic, and that deep unfathomable smell of being a woman.

'It's all right,' Magda said. 'It's what she wanted more than anything. She was tired of waiting for it. She'll be flying round the bay right now, calling out to her old pals.'

'Fuck, fuck, fucky fuck,' choked Jessie. 'That's what it sounds like you all say to me.'

'Oh,' Magda stroked her hair, 'we're not nearly as witty as that.'

Jessie wiped her nose. 'What did she say to you anyway?'

Magda let out a breathy laugh. She was pleased. 'Gave me her batter recipe.'

'She didn't.' Jessie couldn't believe it. 'On her death bed? Heaven's sake.' She didn't know if she was crying or laughing. 'What was it anyway?'

'I'm not telling you,' Magda shook her head. 'Oh no. It's a secret.'

CHAPTER 17

Jessie dreamed she was giving birth in the Ocean Café lavatory. She cleaned the lavatories a couple of times a day, a job she loathed. She was being tended by a blond man who'd flirted with her over his watercress soup a couple of nights before. He told her to push and she swore foully at him, said she was pushing. He said he could see the head, and she said she could feel it and didn't want to push any more, fearing she would break it. She complained that the yellow knobbly carpet was vile and a person in labour should have better quality soft furnishings. The pain woke her. She breathed deeply, scarcely able to believe she was not in pain at all, and ran her hand gingerly over her stomach – just in case. The relief to find it flat, or flattish. She still felt embarrassed at being so intimate with someone she scarcely knew.

'What's wrong?' Dave asked gruffly. He did not want to be awake yet.

'I dreamed I was giving birth,' she told him.

'Christ.' He turned over, keen to get back to sleep.

'You don't understand. It was sore. I was in pain.'

'You were dreaming.'

'I was in agonies in my dream, giving birth.'

'Never mind. Here you are in bed, and the baby you had is still in your dreams. Best kind of kid. It won't grow up to demand cash and slag you off to his chums.' He snorted at his joke.

Telling him he was a stupid bastard who didn't understand, Jessie got up to light a cigarette and smoked it staring out of the window. The depth of her upset shook her; she felt as if she had been crying her eyes out.

'Who the hell do you think you are,' Dave demanded, 'calling me a stupid bastard? Saying I don't understand? I understand. I understand plenty.'

'I don't think you do.' Jessie sounded caustic.

'Babe, you'll never know.'

'Oh you patronising shit. Babe, you'll never know.' She curled her lip, strutted some, imitated him again. 'Babe, you'll never know. What is it I'll never know? The meaning of life? All the butch macho things men know? How to drive a fast car . . . in reverse? How to drink a pint of beer in a oner? How to use big shiny power tools? How to shout louder than anybody else with your big deep voice . . .'

Dave got out of bed, moved across the room to where she was, by the window, put his face up to hers and, using his big deep voice, yelled, 'How about how to take responsibility for yourself?'

She was stunned. 'The hell do you mean by that?'

'I mean what exactly are you doing here, Jessie? Working as a waitress in a seaside café with your money, your education. Are you enjoying yourself mixing with the lower orders? Do we amuse you?'

'No,' she shook her head. 'It isn't like that.'

'What is it about?'

'I'm trying to sort myself out.'

'I get the feeling you're floating above us, Jessie. Looking down, being slightly amused the while. I think we're not really real to you. Just a little distraction whilst you do your running-away-from-life thing.'

'Who the hell are you to criticise people for running away? You're the great Non-existent Dave.'

'Yeah. And when I ran away I made a job of it. You're dealing with a master here. And like I said, you'll never know babe.'

'Oh for heaven's sakes, Dave. Of course I know. You run away all the time . . .'

'If you say, "Where are we going with this relationship, Dave?" Or "I want some kind of commitment, Dave", I'll . . . I'll . . . throw you out the bloody window.'

They stared at each other in surprise. This was absurd; not only would he never throw her out the window because he wasn't the type, the window was too small anyway. More, though, it came as a mutual revelation that neither of them wanted any sort of commitment. And neither of them really cared where they were going with the relationship. Oh the relief. They went back to bed.

They carried Granny Moran to the graveyard. Six pall-bearers in top hats and tail-coats walked slowly along the shore with the coffin on their shoulders. Most of Mareth followed. It was an exquisite day, that summer stillness lay in the bay.

The whole village had come to bid the old lady farewell. In church Reverend Borthwick smiled and nodded. Fourteen years Mareth had been his parish, never before had he seen the place so full. People had come to Mareth from across the world to say goodbye to Granny M. Magda pulled Jessie back as she headed for a seat near the front.

'Front rows are for relatives only.'

Relatives filled the front ten pews. An extra-ordinary amount of them looked just like her. But then, looking round the faces in the rest of the church, half of Mareth bore a resemblance to Granny Moran. Maybe the tales they told about her voluptuous past were true.

'Are you related?' Jessie leaned close to Magda's ear, whispering her question.

'Nah,' she shook her head. 'The Lomaxes are a whole different breed. Though . . .' Though, she was not really a Lomax. She didn't know who her father was. It wasn't her mother's husband, that was for sure. 'You'll not see a funeral like this again,' Magda said.

'They don't take everyone to the graveyard on their shoulders, then?' Jessie asked.

Magda shook her head. 'It's Granny's way. All her friends would have had that. But then most of them went about thirty years ago. She's been a long time alone.'

Jessie looked round at the mourners, barely a dry eye. This was alone? These people know nothing about alone. She could show them alone.

They sang the twenty-third psalm.

Reverend Borthwick said Granny's name, 'Euphemia Maureen Moran, Granny M., Mareth will be an empty place without her . . .'

Jessie watched the grieving faces. She had never seen communal crying before. The church was filled with flowers people had brought from their gardens. Every flag in the village was at half-mast, every curtain was drawn. Visitors to Mareth would find the village closed for the day.

'Mareth does a good funeral,' she said.

'We're good at death,' said Magda. 'Drinking and death.' Freddie Kilpatrick sang 'Yesterday', Granny's favourite song. His rich tenor surprised Jessie. He came and went to and from the Ocean Café in oily dungarees and cap. Who would have thought such a thrilling voice lurked inside him? After the sermon they sang 'Onward Christian Soldiers', hardly funereal, Reverend Borthwick smiled. But Granny Moran always liked it. And when at last they went out into the graveyard, everyone agreed that Granny M. would be well

246

pleased to have her gravestone finished at last. It was a weathered stone.

'Been up twenty-five years,' Magda said. 'Had it put up herself. She didn't trust anyone to do it right.' She nodded, smiling. 'Granny M. had it all figured, did she not?'

'She did that,' Jessie agreed, looking wistfully at the stone.

> Euphemia Maureen Moran, 1898 –
> Time of Her Life.

'Time of her life,' Jessie read. Magda nodded. The envy they felt at Granny Moran's departing glee. Death scared the shit out of them.

The café was closed to the public for the day. Family and friends squeezed in and drank to Greasy Mae, a legend in her time. They had to put away fourteen bottles of whisky, one more than had been drunk at the funeral of Granny Moran's best friend twenty-eight years ago. To fortify the drinkers, Magda brought in a huge platter of battered fish and chicken. Ruby from the Spar held a piece between her fingers and, weeping still from the song and Onward Christian Soldiers, cried, 'Oh, Magda. She passed on the recipe. Now that was grand of her. She was a grand old lady.'

At four o'clock seagulls gathered on the quay. Jessie took some scraps to spread for them. They swooped and fought round her. There you go, there you go. Some for you and some for you and let the little one through. She needs some.

The place was still. Not a car moved. No children played. No ghetto-blasters on the harbour. There was only the aching thrum of Granny's Australian grandson's pipes. A lonely pibroch at the end of the pier.

The first storms came in September. Early, Magda said. They usually came a month later.

'There'll be no more nudy swimming for you.' She wagged her finger at Jessie.

Huge waves galloped in and smashed against the quay. The spray flew across the street and hit the Ocean Café window. Passing cars were drenched, and the fish shed ladies scattered squealing when they clambered from the evening bus.

For two days, four tides, waves boomed, and spray hit the café window. Hardly anybody came, only Lipless and Jarvis for his crêpe and mountain stare.

The wind was incessant, a constant howl. Upstairs in the flat Dave lit a fire, sat staring at the flames. Storms unsettled him. Seagulls rode the waves or lined the quay. Morning and evenings Jessie fed them.

'Come on now. Some for you. Here you are Granny M., chocolate doughnut. Can't resist it, can you? Come on then . . .'

The wind whipped round her, flapped her coat. Gulls snatched and gobbled. 'Now you, that's enough of that . . .'

Dave watched from the window.

'Here little one . . .'

'Jessie?' A familiar voice.

She turned. 'Alex.'

'Dare I ask what you're doing?' He came close, shouting above the storm.

'What do you think I'm doing? Feeding the gulls.' She was soaked. Her hair was plastered to her head, mascara ran down her cheeks. There was so much rain she could hardly see.

'But it's lashing rain. Won't it wait?'

'No.' She continued tossing lumps of bread and doughnut.

'Can we talk?'

She was deeply tempted to say no again. But nodded toward the café.

'No. I want to talk,' Alex insisted.

Reluctantly, fearing a confrontation with Dave, she led him upstairs to the flat. Her espadrilles squelched as she walked. She'd been standing in a puddle. Dave wasn't there. No sign of him at all. She looked round for him. Seconds ago he'd been at the window, now he'd vanished. He wasn't keen on confrontations either.

Alex hung his damp coat in her hall then sat in front of the fire. 'Cosy,' he said, trying to hide his horror. He still found cosy offensive. Jessie nodded. So it was.

'I'll make some tea,' Jessie offered.

Alex nodded, 'That would be good.' He pulled out his wallet. Handed her a cheque. 'I've brought you some money. I would have had it transferred to your bank account but I don't know if you have one.'

'I have one at the local bank. It's got less than a pittance in it.'

'Well here's half the profit I made on the house. A bit more as a matter of fact. It'll see you through for a while if you don't go wild. But I'd invest it.'

'Yes. You would.'

They stared at each other. So much to say, but how to start?

'Jessie. I can't bear to see you living here. I can't bear it.' He was a knight in a shiny little sports Mazda. He could rescue her. He gripped her arms, 'We could go back to Italy. Take the car. Fill the boot with decent wine and olive. We could visit old haunts. Lucca.' He was enthusing, convincing himself as much as her that this would solve everything. He took her hands as if they could just run out into the night, get into their little red car and drive into the night, forgetting everything. 'You always used to complain that we never did anything on impulse. I always planned too much. Think of it, Jessie. Italy. The light. The smells. The shoes . . .'

He was a man for buzz words. Shoes got her.

'Italy.' She remembered. 'The shoes. Oh the shoes . . .' When had she last shopped for decent shoes?

'Visit the late-night street markets. Buy books.' He was getting carried away.

'Alex, stop it. You're doing what you always do. Building up a glowing picture . . .' She sighed, 'Let's drive to Italy, Alex. Let's get caught up in the traffic in Rome, Alex. Let's get hysterical yelling at each other. Let's fight over my map-reading. Or my driving. You know, with you stamping the floor shouting brake, brake. Let's get sick eating squid . . . Life is not a series of perfect moments, Alex, no matter how hard you try.'

'You could still come back. We had a marriage.'

She shook her head, 'No we didn't and you know it. We had a shampoo-ad relationship that got soured by reality.'

That hurt. He let go of her and turned away. 'If we're talking superficial, you're the one turned on by shoes.'

'You of course don't need accessories. You're so perfect, you're your own accessory.'

He shook his head. 'What's happening to you, speaking to me like this? Standing out there in the rain talking to the gulls?'

'I don't know,' said Jessie. 'Why don't you leave me alone? Please go.'

Without a word he rose, took his coat and made for the door. 'If you're passing the café, would you go in and tell Magda I won't be back tonight. I don't feel well,' Jessie called, then considered the state of her health. 'Actually, I really don't feel well. I think I'm going to be sick.' Alex hovered in the doorway. If she was going to be sick he should do something. What?

'Please,' Jessie said.

He needed a drink. Went into the café. Edie and Magda stopped their conversation and looked at him.

'Sorry,' he said. Aware that he was not wanted. 'Could I have a whisky? And Jessie says she won't be back she's not well. Actually, she's sick.'

Lipless hoped she'd be better soon. 'I like Jessie,' he told Magda. 'She's got manners.'

Magda laughed, 'Not like me. Well, you know me, Lipless. Manners are a pain in the arse. They'll always get you exactly where other people want you to be.' She handed Alex his whisky. The wind battered the windows, waves crashed against the quay, a great wall of water heaved into the air, battered to the ground and sucked back, leaving a debris of pebbles, dulce and sand.

'Some weather,' Alex said, staring out. It was warm here, windows steamed, somehow the world seemed far away. He sat in the far corner and asked to see a menu.

He had cream of potato and tomato soup and a bottle of Sancerre, and did Magda know what was up with Jessie? Edie nodded. Sancerre, typical September visitor.

'She's sorting herself out. Leave her to it.'

Alex shook his head. 'So much pain,' he said.

'Yep,' Magda agreed. 'Life's a bitch. Mind you,' she never could resist making judgements, 'if you ask me, and I know so far you haven't, if there's pain going about you caused a fair bit of it.'

'I hurt too. It was my baby too,' Alex said. Speaking about it always made him grumpy.

'Tell me about it. You lost interest after the conception,' Magda said, removing his empty plate. 'There's only steak on the menu.'

'I'll have it. Nobody asked me if I wanted a baby. I'd only just got used to the idea of being a dad when it died.'

Magda nodded. 'You felt guilty when it died too, then?'

Alex nodded. 'Yeah, of course I did.'

Magda glared at him intently. 'Why are you staring at me?' he asked, wincing under the scrutiny. 'I just came in for a drink. I didn't ask for this.'

'That's OK,' Magda assured him. 'I don't charge extra for criticism. Or for sorting folks out.' She sat down and gave him the full piercing, all-seeing look. 'You didn't want a baby. You didn't want to share Jessie. You didn't want the mess. When it died for a moment you were glad. It wasn't a big moment, but it was there that moment. And after it you couldn't bear to be with Jessie, you felt so bad. You couldn't stand it. That's it, isn't it?'

Alex stared out the window. 'Could I just have my steak, please?'

Magda rose and went to the kitchen.

'She's a cow,' said Lipless. 'She does that to everybody. She feeds you. She figures out your life. Then she gives you the bill. Don't know why people put up with it.'

253

'She dishes up food and the truth. Who could resist it?' Alex reflected.

Magda stuck her head round the kitchen door. 'Lots of men feel like that,' she said. 'You can congratulate yourself on being normal.'

She liked his suit. Mareth men didn't wear suits, except for weddings and funerals, or unless they were the doctor, lawyer or bank manager. Or unless, she continued her muse, they were off to see the bank manager for a loan. She thought she would have Alex. She always wanted something of Jessie's. Alex no longer felt hungry. Hated to be reminded of when the baby died. Looking back he had a vision of himself running around for weeks with his palms spread, mouthing incoherently, lips opening and shutting, like a goldfish. He remembered himself as wearing a permanent bewildered and pained expression. The weeks immediately after the death had been the worst in his life. He thought he behaved quite well but didn't dare ask what other men did in the same circumstances lest he discovered he'd been a prat.

Magda brought him a peppered steak in Madeira sauce. She leaned on the bar watching him eat.

'I see you looking at him,' Lipless muttered into his beer. 'City shite.'

'Oh yes, he's that,' Magda agreed, and went to fetch a tarte tatin. Alex ordered another bottle of wine. It was funny, folks here thought city men to be wankers.

'Blokes like that,' Lipless said, 'are just women. Can't hold their drink.'

'What do you mean, just women?' Magda said. She sounded glum. She could feel an argument coming on and didn't feel up to it. This storm was draining enough.

'Just women. They can't do much, can they? Like hold their drink. City shites are women when they drink.'

'I can drink you under the table any night, Lipless,' Magda sneered.

'Yes, I'll give you that.'

'And I can cook, run a restaurant, care for a family and—'

'Oh I know, 'cos I'm a wooooooman,' Lipless burst into song. His flat, lifeless singing was surprising.

'Oh, I can't stand that stuff,' Magda scorned, before singing her own life's song. 'I get up five in the morning, scrub miners' backs in the tub outside, feed the bairns, discover a cure for cancer, do a milk round, take hot meals to housebound old folks, give my man a blow job and never give a sod about myself. 'Cos I'm a wooooooman . . .' Her song stopped. In the light of not being able to think of a single thing to say, Lipless made a dismissive face.

Magda's song went on, 'Or should it be, 'Cos I'm stooooooooopid?'

'Still think city shites can't hold their drink,' Lipless muttered. He glared at Magda triumphantly. As far as he was concerned he'd won the argument.

255

But this city shite could hold his drink. He could hold quite a selection of alcohol. He'd had one and a bit bottles of wine and several whiskies and was still standing. Well, Magda thought, he's not going anywhere tonight.

At nine Edie went home. She needed an early night and she wasn't needed to look after two customers, only one of whom was eating. Lipless drank on. Alex drank whisky with his coffee. Magda cleaned the kitchen. Outside the Harrys complained about the weather. 'You're not coming in here,' Magda told them.

Lipless left at ten, 'Where is everybody? It's dead in here tonight.'

Magda smiled. She was wondering when to charge Alex – before or after? Before. It would be easier to take his money before sex; there was something lurid about after even though he owed her for the meal.

Upstairs Jessie lay in her darkened bedroom sweating and nauseous. She'd caught a chill feeding the gulls.

She visited her past. She saw it so clearly, her old house, the Smallbone kitchen with french windows leading to the garden where she'd walked serenely pregnant. She reached out into the dark, as if her life were out there to be touched, waiting for her to come back to it. But the house was sold, husband sent packing; everything was gone. Nothing left, she said. Nothing left. Outside the wind blasted relentlessly.

Magda locked the café door. 'Enough's enough,' she said. 'If anybody wants fed tonight they can go somewhere else.'

'They're missing a lot,' said Alex.

Magda brought a bottle to the table. But only half-filled his glass, 'You've had enough already.'

He kissed her. His tongue in her. She moved her hand on the back of his head. Liked the short hairs against her palm. He pulled her to him, knocking over her chair.

'I have to switch off the lights,' Magda said. Before she did, kissed him again. Let her body move against his. He pulled her to him, lips on hers. She loved the feel of mouths. Unbuttoned his shirt. Not wanting to stop, each scared lest the other came to their senses and say no, they collapsed to the floor. Mauling each other, pulling off clothes. Kissing. Moaning. He took her breast in his hand. Sucked it. She wrapped her legs round him. Another chair toppled. Above them the bottle on the table fell over, vodka poured out, flooded the floor.

'Please,' Magda thought, 'don't let that put him off.'

'Please,' he thought, 'don't let her stop to clean it up.'

Love oh love oh clumsy love. Afterwards they moved to the bashed sofa in the office. Magda threw back her head and laughed and yelled. His face twisted with ecstasy. He pounding into Magda as if it would dispel the guilt and pain of the rest of the evening rather than add to it. Neither of them thought about Jessie.

They lay afterwards amidst the mess, nothing to say. After a while Alex got up, stuffed his shirt-tail into his trousers and collected his coat. He did not look at Magda. As he left he laid money beside the till. 'For the meal,' he said shortly. 'I owe you.'

Magda nodded. She was sitting at the table. Head bowed as she ran her fingers through her hair. She did not look at him. When he finally walked through the door they did not bid each other goodbye.

'You shouldn't have done that, Magda,' she said out loud. She thought of Jim and her children at home sleeping whilst she got up to mischief. She was too old to behave like this. When she set out to seduce Jessie's husband, she hadn't considered how guilty she'd feel afterwards. Sometimes she was like a child stripping off her clothes and rushing into the sea, sometimes she was like that with sex. She didn't stop to think she was getting in too deep.

'You stupid cow,' she chastised herself. 'Stupid. Stupid. Stupid.'

She picked up an ashtray and threw it at the wall. But she was tired. It sailed weakly for a short distance, trailing ash and cigarette butts before sinking to the floor. More mess. She hated herself. But checked herself for bites and scratches, though she knew a man like Alex would be incapable of both. She tidied her hair and went home.

Jim was up. 'Where have you been?'

'At the café.' She feared she smelled of sex.

'What have you been doing till this time?'

Magda shrugged. She wasn't going to answer that. 'What's the point of coming home these days?'

Jim didn't answer that. 'They're selling me off in three weeks. Everything in the yard has to go.'

Magda reached for his arm. She should have been here earlier.

'Magda, I feel like they've stripped the skin from my bones and snipped it into little bits to feed to anybody that's passing.'

Magda's eyes filled with tears. She hated seeing him like this. 'They can't touch you. Not you.'

'They're taking my life and selling it off. Just like that. Have this, two pounds, take that fourteen pounds fifty. That's me they're fucking.' He turned away from her. He was crying.

'No,' Magda said. 'They can't do that. They can't ever do that.' She cradled his head against her. Could feel his tears dampen her shirt. Her favourite pink denim too. He unbuttoned it, took her nipple in his mouth. Such comfort. She sat on him. Hoped he wouldn't notice she'd come home without knickers. Opened his fly and moved him into her.

'It's all right,' she said. 'Everything will be all right. I won't let them hurt you. I won't let them.' And he gasped, slow pleasure. Thank heavens for

259

good old-fashioned well-made sturdy kitchen chairs.

Edie got to the café first. She looked round and knew what Magda had been up to. And disapproved.

'You're a bitch, Magda Horn. A hussy and a bitch . . .' she blistered when Magda arrived.

'Oooooh,' Magda wasn't going to let her shame show.

'That was Jessie's husband you did that with.' Edie pointed at the mess on the floor, overturned chairs, spilled booze.

Magda dismissed the accusation. 'So what? They're not getting back together.'

'Makes no difference.' Edie shook her head and set about working off some of her shock cleaning up. Magda laughed. Didn't mean to but Edie's moral stand amused her. Aggression passed Edie by. She didn't carry anger well. Magda always wanted to cuddle her when she raged, which always made her angrier.

'Don't you go laughing at me. You did a terrible thing last night. And you know it.' She pointed at the ashtray. 'You took a little tantrum and you threw that. You always throw things when you're mad at yourself, Magda Horn.'

Magda smirked at her. 'Oh well done, Sherlock. It was almost worth it, though.' Disapproval brought out the worst in Magda. 'In fact, he was quite good. Better than some of the blokes round here . . .'

'How are you going to look Jessie in the eye?'

'. . . But then, what's sex to them? A swift twenty-second blast followed by ten hours' sleep and a plate of Cocopops . . .'

'She'll know.'

'. . . And foreplay . . . ?'

'You can clean up your own mess in the office.'

'. . . Brace yourself, lass. That's foreplay round here . . .'

Edie threw down her duster, 'That's enough of that.'

Magda put on The Rolling Stones full blast. A jangle of guitars and harmonica roared out. Boomed from the café over the bay.

'What do you mean, look me in the eye?' Jessie walked in.

Magda smiled. Edie looked guilty.

'What's going on?' Jessie looked at the mess on the floor and immediately understood. She sat down, stunned. 'You've shagged Alex,' she said. Magda nodded.

Jessie took her time considering this. 'How was it for you?' she asked.

'Not bad. Better than some I've had. Not as good as Dave.'

'Oh come on, Alex has his moments.' Jessie was surprised at how little she cared. Or how she was giving the impression of caring little.

'He had one last night. In fact I'd say he had quite a moment.'

They laughed. Shrieked together. Women are such bitches.

'I'm shocked. The pair of you, listen to you. Poor bloke,' Edie went off to the office tutting, shaking her head, a can of Sparkle in one hand, a bright yellow duster in the other. Her ineffectual rage made Jessie and Magda laugh even harder.

'Tumblin' Dice' howled out. Jagger hollered loud enough to let Mareth know Magda had been up to no good last night.

Alex woke. He was crumpled and sore. Last night, after Magda, he had driven down the coast road. Fearing he was still drunk, he stopped in the clifftop car park in the neighbouring village and fell asleep crumpled in the driving seat, face pressed against the window.

He leaned on the steering wheel. He was shattered, raw, utterly alone and very cold. The damp seeped into his bones. It hurt to move. His head ached. He felt as if a layer of skin had been ripped from the back of his throat. The light seared against his eyelids. Soon he would have to open his eyes. He dreaded the moment.

The sun came exquisitely up, black against a glowing sky. Seagulls laughed, tumbled freefall. Alex had tears in his eyes.

That woman, the sort of woman he would normally dismiss out of hand – too fat, too common, too honest, too tiring – had taken one look at him and had seen his secret right away. When the baby died, for one small spark of a moment, before the grief set in, he'd been relieved. He could have Jessie to himself again. After that betrayal, what did it matter if he slept with another woman? Or two?

He snorted. There was no doubt that Magda would tell Jessie what had happened. He'd lost Jessie now for sure. There was no going back.

'A shampoo-ad relationship,' he muttered, starting up the car. The sky turned from night to day, white where the chilled haze met the sea. A cormorant keened across the top of the waves.

'Shampoo ad,' he said again, and shrugged. He put the car into reverse and screeched back across the car park, skid marks in the grit. He shoved it into first, swung out into the road, snapped some Verdi into the cassette deck and, gunning through the gears, roared away.

'Shampoo ad. There are some pretty bloody good shampoo ads out there, baby.'

CHAPTER 18

John Lomax could hardly bear to touch his wife. She was more than just thin, she was frail, suddenly old. When he reached for her in bed it was bones he touched. When he took her hand as they climbed the stair at night, it was a skeletal thing he held – long fingers, deep veins. It looked as if her very skin had given up on her. He called the doctor.

'Dr MacKintyre,' Mary blushed when she opened the door to him. For goodness' sakes, surely he had more important things to do than come to see her. 'What brings you here?'

'John's worried about you.' The doctor came in.

'About me? For crying out loud. That man . . .'

'We don't see you about these days.' He watched her face.

Mary dismissed this. 'I'm just biding my time. When things are right . . .' She tailed off.

'But you feel well?'

'A touch of indigestion. What else can you expect at my age?'

Dr MacKintyre brought out his stethoscope. 'Can I listen?'

'If you must. But I don't know what you mean about not getting about. Only the other week I was in London. All that way. Went to see *Cats*. Lovely. It was lovely, Doctor. Oh you should go . . .'

He gently listened to Mary's heart. A pale and ailing thing fluttering in there. 'I think you should drop by the surgery sometime soon, Mary.'

'And I got the loveliest of frocks. Beautiful. Of course it's not the sort of thing you can wear anywhere. Not for everyday use. I'm saving it for good.'

'I think we'll make a wee appointment for you to see someone. A specialist. Would you do that, Mary? Put on your red dress.'

'I can't wear it to a hospital. Hospital's not good.'

'When is good then?' Dr MacKintyre was intrigued.

Mary looked at him. Couldn't answer. When was good, then? She turned pale wondering. Damned if she knew.

'You could close down the café.' Ginny Howard's eyes gleamed. Power. 'You could shut the café and you could have their house, too.' She got wet thinking about it. She hated Magda Horn. 'They'd have to leave Mareth.'

'Where would they go?'

Ginny didn't know. Didn't care.

'Ginny,' Jarvis sat back in his chair. 'Where would Mareth be without the Ocean Café?'

'Oh food. Who needs it?'

'Why do you hate the place?'

'It's horrible. Full of old drunks. That Lipless. And it needs refurbishing. I mean, that Alpine scene. And Magda Horn is always mincing about in those shoes of hers. And her skirts are too short. You can see her knees. I ask you – knees on a woman that age.'

'She brings in tourists. She feeds children.'

'She's a whore.'

'Cats, she feeds cats.'

'She's a cow.'

Jarvis had never seen his wife so animated. She was luminous with loathing. He had thought the tragedy of his life was that the lustful willing woman who had moved, shuddered under him all those years ago had turned into an overly moti-vated bossy shrew. All that passion had been denied him and searingly redirected into a series of petty causes. He knew her passion scared her. She denied it. But here it was in the living room with him. He saw again the torrid woman he'd fallen in love with. And saw that the true tragedy of his life was that she'd turned into a bitch right under his eyes. He'd done nothing about it.

Now that he had something she desperately wanted, he could have her. Right now he could take her upstairs to bed. She would writhe again for him and scream for him. He owned the lease to the Ocean Café and she wanted it. He got up, poured a drink.

Granny Moran was his aunt. Granny Moran was auntie to half Mareth. But she had left the lease of the Ocean Café to him. He could close it down.

'We could open a shop. We could sell paintings and souvenirs. Tasteful things, of course.'

Oh but Magda made such crêpes. And as her landlord . . . well . . . he could get the best. He didn't want to fuck Magda. But power over her – that was something else. A small, and unheeded voice told him that nobody had power over Magda.

He imagined himself being brought the best. Salmon with balsamic butter, or maybe dill sauce, warm wood-pigeon salad, a plain perfect steak with Madeira sauce, chocolate Bavarian cream. Oh yes. Lovely. He'd sit by the window and demand that Magda keep the Alpine scene for ever.

'Granny Moran asked me to try to keep the café going.'

'Granny Moran's dead,' Ginny enthused. 'We could . . . you could . . .'

Yesterday on the golf course – Mareth had a golf course; the golf curse, they called it, nine hellish holes (anybody wanting a full round had to go on twice) – Dr MacKintyre had given him the works.

'Frankly, Jarvis, if you close down the café, you close down Mareth. Or at least a very important part of it.' He had selected a five iron, swung wildly at his ball, hit it and sent it singing into the sea. Small splash. 'Bugger.'

Jarvis whacked his ball and it whistled through the air, easily easily on to the sixth green.

'Nice one, Jarvis,' the doctor nodded in admiration. 'You've certainly got the hang of the course.' Then, as they strode together towards Jarvis's ball, 'It'd be a pity to see it close down.'

'Close down?'

'Well, if the tourists stop coming –' he let Jarvis have a few minutes alone with his imagination – 'if the café closes, if the children stop getting their breakfast, if the school starts showing the results it would have with unfed infants, if the Ocean Café's reputation didn't bring in odd gourmets and . . . well, just if . . . Jarvis . . . let me see. Now my ball went into the sea. Will you concede that it might have landed here. And I'll try and get it up from the beach?' Jarvis nodded. 'Good man. I think I must owe you a lunch. Where do you want to go? Is there anywhere else you'd consider going, Jarvis? Can I treat you to a crêpe?'

'You don't have to let me win to make your point,' Jarvis said. 'Someone with your handicap. You're so bloody obvious. Did you know that?' He whacked his ball, watched it rise, clear against the blue and tumble into the sea.

People were getting at him. He couldn't stand it. He could almost convince himself that he held the future of the village in his hands. But he knew that wasn't true. He'd lived too long. He'd seen too much. Mareth would survive. The people would live on. Their children would still grow up here, on hot days they'd jump off the harbour wall into the sea, on cold days they'd wrap up, walk, bent against the wind, up the cobbled wynd to school. He could die tomorrow and life would go on. That was the way of it. Life would go on with or without Magda's crêpes. He'd prefer with. Crisp and perfect batter, creamy hot insides, oh yes. And an Alpine scene to gaze at, dream into. That was for him.

So, Magda had slept with Alex. Well, not slept exactly. They had done it. Jessie sat at the window table of the café drinking coffee.

'I have been betrayed,' she thought. 'Betrayed.' Sometimes she tortured herself with it, and sometimes she dismissed it. If she thought of the act as a swift bonk, she could live with it. A bonk, nothing more, nothing less. I've done that. They probably hardly took their clothes off, didn't touch, didn't even really look at each other. I'm mature, I'm sophisticated. I can handle that. She would shrug, things happen.

But if she thought, 'They made love. They touched. They whispered each other's names. He stroked her face and kissed her. They moaned in exquisite pleasure and afterwards lay talking in quiet voices . . . about me. I hate them. How could they?' If she thought that she felt her throat tighten. She wanted to defend herself against the hurt they were causing her. Or at least do them some damage. She gripped a fork. Alex was long gone; she could not stab him. She dared not stab Magda. She thought she might plunge it savagely into her own wrist. That would show them.

She thought she was alone. But Edie was across the café emptying ashtrays into a pink plastic bucket and wiping them out with deft and vibrant movements. She watched Jessie clutching a blunt fork, staring wildly at her arm. 'That'll do it?' she said. Her voice was clipped, eagerly correct.

Jessie looked up, alarmed. She was abashed that her stupidity had been observed.

'That'll do it every time,' Edie went on, waving her fingers at the fork. 'That's a well-known cure for adultery, stabbing yourself in the arm with a fork.'

Jessie put it down. 'I was . . .' She could not think of anything to say. 'I was . . .'

Edie watched. Jessie's embarrassment interested her. 'You were just realising that your husband has been with Magda,' Edie guessed.

Jessie nodded. Been with? Yes, she could live with that. It sounded more social than passionate. There was something dutiful about it. Yes, yes, they'd been with each other.

'It's hard to bear,' Jessie said.

'I know,' Edie nodded.

'My Fred was a terrible one for women. He was a terrible trouser-dropper, if I say so myself. I felt such a fool. I was inadequate. I wasn't enough for him.'

'Oh no,' Jessie rushed to comfort Edie. 'Not you.'

Yet, she felt that if she was inadequate, Magda would now know it. Didn't matter what word she used – screwed, had, made love, humped – it was all the same. Magda knew Alex now, and knew something deeper and more secret about her than she knew about Magda.

'I'll tell you what it is,' Edie offered. 'You're jealous.'

'Jealous?' she wondered. 'Me. Oh no. Jealousy's not in my life's remit.'

'Oh rubbish,' Edie flapped her hands, shooing away this sophisticatedly ludicrous claptrap.

'Of course you're jealous. But you're not jealous of Magda having your husband. You're jealous of your husband having Magda.'

Edie busily took her bucket of cigarette stubs and ash through the kitchen to the bins at the back door. Jessie heard her enthusiastically mulling over her analysis of the situation.

'Yep,' she said, bang of bin lid. 'Hmm-hmm. That's it.'

She came back. Started clearing a table, removing the cloth and shaking it feverishly. 'Oh yes. You want Magda to yourself. You don't want your husband to have any part of her. She's your friend.'

Jessie turned pale. Edie's deftly delivered truth stunned her.

'And if you ask me – and it's only an opinion, mind,' Edie's active little face became briefly earnest as she spoke, 'none of it is worth jabbing your arm with a blunt fork for. Of course, that's only what I think. And who listens to me round here?'

Eleven o'clock in the Ocean Café and the last customer had long gone. Magda was sitting with Jessie listening to Aretha Franklin.

'She's the best.' Magda tipped her glass toward her tape deck.

'Absolutely,' Jessie said. 'Nobody better. Nobody.'

Joe burst in, grinning wildly, smelling boozy. He had with him four drunken, baggily clothed friends. They all wore baseball caps. They looked like a group of pleasantly maladjusted youths out on day release. They moved sheepishly behind Joe, avoiding Magda's eye. Joe pointed to the kitchen and raised his eyebrows. Could he . . . ?

'OK,' Magda said. 'Only . . .'

'I know,' Joe smiled. '. . . Only don't.'

Magda looked at him. Somehow along the line, and she was sure she hadn't taught him this, he'd become charming. He knew if he smiled in such a way, people, especially female people, would let him do anything.

'That's the thing about men,' Magda said to Jessie, 'they seem to know you want them to like you. I hate them for that.' She went for a pee. In the lavatory she looked glumly at her face, 'This is me,' she told herself. 'Old face, hello old face.' Vodka swirled through her brain. And from nowhere the mystery of the omelette pan came to her.

'I know,' she yelled out. 'I know who did my pan.'

She burst out of the lavatory and hurled herself into the kitchen. Her sudden intuition served her well. Joe had her best pan on the burner. It was filled with fat, mushroom, tomatoes, eggs and bacon.

'My pan. You little shit,' Magda howled. 'My best pan.'

Joe shrank back. 'It's only a pan,' he weakly suggested. 'You have others.'

Magda reeled and raved. Joe thought in horror she was going to burst or have some kind of fit.

'It came to me,' Magda shouted, 'truth always dawns when you're not thinking about it. You're using my pan. Have you any idea? Any idea . . . ? This pan took years. Years. You don't just get a pan.'

Saying nothing, Joe approached Magda slowly, hands spread. He had some simplistic notion he could calm her down.

'Enough,' Magda shrilled. 'Enough. You have taken enough.'

Joe laughed. 'What do you mean?'

'I mean enough. That's all. Enough.'

Joe cocked his head sideways, indicating that he didn't understand. He did, of course, understand. He was just testing Magda. How far could he go?

'It's only a pan,' he suggested again.

'Don't be boring,' Magda said, tired voice. 'You know what I mean. You rummage through my

273

clothes to see if there's anything you fancy. And if there is, you take it.'

'Oh,' said Joe. He didn't know she knew he did that. He put his hand guiltily on the pink denim shirt he was wearing. He was a fool to think she wouldn't notice.

'You take clothes, records, money, anything. Enough. Leave me something. You know me. Me. Me. Me. You think you can do anything. But you can't. Just because your mother loves you doesn't mean you can bugger up her pans.'

Joe stepped back, sensing another outburst. Did Magda know about the moisturising cream he plastered on when he shaved and the money he took from her purse? Magda picked up the pan. Hot fat and food tumbled out on to the floor. She held it a moment, viciously eyeing her son. He seized a knife.

'Oh that's right, protect yourself with one of my good knives. Ruin that too.'

'What do you expect me to do? Get bashed with a pan?'

She quietly picked up a potato peeler. Handed it to him, 'Use that.'

He took it from her, turned it round and round in his hand. Then left, still holding it.

Magda waited, eyes shut. 'Me,' she whispered. 'Me. Me. Me.' Every time she said the word, she said it louder. 'Me. Me. Me,' shouting now. She beat her chest, fists clenched. 'Me. Me. ME. ME.' Yelling, eyes bulging, throat throbbing, voice cracking. '*ME.*'

Out in the yard the Harrys scattered. When she returned to the café to finish her drink, everyone had gone.

'Oh,' she said. How strange. She had forgotten people were out here, hadn't realised they could hear her. Besides, it was her anger, why should other people be so bothered by it?

Everybody knew about Jarvis. It was the rumour of the moment. The bank had told him it was reconsidering its position on rural managers. The new policy was to invest in young people and at forty-three he was considered too old . . .

'What does it mean?' Ginny wanted to know.

'I've been made redundant,' Jarvis told her flatly.

Out in the village the news spread wildly. It started with Duncan the postman, but the clerks in the bank had already guessed.

'Irony,' Magda said. 'That's all there is to it. There's always irony.'

Jarvis took it well. He worked a month's notice, giving as many personal loans as possible. He walked round the harbour to tell Willie Patterson and Joe Boyle who worked the creels bringing in lobsters to come in and borrow the money for their next tax payment before he left. The new policy from head office was not to lend money to fishermen to use to pay taxes. During his final fortnight, Jarvis stopped wearing his suit and tie. He sat at his desk, feet up, swigging cans of Bud in jeans and a sweater. His final week he spent at the harbour, chatting to Willie and Joe and finally worked on their boat with them.

He could remember what it was like to be a boy. The smell of it. Sitting on the harbour wall clutching his knees. He stood staring at a cormorant flying low across the surface of the water. If he reached back far enough into his past he would remember the smell of his knees.

He had known every rock round the bay where the lobsters hid when the tide went out. Once he was able to go to their secret crevices and hook them out, a triumphant boy in short pants taking lobster home for tea. They were beautiful beasts, dark blue and brown before cooking turned them red. And they were sweet, so sweet. He put his hands to his face, remembering like this shook him. When he was a boy, Willie Patterson's dad had fished these waters. They'd brought in crab and lobsters in such quantities local kids got tired of them. 'What's for tea? Aah Mum, not lobster again.' 'What've you got in your lunch box?' He'd had a Lone Ranger lunch box – where was it now? 'Lobster sarnies.' 'Oh no, not that. We want meat paste.'

'I think I'll get a boat,' he said to Willie Patterson. Willie said, 'Oh aye.' Jarvis smiled hugely. He knew Willie would get up before him in the morning to rob his creels. Willie caught the grin. He knew Jarvis knew he would get up before him to check the creels It was the Mareth way.

'Well, that would be fine.'

The rhythm of not working at the bank was easy. Jarvis took his boat out, laid down his creels and waited for the next tide so that he could go out again and haul them up, take in his catch, bait the creels again and leave them. Between tides he sat in the Ocean Café drinking coffee and whisky. He only sometimes looked over at the Alpine scene.

'No need of it now,' Magda said. 'You took off and flew.'

'I was pushed,' Jarvis told her.

He had his pay-off from the bank, and his rent money from the Ocean Café and Granny Moran's old flat. He was giving the flat a deal of thought. Jessie would hear him go to it. Stay a while. When he went back down to the harbour, Lipless and his crew loading the council lorry on their way home always called to him and he always called back. It seemed to Jessie he said, 'Fuck. Fuck. Fucky. Fuck.'

Magda shut her kitchen door and stood quite still, feeling the atmosphere. Something was wrong, it was in the air. She didn't know what it was, this wrongness. But she could smell it.

She wandered through the house. There was, it seemed, nobody home and nothing was missing. She stood motionless, felt the hairs on the back of her neck rising. Yes, something was going on in this house. A long low swoon drifted from her bedroom.

Magda looked up, fiercely peering at the ceiling. If she peered hard enough she might just see right through it, see what was going on. Not that she had to do that, she had a very good idea what was going on. She just wanted to know who was doing it and with whom. She climbed the stairs, holding her breath as if her very breathing would disturb the noisemaker. Though she knew it wouldn't, the swoons were getting longer and louder. Furthermore she recognised the voice. That was Janis in her bed. She was, no doubt, with one of those horrendous shore boys.

Even before she burst into her bedroom, Magda could see the scene vividly. They'd be naked, the pair of them, in her bed writhing and tumbling, skinny white teenage bodies; and on the floor by the bed there'd be a heap of clothing, grubby jeans, bashed trainers, T-shirts, socks and discarded underwear. She'd kill them.

She quietly opened her bedroom door. Janis lay sprawled on top of the bed, a slow smile on her face; she gazed dreamily at the ceiling. One hand was spread over the pillow, the other held the head between her legs. Magda recognised that bum, that back, that head . . .

'Dave. You bastard.' Magda was shocked. 'How could you?'

He turned to her, grinning. 'Easy,' he said.

Magda slammed the door and went downstairs to the kitchen. She was sitting at the table staring

278

fixedly at the oven when Dave came down. She did not look at him. Her anger scared her.

'She's only a child. Sixteen,' she said. 'What sort of pervert are you?'

Dave looked past her, 'Oh come on, Magda. She's a big girl now.' Then he said, 'Don't give me any crap about ruining her. She ruined herself long ago.' He stuck his hands in his pockets. 'I won't say town bike . . . but . . .'

Magda got up. 'How dare you speak about my daughter like that? How dare you?'

'Because it's true. Like mother . . . like daughter.' He grinned at her. 'Huh?'

Feeling for the first time in his life he had the edge over Magda, Dave went on. 'Such a sweet young cunt. I love it.' He leaned forward, nudged Magda. 'She loved it too. She's not a goer like you. You're still better. But oh boy, give her a year or two . . .'

Magda hit him so hard she felt the blow jar right up her arm. Her hand hurt for hours after. Dave's head reeled, for a moment his vision blurred. He rubbed his cheek, looked at Magda, said, 'Yep.' And left. Magda covered her face with her hands.

'Oh Janis. Janis. Janis,' she cried for her daughter.

The roup was held on 15 September at ten-thirty at Jim Horn's boatyard. It had been advertised in the local press. Most of Mareth went. They gathered early to stop strangers getting near the front, though the view had been the day before.

Jim refused to watch. He went swimming at Ardro Bay, then came shivering back to Magda at the café. She gave him whisky and sat with him and Janis at the table furthest from the door. They didn't want to hear the goings-on.

Janis was, at Magda's insistence, working at the café. 'I have to keep an eye on you. You stupid bitch.'

The three sat in silence. Jim drumming his fingers, Magda staring ahead, Janis twirling a fork.

'You were sick again this morning, weren't you?' Magda said. Janis nodded glumly.

'You're pregnant, aren't you?' Magda accused. If things were going to be bad, they might as well get it all over now. Janis sniffed and said she thought so, in fact she knew so. Yes. Yes she was pregnant.

'Christ,' said Jim. 'I don't believe it.'

'You better,' Magda told him. 'It gets worse. It's Dave, isn't it?'

Janis nodded.

'I'll kill him.' Jim looked wildly round. If Dave was about he could do it now.

'How long have you been seeing him?' Magda asked.

'Dunno,' said Janis. 'Since he came back.'

'I thought Dave was seeing Jessie.' Jim was incensed. The intricacies of people's affairs amazed him. He was Jim. He lived with Magda. He used to go to the fishing. Now he fixed boats. That was him. He and Magda exchanged despairing glances and sank privately into themselves. When they worried, they worried alone.

Along the quay the sale went on. A couple of the boats Jim had renovated went to visitors. Then the locals took over. Jarvis bought the remaining boat. Freddie Kilpatrick took up the bidding for Jim's tools and eventually got them. Edie bought the computer he'd bought recently to do his accounts. Ruby from the Spar surprised everyone by buying Jim's trailer and winch. And so it went on: the local people moved in, stopping outside buyers from bidding successfully.

The auctioneer had seen it before. It was protectionism. People looked after their own, and in the process looked after themselves. If locals got together to buy up the boatyard they could keep Mareth the way they wanted it, the way it had been all their lives. When the news spread that Jarvis had bought the yard, others came forward to buy whatever they could afford. Now the boatyard at the harbour would stay a boatyard at the harbour. Nobody would build a supermarket, or a hotel or a block of flats. Mareth would continue to be Mareth. Nobody would undercut Ruby's prices at the Spar, or Freddie Kilpatrick's or Frankie's at the ironmonger's. There wouldn't be a new restaurant in opposition to the Ocean Café. Life went on.

The *Sad-Eyed Lady* came up. Fishing boat, built 1958, currently under renovation. It had been undergoing renovations since Jim bought it fifteen years ago. Jessie brought her chequebook along, intending to buy it. But she couldn't bid. Couldn't buy Jim's dream and hand it sweetly back. That would tarnish it. Jarvis bought the boat. He would work on it with Jim. Jim would add bits, then Jarvis. In time they wouldn't know or care whose it was. And maybe they'd take it out, catch fish for the café. And maybe they wouldn't. Only the chat and the planning mattered.

'Would buyers please settle up and collect their goods before leaving?' the auctioneer called, disappointed the *Sad-Eyed Lady* hadn't gone for more. It was always the same in these little towns. Local people stopped serious buyers by moving in front of them. Today the person most interested in the *Sad-Eyed Lady* had been bidding well when someone had pointed out that his Mercedes was slipping slowly off the end of the harbour. God dammit.

Freddie paid for his tools. 'I'll just leave them here for now,' he said. 'I've no need for them at the minute.'

Ruby laughed out loud at the suggestion she remove the trailer and winch. 'I can't be working with stuff like that. Oh my no.' Edie refused to take the computer. 'I've my eye on something a bit bigger. Something with a really, really big memory.' She spread her arms wide, explaining.

'I thought for a moment you were going to buy the *Lady*,' Jarvis said.

Jessie shrugged, 'I'm not local enough for that. Or rich enough. No matter what I do, I'm going

282

to need all my money. If I stay in Mareth, or go back where I came from, I'm going to need all my money.'

It was over by noon. Everything was sold and, apart from a couple of boats and odds and ends, everything lay untouched.

Three days later, Jarvis asked Jim in the Ocean Café if he'd do some work on the boat he'd bought. Jim said why not? They'd gone back to the yard, picked up the tools and started.

'Did you know I'm to be a grandad?' Jim said.

'I heard,' Jarvis nodded.

'Bloody children,' Jim said.

By the end of the week, Jim Horn's boatyard was back in business. This time it wouldn't close, couldn't close. Who the hell owned it?

Dave disappeared slowly. He did not just go. He went away in stages. His first vanishing was the night Alex came to see Jessie. He was away a week.

'Where does he go?' Jessie asked Magda.

'Who knows? We used to wonder if he had another life somewhere else. A wife, children. But I don't think so. When the weather's good he walks. He just walks and walks. He takes his tent, sleeps out. In the winter . . .' she shrugged.

Wiping himself off the face of the earth had been a wheeze for Dave. Then when it was done he couldn't cope. He had to move, movement helped. Hitching rides was OK but actual movement was best. Walking. The last Jessie heard of him was after he had walked his first hundred miles away from her. He phoned to see how she was.

'Fine,' she said. Would she ever say anything else? 'I'm fine. How are you?'

'Great. I saw an eagle today, really close. Huge bugger. You should come. I'll show you.'

But he never did say where he was.

CHAPTER 19

The year moved on. Janis worked at the café and got fatter. Jessie watched, not knowing if she was jealous or relieved. She had for a while ached to be pregnant again. She longed for a baby.

Recently, though, she had been feeling vulnerable. If she had a child now, she had a child on her own. More than that, she did not feel able to cope with the nine months of worry a pregnancy would bring. She would, she knew, be constantly monitoring her body for signs of life, waiting for the child to move. She would be thrown into a panic if there was too long a pause between little kicks and dunts from within, imagining all sorts of dire things if they didn't come. No, she was not ready to brave any more pain. But one day. Definitely one day.

October evenings were busy. Jessie had no help with the tables. Edie had gone on holiday and Janis wasn't allowed out front for fear of what she might say. She wasn't taking her pregnancy well.

'I hate this,' she whined, slumping into a chair, legs apart. 'It's horrible. Look at me. I'm horrible.'

Then turning on Magda, 'You bitch. You didn't tell me having a baby was like this. You think it's funny. I hate you.'

Magda, resigned to Janis's outbursts, said that a little bit of hate gets you through the day. Not getting the reaction she wanted Janis screamed, 'It's all your fault that I'm expecting a baby.'

'Don't be absurd,' Magda said. She had been accused of many things, but this was a first.

At the end of every working day, Jessie's legs ached. Her feet swelled. She soothed them by sticking them out of the window. The chill evening air was wonderful. Night after night Jessie sat, feet jutting one floor up into the night, drinking vodka, smoking Marlboro Lights and considering her fate.

She wasn't good at decisions. The only time she had instantly made up her mind about something was when she decided to come to live in Mareth. Usually she pondered, she debated with herself, squirming at any sort of commitment. She even went through this tortuous routine when in the baker's shop, choosing between a slice of carrot cake and a fudge doughnut.

She thought about the life she had left behind. Trish and Lou would be there now in bars, at dinner parties, laughing, flirting, sitting in each other's kitchens complaining about their love lives, making judgements about other people and other people's lives. Here she was sitting alone in this God-awful flat with her feet out the window swigging vodka straight from the bottle. This wasn't right.

Trish and Lou were her friends and she missed them, their chat. She just didn't know if she missed them more than she would miss Mareth and Magda if she went back. Trish ran her own press-cuttings business; recently she had moved into video. She scanned the world's media on behalf of several huge corporations. If they were mentioned anywhere from Bangkok to Birmingham she would find it, repackage it glossily, send it to the corporation in question and charge them a huge amount of money. She employed six people including a p.a., and had the messiest private life imaginable She'd been married twice, and had a child that lived with her mother, 'I'm just not good at the maternal thing, darling.'

She kept a shifty eye on the door in bars and restaurants, there were so many people she had to avoid. Mostly male, mostly because she'd slept with them and, that done, didn't want to see them again.

'One day she's going to run out,' Jessie said aloud to the empty room. She knew Trish had slept with Alex and for a couple of months afterwards she too had been on the avoidance list.

'What it is,' Trish once explained, 'is I dread meeting a man I like. I can cope with love. It only breaks your heart. But if a man you like rejects you then he's not just rejecting your body and your sex, he's rejecting all of you. I can't face that.' Trish had been hurt a lot.

People had long since stopped going to Trish's flat. Not that they didn't care for her. It was the dysentery aspect kept them away. It was no longer a joke that the mould in Trish's bread bin and fridge should be donated to science. Trish had loaves that were into the fifth or sixth degree of growth. 'Look,' she enthused. 'It goes green, then brown, then it has wonderful spindly stuff like a spider's web. It's quite exquisite.'

Jessie disagreed. 'It's quite revolting.'

Mould infestations in Trish's life were a sign of broken affairs. The only people that brought food into her kitchen were lovers. Trish would fall on the supermarket bags with childish glee.

'Look bacon. And eggs. How super, we could have breakfast.' Men fussed over Trish. Once Jessie had been in her kitchen when a rancid egg exploded.

'How long have you had that?' Jessie asked.

'Oh,' Trish looked at it mildly. 'These eggs were Steve. He was four months ago.' Dysentery looms, Jessie thought. But oh she envied her.

Lou was the opposite. Her flat was perfect, everything painstakingly chosen and placed. Lou had been engaged to the same man for ten years. She saw nobody else. Her weirdness was skin deep only. Ordinary weird, Jessie thought. Black fingernails, pale skin sort of thing. Lou was the first to bleach her hair and have it cropped. Lou worked in an art gallery.

Jessie wondered what she and Trish were doing

now. Sometimes she longed for the city. That boozy waft from pubs, swift blasts of this week's hero in the pop charts humming from shops, international smells – Italian, Chinese, Indian – oozing from restaurants. She missed the noise and clatter, the rush and hum. Then again she didn't miss it at all.

Realising her feet had become numb with cold she shut the window and crawled into bed. She dreamed the dream that had been recurring since she was twenty. Recently she'd been having it once, sometimes twice a week. She lived in a large house. In the middle of the ground floor was a wide staircase, yet she never climbed it. It was carpeted with plush green Wilton. One day she went up the stairs, into a huge room filled with shiny treasures in glass cases. She moved among them in wonder; all this was hers, yet she hadn't as much as visited any of it and couldn't under-stand why. In the morning, feeling as if she hadn't slept at all, she went to work.

'Do you know,' she said to Magda, 'I was thinking about my friends last night and I realised they're just ordinary. Just like anybody else.'

'It's taken you a while,' Magda said. 'What a pressure you put on them to be more than that.'

Jessie said nothing. Later she phoned her mother. She wanted to ask her what to do. She had forgotten about the tiny world her mother in-habited. Her only decisions were if she should put on her blue blouse with the pink floral print or her plain navy. Or if she should make an apple crumble for supper. Or not. 'How are you dear?' her mother asked.

'Fine,' Jessie couldn't say anything else. In her entire life she'd never answered anything other than fine to that question. She wondered how to broach the subject of her dilemma.

'Your father fell down on the garden path yesterday and has such a big bruise on his leg. He tripped on the step. Oh I don't know. What time is it? Goodness me. I've missed lunch. I think I'll just have a banana. I had a cheese sandwich yesterday and it gave me indigestion. I have to be careful these days . . .'

Jessie listened. She had forgotten, too, how her mother had turned small talk into an art form. She remembered her father's business friends coming for dinner and having their discussion on South African politics interrupted by her mother. They listened, frozen by suburban politeness, as her mother took half an hour to tell them how she'd seen a weed growing amongst her pansies and had kneeled down to pluck it out.

'. . . I only had a bit of toast for breakfast, I thought I was feeling a bit hungry.'

Jessie felt her neck stiffen. She rolled her head around to loosen it up.

'. . . I'm not making jam this year. Well, I didn't last year come to that. Or the year before. It's just your father and me now and we just don't eat the stuff like we did when you were home . . .'

Jessie held the receiver away from her ear, 'I don't know what to do,' she whispered. 'I don't know what to do.'

'Mrs Thomson across at number ninety-four makes it all the time. Goodness knows what she does with it. You're awfully quiet, Jessica. Is anything wrong, dear?'

Jessie said that no nothing was wrong. She was fine. And rang off. Put back her head. And screamed, 'Aaaaaaaaaaah.'

As her pregnancy developed, Janis got grumpier and grumpier.

'I thought the baby moved,' she complained, bent over clutching her stomach. 'This isn't moving. This is boogying. This is jumping around. I hate this baby.'

Magda said she shouldn't read romantic literature usually written by poetic men about pale winsome women being with child. Janis told her to bugger off what the hell did she know about having a baby? Magda gave her the Look. Ignoring it, Janis continued to complain, 'It feels like it's having a party. What's it finding to do in there?'

'It has invited all the other foetuses from the ante-natal clinic round for a rave,' Magda offered.

'Another thing.' Janis was whining so much she was beginning to permanently speak through her nose. 'I thought babies lay in the foetal position. This one is lying diagonally, leaning his elbow on my ribs and spends all day idly kicking my bladder. I hate this baby. I hate him. And I don't want him. I'm going to call it Wayne. Serves him right for kicking about inside me.'

They decided Janis was expecting a boy. Dave, it was agreed, could not possibly have a female chromosome in him.

'It'll probably come out with a tattoo on each arm,' Jessie said.

'And needing a shave.' Magda sighed. 'If only it was non-existent.'

On the day the first geese flew over Mareth on their way to the marshes past Ardro Bay, clattering and honking, V-ing across the sky, Mary Lomax died. She was walking across the living room when the pain hit her. She went white, turned to John, said, 'Oh my God.' And dropped dead before he could reach her.

Magda was in the Ocean Café at the time. She turned to Edie, said, 'Oh no.' She dropped her best knife and ran out into the late autumn chill wearing only her thin blouse, absurd skirt and baseball cap. Even though it was a non-police day in Mareth and Jim's BMW was at the door, she ran all the way to her parents' house and found her father on the living-room floor cradling her mother's head, crying, 'Oh no. Oh no. Oh no.'

They buried her three days later. Magda cried as she stared bitterly into the grave, 'The silly bitch.

Silly silly bitch. She broke her own heart. Bloody stupid cow, she'd no right dying.'

John put his arm round her. 'Maybe she's happy at last.' He sighed deeply, 'She's got on her red dress. First time she wore it was to her own funeral.'

The first fistfuls of earth rattled as they hit the coffin.

'Now she won't ever take it off,' Magda said.

Mary Lomax lay in her coffin, first peaceful expression on her face for months and months, wearing her red dress. She had something to wear when good finally came.

Friends and relatives gathered in the Ocean Café after the burial. John did not eat. He drank. It was hard when someone you loved ached and finally died for something you could not give them. Achingly, then, as the whisky in his glass dwindled, his slow tuneless voice seeped through the afternoon's small talk and expressions of sympathy and grief.

'Put on your red dress, baby.'

'I didn't know my Dad knew any blues,' Magda looked shocked. Sometimes it was hard even at Magda's age to realise that parents were, after all, only folk.

And still in childish revolt, she protested, 'That song isn't meant to be sung like that.'

Jim put his arm round her. 'Magda, you especially must know you can sing the blues any way you want.'

★   ★   ★

293

For weeks Magda visited the grave every day. Jessie came across her sitting in the graveyard throwing pebbles at her mother's tombstone. Mary Lomax, aged sixty-four years, beloved wife of John. Good finally came.

'Do you know, Jessie, I miss her. Who would have thought it? I want the old bag back so I can tell her what an arse she was. I feel cheated. She got away with being stupid. I'm so bloody angry with her. Christ, what a waste.'

'Her life wasn't a waste, Magda. Look at the time she had, all those Elvis songs she knew. She was fine. You should meet my mother. She and Dad bought their house in 1946, just after the war. They bought it, then they sat in it for the rest of their lives. My mother is lost in trivialities. I don't think she's ever really enjoyed herself ever. I don't think she knows how. I don't think she liked sex much. She has spent every day of her life in that house in that street of houses waiting for my father to come home. She's been alone all that time.'

'Some women,' said Magda, 'are never alone. They always have their own mother standing, arms folded, tutting and disapproving in the dark of their minds.'

Jessie said nothing. She didn't want this to be true. She was not ready yet to forgive her mother for being so trivial.

'Maybe your mother was so obsessed with her mother she wasn't able to take you seriously. Here you are, despairing, about her, but you don't feel any guilt about her. Maybe, Jessie Tate, that gives you more freedom than any of us.'

Just before Christmas, Jarvis Howard came to live in Granny Moran's flat. Deciding he was the source of too much mess, dirty socks, crumpled newspapers, Ginny threw him out. Besides, she didn't want to be married to a fisherman, she wanted to be the wife of a bank manager. Jarvis sat on Granny's chair, looked about the room at the huge bits of antique furniture, and felt the silence. There was a calming silence within the flat, heightened by the noises, cars, workmen's shouts, gulls, without. It was different from the tense silence at home which had unnerved him. He was so overcome with relief that, had he known how, he would have cried.

Next day he went with Jim to shoot geese. They got four. One for him, one for Jim and two for Freddie Kilpatrick to repay him for the loan of the gun and the new water pump he'd put into Jim's car. Magda would cook one with brandy and prunes and hand it in on Christmas Eve.

In the off-season the Ocean Café served several meals a week that were not charged. They were payment to the plumber, the electrician; anybody who had done some work for the Horns. Mareth had a healthy, seething black economy that was recession-resistant. Two meals with wine at the Ocean Café paid the electrician for rewiring Jim's garage. Lobsters and crabs kept Jarvis in crêpes, and a glass of malt of an evening helped him turn a blind eye when rent on the lease was late.

When Jarvis caught a particularly large lobster he handed it to Magda: there were three lunches at least in that he reckoned. Jim requisitioned it to give to Frankie the ironmonger for some tins of paint, Frankie had given it to the plumber for plumbing in his new washing machine, the plumber had given it to Ruby at the Spar to pay off at least some of the huge grocery bill he had run up whilst business was slow, and she'd given it to young Paula Kilpatrick to come do her hair. It was a prize, this lobster. Its life as an item of currency was long. By the time it was cracked open it was too rancid to eat.

Jarvis cooked his goose with chestnut and apple stuffing and invited Jessie in on Christmas Day to share it. She brought the pudding and a bottle of champagne which they opened before they ate. Jarvis reminded her of Alex, he was so efficient in the kitchen. Alex had done most of the cooking and cleaning. Looking round his immaculate flat, she felt guilty about her flat: the dirty heaps of laundry on her bedroom floor, unwashed dishes cluttering the sink and scatterings of newspapers and coffee cups. Shoving some pine-scented stuff down the lavatory was the only housework she did. She no longer straightened her bed, had mastered the art of making it at night whilst in it, just before she went to sleep. She arched her bum and smoothed the sheet beneath her, then sorted out the rest of the bed with her feet. It worked well enough.

'I don't expect you miss the bank,' she said.

'Of course I do,' he told her. 'I miss the respect. The order. I miss the big desk. I even sometimes miss the suit. Life isn't that black and white.' He leaned towards her, 'I miss the power.'

His honesty shook her. Of course, she knew bank managers had power. It was a surprise to her that they enjoyed it.

'You could do something else, surely. You must have qualifications.'

'I'd have to leave Mareth and that would be hard. My family's here. I was brought up here. Everybody knows me here. I belong. It's home. But yes, you're right, in time when I'm ready, I will do something else. I am the worst fisherman in the world. But for the moment it pleases me.'

He poured some more champagne. She worried him. She had what he had come to call the privet-hedge mentality, typically suburban. She thought people led separate lives in separate houses cut off from each other by a neatly trimmed boundary of privet. Here in Mareth, people's lives were grit-tily entwined. They were a tangle of inter-relations and shared experience. The notion of separate and secret lives would bore them witless. What would they gossip about?

Jessie was so embroiled in the absurd business of being Jessie, it seemed to escape her that everyone round her was similarly embroiled in the absurd

297

business of being themselves. If any religion was instilled in Jessie, it was the glorification of niceness. Jessie thought that being nice mattered. Why, she was almost fanatically nice. Jessie got up in the morning and spent the day being nice to people, and no matter how nasty they were to her, she would wake next day, vision of niceness renewed. It was odd, a woman like Jessie must have examined and rejected all sorts of beliefs, but that great suburban creed of niceness, the blandness of it, was so inherent in her, so deep in there, she hadn't thought to reject it. God, he didn't want his children to be hard or cold, but he hoped they would grow up with more savvy than Jessie Tate, for if they did, that would mean they would grow up with more savvy than him. 'I do believe our goose is ready,' he said, refraining from saying that their goose was cooked.

They did the Christmas thing. Ate too much, pulled crackers, told jokes and worked hard at having a day away from the world. Only once did Jarvis ask, 'Do you know what you are going to do? Are you going to stay or are you going to leave us?'

'Yes,' said Jessie. 'One of those.'

He nodded. Decisions were a bitch.

'I have some money from the sale of the house. It isn't that much. But I could perhaps buy some place. I could get a computer and do some freelance work from here. I can't keep working as a waitress. There are things I could do. I just have to make up my mind.'

At four Jarvis left to visit his children and hand over his presents. He walked up the wynd from the shore, across the High Street then up to the large Victorian houses on top of the hill. Every now and then he turned to look back over the village rooftops to the sea. When dusk came down it spread grey over the water up through the day, a real colour, like a fine curtain; he always thought he might just be able to get a fistful of it. Smoke rose straight from chimneys. There was nobody about. In a garden a blackbird called. The sea was empty today, no boats out. A pale half moon was scratched on to the sky. That same moon had risen on these same rooftops for years and years before he was born, and would rise long after he was gone.

'Hold on to this moment, Jarvis. It's the nearest you'll get to for ever.'

He imagined the scene at home. It wasn't hard. He'd been through twelve Christmases with Ginny already, every one the same as the one before. His in-laws would be there, sitting on the grey velour sofa in the overheated living room. There would be a fake silver Christmas tree, and cards strung up on the walls. The television would be on. His children would take their presents, open them, then ignore him. Handing him a sherry, Ginny would stiffly say, 'Merry Christmas, Jarvis.' There would be no disguising how disappointed in him she was. His mother-in-law would look at him with loathing, and his father-in-law with envy. Ah well.

Jessie went back to her flat. This was the first time in her life that she had spent time alone at Christmas. She phoned Alex.

'Merry Christmas,' she said. 'I just wondered how you were.' She could hear voices and laughter in the background. He was not alone.

'I'm fine. How are you?'

'Oh, fine.' Would she *ever* say anything else? They hung on in silence for a couple of minutes before Alex asked, 'Are you sure you're all right?' He sounded as if he actually cared.

'Of course I am. I'm fine. Really fine.' She hung up.

Jessie stared into the fire. Lining the mantelpiece were cards from all her friends, old and new, Trish and Lou, Magda, Lipless and Edie. She still didn't know what to do. If she didn't go back soon there would be very little to go back to. Her friends would get on with their lives and leave her behind; they'd have nothing in common to talk about. She'd lose her place on the career ladder. Though she suspected she had lost that already. Lost ground was always hard to make up. Her home had been sold. She didn't want to go back to her folks. She sat in front of the fire, Black Harry on her knee, a comfortable weight. She contemplated her new situation. She no longer knew where home was.

She thought she might stay in Mareth a while. She could try to buy this little flat. She could redecorate. If she stayed in Mareth she'd spend time staring out the window, wondering what her friends were up to, and if she went back to her old life she'd spend time with her nose pressed against the windowpane dreaming of Mareth.

CHAPTER 20

On 25 February, with a deal of shouting, swearing and screaming, Janis gave birth to a boy. When the doctor laid the new-born infant on her stomach, Janis leaned forward and took it and wept. She cradled it and loved it, and was reluctant to give him to the nurse to get him cleaned up, checked and weighed.

'I'll be a better mother than you,' she said to Magda. 'I won't be off cooking and shouting and having affairs like you.'

'Well, I hope so,' Magda said quietly. 'I hope so.' She took the child in her arms and watched his tiny crumpled face, 'Well, aren't you beautiful,' she said gently. Janis watched her.

'Nobody told me this,' she complained later, not sounding in the least nasal. 'I didn't know I would love him. Not like this.' She took the baby, held her cheek against his head and crooned to him softly. Her eyes damp, voice stretched and ruined from yelling bastards at the doctor and midwife, 'Hello, little one,' she said. 'This is me, your mummy, Janis.'

It was the first birth Magda had witnessed. She

had, of course, been there when her own children came into the world, but always complained she was at the wrong end to see what was going on. When she entered the delivery room, Janis was at full screech, yelling and swearing foully.

Magda thought, shamefully, 'That's what I'm like normally, never mind giving birth.' But she did not vow to change.

She saw the baby's head appear, tiny damp. Little wrinkled puckered bewildered face, waiting on the brink of the world for life to begin.

'Don't push,' the midwife bossed. 'Now push.' And here he was. First breath. First bawl. It had begun.

'Oh God, Janis,' Magda cried in amazement. 'It's a baby.' She stood in wonderment, 'I didn't know. I didn't know.' She didn't know she would feel this rush of joy to see a new person, child of her child, enter the world.

She was shaken more by this birth, this moving on of generations, than she had been by the birth of her own children. But back then she had been too overcome with her own maternalism and pain. Now all she wanted to do was find a quiet corner, bury her head in her hands and weep.

'What are you going to call him?' she asked cautiously. She didn't really want to know. Last week Janis was going to call her baby Fast Eddie, after Paul Newman in *The Hustler*. The week before Flavor Flav after one of her heroes. She had also considered Slash and, briefly, Snake.

'Well,' Janis said firmly. 'I'm not having all this Jim nonsense. He has to have his own identity. I'll call him James.'

Edie festooned the outside of the café with balloons and put notice of the baby in the window in the menu holder. A boy, James, 7lbs 3oz, at five o'clock in the morning, adding, at Magda's insistence, mother and guilt complex doing well. It was a day of free drinks at the Ocean Café. Everybody asked Magda what it was like to be a granny.

'Exactly the same as not being a granny only older and wiser and with one more birthday to remember,' she said. But they could tell it meant more than that. She just wasn't letting on.

Six weeks later, Janis was fully in charge of her emotions once more. She dyed her hair purple, 'For a change,' she told Magda. She sat in the Ocean Café, legs seeming skinnier than ever in leopard-skin leggings, vast steel-capped workman's boots on her feet.

'They keep her from blowing away,' Magda said, looking through the kitchen door at her daughter. Janis was feeding James, tits hanging out of the collarless shirt she'd found in her grandfather's wardrobe.

'You got a problem with this?' Janis asked a couple who were eyeing her as they drank coffee and ate some raspberry shortbread. They shook their heads, 'No, they hadn't a problem.'

'Hey Mags,' Janis yelled. 'Do you think it'd spoil the baby's feed if I got my nipple pierced?'

'Does the term garden sprinkler mean anything?' Magda hollered back.

Thirty years on, Miss Clarkson's face was still terrifying. It didn't look any different. It must have reached wrinkle peak when she was teaching and stopped developing. 'Well,' thought Magda, 'is there room for any more?' Maybe, though, the eyes were more watery, less piercing. She still came to the Ocean Café every week after she'd returned her library books. She sat in the window drinking cappuccino, eating maybe a slice of apple cake, maybe a chocolate croissant. She didn't like to be too predictable.

'I know you've been overcharging me for years, Magda Horn,' she accused.

'Me?' Magda arranged her features into a semblance of innocence. 'Who, me?'

'Oh, don't do that innocence trick with me. I'm too old.'

Magda didn't know what to do. With Miss Clarkson she would always be a scared child with a grubby jotter and a spelling problem. Miss Clarkson was the only person in the world who made her doubt herself.

'What have you been doing with the money? I know you. You're a terrible woman. You have

305

been too busy being yourself to notice half of what goes on around you. But you are honest. And I want to know what happened to my money.'

'I gave it to charity,' Magda told her.

'I won't ask which one. I don't want to know,' the old lady spoke crisply.

Jessie cleared a table nearby and took the dirty dishes to the kitchen. For a second, only a second, Miss Clarkson stopped speaking, stopped thinking to watch her go. Magda caught the look. A tiny tiny fleeting moment in their lives that was over almost before it happened. The teacher suddenly gathered her handbag and picked up her crumpled, over-used Safeway bag full of library books. 'I trust I'm donating to something worth-while and not one of your absurdities, Magda Horn,' she said crisply. And left.

Magda turned to Edie and said, 'Well me. Did you see that?'

'See what?' Edie said. 'I didn't see anything.'

'The way she looked at Jessie, just then – a moment ago. The longing in her eyes. She's not a demon. She's just a lonely, insecure old lady. Like me.'

'Oh rubbish,' Edie dismissed her. 'You live in your head, imagining things.'

'All those years, Edie. She's been by herself all those years. Edie, I think she's even unhappier than I am.'

'The drivel you talk, Magda Horn. Unhappy.

You don't know the meaning of the word. There is not a person you know doesn't care about you.'

Magda went huffily to the kitchen. Edie heard her furiously chopping some chives and parsley. Heard Magda say, Oh sod it. Sod the lot of you.

CHAPTER 21

March came round again. Jessie looked out, hoping to see porpoises.

'You're lucky to have seen them the once,' Magda said. 'Some folks never do.'

Jessie was looking for a sign. As a child she'd believed in signs. If I can beat the bus to the end of the street, everything will be all right, little hurtling figure in a blue dress steaming up the pavement. Bus drivers who still had some of their childhood in them knew the symptom and slowed deliberately to let her charge past the winning post. She'd grin. The joy of triumph. Everything would be all right. Jump the cracks on the pavement, step over the lines. Stand on a line you'll break your spine, stand on a crack you'll break your back. She would never risk anything as dire as that.

Hold your breath from the school gate to the classroom and everything will be all right. If it takes three hundred steps from the bus stop at the end of the street to her front door, everything will be all right. If she can do a proper handstand and hold it for ten, everything will be all right. If her mother doesn't make fish for tea, everything will be all right. If she sees porpoises out of the window again, everything will be all right.

When no porpoises passed, Jessie looked for another sign. She read old horoscopes in the dentist's waiting room, watched the sky for shooting stars. Nothing. On her day off she drove out to Ardro Bay. She was wearing her long black coat and big boots. It was cold, the sea was icy calm.

'You'd not last four minutes in it this time of year,' Jarvis told her. Gannets flew in a long line and out on the rocks cormorants hung themselves out to dry. It was four o'clock, getting dark. She strode the length of the bay, torturing herself with every step. What should she do? This was her life, she couldn't let it slip away. If she stayed she'd wonder what her old friends were doing without her. And if she went she'd miss Mareth. She could imagine herself working in some tidy office, plants and books and Apple Mac, dreaming of Mareth, a distant sparkle. Without her Mareth would carry on, no doubt about it.

She found a perfectly round flat black stone and took off her glove to pick it up. It was a good skimmer, this stone. She stepped towards the shore. If she could get it to jump over the surface four times, four bounces, she would stay.

'Ah, but,' she thought, 'I'll never manage four. Three. If I can get it to skim three times I'll stay in Mareth.'

She leaned down, took aim and threw. The stone

flew out over the water, bounced. Once, twice, three times, four times.

'Damn,' Jessie said. 'Now I'll have to do it again.' She'd promised herself three skims to stay in Mareth and couldn't renege on that. She found another stone. It skipped twice on the water. The next once. Then twice again. It got darker. There was one star in the sky. One star, didn't that mean a wish? She shut her eyes: wishes don't happen for wishers with open eyes. How childish could she get, she wondered?

'I wish I could find another stone and get three skims.'

Was that two wishes? She didn't know. Maybe she wouldn't get any for being greedy. She was being silly, and knew it. But still she looked around and found another flat stone. Yes, her wish was answered. Now she could get three skims and go home. It was cold here. It skimmed one long beautiful bounce.

'Damn. Damn. Bugger and damn.'

She cast around for another stone, couldn't see one. 'Oh fart.'

She went up the beach to the stony patch on the softer sand and gathered as many flat stones as she could find. It was dark, her nose was running, her hand numb. She was stumbling about. Her scarf kept unfurling and her woolly hat fell over her eyes.

'Oh sod this. What a stupid, adolescent way to behave.'

Carrying a pile of stones suitable for skimming,

she lumbered down the beach to the shore. The tide was going out. A gull called.

'Oh God,' she sighed. 'Three skims. This could take for ever.'